Spinal Fusion

J.M. Cotler H.B. Cotler
Editors

Spinal Fusion

Science and Technique

With a Foreword by A.F. DePalma

With 317 Illustrations in 570 Parts

Springer-Verlag New York Berlin Heidelberg
London Paris Tokyo Hong Kong

Jerome M. Cotler, M.D.
Professor and Vice Chairman, Department of Orthopaedic Surgery, Jefferson Medical College of Thomas Jefferson University, Philadelphia, PA 19107, USA

Howard B. Cotler, M.D.
Assistant Professor of Surgery, Division of Orthopaedic Surgery, The University of Texas Medical School at Houston, Houston, TX 77030, USA

Library of Congress Cataloging-in-Publication Data
Spinal fusion: science and technique /Jerome M. Cotler, Howard B. Cotler, editors; with a foreword by A.F. DePalma.
p. cm.

ISBN-13: 978-1-4612-7944-0 e-ISBN-13: 978-1-4612-3272-8
DOI: 10.1007/978-1-4612-3272-8

1. Spinal fusion. I. Cotler, Jerome M. II. Cotler, Howard B.
[DNLM: 1. Spinal Fusion. WE 725 S7563]
RD768.S653 1990
617.3'75059—dc20
DNLM/DLC
for Library of Congress 89-21730

Softcover reprint of the hardcover 1st edition 1990

Typeset by Arcata Graphics/Kingsport, Kingsport, Tennessee.

9 8 7 6 5 4 3 2 1

To Florence and Susan

Foreword

As with men in all disciplines, so it is with orthopaedic surgeons concerned with surgery of the spine; every generation as it reaches maturity and its highest peak of performance must objectively take inventory of its accomplishments—both its successes and its failures, compare them with the accomplishments of previous generations and lay down the guidelines for the next generation. This is not a simple task; indeed, it is a monumental task, one that is beyond the capability of one man, one that calls for the best brains and the most knowledgeable in the many fields relating to surgical treatment of disorders of the spine.

To perform this function, the editors have selected those contributors who are truly authorities in their special fields beginning with Drs. Muschler, Lane, and Dawson on biology of spinal fusions; Dr. Wapner on response to metallic implants; Dr. Kane on electrical stimulation of spinal fusions; and Drs. Ferguson, Allen, and Tencer on biomechanical principles of spinal correction.

For me it is rewarding to read the chapter "Assessing Spinal Instability" by Drs. Frymoyer and Grobler, which also sets forth the indications for spinal fusion. This is truly authoritative and impresses one with the extensive clinical experience, the analytical and logical thinking, and the depth of background information that is required to write such a precise and clear treatise. The chapters dealing with techniques of spinal fusion again are written by recognized masters in the field of spinal surgery, including Drs. Jones, Rothman, and Balderston on fusion for degenerative disease; Drs. Frassica, Sim, and Klassen for tumor; Drs. Meyer and Cotler for traumatic injuries; Dr. Smith for spinal infection; Drs. MacEwen and King for pediatric disorders; Drs. Phillips and Hensinger for scoliosis; and Drs. Bradford and Lauerman for adult spinal deformity. Postoperative management is covered by Drs. Yeakley and Harris on imaging of spinal fusions and Drs. Cotler and Star on complications of spinal fusions.

The chapter by Drs. Dvonch and Bunch is a classic. Unwittingly these contributors unveil the old truism—that from one generation to another the pendulum of thinking on a problem may swing from one extreme to another. The truism in this chapter is the consensus of spinal surgeons of only a few decades ago that all scoliotic spine fusions be rigidly protected until a mature fusion is attained. This was then reversed to the belief that internal instrumentation and the development of such constructs as the Luque system were so effective that no postoperative external protection was needed. Now the thinking pendulum is swinging toward the center, and this position is endorsed by Drs. Dvonch and Bunch who wrote, "In the absence of an ideal instrumentation system to contend with all the complexities of spinal problems, postoperative bracing will continue to fill an important role in the effective management of spinal fusions."

The history and future of spinal fusions is covered by Drs. Peek and Wiltse and by Dr. Gartland, respectively.

I truly believe that the editors and the other contributors of this book have for their generation laid another building block to the ever-growing pyramid of knowledge relating to surgical management of disorders of the spine. And for this my congratulations to all these contributors.

Anthony F. DePalma, M.D.

Preface

Spine fusion represents a longstanding, well-ingrained orthopaedic operation. A procedure that was designed originally to control infection and progressive deformity has gradually been extended over the decades. As improved methods of anesthesia and patient support have evolved so has the magnitude of spine fusion. Techniques for spine fusion, per se, have changed little or at least have received little attention in the literature. Parallel with improved patient support has come advancements in surgical indications, spinal biomechanics, biology of spine fusion, improved biomaterials, and new instrumentation systems.

Stimulated by a national interest in broadening of the scientific base for orthopaedic surgery, the editors perceived this work as a preliminary foray into those areas relating to spine fusion. Realizing a thin scientific base is available, we hope to centralize and summarize current data to simplify the approach for those beginning their interest or those with a long-standing interest in spine fusion. In addition it is hoped this work will light the way for others to build and expand the field for future generations. The material is being presented as a forum offering clinical application. The personal bias of the authors and editors is recognized, and we hope this will be accepted as an academic prerogative and not as an attempt to personally delete anyone's contributions in this area.

The editors were fortunate enough to assemble expert contributors who are experienced researchers, educators, and dedicated clinicians. This work is not intended to be encyclopedic in nature, but is meant to assemble a core of knowledge for the clinician. The monograph is divided into sections relating to history, basic science, surgical indications and techniques, complications, and postoperative management, as well as a philosophical chapter relating to the future of spine surgery. It is hoped that history will accept this work in the vein it is intended, which is that of a broad stepping-stone to aid both young and more experienced surgeons in the primary goal for the presentation.

Many individuals, including orthopaedic surgeons, neurosurgeons, and physiatrists have supported the editors' education, clinical practice, and research efforts. It is impossible for us to recognize each and every one by name. For fear of inadvertently omitting anyone, we offer collectively to each and everyone of you our deepest appreciation.

We are most appreciative of the expert assistance we received from Springer-Verlag, particularly the late Dr. Jerry Stone.

The editors owe a great debt of gratitude to their dedicated secretaries, Ann Louise Smith and Dolores Walker, who worked untiringly until the completion of this work.

Finally, it is most appropriate that our respective training chiefs introduce and conclude this work, for without their knowledge, stimulation, educational efforts, and role models in surgery of the spine, this work would not have been possible.

Philadelphia, Pennsylvania — *Jerome M. Cotler*

Houston, Texas — *Howard B. Cotler*

Contents

IV Fusion Techniques

V Postoperative Management

VI The Future

Contributors

Benjamin L. Allen, Jr., M.D.
Chief of Staff, Shriners Hospital for Crippled Children, Greenville, South Carolina 29609, USA

Richard A. Balderston, M.D.
Clinical Associate Professor of Orthopaedic Surgery and Chief, Scoliosis Service, Thomas Jefferson University Hospital, Philadelphia, Pennsylvania 19107, USA

Frank Bonnarens, M.D.
Resident, Department of Orthopaedics, Louisiana State University Medical School, New Orleans, Louisiana 70118, USA

David S. Bradford, M.D.
Professor Orthopaedic Surgery, University of Minnesota, Minneapolis, Minnesota 55391, USA

Wilton H. Bunch, M.D., Ph.D.
Dean of College of Medicine, University of South Florida, Tampa, Florida 33612, USA

Howard B. Cotler, M.D.
Assistant Professor of Surgery, Division of Orthopaedic Surgery, The University of Texas Medical School at Houston, Houston, Texas 77030, USA

Jerome M. Cotler, M.D.
Professor and Vice Chairman, Department of Orthopaedic Surgery, Jefferson Medical College of Thomas Jefferson University, Philadelphia, Pennsylvania 19107, USA

Edgar G. Dawson, M.D.
Director of Spinal Surgery, Division of Orthopaedic Surgery, Professor of Orthopaedic Surgery, University of California at Los Angeles School of Medicine, Los Angeles, California 90024, USA

Anthony F. DePalma, M.D.
Professor Emeritus, Jefferson Medical College of Thomas Jefferson University, 1015 Walnut Street, Philadelphia, Pennsylvania 19107, USA

Victoria M. Dvonch, M.D.
Assistant Professor of Orthopaedics, University of South Florida, Tampa, Florida 33612, USA

Ronney L. Ferguson, M.D.
Director of Clinical Research, Shriners Hospital for Crippled Children, Greenville, South Carolina 29609, USA

Frank J. Frassica, M.D.
Special Fellow in Orthopaedic Oncology, Assistant Professor of Orthopaedic Surgery, Mayo Graduate School of Medicine, Rochester, Minnesota 55905, USA

John W. Frymoyer, M.D.
Chief of Service, Orthopaedics, Medical Center Hospital of Vermont, and Professor, Department of Orthopaedics & Rehabilitation, University of Vermont School of Medicine, Burlington, Vermont, 05401, USA

John J. Gartland, A.B., M.D.
Chairman, Emeritus, Department of Orthopaedic Surgery, Director, Office of Departmental Review, Jefferson Medical College of Thomas Jefferson University, Philadelphia, Pennsylvania 19107, USA

Leon J. Grobler, M.D.
Assistant Professor, Department of Orthopaedics and Rehabilitation, University of Vermont, Burlington, Vermont 05401, USA

John H. Harris, Jr., M.D., D.Sc.
Professor and John S. Dunn Chairman, Department of Radiology, The University of Texas Health Science Center, Houston, Texas 77030, USA

Stephen D. Heinrich, M.S., M.D.
Assistant Professor, Department of Orthopaedics, Louisiana State University Medical School, New Orleans, Louisiana 70118, USA

Robert N. Hensinger, M.D.
Professor of Surgery, Department of Orthopaedic Surgery, University of Michigan Medical Center, Ann Arbor, Michigan 48109–0328, USA

LCDR. A. *Alexander M. Jones,* M.D.
Medical Corp USNR, Oakland, California 94602, USA

Michael G. Kaldis, M.D.
Chief Resident, Division of Orthopaedic Surgery, The University of Texas Medical School at Houston, Houston, Texas 77030, USA

William J. Kane, M.D., Ph.D.
Professor of Orthopaedic Surgery at Northwestern University, Chicago, Illinois 60611; Minnesota Spine Center, Minneapolis, Minnesota 55454, USA

Andrew G.S. King, M.D.
Associate Professor, Department of Orthopaedics, Louisiana State University Medical School, New Orleans, Louisiana 70118, USA

Rudolph A. Klassen, M.D.
Assistant Professor of Orthopaedic Surgery, Mayo Medical School, Rochester, Minnesota 55905, USA

Joseph M. Lane, M.D.
Professor of Orthopaedic Surgery, Cornell University Medical School, New York, New York, 10021, USA

William C. Lauerman, M.D.
John H. Moe Spine Fellow, Twin Cities Scoliosis Center, University of Minnesota, Minneapolis, Minnesota 55407, USA

G. Dean MacEwen, M.D.
Professor and Chief, Pediatric Orthopaedic Surgery, Louisiana State University Medical School, New Orleans, Louisiana 70118, USA

Paul R. Meyer, Jr., M.D., F.A.C.S.
Professor of Orthopaedic Surgery, Northwestern University Medical School, Chicago, Illinois 60611, USA

George F. Muschler, M.D.
Assistant Head, Section of Musculoskeletal Oncology, Department of Orthopaedic Surgery, The Cleveland Clinic Foundation, Cleveland, Ohio 44106, USA

Richard D. Peek, M.D.
Clinical Instructor of Orthopaedics, Department of Orthopaedics, University of California, Irvine, California 92664, USA

William A. Phillips, M.D.
Child Health Center, University of Texas Medical Building, Galveston, Texas 77550–2776, USA

Richard H. Rothman, M.D., Ph.D.
James Edwards Professor and Chairman, Department of Orthopaedic Surgery, Thomas Jefferson University, Philadelphia, Pennsylvania, 19107, USA

Franklin H. Sim, M.D.
Professor of Orthopaedic Surgery, Mayo Medical School, Rochester, Minnesota 55905, USA

Taylor K. Smith, M.D.
Clinical Professor, Department of Orthopaedic Surgery, University of California, San Francisco, California 94118, USA

Andrew M. Star, M.D.
Former Spine Surgery Fellow at Thomas Jefferson University, Philadelphia, Pennsylvania 19107, USA

Allan F. Tencer, Ph.D., P.E.
Associate Professor, Department of Orthopaedic Surgery, Harborview Medical Center, Seattle, Washington 98104, USA

Keith L. Wapner, M.D.
Assistant Professor of Orthopaedic Surgery, Department of Orthopaedic Surgery, Jefferson Medical College, Thomas Jefferson University, Philadelphia, Pennsylvania 19107, USA

Leon L. Wiltse, M.D.
Clinical Professor of Orthopaedics, Department of Orthopaedics, University of California, Irvine, California 92264, USA

Joel W. Yeakley, M.D.
Associate Professor of Radiology, Chief of Neuroradiology, Department of Radiology, The University of Texas Health Science Center, Houston, Texas 77030, USA

The Science of Spinal Fusions

1

History of Spinal Fusion

Richard D. Peek and Leon L. Wiltse

This chapter is intended, not to cover every aspect of the early history of spinal fusion, but to touch on the early landmark advances and interpret the importance of these in light of subsequent developments.

In reviewing the history of spinal fusion, it is exquisitely apparent how dependent we are for each new advance upon the work of those who came before us. Many of the great advances seem to have been ready and waiting to be made. The basic groundwork had all been done, and when the discovery finally came, it often seemed to be accidental or at least serendipitous. Even the remarkable discoveries of Conrad Roentgen[1] and Joseph Barr[2] came only after painfully slow, lesser advances by other workers.

Berthold Hadra,[3] of Galveston, in 1891 had successfully used wires wound around adjacent spinous processes in a case of fracture dislocation of the cervical spine and is credited with the first attempt at stabilization. Incidentally, Hadra[3] modestly gave credit to a certain Dr. W. Wilkins who had performed a similar operation on the twelfth thoracic and first lumbar vertebrae previously, with a successful result. Fritz Lange,[4] of Munich, as early as 1909 tried to stabilize the spine by tying celluloid bars and, later, steel bars to the sides of the spinous processes by using first silk but later steel wire. This was before the days of inert metals, and when metal was used for internal fixation, there was a race between the bony healing and liquefaction of the bone around the internal fixation device. Interestingly, Fritz Lange's idea of using steel rods tied onto the spine with wire is not so dissimilar to modern fusion techniques.

The history of spinal fusion really begins in New York, with Fred Albee[5] (Fig. 1.1) and Russell Hibbs[6] (Fig. 1.2). Both published the results of their spinal fusions in 1911. Many of the early fusions by Albee and Hibbs were for progressive deformities from tuberculosis. Later, these techniques were expanded to scoliosis and fractures. However, it appears that Albee probably antedated Hibbs by a short time. Hibbs' fusion worked well in children, but in adults the rate of pseudarthrosis was distressingly high. In later years, many surgeons added iliac crest to the Hibbs technique to increase the fusion rate. It is these authors' experiences, however, that the incidence of pseudarthrosis using these fusion procedures is still too high.

Albee's method of fusion consisted of obtaining a strip of autogenous tibia, splitting the spinous processes, and laying the strip of tibia between the two halves of the spinous processes. He then sutured the soft tissues together very securely. Albee even designed a sterilizable motor saw to remove the strip of tibia. Hibb's concept, however, was in some ways more advanced. He denuded the laminae and feathered the bone, overlapping the bony strips. He did not use bone graft from other sources until several years later.

Willis Campbell,[7] of Memphis, described his method of trisacral fusion as early as the mid-1920s. In this operation, he tamped bone clear to the tips of the transverse processes of L5. He also used the principle of taking strips of iliac crest for graft. Campbell's method of fusion never caught on, however, because the sacroiliac joint frequently failed to fuse. Later, it became natural to push bone out onto the transverse processes from L4 to S1 in doing lumbar spinal fusions. In a publication by Ghormley[8] in 1933, the use of iliac crest for graft was advocated and henceforth became the procedure of choice for most situations in which autologous bone graft was needed. It was these authors' experience that the fusion rate was increased by 20%. Strangely, it took 35 years after Campbell had described the placing of bone graft out to the tips of L5 before transverse process fusion became commonly used. Many of the older surgeons never stopped using the simple posterior fusion as described by Hibbs, perhaps only adding some iliac crest bone. They continued to do this even

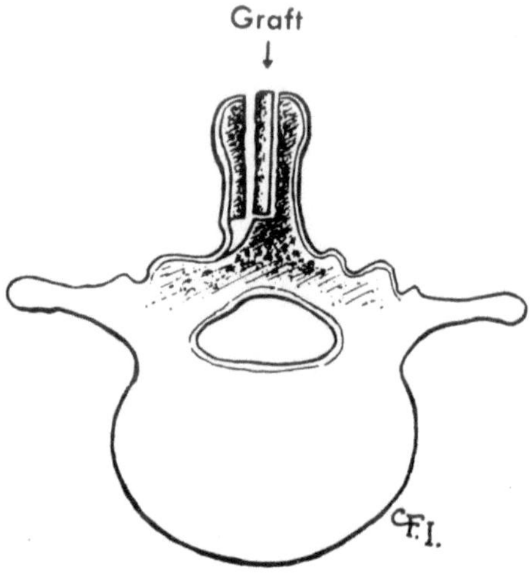

Figure 1.1 Albee's technique of splitting the spinous process followed by insertion of tibial graft is pictured. (Reprinted with permission from Edmonson AS. Campbell's operative orthopaedics. 6th Ed. St. Louis: Mosby, 1980:1992, Fig. 21-53.)

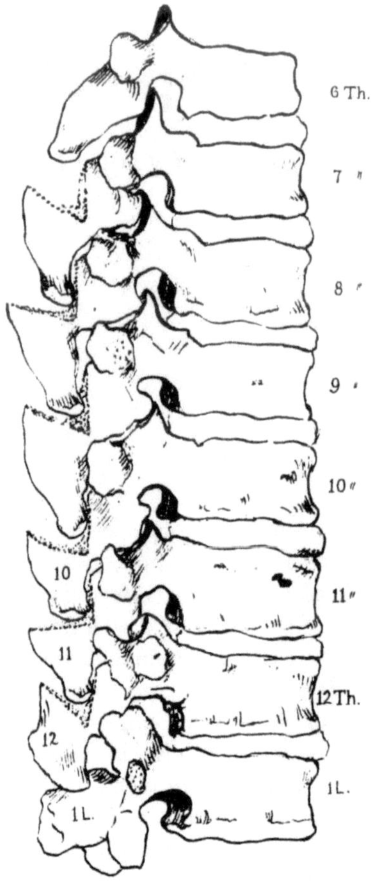

Figure 1.2 The original diagram of Hibbs, who partially fractured the spinous processes, using them to bridge the gap between the vertebrae. (Reprinted with permission from Hibbs R. An operation for Pott's disease of the spine. JAMA 1911;57:885, Fig. 1.)

though including the transverse processes improved the fusion rate remarkably.

In 1948, Cleveland and Bosworth[9] recommended repairing pseudarthrosis by going through the midline, exposing the transverse processes on only one side, and putting autologous iliac strips over this area. For some reason, they did not place graft on both sides. Obviously, using both sides was a simple progression of the technique.[10] Reading their articles emboldened me (LLW), for one, to start pushing bone graft out onto the transverse processes.

Melvin Watkins,[11] in 1953, published his first article recommending approaching the transverse processes from the far lateral position. He approached the spine completely lateral to the sacrospinalis group of muscles. He first recommended denuding the transverse processes and the lateral masses, then laying a large slab of iliac crest along this area and fixing this slab of bone with screws. Watkins was the first one to recommend using this particular far lateral approach. However, Mathieu and Demirleau,[12] two French surgeons, as early as 1936 had advocated far lateral grafting. They recommended driving a peg through a hole in the wing of the ilium and on over the transverse process. A small hole had to be made in the slab of graft to admit the transverse process. This operation never gained popularity. It was technically difficult and fairly dangerous to the spinal nerve, which passes just anterior to the transverse process. The fact that such an operation could be done encouraged others to go out far laterally. Later, the sacrospinalis was split longitudinally in the cleft between the multifidus and the longissimus to reach the transverse processes and the lateral masses.[13] Moe, et al.[14] have refined, expanded, and popularized nearly all the previously described techniques for fusion and instrumentation.

Remarkable studies have been made in an effort to determine the effectiveness of spinal fusion in the relief of back pain. The work of DePalma and Rothman,[15] in Philadelphia; Young,[16] at the Mayo Clinic; and Frymoyer,[17] at the University of Vermont; should be mentioned. A study by DePalma and Rothman revealed that, whether solid arthrodesis or pseudarthrosis was present, there was no significant difference in the clinical result. Young indicated patients did slightly better, but not significantly better, with fusion after discectomy. Hence, the large number of fusions done in the 1950s declined by the 1960s, and there were even fewer performed in the 1970s. It was not until the 1980s, with better understanding of the nature of instability, that the number of fusions again increased.

Grafting Materials

Initially, only facet bone was used for grafting. Grafting with iliac crest was then used to enhance the rate of solid fusion. However, because patients often had inadequate reserves of iliac crest donor bone for these extensive procedures, the need arose for supplemental graft material. Xenograft was used in the 1960s, but this was abandoned because of the high incidence of infection and pseudarthrosis. Since then, allograft has progressively gained popularity.

Allograft has been used safely in all types of spinal surgery without increased infection. Although allograft does not have the osteogenic potential of autograft, it is still effective in anterior cervical, lumbar, and scoliosis surgery.* There have however, been some reports of poor results with the use of cortical allograft for cervical spine surgery in children.[22]

Many other graft supplements and augmentations are currently under investigation. Hydroxyapatite and tricalcium phosphate are bioresorbable ceramic materials that appear promising for future use. Bone morphogenic proteins afford osteogenic potential but lack scaffolding for bone ingrowth. Electrical stimulation is also being used with increased frequency. Consequently, it is possible that the greatest breakthrough in spine fusion will be augmentation with grafting material and electrical stimulation rather than surgical technique.

Metallic Implants

Until the mid-1930s, surgeons had struggled with various materials for internal fixation. Gold did not produce electrolysis, but was too soft and too expensive. Nothing worked well. Most devices had to be removed before they had really done their work.

In 1939, Venable and Stuck,[23] of San Antonio, Texas, published their brilliant work on the use of vitallium for internal fixation. Vitallium, a chrome-cobalt alloy, had been developed by dentists for braces used in the mouth because other metals caused electrolysis with the result that fillings would loosen. The discovery that vitallium could be used in the spine was a remarkable step forward because it made internal fixation really feasible.

Stainless steel was developed in the late 1930s, and of course other metals such as titanium and tantalum are now used. Methylmethacrylate, other plastics, and ceramics have been introduced in the past 30 years.

* 11, 18–21, 50.

Internal Fixation

Hadra, Wilkins, and Lange used internal fixation in the spine around 1900. Albee's graft was a form of internal fixation using a slab of tibial bone. During the 1930s, Phillip Wilson, Sr.[24] published his method designed for fractures and arthrodesis and described the use of a plate that he bolted to the spinous processes, usually with a graft on one side and the plate on the other. This system was never very successful. The next step in the use of internal fixation of the lumbar spine was also made during the late 1930s by Don King,[25] of San Francisco (Fig. 1.3). He recommended using screws through the facets, first publishing his work in 1944. Boucher,[26] of Vancouver, B.C., in 1959 improved on Don King's operation by aiming the screws more medially so they went down into the pedicles, and if driven further, would come out anterior to the base of the transverse processes. The plan, of course, was to keep the screws inside the bone. These techniques did increase fusion rates but did not gain popularity because the use of transverse process fusion was expanding about this time.

The next great advance in spinal internal fixation was made by Harrington[27] for treatment of scoliosis. Knodt[28] rods were developed in the 1950s and are used in the lumbar spine. The Luque system,[29,30] developed during the 1970s, consists of sublaminar wires and posterior rods for scoliosis. R. Judet,[31] since 1964, Roy-Camille,[32] since 1970, and Rene Louis,[33] of France, since 1972, have pursued the idea of pedicle screws and plates. Magerl,[34] in the late 1970s, developed a system in which he inserted Schanz screws into the pedicles either percutaneously or by direct vision. The screws are held in place by an external fixator resembling a Hoffman apparatus. This system has been modified by Dick[35] and others so that the fixator is internalized. Since 1983, Arthur Steffee[36] of Cleveland, Ohio, has also been working on a system of internal fixation by pedicle screws and plates. Krag,[37] working in Frymoyer's laboratory, developed the Vermont system, which uses pedicle screws and connecting bars. The Edwards[38] system uses sacral screws fastened to Harrington-type rods. Marc Asher[39] has developed a plate that fastens to the sacrum by screws into the sacral pedicles. This plate serves as an anchor for Harrington-type rods. Zielke[40] has modified his screws slightly so they can be used in the pedicles and be attached to his standard rods. Cotrel and Dubousset[41] have developed pedicle screws that can be attached to their posterior fixation rods; these are also valuable for reduction of scoliosis. Kaneda,[42] of Japan, has developed pedicle screws that fasten to posterior rods. Wiltse[13] has developed a pedicle screw that attaches to posterior rods by a saddle/nut assembly.

Anterior Interbody Fusion

In 1933, Burns,[43] of Great Britain, did an anterior interbody fusion on a case of spondylolisthesis in a 14-year-old boy. Burns drove an autogenous tibial peg from the abdominal aspect of the fifth lumbar vertebrae into the sacrum. This successful operation was the first anterior interbody fusion reported. Jenkins[44] of New Zealand, in 1935 reported a case similar to that of Burns, but he attempted to reduce the spondylolisthesis by extension and traction, then fusion. Walter Mercer,[20] of Edinburgh, reported his experiences in 1936. To a large extent, he was doing the same type of work as the surgeons previously mentioned.

In the years since these surgeons, many modifications have been made. For instance, the retroperitoneal approach described by Harmon[45] has valuable advantages. For cases of high-grade spondylolisthesis, Freebody, et al.[46] reported that, instead of a tibial peg, a large iliac crest graft was used that nearly filled the bodies of L5 and S1. In most surgeons' experience, the Freebody operation has worked very well. It has the disadvantage that the patient must be kept horizontal in plaster shells for 6 weeks because the graft is soft. For cases of spondylolisthesis where there is virtually no slip, or for disc disease, the use of a hole saw and plugs has been reported. Paul Harmon,[45] in particular, has used this technique. More recently, Harry Crock,[47,48] of Australia, developed a very elegant system for interbody fusion using a hole saw and perfectly fitted iliac grafts. His iliac grafts differ from others in that they are removed from the ilium from the crest downward.

Incidentally, even as early as the 1880s, anterior approaches to the vertebral column for the draining of the tuberculous abscesses were fairly common; but it was a Japanese surgeon, Professor Ito,[49] who in 1934 refined the approach to the vertebral bodies to excise tuberculous tissue. His approach laid the groundwork for future, more complex procedures. Another surgeon who has been prominent in the development of the anterior interbody fusion is Hodgson,[50,51] of Hong Kong. He started his work with tuberculosis but extended it to intervertebral disc disease.

The use of horseshoe-shaped grafts from the iliac crest for interbody fusion was first described by Mercer[20] and has also been described by Goldner[52] and others. These succeed well only if at least four or five grafts can be placed in the interbody space. They can best be used for disc disease or low-grade spondylolisthesis because two large opposing vertebral surfaces are necessary. Obviously, cases of high-grade spondylolisthesis are not suitable. Fibular pegs are very successful when put in the vertical position under heavy pressure. If fibular pegs tip over onto their sides, however, the fusion usually fails.

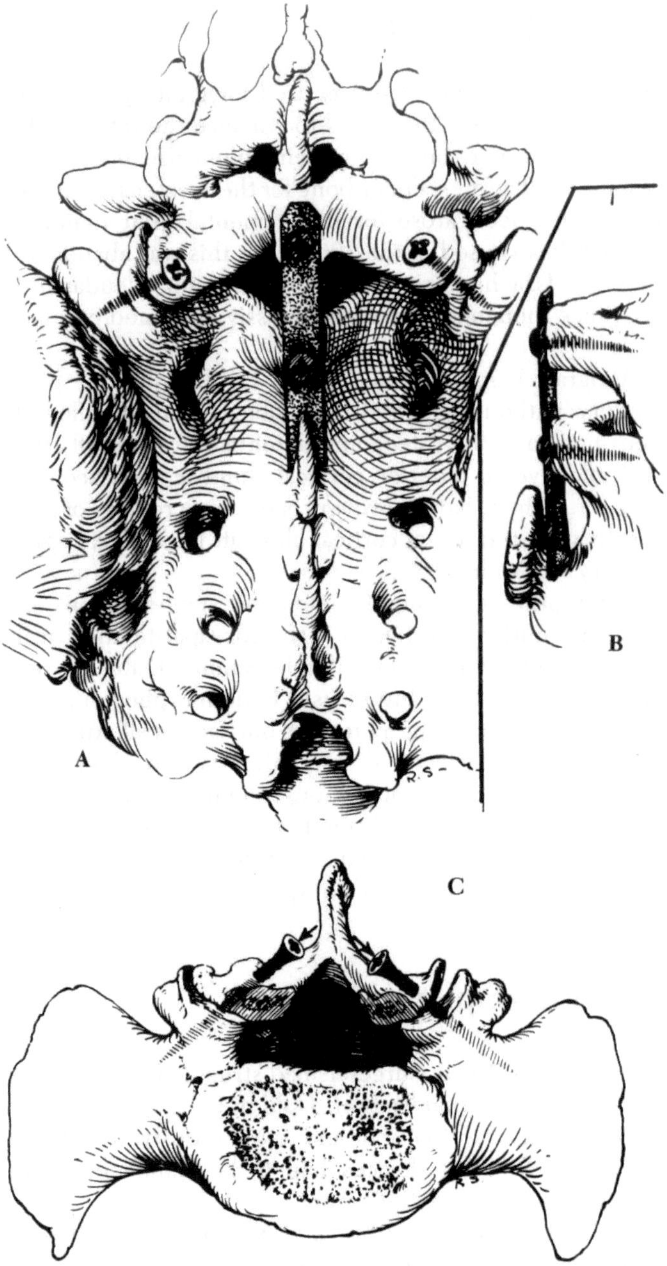

Figure 1.3 **A.** King's original procedure of using screws through the facets; posterior view of lumbosacral joint with screws through lateral articulations and tibial graft screwed to spinous processes. **B.** Lateral view showing tibial graft. (Reprinted with permission from King D. Internal fixation for lumbosacral fusion. Am J Surg Arch 1944;66:357. **C.** From above, illustration of direction of screws through sacrum and arch of fifth lumbar vertebra. (Reprinted with permission from King D. Internal fixation for lumbosacral fusion. Am J Surg Arch 1944;66:357.)

Frank Raney,[53] of San Francisco, during the middle 1950s, described his technique of using a large rectangular iliac graft in the posterior portion of the interbody space, adding fibular struts anteriorly. This technique succeeded well.

Humphries,[54] of Cleveland, was the first to use a plate

for anterior interbody fusion. During the 1950s, he designed a compression plate that was fastened by screws onto the anterior surfaces of the vertebrae. These plates, used especially at the lumbosacral joint, have not been used to any extent because of difficulty of application and possible danger to the great vessels.

Rene Louis[33] recently described a technique using the anterior approach in which a compression screw is placed across the two vertebrae to be fused.

Posterior Lumbar Interbody Fusion

The first published report on posterior lumbar interbody fusion was by Briggs and Milligan[55] in 1944. In the early 1940s, these surgeons began to pack bone between the vertebral bodies after discectomy. Fusion failed, however, so they combined their procedure with a posterior fusion and were then able to obtain solid fusion in most cases.

Cloward[56,57,58] reported that he had done a classic posterior lumbar interbody fusion in 1940 but then did not do another until 1943. Irwin Jaslow[59] in 1946 published his experiences with posterior lumbar interbody fusion, and thus began the PLIF, as it is called. The problem with Jaslow's operation, and others in which fragments of local bone were tamped in, was that solid arthrodesis usually failed to occur. The insertion of these bone fragments probably provided no better relief of pain than an ordinary discectomy, and further added the disadvantage that these pieces of bone might migrate posteriorly.

There have been several other modifications of the posterior lumbar interbody fusion since Briggs and Milligan made their report. These include the use of large autologous iliac crest grafts, large homologous iliac crest or tibial grafts, and even small grapenut-like cancellous autologous or homologous grafts. Plug cutters were used posteriorly by Wiltberger[60] as early as 1957, and more recently Ma and Paulson[61] advocated box chisels to place grafts in the interbody area from the posterior route. Selby[62] has since adapted the Crock system for use from a posterior approach.

In conclusion, the development of spinal fusion has been the progressive addition of blocks of information, inventions, and approaches used to build a pyramid of knowledge. This pyramid is by no means completed, but does establish a solid foundation for the future.

References

1. Roentgen C. In: A biographical history of medicine by Talbott. New York: Grune and Stratton, 1970:993.
2. Barr JS. Lumbar disc lesions in retrospect and prospect. Clin Orthop 1977;129:4.
3. Hadra BE. Wiring of the spinous processes in Pott's disease. Trans Am Orthop Assoc 1981;4:206.
4. Lange F. Support of the spondylolitic spine by means of buried steel bars attached to the vertebrae. Am J Orthop Surg 1910;8:344.
5. Albee FH. Transplantation of a portion of the tibia into the spine for Pott's disease. JAMA 1911;57:885.
6. Hibbs RH. An operation for progressive spinal deformities. NY J Med 1911;93:1013.
7. Campbell WC. An operation for extra articular arthrodesis of the sacroiliac joint. Surg Gynecol Obstet 1927;45:218.
8. Ghormley RK. Low back pain with special reference to the articular facets with present attention of an operative procedure. JAMA 1933;101:1773.
9. Cleveland M, Bosworth D, Thompson F. Pseudarthrosis of the lumbosacral spine. J Bone Joint Surg 1948;30A:302.
10. McElroy, KD. Lumbosacral fusion by bilateral lateral technique. Proceedings of the American Academy of Orthopaedic Surgery. J Bone Joint Surg 1961;43A:918.
11. Watkins MB. Posterolateral fusion of the lumbar and lumbosacral spine. J Bone Joint Surg 1953;35A:1014.
12. Mathieu P, Demirleau J. Surgical therapy of painful spondylolisthesis. Rev Chir Orthop 1936;23:352.
13. Wiltse LL, Bateman JG, Hutchinson BH, Nelson WE. The paraspinal sacrospinalis splitting approach to the lumbar spine. J Bone Joint Surg 1968;50A:919.
14. Moe JH, Bradford DS, Lonstein JE, Ogilvie JW, Winter RB. Moe's textbook of scoliosis and other spinal deformities. Philadelphia: Saunders, 1987.
15. DePalma A, Rothman R. The nature of pseudarthroses. Clin Orthop 1968;59:113.
16. Young H, Love J. End results of removal of protruded intervertebral discs with and without fusion. American Academy of Orthopaedic Surgeons Instructional Course Lecture, Vol. 16. St. Louis: Mosby, 1956:213.
17. Frymoyer JW, Hawley E, Howe J, Kuhlmann D, Matteri R. Disc disease and spine fusion in the management of low back disease: A minimum ten-year follow-up. Spine 1978;3:1.
18. Brown MD, Malinin TI, Davis PB. A roentgenographic evaluation of frozen allografts versus autografts in anterior cervical fusions. Clin Orthop 1976;119:231.
19. McCarthy RE, Peek RD, Morrissy RI, Hough AJ. Allograft bone in spinal fusion for paralytic scoliosis. J Bone Joint Surg 1986;68A:370.
20. Mercer W. Spondylolisthesis. Educ Med J 1936;43:545.
21. Urist MR, Dawson E. Intertransverse process fusion with the aid of chemosterilized autolyzed antigen-extracted allogeneic (AAA) bone. Clin Orthop 1981;154:97.
22. Stabler CL, Eismont FJ, Brown MD, Green BA, Malinin TI. Failure of posterior cervical fusions using cadaveric bone graft in children. J Bone Joint Surg 1985;67-A:370.
23. Venable CS, Stuck WG. Electrolysis controlling factor in the use of metals in treating fractures. JAMA 1939;3(1):349.
24. Wilson PD, Straub LR. American Academy of Orthopaedic Surgeons instructional course lecture, Vol. 9. Ann Arbor, 1952.
25. King D. Internal fixation for lumbosacral spine. Am J Surg 1944;66:357.
26. Boucher HH. A method of spinal fusion. J Bone Joint Surg 1959;41B:248.

27. Harrington PR, Dickson JH. Spinal instrumentation in treatment of severe spondylolisthesis. Clin Orthop 1976;117:157.
28. Knodt TH, Larrick R. Distraction fusion of the lumbar spine. Ohio State Med J 1964;62(12):140.
29. Luque E. Interpeduncular segmental screw fixation. Clin Orthop 1986;203:54.
30. Luque E. The anatomic basis and development of segmental spinal instrumentation. Spine 1982;7(3):256.
31. Judet R. Osteosyntheses: Material, techniques, complications, actualities. De chirugie orthopedique de L'Hopital, Raymond Pain Care, Vol. VII. Paris: Masson and Cie, 1970:196.
32. Roy-Camille R. Internal fixation of the lumbar spine. Clin Orthop 1986;203:7.
33. Louis R. Fusion of the lumbar and sacral spines by internal fixation with screw plates. Clin Orthop 1986;203:18.
34. Margerl F. External skeletal fixation of the lower thoracic and lumbar spine: Current concepts of external fixation of fractures, Uhthoff HK, ed. Berlin and Heidelberg: Springer-Verlag, 1982:353.
35. Dick W. The "Fixator Interne" as a versatile implant for spinal surgery. Spine 1987;12(9):882.
36. Steffee A. Segmental spine plates with pedicle screw fixation: A new internal fixation system for disorders of the lumbar and thoracolumbar spine. Clin Orthop 1986;203:45.
37. Krag MH, Beymmon BD, Pope MH, Frymoyer JW, Haugh LD, Weaver DL. An internal fixator for posterior application to short segments of the thoracic, lumbar or lumbosacral spine: Design and testing. Clin Orthop 1986;203:75.
38. Edwards CC. The sacral fixation device: a new alternative for lumbosacral fixation. Paper read at the meeting of the North American Spine Society, Laguna Niguel, July 1985:882.
39. Asher M, Srippgen W. Anthropometric studies of the human sacrum relating to dorsal transacral implant design. Clin Orthop 1986;203:58.
40. Zielke K, Strempel AV. Posterior lateral distraction spondylodesis using the twofold sacral bar. Clin Orthop 1986;203:151.
41. Cotrel Y, Dubousset J, Gaillaumat M. New universal instrumentation in spinal surgery. Clin Orthop 1988;227:10.
42. Kaneda K. Personal communication. October 1985.
43. Burns BH. An operation for spondylolisthesis. Lancet 1933;1:1233.
44. Jenkins JA. Spondylolisthesis. Br J Surg 1936;24:80.
45. Harmon PD. Anterior extraperitoneal lumbar disc excision and vertebral body fusion. Clin Orthop 1960;18:169.
46. Freebody D, Bendall R, Taylor RD. Anterior transperitoneal lumbar fusion. J Bone Joint Surg 1971;53B:617.
47. Crock HV. Isolated disc resorption as a cause of nerve root canal stenosis. Clin Orthop 1976;115:109.
48. Crock HV. Isolated lumbar disc resorption as a cause of nerve root canal stenosis. Clin Orthop 1976;115:102.
49. Ito H, Tsuchiya J, Asami G. A new radical operation for Potts disease. J Bone Joint Surg 1934;16:499.
50. Hodgson AR, Wong SK. A description of a technique and evaluation of anterior spinal fusion for deranged discs and spondylolisthesis. Clin Orthop 1968;56:133.
51. Hodgson AR, Stock FE. Anterior spine fusion for treatment of tuberculosis of the spine. J Bone Joint Surg. 1960;42A:295.
52. Goldner JL, McCollum DE, Urbaniak JR. Anterior disc excision and interbody spine fusion for chronic low back pain. American Academy of Orthopaedic Surgery symposium on the spine. St. Louis: Mosby, 1969.
53. Raney FL, Jr., Adams JE. Anterior lumbar disc excision and interbody fusion used as a salvage procedure. J Bone Joint Surg 1963;45A:667.
54. Humphries AW, Hawk WA. Anterior spine fusion using an internal fixation device. J Bone Joint Surg 1959;41A:371.
55. Briggs H, Milligan P. Chip fusion of the low back following exploration of the spinal canal. J Bone Joint Surg 1944;26:125.
56. Cloward RB. History of posterior lumbar interbody fusion. Springfield: Thomas, 1982:58.
57. Cloward RB. New treatment of ruptured intervertebral discs. Paper read at annual meeting of the Hawaii Territorial Medical Association, May 1945.
58. Cloward RB. The treatment of ruptured intervertebral di s by vertebral body fusion. Ann Surg 1952;136:987.
59. Jaslow I. Intercorporeal bone graft in spinal fusion after disc removal. Surg Gynecol Obstet 1946;82:215.
60. Wiltberger BR. The dowel intervertebral body fusion as used in lumbar disc surgery. J Bone Joint Surg 1957;39H:284.
61. Ma G, Paulson. Paper presented at meeting of the Western Orthopaedic Association, 1982.
62. Selby D. A modification of the Crock interbody fusion. Instruments for use in P.L.I.F. Personal communication, November, 1985.

■2■

The Biology of Spinal Fusion

George F. Muschler, Joseph M. Lane, and Edgar G. Dawson

Introduction

This chapter is devoted to the discussion of the biology and biological principles of spinal fusion. Successful fusion is a critical element in the successful treatment in a large percentage of patients undergoing spinal surgery.[1–7] Failed spinal fusions result in significant morbidity of spinal surgery patients. The incidence of pseudarthrosis ranges from 5% to 34% in large series,[3,7,8] although generally lower in fusions for idiopathic scoliosis.

Advances of the last decade in diagnostic techniques, internal fixation of the spine, and bone banking have transformed spinal surgery. Intraoperative monitoring and powerful techniques for instrumentation often allow aggressive correction of severe deformity with relative safety. Since the late 1970s, the basic techniques of fusion have remained relatively constant, but this is not so for the next decade. Advances in the understanding of bone healing and bone grafting materials are already occurring in clinical application.

The results of any fusion attempt will depend on three major factors: the surgical preparation of the fusion site, the ability of the graft material to potentiate a bone-healing response, and the influence of systemic and local factors. The following discussion is a mixture of established principles, biological facts, experimental findings, and speculation. There is room for a variety of views. However, we hope it will serve as a platform from which readers can further refine their conceptions about spinal fusion biology and translate that into better clinical solutions for their patients.

Fusion Site

Regardless of the anatomical site of the intended spinal fusion, the basic constituents of the tissue bed are the same. Unless there is systemic or regional pathology, the quality of the tissue bed is entirely in the hands of the surgeon.

The contribution of the tissue bed in which a fusion is desired cannot be understated. Because the entire process of bone healing is the work of living cells and few of the osteocytes transplanted in an autogenous cancellous graft survive,[9] the tissue bed itself must be the source of almost all the active processes of the healing response. Included in the tissue bed are the local blood supply, including the initial hematoma, the cells of the inflammatory response, and all other cells in the bone healing response not included in the graft.

Blood Supply

Good surgical technique dictates tissue handling that minimizes surgical trauma. All avascular or severely traumatized tissue should be removed from the host bed because such tissue can only inhibit vascularization of the fusion site, limit the bone healing response, and enhance the likelihood of infection.

Hematoma

The contribution of the initial hematoma has been debated. Current thinking is that it is probably not a critical factor in the healing response but may serve partly as an osteoconductive vehicle to distribute the healing response throughout the tissue volume in which it occurs.[10] Many surgeons do not drain dorsal spinal wounds, but to our knowledge no study has ever indicated a difference in fusions performed with or without postoperative drains.

Inflammatory Response

The inflammatory response that occurs in the first few days after surgery represents the summed response of the local tissue bed interacting with macrophages, monocytes, lymphocytes, and polymorphonuclear cells which migrate into the site. The activity of these cells is directed to a great extent by local chemical messengers (e.g., prostaglandins) or growth factors that influence the migration, differentiation, and functional activity of each cell. Regional blood flow and local angiogenesis are also mediated by local messengers. These factors profoundly influence induction and progression of events in the healing response. In fact, the events of the first few days may actually determine the outcome of the healing response.

Modification of the inflammatory response can influence bone healing. It has been shown, for example, that if indomethacin is given for the first 6 days of healing, the onset of mineralization is delayed. However, total bone formation is not altered.[11] The efficacy of early postoperative radiation in limiting heterotopic bone formation is a likely example of interference with the inflammatory phase of healing.[12]

Osteogenic Cells

The origin of the critical cells of the bone healing response is a very active area of research. Osteogenic cells (i.e., cells capable of producing bone) can be found in bone, bone marrow, muscle, and possibly even in the general circulation.[13–17] The normal spinal fusion site is, therefore, rich in potential bone-forming cells. An effort should be made to maximize the population of these cells by decortication of all bone surfaces where fusion is desired, and by maintaining healthy viable muscle to cover the fusion site. In addition, on theoretical grounds, the intramedullary space of the vertebral bodies, pedicles, lamina, or transverse processes can be opened to expose the local bone marrow to the fusion site, provided it can be done safely and the mechanical integrity of the sites of internal fixation was not weakened in the process. The issue of how to optimize the recruitment and maturation of these cells is one of the hottest topics in orthopaedic research, and is discussed later in this chapter.

Preparation of Local Bone

The method of preparation of the bony surface is largely a matter of preference, but may also be dictated by the method of internal fixation. Several distinct techniques have been described for posterior decortication in scoliosis fusions.[18–20] Regardless of the technique, the goal is the same, to maximize the area of viable vascular bone.

There has been debate, based on the risk of thermal necrosis, about the decortication using a power burr versus using a simple osteotome or ronguer. Thermal necrosis can and does result from the use of power tools. This can be limited by the use of continuous irrigation and by avoiding prolonged contact of the burr on one site. We know of no study showing an advantage of one method over the other.

Surface Area of Fusion

In general, the larger the surface area available for fusion the better. The larger area will expose more potential osteogenic cells and improve the final mechanical result. If the available surface is not sufficient to support a bone bridge large enough to carry the expected mechanical loads, the fusion will fail. Therefore, any fixation device used must not cover all surface area available for fusion.

With regard to surface area, anterior fusions may have a more favorable biological setting than posterior fusions. This may account for much of the success of allograft bone used anteriorly[21,22] compared to posterior fusions. Decreased surface area may be the greatest contributor to the lower fusion rates seen in myelomeningocele,[23] although the difficulty of fixation and increased infection rates probably also contribute.

Graft Materials

A bone graft material can add essentially three properties to the host tissue bed to enhance the bone healing response: osteogenic potential, osteoconductive potential, and osteoinductive potential[24] (Table 2.1).

Osteogenic potential is the specific ability of the graft material to make bone. This is, therefore, a property only of graft materials that contain viable cells with the ability to make bone or the potential to differentiate into bone-forming cells. Both autogenous bone and bone marrow are osteogenic graft materials.

Osteoconductivity can be defined as a property of the graft material that facilitates the bone healing response so that the response is distributed uniformly over the tissue volume in which the graft is placed. This has been compared to a scaffolding by which the healing response is supported but not directly stimulated. Materials which are osteoconductive include purified fibrillar collagen,

Table 2.1. Outline of properties of available graft materials

	Osteoinductive	Osteoconductive	Osteogenic
Autogenous bone	X	X	X
Alloimplant bone	X	X	
Bone marrow	?		X
Bone matrix	X	X	
Collagen		X	
Ceramic		X	
BMP[a]	X		

[a] BMP, bone morphogenetic protein.

bone and bone matrix, and some ceramics such as hydroxyapatite and tricalcium phosphate.

Induction is a concept arising from the field of embryology. Spemann was given the Nobel Prize in 1935 for his work which defined this type of event. Induction is the process by which some stimulus "induces" a pluripotential stem cell to differentiate into a specific cell type. The concept of osteoinductive potential has entered the orthopaedic literature through the work of Dr. Urist and others with demineralized bone matrix and fractionated matrix proteins. It is clear that at least one protein in bone matrix, bone morphogenetic protein (BMP), has this property of inducing undetermined osteoprogenitor cells to differentiate into bone.

Autogenous Cancellous Bone

Autogenous cancellous bone is currently the most successful bone grafting material. It combines osteogenic, osteoconductive, and osteoinductive properties by virtue of the surviving bone cells, bone collagen and mineral, and bone matrix proteins. In addition, there is a large trabecular surface area that can be linked together as new bone forms, a property that has been called "connectivity."

There are disadvantages of autogenous cancellous bone, however. Graft harvest adds operative time, blood loss, and operative trauma. There is morbidity from pain and potential for deformity or infection. Increased need for perioperative transfusion adds risk of transfusion reaction or transmission of hepatitis B or HIV. Finally, the amount of autogenous bone is limited. The surgeon is often left wishing he or she had more graft.

Autogenous Cortical Bone

Cortical bone grafts have traditionally been found to be less successful than cancellous grafts,[25] probably because of a number of factors. Fewer osteoblasts and osteocytes are present in cortical bone than trabecular bone, and those cells that are present are less likely to survive because they are buried in the cortical matrix, which limits the diffusion of nutrients. Therefore, the osteogenic potential of cortical bone will be less than that of cancellous bone. Cortical bone also has less surface area per unit weight. That means that not only is there less surface for new bone to grow on, but there is also less surface for inductive proteins to elute from. Furthermore, cortical bone represents a formidable barrier to both vascular ingrowth and bony remodeling. Both of these processes are critical for bone healing and the development of optimum mechanical strength. Absence of marrow cells from cortical grafts further limits osteogenic potential. By contrast, autogenous cancellous bone grafts contain as much as 70% marrow. The only advantage of cortical bone over other graft materials is its mechanical strength, which may be very important in many applications.[26]

Vascularized Autogenous Grafts

Vascularized bone grafts are now used extensively in many centers for musculoskeletal reconstructive procedures. High rates of vascular patency are routinely achieved by experienced microsurgeons. Numerous studies have shown the clear advantages of vascularized grafts.[27–30]

In the setting of anterior spinal fusions, donor vessels are available to support a vascularized bone graft. Suitable grafts with excellent mechanical strength are available from the anterior iliac crest or fibula.[31] An iliac graft pedicle flap on quadratus lumborum has also been described.[32]

Alternatively, in intrathoracic procedures, vascularized rib graft may be mobilized on its intercostal pedicle with limited additional morbidity and in much less time than a free vascularized graft.[33,34] However, a rib graft does not have the mechanical strength of the iliac crest[35] or fibula, and must usually be mechanically supplemented by other cortical bone or internal fixation.

Although the increased operative time, technical difficulty, and added morbidity of this type of graft is a significant limitation to routine use, the improved incorporation of these grafts may make them highly desirable in some settings. For example, avascular grafts incorporate very poorly in an area of radiation-induced fibrosis or when radiation therapy is given in the early postoperative period. Vascularized grafts survive the insult of radiation quite well and will generally incorporate despite irradiation.

Bone Marrow

Goujon made the first observations of the osteogenic potential of transplanted bone marrow in 1869,[36] followed by Senn in 1889.[37] Pfeiffer observed bone formation in the anterior chamber of the eye secondary to bone marrow transplantation in 1948.[38] By 1964, Burwell had speculated about the existence of primitive bone precursor cells in bone marrow.[39,40] In recent years, the follow-up on these preliminary reports by Freidenstein,[13,15,41] Urist,[42–59] Owen,[60] Reddi,[61–69] and others[40,70,71] has made the bone precursors in marrow into a hotbed of interest and research. Bone marrow transplantation has been shown to result in bone formation in a number of experimental sites including muscle, subcutaneous tissue, and the peritoneal cavity.

Although not universally accepted, current data suggest that the bone precursor cells in bone marrow can be divided into two groups: determined osteogenic precursor cells (DOPCs) and inducible osteogenic precursor cells (IOPCs). Determined osteogenic precursor cells are primitive cells that are already destined to become bone-forming cells if transplanted. The signal for differentiation of these cells is uncertain, but we do know that it seems to be ubiquitous in the inflammatory response because marrow will produce bone in almost any site. Inducible osteogenic precursor cells, on the other hand, are pluripotential cells capable of differentiation into any connective tissue phenotype. These cells require contact with an "inducing" agent before they become determined to differentiate as osteogenic cells. Bone morphogenetic protein (BMP) is presumed to be the osteoinductive material that acts on these cells.

There have been many studies using bone marrow as a graft material. Werntz, Lane, et al.[71] found that bone marrow used alone to graft a segmental femoral defect in the rat is equivalent to cancellous bone in both radiographic result and mechanical properties. Burwell[72] has summarized the data on experimental and clinical efficacy of bone marrow. Bone marrow is currently being used in a variety of clinical situations as an adjunctive graft material or as a pericutaneous injectable graft.

Allograft Bone

An allograft is tissue transplanted from one individual to another member of the same species. This term is generally misused in the case of bone, because a "graft" is a transfer of living tissue. The correct term for frozen or freeze-dried bone is "alloimplant."

Much work during the past 30 years has investigated and characterized the biological behavior of bone alloimplants. Use of alloimplant bone avoids the morbidity of bone harvest. Blocks or chips of cortical or cancellous bone can be obtained in a relatively unlimited quantity from an increasing number of well-run regional bone banks.

The paramount issue for the surgeon and the bone bank are sterility,[73] immunogenicity, and maintenance of the osteoconductive and inductive properties of the graft. Several methods of preparation of the grafts are currently in use. Although fresh osteochondral shell allografts have been used in the hip and knee, fresh allografting does not have a role in spinal surgery. Freezing and freeze-drying are the most commonly used methods of preparation.

Cells are the most immunogenetic material in bone. Therefore, processing of the bone removes as many cells as possible from the graft. Immunogenicity is further decreased, although not eliminated, by freezing to −20°C.[74–82] Freeze-drying is even more effective, but may result in as much as 50% reduction in mechanical strength.[74,83] Finally, matching donor and host for major histocompatibility loci has been investigated. Stevenson[84,85] and others[86] have shown in the canine model that the immunological behavior of the grafts is clearly improved by matching. However, this has not yet been clearly shown clinically.[87] Regardless, at present the expense of testing and availability of graft material makes this approach infeasible in general practice.

Sterility of most frozen alloimplants is assured through rapid postmortem harvesting using sterile surgical technique and multiple cultures. Ethylene oxide sterilization has been investigated by Urist and others and shown not to interfere with inductive properties if properly aerated. However, Cornell found a 70% decrease in bone induction when demineralized bone powder was sterilized using ethylene oxide, despite aeration.[88] Other methods such as heating bone to more than 60°C, autoclaving, or radiation are disruptive to matrix proteins and are generally avoided.

Urist has developed a protocol for preparation of chemosterilized, autolysed, antigen-extracted allogeneic (AAA) bone to maximally limit immunogenicity without loss of inductive properties. This includes prompt harvest, chloroform : methanol extraction, 0.6 *N* hydrochloric acid extraction of soluble proteins with partial demineralization, and neutral phosphate autodigestion. Use of this preparation in 40 patients undergoing posterolateral lumbar spinal fusion has been reported with an 80% success rate and a 12% pseudarthrosis rate.[89]

Results from other clinical and experimental studies using alloimplant bone in spinal fusions have been mixed. Some authors report that results using alloimplants are significantly inferior to autogenous bone grafting,[21–22,90–92] and others find little or no difference between them.[21,33,93–99] Xenoimplant ("xenograft") bovine bone has also been used with both favorable[100,101] and unfavorable[102,103] results. It should be noted that the preparation techniques and the use of supplemental autogenous bone or marrow used in these studies varied widely, making comparison of individual success rates difficult. One is also reminded in reviewing these studies that clinical success (e.g., pain relief) and successful arthrodesis are not always synonymous; either may occur without the other. Although a successful fusion does have a higher likelihood of success, an asymptomatic pseudarthrosis may give a very satisfactory clinical result. With regards to success of fusion, it is clear that allograft bone is not equal to autogenous bone as a graft material, although under some conditions the results may be similar.

One clear indication for alloimplant bone in the spine may be in settings where the graft material must serve a significant mechanical function, such as anterior vertebral body struts or bone–wire fixation constructs in the cervical spine.[104] Rib, fibula, tricortical iliac crest, and tibial hemicortex grafts have all been used. However, with each of these grafts, there can be significant donor site morbidity, especially the tibial cortical grafts. This morbidity can be eliminated by the use of alloimplant bone rather than autograft cortical bone. In this setting alloimplant bone can probably be used with little loss in biologic efficacy in terms of incorporation provided autograft cancellous bone or bone marrow[25,90,105] are used to supplement the fusion site.

Demineralized Bone Matrix

A subset of alloimplant bone, use of demineralized bone matrix as an implant material, has been an active area of research. The preparation and demineralization of bone serves to reduce antigenicity and uncovers BMP and other bioactive proteins in the bone matrix, making them available to augment the healing response. These materials have been used to induce bone formation and heal a wide variety of bony defects in animal models.[106–113] Glowacki[114–117] and others[118] have reported some applications in craniofacial reconstruction with some success. No spinal applications have been reported to date. These materials have no capacity for mechanical function and handle very differently in the operating room than the graft materials surgeons are accustomed to using. However, they have significant potential as a supplemental stimulant to autogenous bone or marrow grafts.

Ceramic

Calcium phosphate ceramics have been extensively utilized in oral and maxillofacial surgery. They are characterized by a high degree of biocompatibility and are considered osteoconductive in that osteoblasts will form bone directly on the ceramic surface.[119–122] Ceramics are generally brittle materials with low impact and fracture resistance. Preparations may vary in their composition, crystal size, and crystal perfection, as well as structural form, size, and shape. Each factor has an impact on their major biological difference, resorbability. For example, dense nonporous materials exhibit decreased resorption as compared to porous implants because of reduced surface area.[121]

Beta tricalcium phosphate (TCP) and hydroxyapatite (HA) have been the materials most frequently used. Pure commercially available HA has been shown to be resorbed very slowly, if at all, under normal physiological conditions.[121–124] In contrast, TCP is significantly resorbed by 3 to 6 weeks after implantation.[120–122,124,125]

The efficacy of ceramics as a graft material or as a component in a composite graft is not clearly established. Neither are the relative merits of using a resorbable or nonresorbable ceramic. Cook, et al. used both resorbable and nonresorbable implants in a canine cervical spine fusion model and found no differences between them. Cook did note a high incidence of implant fracture in both materials, however.[126] Others have reported TCP to be superior to HA.[127]

On theoretical grounds one can speculate that a resorbable material would be preferred because remodeling is necessary for newly formed bone to acquire optimal mechanical strength. A nonresorbable material may impede remodeling and prolong the mechanical deficiency of new bone[121,128] or leave permanent stress risers in the fusion mass. This is supported by the findings of Muschler and Lane, et al.[129] that the presence of ceramic granules in a collagen and marrow graft to a segmental femoral defect in the rat decreased the stiffness of the healed defects by 50% at 12 weeks. Moore, et al.[130] also found a 50% reduction in total energy to failure when canine ulna segmental defects were grafted with a mixture of HA/TCP ceramic granules and autogenous bone compared to autogenous bone alone.

Bioactive Substances

The biological events leading to surgical spinal fusion can be thought of as a complex interplay between the host tissue bed and the graft material that generally parallels the events of fracture healing. The end result of a successful fusion represents a complex cascade of cellular events mediated by cell–cell interactions and chemical messengers that direct the activity of cells in growth, differentiation, or phenotypic expression through specific receptors. Bone morphogenetic protein (BMP) is probably the most widely known of these substances in the orthopaedic community. There are several excellent reviews that define many of these substances.[131,132]

Some of the local hormones that orchestrate this process have been extracted from bone matrix or other tissues. In addition to BMP, these include osteoinductive factor (OIF), insulin-like growth factor I (IGF-I), transforming growth factor beta (TGF-β), fibroblast growth factor (FGF), and platelet-derived growth factor (PDGF), as well as some less well characterized angiogenic factors. Most of these factors are proteins between 14 to 40 kdaltons. A few of these proteins are already available through recombinant DNA technology. As roles of these messengers become known and means of effective local delivery are developed, they will become powerful clinical tools that may revolutionize our approach to bone grafting and spinal fusion.

Bone Morphogenetic Protein

Bone morphogenetic protein (BMP) is an 18,500-dalton matrix-bound protein that has demonstrated the ability to induce undifferentiated perivascular mesenchymal-type cells (pericytes) to differentiate into cartilage and then normally remodeling bone.[133] It has been extracted from bone matrix of the rat, rabbit, dog, cow, and human; it has been shown to comprise only 0.1% by weight of all bone protein and is most abundant in diaphyseal cortical bone.

Bone morphogenetic protein has been shown to heal otherwise nonhealing diaphyseal defects,[134,135] trephine defects[136] in rodents, and canine ulnar defects.[59] The amount of new bone formed is proportional to the amount of BMP implanted[49,133,137,138] and is dependent on the presence of host bed marrow.[134,136]

Lovell and Dawson[139] have reported the use of BMP in a canine segmental spinal fusion model (Fig. 2.1). In this study, four individual spinal segments were separately isolated in each animal. Laminae on adjacent vertebrae were decorticated and onlay grafts were placed. No fixation was used, and no facet excision was performed. Experimental groups included control; corticocancellous bone strips, 50:50 bone strips plus BMP; impregnated polylactic acid (PLA) strips; and bone strips and PLA alone. Bone morphogenetic protein resulted in fusion of five of seven segments and two to three times more bone formation than the other groups. Only one of seven sites fused using autogenous bone alone.

Bone morphogenetic protein has been used clinically to augment autogenous bone graft in patients with failed spinal fusions. Eight patients have undergone posterior spinal fusion procedures for pseudarthrosis. This group includes six females and two males, aged 24 to 54 years with one to three prior fusion attempts. In seven of the eight patients, only local bone graft was used in the repair. One patient received supplemental iliac crest bone. The fusion was performed in each case using PLA strips impregnated with 100 mg of human BMP, followed by an average of 16 weeks of external immobilization. Seven of eight patients had radiographic evidence of fusion (Figs. 2.2A and 2.2B), which was apparent at 6 months in six of eight patients. One patient was fused at 12 months; another patient has an indeterminant result at 18 months. No complications were noted. Although this is a preliminary report, the use of BMP in spinal surgery is clearly promising.

Systemic Factors

Many systemic factors can be shown in the laboratory, to influence the bone healing either positively or negatively. A partial list of these factors is presented in Table 2.2. A similar but more detailed list has been compiled by Cruess.[10] Based on clinical experience, however, it is likely that within physiological limits most of these factors do not result in significant alterations in fracture healing. Many of these variables can be modified in clinical practice and, if poorly managed, can significantly affect the clinical outcome. The attending surgeon should attempt to optimize every factor where possible, not the least of which is maintenance of optimal nutritional status.

Nutritional status has been shown repeatedly to impact on clinical outcome of surgical procedures[140] and bone healing.[141] Several recent reports emphasize the importance of nutritional support for the orthopaedic patient. Identification of a nutritional deficit using anthropometric measurements, serum albumin and transferrin levels, lymphocyte count, skin-antigen testing, and nitrogen balance studies can be very important in selected patients. Recent weight loss, anergy to skin testing, serum albumin levels less than 3.4 mg/dl, and/or a total lymphocyte count of less than 1500, should be clinical red flags indicating the need for a careful nutritional evaluation and a possible need for nutritional support.[142]

Several lines of evidence suggest that the critical period that may determine the ultimate success or failure of a fusion attempt is the first 3 to 7 days of healing. For example, Urist has shown that BMP need only be present for several hours for induction to occur. Thereafter, the

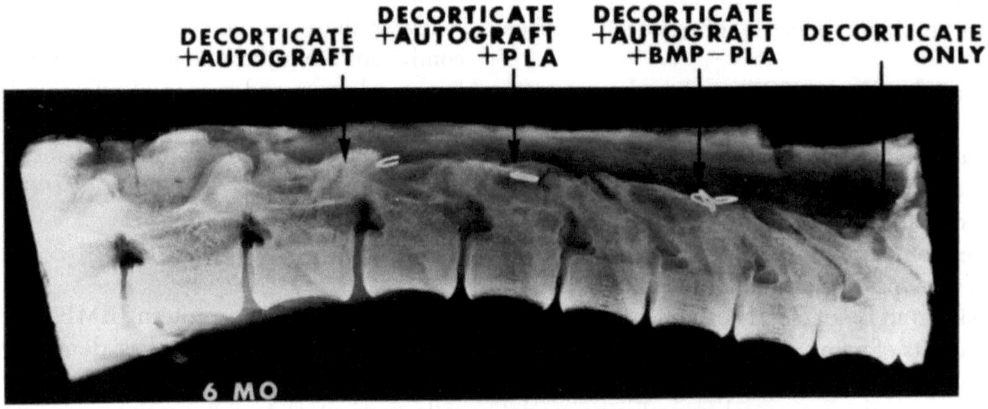

Figure 2.1. Canine segmental spinal fusion model. At 6 months, area implanted with BMP shows increased bone formation as compared to control areas. PLA, polylactic acid strips, used as degradable carrier for BMP.

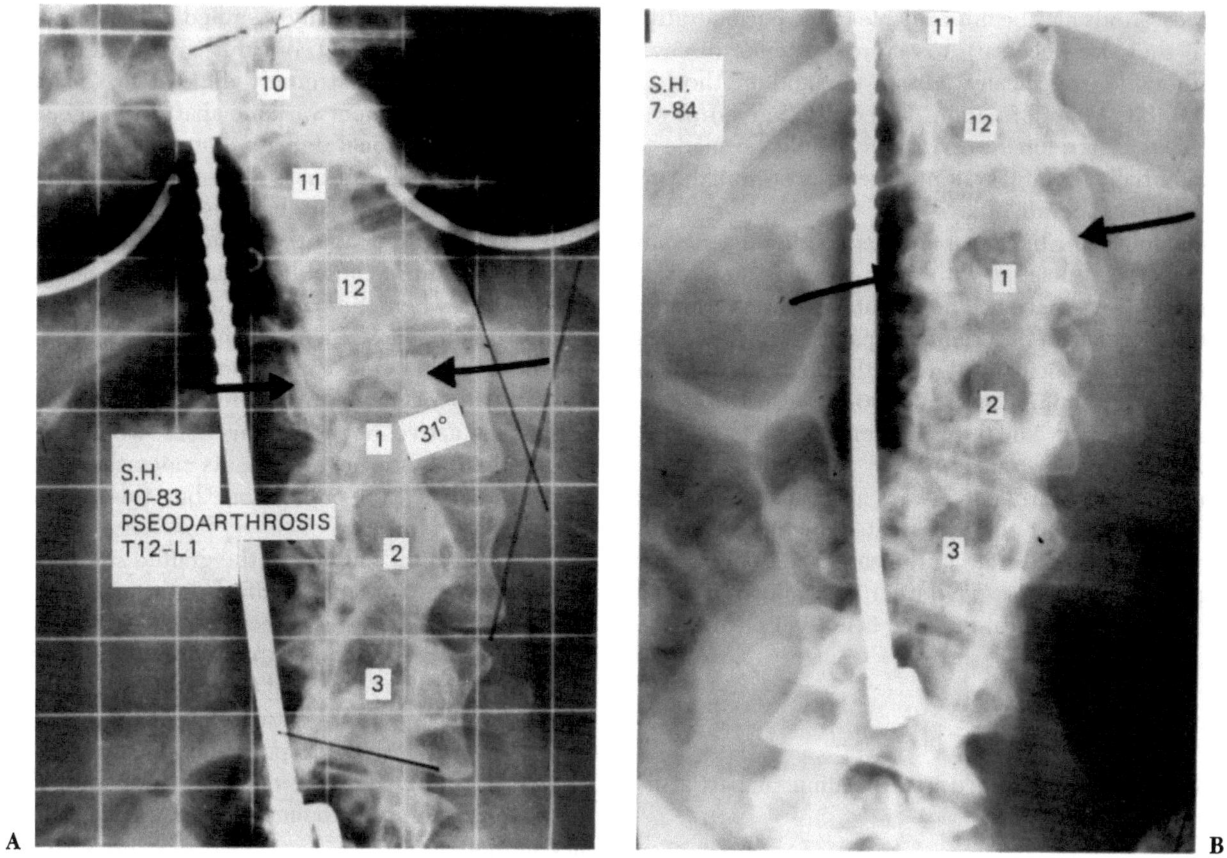

Figure 2.2. Treatment of pseudarthrosis with BMP. **A.** Preoperative radiograph showing nonunion at T12–L1 (*arrow*) with open facet joints. **B.** Nonunion is no longer evident (*arrow*) 6 months after implantation of BMP.

process is independent of further stimulation. Nilsson et al.[11] have shown in the rat abdominal wall that indomethacin inhibits bone formation if given in the first week. If given after the first week, no effect is seen. If given continuously from the onset, the effect is only a delayed normal mineralization. By 10 weeks, bone formation with continuous indomethacin was the same as controls. Likewise, when radiation is used prophylactically to prevent heterotopic ossification, it must be given in the immediate postoperative period to be effective.[12]

Table 2.2. Systemic factors affecting the bone healing response

Positive factors	Negative factors
Insulin	Corticosteroids
Insulin-like growth factor (and other somatomedins)	Vitamin A intoxication
	Vitamin D deficiency
	Vitamin D intoxication
Testosterone	Anemia: iron deficiency[162]
Estrogen	Negative nitrogen balance
GH[a]	Calcium deficiency
Thyroxine	Nonsteroidal antiinflammatory drugs
PTH[a]	Chemotherapy: adriamycin, methotrexate
Calcitonin	Rheumatoid arthritis
Vitamin A	Sepsis
Vitamin D	Syndrome of inappropriate ADH[163]
Anabolic steroids	Castration
	Smoking[164]

[a] GH, growth hormone; PTH, parathyroid hormone.

Corticosteroids may be unavoidable in the perioperative period if they are necessary to control systemic disease. Chemotherapy, specifically adriamycin and methotrexate,[143] inhibits bone formation, especially if given in the first 10 days. Therefore, every effort should be made to avoid potentially harmful systemic agents or stimuli during the first 10 postoperative days.

Rheumatoid arthritis (RA) is another condition generally thought to be associated with complications and fusion failures. Clinical experience bears out this observation.[144] However, here again one cannot separate a physiological fracture healing deficit in RA from the adverse effects of the difficulty in obtaining optimal fixation because of associated osteopenia[145,146] or the concomitant effects of corticosteroids or methotrexate.

Systemic factors are not always negative. There are some data to support the idea that induction of a mild transient hyperthyroid state in the early stages of fracture healing is beneficial.[147–150] Whether this concept is worth incorporating into clinical practice is not yet clear.

Local Factors

Many local factors influence bone healing. A partial list is given in Table 2.3.

Table 2.3. Local factors affecting the bone healing response

Positive factors	Negative factors
Larger surface area	Osteoporosis
Local bone marrow	Radiation scar
Electrical stimulation	Radiation
Mechanical stability	Denervation
Mechanical loading	Tumor
BMP[a]	Primary
Local growth factors[a]?	Metastatic
IGF	Myeloma
PDGF	Lymphoma
FGF	Marrow packing disorders
BDGF	Thalassemia
TGF-β	Sickle cell
EGF	Infection
CDGF	
TGF-α	
OIF	
Angiogenic factors?	Local bone disease
	Paget's disease
	Fibrous dysplasia
	Mechanical motion
	Bone wax

[a] BMP, bone morphogenic protein; IGF, insulin-like growth factor; PDGF, platelet-derived growth factor; FGF, fibroblast growth factor; BDGF, bone-derived growth factor; TGF-β, transforming growth factor-β; EGF, epidermal growth factor; CDGF, cartilage-derived growth factor; TGF-α, transforming growth factor-α; OIF, osteoinductive factor.

Osteoporosis is generally assumed to be an undesirable factor in fracture healing, but this is without direct scientific evidence. It is extremely difficult to separate bone mass as an independent variable apart from age and other systemic or nutritional deficits that may be present. The quality of internal fixation is also significantly affected by bone mass. It is likely that, besides bone mass, the quality of the bone marrow and the number of osteogenic stem cells is deficient in the elderly patient with low-turnover osteoporosis when compared to a young person. In fact, marrow quality may be a more important factor than absolute bone mass. One could speculate that osteoporotic patients with high bone turnover rates and greater concentrations of active bone-forming cells would heal more readily than low-turnover patients since there is a larger local osteogenic cell population, but this has not been tested.

The mechanical stability of the grafted site is one factor that is under the surgeon's control. Internal fixation clearly enhances union rates by decreasing the motion in the grafted level or segment. Anatomical site, the patient's weight and activity level, and the use of external immobilization are all important factors. The higher-than-average fusion rates reported for patients with spinal muscular atrophy[151] and Duchenne muscular dystrophy[152,153] may be the result of improved mechanics from decreased voluntary motion.

Local tumor invasion will weaken bone and replace normal marrow, and may directly invade the fusion site. These problems can be partly overcome by use of specialized fixation techniques[146] and by appropriate use of radiation therapy and systemic chemotherapy, depending on the individual tumor. Use of autograft or autogenous bone marrow is desirable, but the harvest must be maintained as a completely separate surgical field to prevent tumor seeding in the donor site.

Marrow packing disorders such as thalassemia major or sickle cell disease may also decrease the osteogenic potential of marrow by the overgrowth of the hematopoietic elements at the expense of osteogenic stem cells. Similarly, local bone disease such as Paget's disease or fibrous dysplasia can replace normal marrow or gradually replace the bone in a successful fusion with structurally weak bone.

Radiation is a very adverse factor. We have mentioned the acute effects of radiation on bone healing, especially in the first 2 weeks. These may be caused by direct cytotoxic effects on the proliferating cells or be related to the intense vasculitis induced by radiation injury. Long after the acute phase, radiation-induced osteonecrosis and the dense hypovascular scar left in the radiation bed make it a poor biological environment for fusion. In some cases it may be desirable to use free vascularized grafts and donor vessels outside the area of previous radiation to enhance the vascularity of local tissue and the likelihood of a successful fusion.

Electrical stimulation has been shown in many studies to offer some benefit in treatment of nonunions,[154,155] failed arthrodeses,[156,157] and congenital pseudarthroses.[158] There is some evidence that it may also be useful in spinal fusions. In one study,[159] 13 patients with failed posterior interlumbar spinal fusions (PLIF) at least 18 months post-fusion were treated in an uncontrolled fashion with pulsating electromagnetic fields (PEMF). It was found that 77% (10 patients) then fused. Animal studies have also shown some benefit. Kahanovitz et al.,[160] using an instrumented segmental canine spinal fusion model, found accelerated bone formation with PEMF at 4, 6, and 9 weeks, but no difference at 12 and 15 weeks after fusion. Constant current electrical stimulation has also been shown to enhance bone formation.[161]

Future Considerations

The potential for advancement in the area of spinal fusions is tremendous. We have at our disposal many exciting and powerful tools for clinical evaluation and treatment, as well as the benefits of basic science research. Diagnostic modalities, surgical techniques, methods of internal fixation, monitoring technology, and anesthesia will continue to be developed and refined.

In the next decade, the clinical potential of electrical stimulation will be clearly defined in blind studies. The indications and limitations of stimulation will be defined, and better methods of delivery will be developed. Short-term systemic hormonal manipulation may also prove to be useful in augmenting the healing response.

Beyond these areas, the most exciting work in the next two decades will be the translation of our growing knowledge of connective tissue biology into clinical practice. Bone banking techniques will allow a variety of customized bone grafting products to be developed from allogeneic bone. Each material will have a defined and predictable biologic and mechanical behavior for use in a specific clinical setting. In addition, we will see synthetic bone grafting materials brought into the clinical arena. Purified growth factors and other bioactive substances will be incorporated into composite synthetic materials, which, in the presence of an appropriate target cell population, will be far more efficacious than current autogenous bone grafts. Timed sequential release of these growth factors will optimally initiate and drive the bone healing response to suit the clinical situation.

References

1. Burton CV. The role of spine fusion—Question 4. Spine 1981;6:29.
2. Burton CV. Causes of failure of surgery on the lumbar spine. Clin Orthop Rel Res 1981;157:191.
3. Eie N, Solgaard T, Kleppe H. The knee-elbow position in lumbar disc surgery: a review of complications. Spine 1983;8:897.
4. Farger CA, Freidberg SR. Analysis of failures and poor results of lumbar spine surgery. Spine 1980;5:87.
5. Frymoyer JW. The role of spinal fusion—question 3. Spine 1981;6:284.
6. Heithoff KB, Burton CV. CT evaluation of the failed back syndrome. Orthop Clin North Am 1985;16:417.
7. Lehman TR, LaRocca HS. Repeat lumbar surgery—a review of patients with failure from previous lumbar surgery treated by spinal canal exploration and lumbar spinal fusion. Spine 1981;6(6):615.
8. DePalma AF. The nature of pseudarthrosis. Clin Orthop 1968;59:113.
9. Burwell RG. The fate of bone grafts. In: Apley AG, ed. Recent advances in orthopaedics. London: Churchill, 1969:115.
10. Cruess RL. Healing of bone tendon and ligament. In: Rockwood CA, Green DP, eds. Fractures. Philadelphia: Lippincott, 1984:153.
11. Nilsson OS, Bauer HCF, Brosjo O, Tornkvist H. Influence of indomethicin on heterotopic bone formation in rats. Importance of length of treatment and of age. Clin Orthop 1986;207:239.
12. Coventry MB, Scanlon PW. The use of radiation to discourage ectopic bone: a nine-year study in surgery about the hip. J Bone Joint Surg [Am] 1981;63:201.
13. Freidenstein AJ. Determined and inducible osteogenic precursor cells. In: Sognaes R, Vaughan J, eds. Hard tissue growth, repair, and remineralization. Ciba Foundation Symposium II, New York: Elsevier, 1973:169.
14. Freidenstein AJ. Precursor cells of mechanocytes. Int Rev Cytol 1976;47:327.
15. Freidenstein AJ, Chailakhyan RK, Latsinik NV, et al. Stromal cells responsible for transferring the microenvironment of the haemopoietic tissues. Transplantation 1974;17:331.
16. Freidenstein AJ, Petrakova KV, Kurolesova AI, Frolova GP. Heterotopic transplants of bone marrow. Analysis of precursor cells for osteogenic and haemopoietic tissues. Transplantation 1968;6:230.
17. Urist MR. Bone and bone transplants. In: Urist MR, ed. Fundamental and clinical physiology of bone. Philadelphia: Lippincott, 1980:131.
18. Goldstein LA. Surgical management of scoliosis. J Bone Joint Surg 1966;48A:167.
19. Hibbs RA. An operation for progressive spinal deformities. NY State J Med 1911;93:1013.
20. Moe JH. Methods of correction and surgical technique in scoliosis. Orthop Clin North Am 1972;2:17.
21. Brown MD, Malinin TI, Davis PB. A roentgenographic evaluation of frozen allografts versus autografts in anterior cervical fusions. Clin Orthop 1976;119:231.
22. Curtis BH. Orthopaedic management of muscular dystrophy and related disorders. American Academy of Orthopaedic Surgeons Instructional Course Lecture, Vol. 19, St. Louis: Mosby, 1970:78.

23. Allen BL, Ferguson RL. The operative treatment of myelomeningocele spinal deformity—1979. Orthop Clin North Am 1979;10:845.
24. Prolo DJ, Rodrigo JJ. Contemporary bone graft physiology and surgery. Clin Orthop 1985;200:322.
25. Espersen JO, Buhl M, Eriksen EF, et al. Treatment of cervical disc disease using Cloward's technique. I. General results, effect of different operative methods and complications in 1,106 patients. Acta Neurochir (Wien) 1984;70(1–2):97.
26. Takeda M. Experience in posterior lumbar interbody fusion: unicortical versus bicortical autogenous grafts. Clin Orthop 1985;193:120.
27. Weiland AJ, Moore JR, Daniel RK. Vascularized bone autografts: experience with 41 cases. Clin Orthop 1983;174:87.
28. Dell PC, Burchardt H, Glowczewskie FP. A roentgenographic, biomechanical, and histological evaluation of vascularized and non-vascularized segmental fibular canine autografts. J Bone Joint Surg 1985;67A:105.
29. Shaffer JW, Fields GA, Goldberg VM, Davy DT. Fate of vascularized and non-vascularized autografts. Clin Orthop 1985;197:32.
30. Weiland AJ, Phillips TW, Randolph MA. Bone grafts: a radiologic, histologic, and biomechanical model comparing autografts, allografts, and free vascularized bone grafts. Plast Reconstr Surg 1984;74:368.
31. Hubbard LF, Herndon JH, Buonanno AR. Free vascularized fibula transfer for stabilization of the thoracolumbar spine. A case report. Spine 1985;10:89.
32. Hartman JT, McCarron RF, Robertson WW. A pedicle bone grafting procedure for failed lumbosacral spinal fusion. Clin Orthop 1983;178:223.
33. McBride GG, Bradford DS. Vertebral body replacement with femoral neck allograft and vascularized rib strut graft. A technique for treating post-traumatic kyphosis with neurologic deficit. Spine 1983;8(4):406.
34. Rose GK, Owen R, Sanderson JM. Transposition of rib with blood supply for the stabilization of spinal kyphosis. J Bone Joint Surg 1975;57B:112.
35. Bradford DS. Anterior vascular pedicle bone grafting for the treatment of kyphosis. Spine 1980;5:318.
36. Goujon E. Recherches experimentales sur les proprietes physiologiques de la moelle des os. Journal de l'Anatomie et de Physiologie Normales et Pathologiques de l'Homme et des Animaux 1869;6:399.
37. Senn N. On the healing of aseptic cavities by implantation of antiseptic decalcified bone. Am J Med Sci 1889;98:219.
38. Pfeiffer CA. Development of bone from transplanted marrow in mice. Anat Rec 1948;102:225.
39. Burwell RC. Studies on the transplantation of bone. VII. The fresh composite homo-autograft of cancellous bone. An analysis of factors leading to osteogenesis in marrow transplants and in marrow containing bone grafts. J Bone Joint Surg 1964;46B(1):110.
40. Burwell RC. The function of bone marrow in the incorporation of a bone graft. Clin Orthop 1985;200:125.
41. Freidenstein AJ, Chailakjan RK, Lalykina KS. The development of fibroblast colonies in monolayer culture of guineapig bone marrow and spleen cells. Cell Tissue Kinet 1979;3:393.
42. Urist MR. Bone: formation by auto induction. Science 1965;150:893.
43. Urist MR. Surface-decalcified allogeneic bone (SDAB) implants. Clin Orthop 1968;56:37.
44. Urist MR. New bone formation induced in post fetal life by bone morphogenetic protein. In: Becker RD, ed. Mechanisms of growth control. Springfield: Thomas, 1981:406.
45. Urist MR, Hay PH, Dubuc F, et al. Osteogenic competence. Clin Orthop 1969;64:194.
46. Urist MR, Iwata H, Cecotti PL, et al. Bone morphogenesis in implants of insoluble bone gelatin. Proc Natl Acad Sci USA 1973;70:3571.
47. Urist MR, Huo YK, et al. Purification of bovine bone morphogenetic protein by hydroxyapatite chromatography. Proc Natl Acad Sci USA 1984;82:371.
48. Urist MR, Lietze A, Dawson E, et al. Beta-tricalcium phosphate delivery system of bone morphogenetic protein. Clin Orthop 1984;187:277.
49. Urist MR, Lietz A, Mizutani H, et al. Bovine low molecular weight bone morphogenetic protein (BMP) fraction. Clin Orthop 1982;162:219.
50. Urist MR, Mikulski A, Lietz A. Solubilized and insolubilized bone morphogenetic protein. Proc Natl Acad Sci USA 1979;76:1828.
51. Urist MR, Nakagawa M, Nakata, et al. Experimental myositis ossificans. Arch Pathol Lab Med 1978;102:312.
52. Urist MR, Nogami H. Morphogenetic substratum for differentiation of cartilage in tissue culture. Nature (London) 1970;225:1051.
53. Urist MR, Silverman BF, Buring K, et al. The bone induction principle. Clin Orthop 1967;53:243.
54. Nogami M, Urist MR. Substrate prepared from bone matrix for chondrogenesis in tissue culture. J Cell Biol 1974;62:510.
55. Sato K, Urist MR. Induced regeneration of calvaria by bone morphogenetic protein (BMP) in dogs. Clin Orthop 1985;197:301.
56. Takagi K, Urist MR. The role of bone marrow in bone morphogenetic protein-induced repair of femoral massive diaphyseal defects. Clin Orthop 1982;171:225.
57. Van de Putte, KA, Urist MR. Osteogenesis in the interior of intramuscular implants of decalcified bone matrix. Clin Orthop 1966;43:257.
58. Lakasi K, Urist MR. The reaction of the dura to bone morphogenetic protein (BMP) in the repair of skull defects. Ann Surg 1982;196:100.
59. Nilsson OS, Urist MR, Dawson T, et al. Bone repair induced by bone morphogenetic protein in ulnar defects in dogs. J Bone Joint Surg 1986;68B:635.
60. Owen M. The origin of bone cells in the post natal organism. Arthritis Rheum 1980;23:1074.
61. Reddi AH. Bone matrix in the solid state—geometric influence on the differentiation of fibroblasts. In: Lawrence JH, Gotman JW, eds. Advances in biological and medical physics, Vol. 15. New York: Academic Press, 1973:1.
62. Reddi AH. Cell biology and biochemistry of endochondral bone development. Coll Relat Res 1981;1:209.
63. Reddi AH. Extracellular matrix and development. In: Piez KA, Reddi AH, eds. Extracellular matrix biochemistry. New York: Elsevier, 1984:375.

64. Reddi AH. Extracellular matrix dependent local induction of cartilage and bone. J Rheumatol 1983;11:67.
65. Reddi AH, Anderson WA. Collagenous bone matrix-induced endochondral ossification and hemopoieses. J Cell Biol 1976;69:557.
66. Reddi AH, Higgins CB. Biochemical sequences in the transformation of normal fibroblasts in adolescent rats. Proc Natl Acad Sci USA 1972;69:1691.
67. Sampath TR, De Simone R, Reddi AH. Extracellular matrix derived growth factor. Exp Cell Res 1982;142:460.
68. Sampath TR, Reddi AH. Role of extracellular matrix components in cartilage and bone induction. UCLA Symposia on Molecular and Cellular Biology 1985;25:293.
69. Weiss RE, Reddi AH. Role of fibronectin in collagenous matrix-induced mesenchymal cell proliferation and differentiation in vivo. Exp Cell Res 1981;133:243.
70. Ashton BA, Allen TD, Howlet CR, et al. Formation of bone and cartilage by marrow stromal cells in diffusion chambers in vivo. Clin Orthop 1980;151:294.
71. Werntz J, Lane JM, Piez, et al. The repair of segmental bone defects with collagen and marrow. Transactions of the 32nd Orthopaedic Research Society Meeting, 1986:108.
72. Burwell RG. The function of bone marrow in the incorporation of a bone graft. Clin Orthop 1985;200:125.
73. Tomford WW, Starkweather RJ, Goldman MH. A study of the incidence of infection in the use of banked allograft bone. J Bone Joint Surg 1981;63:244.
74. Friedlaender GE, Mankin HJ. Bone banking: current methods and suggested guidelines. In: Instructional course lectures, Vol. 30. The American Academy of Orthopaedic Surgeons. St. Louis: Mosby, 1981:36.
75. Bos GD, Goldberg VM, Zika JM, Hieple KG, Powell AE. Immune responses of rats to frozen bone allografts. J Bone Joint Surg 1983;65A:239.
76. Chalmers J. Transplantation immunity in bone homografting. J Bone Joint Surg 1959;41B(1):160.
77. Friedlaender GE, Strong DM, Sell KW. Studies on antigenicity of bone. I. Freeze-dried and deep frozen allografts in rabbits. J Bone Joint Surg 1976;58A:854.
78. Halloran PF, Lee EH, Ziv I, et al. Orthotopic bone transplantation in mice. II. Studies of the alloantibody response. Transplantation (Baltimore) 1979;27:420–426.
79. Langer F, Czitrom A, Pritzker KP, Gross AE. The immunogenicity of fresh and frozen allograft bone. J Bone Joint Surg 1975;57A:216.
80. Muscolo DL, Kawai S, Ray RD. Cellular and humoral immune response analysis of bone-allografted rats. J Bone Joint Surg 1976;58A:826.
81. Friedlaender GE, Strong DM, Sell KW. Studies of the antigenicity of bone. II. Donor-specific anti-HLA antibodies in human recipients of freeze-dried allografts. J Bone Joint Surg 1984;66A:107.
82. Lee EH, Langer F, Halloran P, Gross AE, Ziv I. The immunology of osteochondral and massive allografts. Transactions of the 32nd Orthopaedic Research Society Meeting, 1986;4:61.
83. Pelker RR, Friedlaender GE, Markham TC. Biomechanical properties of bone allografts. Clin Orthop 1983;174:54.
84. Stevenson S. The immune response to osteochondral allografts in dogs. J Bone Joint Surg 1987;69A:573.
85. Bos GD, Goldberg VM, Powell AE, Heiple KG, Zika JM. The effect of histocompatibility matching on canine frozen bone allografts. J Bone Joint Surg 1983;65A:89.
86. Stevenson S, Hohn RB, Templeton JW. Effects of tissue antigen matching on the healing of fresh cancellous bone allografts in dogs. Am J Vet Res 1983;44:201.
87. Muscolo DL, Caletti E, Schajowicz F, Araujo ES, Makino A. Tissue typing in human massive allografts of frozen bone. J Bone Joint Surg 1987;69A:583.
88. Cornell CN, Lane JM, Nottebaert M, et al. The effect of ethylene oxide sterilization upon the bone inductive properties of demineralized bone matrix. Transactions of the 32nd Orthopaedic Research Society Meeting, 1986.
89. Urist MR, Dawson E. Intertransverse process fusion with the aid of chemosterilized autolyzed allogeneic (AAA) bone. Clin Orthop 1981;154:97.
90. Oikarinen J. Experimental spinal fusion with decalcified bone matrix and deep-frozen allogeneic bone in rabbits. Clin Orthop 1982;162:210.
91. Bowen JR, Angus PD, Huxster RR, MacEwen GD. Posterior spinal fusion without blood replacement in Jehovah's Witnesses. Clin Orthop 1985;198:284.
92. Stabler CL, Eismont FJ, Brown MD, Green BA, et al. Failure of posterior cervical fusions using cadaveric bone graft in children. J Bone Joint Surg 1985;67A(3):371.
93. Collis JS. Total disc replacement: a modified posterior lumbar interbody fusion. Report of 750 cases. Clin Orthop 1985;193:64.
94. Aurori BF, Weierman RJ, Lowell HA, et al. Pseudarthrosis after spinal fusion for scoliosis. A comparison of autogeneic and allogeneic bone grafts. Clin Orthop 1985;199:153.
95. McCarthy RE, Peek RD, Morrissy RT, Hough AJ. Allograft bone in spinal fusion for paralytic scoliosis. J Bone Joint Surg 1986;68A:370.
96. Malanin TI, Rosomoff HL, Sutton CH. Human cadaver femoral head homografts for anterior cervical spine fusions. Surg Neurol 1977;7:249.
97. Schneider JR, Bright RW. Anterior cervical fusion using preserved bone allografts. Transplant Proc 1976;8(Suppl 1):73.
98. Gepstein R, Nakamura K, Latta M, et al. Posterior spinal fusion with various types of bone grafts. Transactions of the 32nd Orthopaedic Research Society Meeting, 1986; 11:203.
99. Nasca RJ, Whelchel JD. Use of cyropreserved bone in spinal surgry. Spine 1987;12:222.
100. Siqueira EB, Kranzler LI. Cervical interbody fusion using calf bone. Surg Neurol 1982;18(1):37.
101. Salama R. Xenogeneic bone grafting in humans. Clin Orthop 1983;174:113.
102. DeBowes RM, Grant BD, Bagby GW, et al. Cervical vertebral interbody fusion on the horse: a comparative study of bovine xenografts and autografts supported by stainless steel baskets. Am J Vet Res 1984;45(1):191.
103. McMurray GN. The evaluation of Kiel bone in spinal fusions. J Bone Joint Surg 1982;64B(1):101.
104. Whitehill R, Wilhelm CE, Moskal, et al. Posterior strut fusions to enhance immediate postoperative cervical stability. Spine 1986;11:6.

105. Bradford DS. Instrumentation of the lumbar spine. An overview. Clin Orthop 1986;203:209.
106. Tuli SN, Singh AD. The osteoinductive property of decalcified bone matrix. An experimental study. J Bone Joint Surg 1978;60B:116.
107. Harakas NK. Demineralized bone matrix-induced osteogenesis. Clin Orthop 1984;188:239.
108. Bolander ME, Balian G. The use of demineralized bone matrix in the repair of segmental defects. J Bone Joint Surg 1986;68A:1264.
109. Einhorn TA, Lane JM, Burstein AH, et al. The healing of segmental bone defects induced by demineralized bone matrix. A radiographic and biomechanical study. J Bone Joint Surg 1984;66A:274.
110. Gepstein R, Weiss RE, Saba K, Hallel T. Bridging large defects in bone by demineralized bone matrix in the form of a powder. J Bone Joint Surg 1987;69A:984.
111. Lindholm TS, Nilsson OS, Lindholm TC. Extracellular and intraskeletal new bone formation induced by demineralized bone matrix combined with bone marrow cells. Clin Orthop 1982;171:251.
112. Wittbjer J, Palmer B, Rohlin M, Thorngren KG. Osteogenic activity in composite grafts of demineralized compact bone and marrow. Clin Orthop 1983;173:229.
113. Muthukumaran N, Reddi AH. Bone matrix-induced local bone induction. Clin Orthop 1985;200:159.
114. Glowacki J, Kaban LB, Murray JE, et al. Application of the biological principle of induced osteogenesis for craniofacial defects. Lancet 1981;1:959.
115. Glowacki J, Altobelli D, Mulliken JB. Fate of mineralized and demineralized osseous implants in cranial defects. Calcif Tissue Int 1981;30:71.
116. Glowacki J, Mulliken JB. Demineralized bone implants. Clin Plast Surg 1985;12(2):233.
117. Mulliken JB, Glowacki J. Induced osteogenesis for the repair and reconstruction of the craniofacial region. Plast Reconstr Surg 1980;65:553.
118. Mulliken JB, Kaban LB, Glowacki J. Induced osteogenesis—the biologic principle and clinical applications. J Surg Res 1984;37:487.
119. Flatley TJ, Lynch KL, Benson MD. Tissue response to implants of calcium phosphate ceramic in rabbit spine. Clin Orthop 1983;179:246.
120. Ferraro JW. Experimental evaluation of ceramic calcium phosphate as a substitute for bone grafts. Plast Reconstr Surg 1979;63(5):634.
121. Jarcho M. Calcium phosphate ceramics as hard tissue prosthetics. Clin Orthop 1981;157:259.
122. Jarcho M, Kay JF, Gumaer KI, et al. Tissue cellular and subcellular events at bone-ceramic hydroxyapatite interface. J Bioeng 1977;1:79.
123. Holmes RE, Bucholz RW, Mooney V. Porous hydroxyapatite as a bone graft substitute in diaphyseal defects: a histometric study. J Orthop Res 1987;5:114.
124. Rejda BV, Pellan JGJ, de Groot K. Tricalcium phosphate as a bone substitute. J Bioeng 1977;1:93.
125. Hoosendoorn HA, Renooji W, Akkermans LMA, et al. Long-term study of large ceramic implants (porous hydroxyapatite) in dog femora. Clin Orthop 1984;187:281.
126. Cook SD, Reynolds MC, Whitecloud TS, et al. Evaluation of hydroxyapatite graft materials in canine cervical spine fusions. Spine 1986;11(4):305.
127. Waisbrod H, Gerbershagen HU. A pilot study of the value of ceramics for bone replacement. Arch Orthop Trauma Surg 1986;105(5):298.
128. Patka P. Bone replacement by calcium phosphate ceramics: an experimental study. Thesis, Univ. of Amsterman. Amsterdam: Free University Press, 1984.
129. Muschler GM, Lane JM, Werntz J, et al. The use of composite bone graft materials in a segmental femoral defect model in the rat. Inaugural Meeting of the International Society for Fracture Repair, Helsinki, September 2, 1987.
130. Moore DC, Chapman MW, Manske D. The evaluation of a biphasic calcium phosphate ceramic for use in grafting long-bone diaphyseal defects. J Orthop Res 1987;5:356.
131. Canalis E. Effect of growth factors on bone cell replication and differentiation. Clin Orthop 1985;193:246.
132. Canalis E. The hormonal and local regulation of bone formation. 1983; Endocr Rev 42:62.
133. Urist ME, Delange RJ, Finerman GAM. Bone cell differentiation and growth factors. Science 1983;220:680.
134. Lindholm TS, Urist MR. A quantitative analysis of new bone formation by induction in composite graft of bone marrow and bone matrix. Clin Orthop 1956;150:288.
135. Takagi K, Urist MR. The role of bone marrow in bone morphogenetic protein-induced repair of massive femoral diaphyseal defects. Clin Orthop 1982;171:224.
136. Takagi K, Urist MR. The reaction of the dura to bone morphogenetic protein (BMP) in repair of skull defects. Ann Surg 1982;196:100.
137. Urist MR. Bone formation by auto-induction. Science 1965;150:893.
138. Urist MR, Granstein L, Nogami H, Swenson L, Murphy R. Transmembrane bone morphogenesis across multiple walled chambers. New evidence of a diffusible bone morphogenetic property. Arch Surg 1977;112:612.
139. Lovell T, Dawson EG. BMP augmentation of experimental spinal fusion. Transactions of the 32nd Orthopaedic Research Society Meeting, 1986.
140. Dickhaut S, DeLee JC, Page CP. Nutritional status: importance in predicting wound-healing after amputation. J Bone Joint Surg 1984;66A:71.
141. Einhorn TA, Bonnarens F, Burstein AH. The contributions of dietary protein and mineral to the healing of experimental fractures. J Bone Joint Surg 1986;68A:1389.
142. Jensen JE, Jensen TG, Smith TK, et al. Nutrition in orthopaedic surgery. J Bone Joint Surg 1982;64A(9):1263.
143. Nilsson OS, Bauer HCF, Brostrom L-A. Methotrexate effects on heterotopic bone in rats. Acta Orthop Scand 1987;58:47.
144. Conaty JP, Mongan JL. Cervical fusion in rheumatoid arthritis. J Bone Joint Surg 1981;63A(8):1218.
145. Bryan WJ, Inglis AE, Sculco TP, Ranawat CS. Methylmethacrylate stabilization for enhancement of posterior cervical arthrodesis in rheumatoid arthritis. J Bone Joint Surg 1982;64A:1045.
146. Clark CR, Keggi KJ, Panjabi MM. Methylmethacrylate stabilization of the cervical spine. J Bone Joint Surg 1984;66A(1):40.
147. Koskinen EVS. The effect of growth hormone and thyrotro-

pin on human fracture healing. Acta Orthop Scand (Suppl) 1963;62:7.
148. Udupa KN, Gupta LP. The effect of growth hormone and thyroxine in healing of fracture. Indian J Med Res 1965;53:623.
149. Koskinen EVS. The influence of hormonal treatment and orchiectomy, oophorectomy, and thyroidectomy on experimental fractures. Acta Orthop Scand (Suppl) 1965;80:7.
150. Barth R, McDonnell J, Muschler GF, Zimmerman P, Lane JM. The effect of thyroid hormone on bone healing in a segmental defect model. Transactions of the 32nd Orthopaedic Research Society Meeting, 1986.
151. Aprin H, Bowen JR, MacEwen GD, Hall JE. Spinal fusion in patients with spinal muscular atrophy. J Bone Joint Surg 1982;64A:1179.
152. Swank S, Brown JC, Perry RE. Spinal fusion in Duchenne's muscular dystrophy. Spine 1982;7:484.
153. Bunch WH. Muscular dystrophy. In: Hardy JH, ed. Spinal deformity in neurological and muscular disorders. St. Louis: Mosby, 1974:92.
154. Bassett CAL, Mitchell SN, Gaston SR. Treatment of ununited tibial diaphyseal fractures with pulsing electromagnetic fields. J Bone Joint Surg 1981;63A:511.
155. Paterson D. Treatment of nonunion with constant direct current: a totally implantable system. Orthop Clin North Am 1984;15:47.
156. Bassett CAL, Mitchell SN, Gaston SR. Pulsing electromagnetic field treatment in ununited fractures and failed arthrodeses. JAMA 1982;247:263.
157. Bassett CAL. The development and application of pulsed electromagnetic fields (PEMF's) for ununited fractures and arthrodeses. Orthop Clin North Am 1984;15:61.
158. Bassett CA, Pilla AA, Pawluk RJ. A non-operative salvage of surgically resistant pseudarthrosis and non-union by pulsing electromagnetic fields. Clin Orthop 1977;124:128.
159. Simmons JW. Treatment of failed posterior lumbar interbody fusion (PLIF) of the spine with pulsing electromagnetic fields. Clin Orthop 1985;193:127.
160. Kahanovitz, N, Arnoczky SP, Hulse D, Shires PK. The effect of postoperative electromagnetic pulsing on canine posterior spinal fusions. Spine 1984;9(3):273.
161. Nerubay J, Marganit B, Bubis JJ, et al. Stimulation of bone formation by electrical current on spinal fusion. Spine 1986;11(2):167.
162. Rothman RH, Klemek JS, Toton JJ. The effect of iron deficiency anemia on fracture healing. Clin Orthop 1971;77:276.
163. Bell GR, Gurd AR, Orlowski JP, Andrish, JT. The syndrome of inappropriate antidiuretic-hormone secretion following spinal fusion. J Bone Joint Surg 1986; 68A: 720.
164. Brown CW, Orme TJ, Richardson HD. The rate of pseudarthrosis (surgical non-union) in patients who are smokers and patients who are non-smokers. Spine 1986;11:942.

3

Response to Metallic Implants

Keith L. Wapner

Metallic implants have been used in the treatment of fractures for more than a hundred years. Initially fraught with material and mechanical problems, the application of such implants has blossomed in the last few decades through major advances both in metallurgy and in biomechanics. The success of total joint arthroplasty and new fracture fixation devices would suggest an even bigger role for metallic implants in the future.

Most orthopaedic fixation devices in use today are fabricated from three alloy systems: iron-based chromium alloys, collectively called stainless steel; cobalt-based alloys; and titanium-based alloys.[1] Although cobalt-based and titanium-based alloys have largely supplanted stainless steel in the manufacturing of total joint prostheses, stainless steel remains the metal most commonly used for spinal fixation. The composition of these metals is shown in Table 3.1.

Despite efforts to develop corrosion-resistant alloys, research has shown all metallic implants in use today corrode to some degree after implantation.[2] This finding is important as elements released in this corrosion process are known to be biologically active and in some cases potential carcinogens.[3–7] Therefore, it seems useful to examine the actual chemical and physical properties of the products released.

In reviewing studies on total joint prostheses, it must be kept in mind that these are weight-bearing, not weight-sharing, devices. The mechanical wear on these devices can be assumed to increase the rate of metal ion release through such mechanisms as disruption of the passivation layer and mechanical wear leading to crevice corrosion. Spinal instrumentation is performed with weight-sharing devices, and these factors should be minimal.

Toxic Effects of Metallic Elements

Nickel Toxicity

Dermatitis secondary to exposure to nickel was first described in response to industrial nickel dust.[8] Contact dermatitis caused by nickel release from objects that are worn has often been described.[9] The degree of perspiration seems to influence the severity of the dermatitis. Metal alloys are leached from the object, and divalent nickel ions can penetrate the skin to bind with keratin.[10] Eczematous dermatitis from implants of vitallium[11] and stainless steel[12,13] have also been described.

Oral toxicity has been minimal in low-dose studies up to a thousand parts per million.[14,15] Higher dose studies in mice have shown decreased growth rate[14,15] attributed to interference with normal enzymes of the kidney, liver, and heart.[16] High doses of nickel ingestion have led to decreased reproductive capacity in rats[17,18] and has produced hypoglycemia in rabbits.[19]

Intravenous and subcuticular administration has led to acute toxicity in the form of gastroenteritis, tremors, paralysis, and hyperglycemia.[10] Localization of injected nickel salts has been found in the pituitary gland and decreased serum prolactin levels have been detected. Changes in the distribution of serum lactic dehydrogenase (LDH) enzymes have also been reported.[10]

Nickel carcinogenicity was first described in the industrial literature. Inhalation of nickel compounds has been shown to produce acute pneumonitis.[19] Chronic exposure has been implicated in squamous metaplasia of the bronchial epithelium and carcinomas of the upper respiratory tract.[20] Especially implicated were nickel carbonyl,[20,21] nickel subsulfide, and nickel oxide.[21]

Numerous animal studies have shown nickel carcinoge-

Table 3.1 Structure and properties of metal alloys for surgical implants

	Stainless steel ASTM F55 or F56 316 or 316L wrought	CO-CR ASTM F75 ASTM F75 (Vitallium, Zimalloy Vinertium, Allivum, Protasul-2): cast	CO-CR ASTM F90 (Protasul-10:) wrought	MP35N AMS 5758 Vacuum remelt: cast-wrought	Titanium (pure) ASTM F67 cast-wrought	Titanium 6Al-4V Alloy ASTM F136 cast-wrought
Weight %						
Carbon	0.08 max. (0.03 max.)	0.35 max.	0.05–0.15	0.25 max.	0.10 max	0.08 max.
Manganese	2.00 max.	1.0 max.	2.0 max.	0.15 max.	—	—
Phosphorus	0.03 max.	—	—	0.015 max.	—	—
Sulfur	0.03 max.	—	—	0.01 max.	—	—
Silicon	0.75 max.	1.00 max.	1.00 max.	0.15 max.	—	—
Tungsten	—	—	14–16			
Cobalt	—	57.4–65	46–53	30.25–38	—	—
Chromium	17–20	27–30	19–21	19–21	—	—
Nickel	10–14	2.5 max.	9–11	33–37	—	—
Molybdenum	2–4	5–7	—	9–10.5	—	—
Iron	59–70	0.75 max.	3.0 max.	1.0 max.	0.5 max.	0.25 max.
Oxygen				—	0.45 max.	0.13 max.
Aluminum				—	—	5.5–6.5
Vanadium				—	—	3.5–4.5
Titanium				99+	88.5–92	

nicity through intravenous and intramuscular administration of ground nickel complexes,[22–24] as well as through inhalation.[25,26] The mechanisms of nickel carcinogenicity appear to be related to its ability to enter the cell by direct crossing of the membranes, as with nickel carbonyl, or by formation of protein complexes that adhere to the cell and enter via pinocytosis.[10] Once in the cell, nickel ions can inhibit the induction of certain enzymes[27,28] and bind to certain nucleic acids.[29] The proposed mechanism involves alteration of deoxyribonucleic acid (DNA) polymerase to temporarily decrease the fidelity of the DNA replication. Chemical modification of ribonucleic acid (RNA) and nuclear proteins that regulate the DNA template activity may cause expression of normally repressed portions of the genome. Metabolic block at the level of mRNA and inhibition of induction of enzymes involved in metabolic degradation of organic carcinogens also has been described.[10] Myoblasts involved in the repair of muscle injury have shown absorption of nickel protein complexes and have been implicated in causing myoblast neoplastic transformation.

Cobalt Toxicity

Animal studies involving administration of cobalt show that sheep tolerated oral doses as much as 1000 times normal (3 mg per kilogram of body weight) without adverse effects. Doses greater than this produced decreased appetite, loss of body weight, and anemia.[30] Anemia is believed to be related to inhibition of iron uptake because of a common pathway of absorption.[31,32] Single doses of 300 mg/kg of body weight were lethal.[33] Polycythemia has been described secondary to cobalt administration. When given in doses of 10 mg/kg of body weight for 2 weeks, polycythemia was induced, presumably from increased erythropoietin production in the kidneys as a response to local tissue anoxia caused by inhibition of respiratory enzymes. This hypoxic stimulation of the bone marrow led to induced erythrohyperplasia.[34–36]

Cobalt had been previously used for the treatment of anemias[37–39] at a dosage of 20–30 mg per day,[40] but this was discontinued secondary to toxic side effects of thyroid hyperplasia, myxedema, and congestive heart failure.[41,42] Cobalt has also been implicated as a cause of goiters secondary to decreased thyroid activity; it apparently interferes with iodine intake and transfer. Goiters have also been described in people living in geographical areas where the ratio of cobalt and iodine is abnormal. It has been suggested that cobalt is needed for thyroid hormone synthesis.[40] Congestive heart failure and cobalt cardiomyopathy were described in detail following the beer epidemic of 1965–1966; cobalt, which had been added as a stabilizer, led to a unique cardiomyopathy. Retrospective epidemiological studies implicated cobalt in patients that had a triad of findings involving cardiomyopathy, polycythemia, and thyroid hyperplasia. The cardiomyopathy is reversible with nonspecific electrocardiogram (EKG) changes, a high incidence of pericardial effusions, and a low rate of arrhythmia. Histological examination revealed an accumulation of glycogen in the muscles and an accumulation of cobalt in the mitochondria.[41–43]

Cobalt decreases oxygen uptake in the mitochondria by inhibiting alpha ketoglutarate de hydrogenase (α-KGDH) and pyruvate dehydrogenase (PDH). The heart is dependent on high oxygen uptake because of its oxidative metabolism and high energy requirements. Cobalt kelates the disulfate groups of lipoic acid, the coenzyme for α-KGDH and α-PDH. The presence of alcohol, thiamine deficiency, and protein deficiency are needed to induce cobalt cardiomyopathy.[44–47]

Cobalt has also been implicated in the production of local fibrosarcomas[40,43,48,49] and thyroid tumors[50] in animal studies.

Chromium Toxicity

Only 1%–3% of chromium ingested in the normal diet is absorbed.[51–54] Chromium is present in various valence states, the hexavalent form being better absorbed than the trivalent. The mechanism of absorption is unknown but is suggested to be related to the same pathway as zinc.[55,56]

The storage and transport of chromium proposes a difficult problem in relationship to studying its toxic effects. Chromium VI passes through the red blood cell membrane and binds to the globin portion of hemoglobin.[57] Chromium(III) cannot enter the cell and travels in the serum bound to transferrin. Rapid tissue turnover and uptake of chromium have been shown in various studies.[54,58] Whole-body clearance seems to have a three-component half-life of 0.5, 6, and 83 days, respectively. In view of these and other findings, it is suggested that there may not be an equilibrium between body and blood stores of chromium.[57] Therefore, serum measurements may not be a good indicator of total body chromium load.

The subcellular distribution of chromium reveals that most is found in the nuclear portion, less in the supernatant, and least in the mitochondria.[59,60] Organ distribution studies reveal that before exposure chromium is located mostly in the lung, liver, kidney, spleen, pancreas, thyroid, and adrenal glands. After exposure, marked increases have been noted in the respiratory tract, bone, kidney, and tissues of the reticuloendothelial system.[60,61] Chromium is mostly excreted in the urine, but small amounts have also been detected in bile and in the feces. However, there is a poor correlation between blood and urine levels in exposed individuals.[61]

Toxicity of chromium seems to be intimately related to its valence state. In various studies, animals fed large doses of chromium(III) did not seem to show toxic effects. In one study, mice and rats fed 5 parts per million of chromium(III) actually lived longer than the controls.[62] Parenteral administration of chromium(III) can be toxic, but to a much lesser degree than chromium(VI).[63]

Hexavalent chromium has been found to be toxic in many ways. Topical exposure can lead to erosion of the mucosal membranes.[62] When used topically to treat warts, chromium has been described as causing anurea, nephritis, and kidney lesions.[62] Oral ingestion of dichromate has been reported to show gastrointestinal ulceration as well as central nervous system disturbances.[62] In animal studies ingestion of five parts per million of hexavalent chromium caused growth retardation and malignant tumor formation.[64,65] Inhalation of chromium VI has been reported to cause dermatitis, nasal ulcerations, and lung carcinomas.[64,66]

Carcinogenicity of chromium initially was described in industrial exposure.[67–70] Chromium is widely used in metallurgy, brick, glass, ceramic, paint, dye, and tanning industries. Although the multiple valance states have been described, the trivalent and hexavalent are the only forms that exist in nature in an appreciable amount.[70] Chromium(III) is the stable oxidation state and is always present as a coordination complex that tends to hydrolyze and chelate at physiological pH. Although studies would seem to implicate chromium(VI) as the causative agent in most of the toxic effects, it is believed that the trivalent state is the real agent of toxicity and mutagenicity.[71–74] It appears that chromium enters the cell in a hexavalent form but then is rapidly reduced to the trivalent form. It is this trivalent form that ultimately binds to nuclear material and has been shown to induce point mutations and infidelity of DNA replication, as well as chromosomal aberrations and sister chromatid exchanges in mammalian cells.[75–83] Because intracellular chromium is rapidly converted to chromium(III) an intracellular sink is created and a plasma erythrocyte or plasma reticuloendothelial cell equilibrium is never reached.[84]

Aluminum Toxicity

With the advent of titanium alloy prostheses, concern has been raised over the toxic effects of aluminum. It has been demonstrated previously that aluminum is not released from brain tissue after uptake.[85–87] This can lead to a gradual increase in brain burden of aluminum. Changes in the central nervous system following systemic administration of aluminum salts has been described over the years, and it has been implicated as having an epileptogenic effect.[88] Recent concern over aluminum toxicity has increased since its identification as an agent in the dementia of Alzheimer's disease.[85,89,90]

There has also been great concern about the toxic effects of aluminum in renal dialysis patients. Both dialysis dementia[91] and osteomalacia have been seen secondary to toxic effects of aluminum.[92] Animal studies indicate that the quantity of aluminum found in both the blood and brain may be dependent on the preparation of aluminum that is used.[93] Aluminum transfers poorly across the blood–brain barrier. In animal studies, increased blood levels with aluminum gluconate were found only with very high doses. However, this differs from observations in long-term hemodialysis patients in whom high aluminum levels have been observed with blood aluminum levels less than 1 mg per liter.[91,94,95,98] Alterations in several biochemical parameters of the nervous system, particularly in the cholinergic transmission system, have been suggested as the causative agent of these changes of dementia. Aluminum-induced osteomalacia has been reported in as many as 70% of patients with dialysis dementia.[92] These patients have osteomalacia with low bone formation and no fibrosis.[96] They are often symptomatic with spontaneous fractures. The serum calcium values are usually elevated but parathyroid hormone levels are depressed.[97] Treatment with calcitriol and calcidiol has been unsuccessful.[98] Parathyroidectomy leads to deterioration of bone disease in this group.[99]

Vanadium Toxicity

Vanadium has been suggested as being an essential trace element in the body.[100] Although its exact biochemical and physiological function is not known, it has been suggested that it interacts with intracellular components and inhibits certain enzyme functions.[101] Animal studies with high rates of vanadium exposure have shown increased levels in bone, liver, kidney, spleen, and testes, but not in the brain.[102,103] Although the patterns of distribution and metabolism seem to be independent of its oxidation state,[103,104] mortality studies in a number of species have shown the pentoxide to be three- to fivefold more toxic than the trioxide by the pulmonary route.[105] In tissue studies the solubility rather than the oxidation state has been implicated in its toxicity.[106] For equivalent concentrations of the three oxidation states, the observed toxicity on rabbit alveolar macrophages did not vary. Similar results in systemic and subcellular time distribution studies of vanadium have been reported.[100,107] This finding suggests that vanadium is converted either extracellularly or intracellularly to a common oxidation state.

It has been shown that vanadium is poorly stored in the red cells of human blood and is bound mainly to transferrin in plasma.[107] Liver ferritin has also been shown to bind vanadium in animal studies. Cell culture studies have shown an increase in lactate dehydrogenase from cells exposed to particulate vanadium.[108] Histological examination of fibroblasts exposed to vanadium have shown gross necrosis with only cytoplasmic debris and pyknotic nuclei remaining in contact with the metal. However, it should be noted that similar studies using wear debris from a titanium alloy prosthesis showed neither evidence of cell damage by morphological appearance nor any release of lactate dehydrogenase. It is possible that the difference between the exposure to the pure metal and wear debris may be secondary to the effects of the pure metal on cell membranes.[109]

Studies on respiratory symptoms from chronic vanadium exposure in industry have reflected principally the irritative properties of the vanadium oxides.[110] The intensity of these effects has been related directly to exposure concentration and particle size.[111] Tissue culture studies on animal alveolar macrophages have shown that acid phosphatase is inhibited as much as 70% by dissolved vanadium pentoxide. It has been suggested that exposure to vanadium may result in an impairment of the lung's resistance to bacterial infection, secondary to inhibition of macrophage function.

Titanium Toxicity

Studies on the toxic effects of titanium have shown that titanium is usually well tolerated in cell culture experiments.[103,112] Tissue culture studies using human synovial fibroblasts showed slight increases in the release of lactate dehydrogenase above that observed in untreated cells. However, no morphological changes were observed.[113] Investigations using porous titanium fiber metal implanted in animal bone have shown an increased rate of release with increase in porosity. It has been suggested from these studies that titanium may accumulate in the marrow.[114]

This local accumulation of titanium may be secondary to its acidic character. It has limited coordinating capability to representative cellular chelators, and this may decrease its ability to migrate from its point of release.[114] In general, it is believed that titanium is well tolerated in biological systems.

Human Studies

Numerous studies have been reported in the literature analyzing trace element burdening of human tissues from corrosion of hip and knee joint prostheses.[87,115–118] Most of these studies have been done on metal-on-metal prostheses, but recently studies of conventional metal-on-polyethylene prostheses have been performed. Coleman,[119] using neutron activation techniques, demonstrated increased levels of cobalt and chromium in the urine and serum in patients with metal-on-metal prostheses. Schniewind[120] investigated adjacent soft tissues after implantation of vitallium cups, and also found increased metal burdens. This is in agreement with the work of Evans,[121] who showed increased burdens of cobalt and chromium in patients with metal-on-metal prostheses as well as a small increase in patients with metal-on-polyethylene. Jones[122] and Dobbs and Minski[123] also demonstrated increased levels in the urine and various tissue samples. However, normal values have not been clearly delineated for comparison.

Abeln[124] compared serum cobalt and chromium levels in patients who have undergone metal-on-metal as opposed to metal-on-polyethylene prosthetic implants. He showed significant increases in cobalt and chromium for the metal-on-metal prostheses but no significant increases for metal-on-polyethylene. However, no blind data were available for comparison. Mielke[125] reviewed a series of patients who underwent total knee arthroplasties. He demonstrated no increase in serum levels for metals, but did show increased synovial tissue levels. This is also demonstrated by Michel et al.[126] in their evaluation of articular capsules and distant tissue specimens. They have found increases of many orders of magnitude for cobalt, chromium, and nickel in the adjacent capsular tissues, and increases in chromium at a distant site 6 cm from the implant in the fascia lata. All the prostheses in this study were the metal-on-metal polyethylene type. They also found increases in other trace metals, such as zinc, and stated that there may be changes in body metabolism of these other metals secondary to increased burdens of the trace metals released from the prosthesis. However, they concluded that not enough was known about the body's ability to handle the trace element burdening as well as the normal mechanism by which the body metabolizes these elements.

Recently, Bartolozzi and Black[127] and Black et al.[128] have shown increased levels of nickel, cobalt, and chromium in urine and serum in patients who have undergone metal and plastic polyethylene implants. The point that must be stressed in reviewing all these recent studies in patients who have undergone metal-on-polyethylene implants is that, although increased values have been determined, none of these values is outside of normal values reported for these metals. Although there is presently broad disagreement about what represents normal levels, there is no significant evidence to suggest that with the newer metal-on-polyethylene implants tissue burdening is occurring in pathological ranges. Most of these studies have short-term follow-up, and longer term studies are definitely needed. However, there is evidence to support the theory that an equilibrium is reached in the corrosion process such that if the body is capable of handling the level of release, long-term tissue burdening should not be occurring.

A number of recent reports of tumors developing at the site of implants deserve review. The first case reported of malignant tumor at the site of the metallic implant was by McDougall[129] in 1956. He reported a sarcoma presumed to be a Ewing's type at the site of a stainless steel implant, a stainless steel plate that had been placed 30 years previously for fracture of proximal humerus. The plate and screws were composed of dissimilar metals, which would account for an increased rate of corrosion about this implant. There was also a long latency period between the time of implantation and the time of tumor formation, suggesting a causal effect.

Delgato[130] reported a case of a sarcoma that developed about the site of the tibial plate. The etiology of this tumor was obscured as the patient had received radiation therapy to this area for periosteal ossification 2 years after the initial plate was implanted. Additionally, the plate was removed at the time of radiation therapy. One year subsequent to that, a second biopsy revealed a malignant sarcoma. In view of the short latency period after the plating and with the added insult of radiation therapy, a pure causal effect is difficult to establish. In 1972, Dube and Fisher[131] reported a case of the hemangioendothelioma of the tibia at the site of a metal plate used for treatment of a nonunion. In this case, the plate had been retained for 30 years. Evaluation of the plate and screws revealed they were dissimilar types of stainless steel. The plate and six of the screws were 316 stainless steel; two other screws were composed of 304 stainless steel. The belief was that the use of dissimilar metals may have certainly been a contributing factor to the corrosion that was seen, and may have subsequently increased the burden of metal ions, leading to the formation of this tumor.

Taynton[132] reported a case of a Ewing sarcoma at the site of a metal plate made of cast vitallium. The tumor was seen in an 11-year-old girl who was 7.5 years status post subtrochanteric rotational osteotomy. One might suggest a cause-and-effect relationship between the plate and the development of the tumor; however, when this case is evaluated in light of the incidence of Ewing's sarcoma in this age group, a causal relationship between the plate and the sarcoma is less likely. It is possible that the sarcoma would have developed without the plate ever having been inserted.

Dodion et al.[133] reported immunoblastic lymphoma at the site of the infected vitallium bone plate. The initial subcapital fracture occurred in a 49-year-old man after a fall on the street, and after plating the fracture became infected. A subsequent biopsy was positive for immunoblastic lymphoma. It is certainly unusual for an otherwise healthy 49-year-old man to sustain a fracture of the hip. Therefore, the hypothesis entertained by the authors of this study is that the lymphoma was present from the beginning.

Penman and Ring[134] described an osteosarcoma at the site of the metal-on-metal Ring-type uncemented prosthesis. Six years after surgery the patient presented with a grossly swollen right hip and a fracture of the femur around the prosthesis. Biopsy performed revealed a pleomorphic malignant tumor consistent with an osteogenic sarcoma. By history the patient had no evidence of previous radiotherapy, and histological examination failed to reveal any evidence of Paget's disease. Swan[135] also reported on a soft-tissue tumor presumed to be a malignant fibrous histiocytoma around a vitallium all-metal McKee–Farrar prosthesis. The diagnosis was made in a 63-year-old man 3 years after implantation of this prosthetic device. In this case there was no direct contact between the metal and the tumor or between the cement and the tumor, thus making a causal relationship difficult to establish.

Bago-Granell et al.[136] also reported a case of a malignant fibrous histiocytoma at the site of a total hip arthroplasty in a 77-year-old woman who developed this lesion 2 years after her total hip procedure. They hypothesized that the malignant transformation was a consequence of bony necrosis from the acrylic cement. As pointed out in their article, there have been previous reports of a transformation to malignant fibrous histiocytoma at the site of bone infarcts. However, in each case there has been a long latency period between the infarct and the malignant transformation. In this patient there was only a 2-year period, again making a causal relationship difficult to establish. Lee et al.[137] reported a case of a malignant fibrohistiocytoma at the site of plate 14 years after open reduction and internal fixation of a femur fracture in a 44-year-old man. In their review, they failed to mention the composition of the plate. The case is further complicated by osteomyelitis at the involved site, suggesting that perhaps malignant transformation was secondary to this cause rather than to metallic release.

Although one cannot conclusively rule out the relationship between these tumors and the metallic implants, with the exception of the studies by McDougall and by Dube and Fisher, the latency period between insertion of the implant and the development of the tumors suggests that a causative relationship is unlikely. Tumor latency periods derived from industrial studies show an average of 21 years for chromium and 23–27 years for nickel.[138] Of note in these two cases is that dissimilar metals were used, which could lead to a drastic increase of the corrosion rate and release of metallic ions. Laboratory studies have shown that there is a direct dose–response effect in the development of tumors in animals and this may account for the etiology of these lesions. These lesions, however were around the site of a fracture fixation plate.

Primary bone tumors are extremely rare, accounting for only 0.22%–0.25% of all tumors in adults.[139–141] Their incidence is approximately one per million of the adult population. The use of spinal instrumentation has been increasing in the last few decades because of advances in both the strength and designs of the available implants. It is unlikely that there are more than several million patients worldwide with spinal implants. In light of the low intrinsic sensitivity to neoplastic transformation in this relatively small population at risk, implant site tumors would appear to be unlikely to occur.[1]

Conclusion

It has been well established that metallic devices corrode to some degree after implantation. Review of the in vitro, in vivo, and human studies on the effects of metallic ions from corrosion of orthopaedic implants clearly demonstrates a dose–response relationship in toxicity and mutagenicity. The studies showing elevations of these ions in serum, urine, and tissues of patients have not shown them to be beyond the range of normal. The risk associated with these devices at this point appears minimal.

The biological consequences of spinal instrumentation devices must be viewed in terms of their immediate, intermediate, and long-term effects as well as the local systemic and remote effects. To date several human studies have shown increased levels of corrosion products in serum and urine in patients after total hip arthroplasty. In addition, autopsy studies have revealed metal concentrations in numerous organs throughout the body. Investigations using neutron activation technique have revealed increased levels of cobalt and chromium in tissues adjacent to metallic implants. We are aware of no studies of this nature in patients with spinal instrumentation. Evaluation of this data is difficult as there is no clear consensus on what the so-called "normal" levels of these ions in human tissue should be.

Advances in manufacturing technology have led to better passivation of these implants. By adhering to the principles of proper insertion of these devices, the passivation layer should not be disturbed. With the current implants in use, the rate of corrosion should be minimized.

Further studies on the long-term effects of these implants are certainly indicated. With the present widespread use of the implants, there have been no data to suggest that toxic effects are occurring. There are presently a substantial number of spinal instrumentation procedures that have more than a 10-year follow-up with no current evidence to suggest any pathology occurring from metallic ion release. However, this possibility cannot be ruled out until well-organized epidemiological studies are performed.

References

1. Black J. Metallic ion release and its relationship to oncogenesis. Proceedings of the Thirteenth Open Scientific Meeting of the Hip Society. CV Mosby, St. Louis: Mosby, 1985:199–213.

2. Mears D. Materials in orthopaedic surgery. Baltimore: Williams & Wilkins, 1979.
3. Black J. Systemic effects of biomaterials. J. Biomater 1985;5:11–18.
4. Burrows B. Chromium: metabolism and toxicity. Boca Raton: CRC Press, 1983.
5. Clark GCF. Biologic properties of cobalt. In: Williams DF, ed. Systemic aspects of biocompatibility, Vol. 1. Boca Raton: CRC Press, 1981:133–142.
6. Mushak P. Metabolism and systemic toxicity of nickel. In: Nriagu JO, ed. Nickel in the environment. New York: Wiley, 1980:499–524.
7. Smith GK, Black J. Models for systemic effects of metallic implants. In: Weinstein A, et al., eds. Retrieval and Analysis of Orthopaedic Implants. NBS Special Publ. 472. Washington, DC: U.S. Govt. Printing Office, 1977:23–30.
8. Underwood DJ. Trace elements in human and animal nutrition. New York: Academic Press, 1977:159–169.
9. Malten KE, et al: Nickel sensitivity in detergents. Acta Dermatovenu 1969;49:10–13.
10. Venugopol B, Luckey ID. Metal toxicity in mammals. New York: Plenum Press, 1978:293–297.
11. Symeonides PP, et al. An allergic reaction after internal fixation using a vitallium plate. J Allergy Clin Immunol 1973;51:251–254.
12. Barranco DP, Solomon H. Eczematous dermatitis from nickel. JAMA 1972;220:1244.
13. Cramer M, Lucht V. Metal sensitivity in patients treated for tibial fractures with plates of stainless steel. Acta Orthop Scand 1977;48:245–249.
14. Phatak SS, Patwordhon ZN. Nickel sulfate toxicity in the mouse. Indian J. Sci Ind Res 1950;9B:70–76.
15. Phatak SS, Patwordhon ZN. Oral toxicity of nickel sulfate in mice. Indian J. Sci Ind Res 1952;11B:173–175.
16. Webber CW, Reid DL. Nickel toxicity in young growing mice. J Anim Sci 1969;28:620–623.
17. Heath JC, Webb M. Content and intracellular distribution of the inducing metal in primary rhabdomyosarcomata induced in the rat by cobalt, nickel and cadmium. Br J Cancer 1967;21:768–772.
18. Watschewa W, et al. Testicular changes due to long-term administration of nickel sulfate in rats. Exp Pathol 1972;6:116–121.
19. Gordynya RI. The effects of nickel on rabbits. Vopr Ratsion Pitan 1969;5:167–170.
20. Sunderman FW, Selin CE. The metabolism of nickel-63 carbonyl. Toxicol Appl Pharmacol 1966;12:207–218.
21. Anonymous. National Academy of Sciences Committee on Medical and Biologic Effects of Environmental Pollutants; Nickel. DC: NAS, 1975.
22. Gilman JPW. Proceedings of the 6th Canadian research conference on muscle tumorgenesis, Honey Harbor, Ontario. Oxford: Pergamon Press, 1964:209–223.
23. Heath JC, Daniel MR. The production of malignant tumours by nickel in the rat. Br J Cancer 1964;18:261–264.
24. Lau TJ, Hackett RL, Sunderman FW. The carcinogenicity of intravenous nickel carbonyl in rats. Cancer Res 1972;32:2253–2258.
25. Heuper WC. Experimental studies on metal carcinogenesis. Arch Pathol 1958;65:600–604.
26. Sunderman FW. Metal carcinogenesis in experimental animals. Food Cosmet Toxicol 1971;9:105–120.
27. Kasprzak KS, Sunderman FW. The effect of nickel carbonyl^{14}C. Toxicol Appl Pharmacol 1969;15:295–301.
28. Sunderman FW. Inhibition of induction of benzopyrene hydroxylase by nickel carbonyl. Cancer Res 1967;27:950–955.
29. Hotem-Champey S. Affinity of the folic acid for nickel and nickel-induced cancer. CR Acad Sci 1961;253:2791–2792.
30. Becker DE, Smith SE. The level of cobalt tolerance in yearling sheep. J Anim Sci 1951;10:226.
31. Forth W, Rummel. Intestinal absorption of metal ions, trace elements, and radionucleotides. New York: Permagon Press, 1971.
32. Symposium on cardiomyopathy. Can Med Assoc J 1967;97:881–928.
33. Andrews ED. Cobalt poisoning in sheep. New Zealand Vet J 1965;13:101.
34. Davies JT. The clinical significance of the essential biological metals. Springfield: Thomas, 1972:94–101.
35. Fisher JW, et al. Influence of cobalt on sheep erythroporetin and several hormones on erythroporesis in bone marrows of isolated perfused hind limbs of dogs. Blood 1964;23:87–98.
36. Underwood DJ. Trace elements in human and animal nutrition. New York: Academic Press, 1977:132–158.
37. Coles BL. Use of cobalt in common anemias of childhood. Arch Dis Child 1955;30:121–126.
38. Lancet and Anon: cobalt and anemia, Lancet 1955:1:1312.
39. Venugopol B, Luckey TD. Metal toxicity in mammals. New York: Plenum Press, 1963:285–289.
40. Thomas JA, Thiery JP. Production de elective de liposarcoma chez des lapins parles oligollemente zinc et cobalt. CR Acad Sci 1953;236:1387–1389.
41a. Grece AC, et al. Myocardial toxicity of cobalt in the rat. Ann NY Acad Sci 1969;156:184–196.
41b. Kriss JP, Carnes WH, Gross RT. Hypothyroid and thyroid hyperplasia in patients treated with cobalt. JAMA 1955;157:117.
42a. Roby JS, et al. Cobalt-induced myxedema: a report of a case. N Engl J Med 1956;255:955.
42b. Lin JH, Duffy JL. Cobalt-induced myocardial lesions in rats. Lab Invest 1970;23:158–162.
43. Sullivan JL, et al. Tissue cobalt content "beer drinkers myopathy." J Lab Clin Med 1968;71:893–896.
44. Alexander CS. Cobalt in the heart. Ann Intern Med 1969;74:11–13.
45. Bolkhena RJ. Trace element metabolism in animals. London: Livingstone, 1970:426.
46. Derr RF, Aakers H, Alexander CS. Synergism between cobalt and ethanol and rat growth rate. J Nutr 1970;100:521–524.
47. Wiberg GS. The effect of cobalt ions on energy metabolism in the rat. Can J Biochem 1968;46:549–554.
48. Gilman JP. Metal carcinogenesis. II: A study on the carcino-

genic activity of cobalt, copper, iron and nickel compounds. Cancer Res 1962;22:158–160.

49. Heath JC. The production of rat tumors by cobalt. Br J Cancer 1957;10:668–673.
50. Sullivan JL, et al. Myocardiopathy of beer drinkers. Ann Intern Med 1969;70:277–282.
51. Donaldson RM, Barreras RF. Intestinal absorption of trace quantities of chromium. J Lab Clin Med 1966;66:484–493.
52. Hopkins LL, Scwarz K. Chromium. III: Binding to serum proteins, especially siderophilin. Biochim Biophys Acta 1964;90:484–491.
53. Mertz W, Roginski EE. The dependence of chromium transferred into the rat embryo on the chemical form. Am J Physiol 1965;209:489.
54. Visek WJ, et al. Metabolism of chromium[51] by animals as influence by chemical state. Proc Soc Exp Biol Med 1953;10:610–615.
55. Hahn CJ, Evans GW. Absorption of trace metal in the zinc-deficient rat. Am J Physiol 1975;228:1020.
56. MacKenzie RD, et al. Chronic toxicity studies. II: Hexavalent and trivalent chromium administered in drinking water to rats. AMA Arch Ind Health 1958;18:232.
57. Underwood EJ. Trace elements in human and animal nutrition. New York: Academic Press, 1977: 258–270.
58. Hopkins LL. Distribution in the rat of physiological amounts of injected chromium. III: With time. Biochim Biophys Acta 1965;209:731–735.
59. Edwards C, et al. Intracellular distribution of trace elements in liver tissue. Proc Soc Exp Biol Med 1961;107:94.
60. Tandon SK, et al. Distribution of chromium in poisoned rats. Toxicology 1979;13:29–34.
61. International Agency for Research on Cancer. Monograph on the evaluation of carcinogenic risk of chemicals to humans: some metals and metallic compounds, Vol. 23, evaluation of carcinogenic risk. Leone, France: World Health Organization, 1980.
62. Venugopol B, Luckey TD. Metal toxicity in mammals, Vol. 2. New York: Plenum Press, 1978:248–250.
63. Mertz W, Roginski E. Some biologic properties of chromium nicotinic acid complexes. Fed Proc 1975;34:922.
64. Brinton HP, Frazier ES, Koven AL. Morbidity and mortality experience among chromium workers. Public Health Rep 1952;67:835.
65. Schroeder HA, Balassa JJ, Vinton WH, Jr. Chromium, cadmium and lead levels in rats: effects on life span, tumors and tissue levels. J Nutr 1965;86:51–66.
66. Browning E. Toxicity of Industrial Metals. 2d ed. Stoneham, Maine: Butterworths, 1969.
67. Laskin S. Research in environmental science. Washington, DC: Institute of Environmental Medicine, 1972:92–97.
68. Mancuso TF, Hueper WC. Occupational cancer and other health hazards in a chromate plant: a medical appraisal. Ind Med Surg 1951;20:358–363.
69. Meltoni C. Occupational carcinogenesis. Excepta Med Int Congr Ser 1974;322:19–26.
70. Meltoni C. Precursor lesion in exposed populations as indicators of occupational cancer risk. Ann NY Acad Sci 1976;271:444–447.
71. Bianchi V, Levis AG, Saggioso D. Differential cytotoxic activity of potassium dichromate on nucleoside uptake in BHK fibroblasts. Chem-Biol Interact 1979;24:137–151.
72. Bianchi V, Levis AG, Majone F, et al. Mechanisms of chromium toxicity in mammalian cell cultures. Toxicology 1980;17:218–224.
73. Fishbein L. Environmental metallic carcinogens: an overview of exposure levels. J Toxicol Environ Health 1976;2:77–109.
74. Majone F, Levis AG. Chromosomal aberrations and sister chromated exchanges in Chinese hamster cells treated in vitro with hexavalent chromium compounds. Mutat Res 1979;67:231–238.
75. Levis AG, et al. Effects of potassium dichromate on nuclear acid and protein synthesis and on precursor uptake in BHK fibroblasts. Cancer Res 1978;38:110–116.
76. Levis AG, et al. Cytotoxic effects of hexavalent and univalent chromium in mammalian cells in vitro. Br J Cancer 1978;37:386–396.
77. Levis AG, Majone F. Cytotoxic and clastogenic effects of soluble chromium compounds on mammalian cell cultures. Br J Cancer 1979;40:523–533.
78. Mathier AK. Comparative toxicity of hexavalent and trivalent chromium to rabbits. Toxicology 1977;8:53–61.
79. McRae WD, et al. Sister chromated exchanges induced in cultured mammalian cells by chromate. Chem-Biol Interact 1979;26:281–286.
80. Nakamuro K, et al. Comparative studies of chromosomal aberration and mutagenicity of trivalent and hexavalent chromium. Mutat Res 1978;58:175–181.
81. Newbold RF, et al. The cytotoxic mutagenic and clastogenic effects of chromium containing compounds on mammalian cells in culture. Mutat Res 1979;67:55–63.
82. Tandon SK, et al. Comparative toxicity of trivalent and hexavalent chromium: alterations in blood and liver. Environ Res 1978;15:90–99.
83. Umeda M, Nishemura M. Inducibility of chromosomal aberrations by metal compounds in cultured mammalian cells. Mutat Res 1979;67:221–229.
84. Lilien PL, Spival JL, Goldman ID. Chromate transport in human leukocytes. J Clin Invest 1970;49:1551–1557.
85. Crapper DR. Neurobiology of aging. In: Terry RD, Gershon S, eds. Aging, Vol. III. New York: Raven Press, 1976:405.
86. Deboni U, Scott JW, Crapper DR. Intracellular aluminum binding: a histochemical study. Histochemie 1974;40:31.
87. Marquis JK. Aluminum neurotoxicity: an experimental perspective. Bull Environ Contam Toxicol 1982;29:43–49.
88. Kopeloff LM, Barbera SE, Kopeloff N. Recurrent convulsive seizures in animals produced by immunologic and chemical means. Am J Psychiatry 1942;98:881.
89. Hetnarski B, Wisniewski HM, Iqbal JD, Aziedzic and Lajthaj: Central cholinergic activity in aluminum induced neurofibrillary degeneration. Ann Neurol 7:489, 1980.
90. Perl DP, Brody AR. Alzheimer's disease: x-ray spectrometric evidence of aluminum accumulation in neurofibrillary tangle bearing neurons. Science 1980;208:297.
91. Alfrey AC, LeGendre GR, Kaehny WD. The dialysis encephalopathy syndrome. Possible aluminum intoxication. N Engl J Med 1976;294:184–188.

92. Pierides AM, Edwards WG, Cullum V, McCall JT, Ellis HA. Hemodialysis encephalopathy with osteomalacic fractures and muscle weakness. Kidney Int 1980;18:115–24.
93. Leblondell G, Allain P. Blood and brain aluminum concentrations in mice after intraperitoneal injection of different aluminum compounds. Res Commun Chem Pathol Pharmacol 1980;27:3.
94. Cartier F, et al. Encephalopathie myoclonique progressive des dialyses role de l'eau utilisee pour l'hemodialyse. Nouv Presse Med 1978;7:97–102.
95. Flendrig JA, Kruis H, Das HA. Aluminum intoxication: the cause of dialysis dementia. Proceeding of 13th Congress of EDTA, Hamburg, 1976: 355–363.
96. LaBelle FS. Prolactin secretion specifically inhibited by nickel. Nature (London) 1973;245:300–302.
97. Hodsman AB, et al. Vitamin D resistant osteomalacia in hemodialysis patients lacking secondary hyperparathyroidism. Ann Intern Med 1981;94:621–37.
98. Ott SM. Aluminum related osteomalacia. Int J Artif Organs 1983;6:173–175.
99. Felsenfeld HA, et al. Osteomalacia after parathyroidectomy in patients with uremia. Ann Intern Med 1982;96:34–39.
100. Hopkins LL, Mohr HE. Vanadium as an essential nutrient. Fed Proc 1974;33:1773–1775.
101. Simons TJB. Vanadate—a new tool for biologists. Nature 1979;281:337–338.
102. Peabody RA, et al. Metabolism of vanadium-48 in normal and endocrine deficient rats. In: Hemphill DD, ed. Trace Substances and Environmental Health, Vol. 10. Columbia, Missouri: University of Missouri Press, 1976:441–450.
103. Sabbioni E, Marafante E. Metabolic patterns of vanadium in the rat. Bioinorg Chem 1978;9:383–407.
104. Sabbioni E, Marafante E. Relationships between iron and vanadium metabolism: in vivo incorporation of vanadium into iron proteins of the rat. J Toxicol Environ Health 1981;8:419–429.
105. Roshchin IV, et al. Effects on organisms of vanadium trioxide. Fed Proc (Suppl.) 1965;24:611–613.
106. Waters MD, Gardner DE, Coffin DL. Cytotoxic effects of vanadium on rabbit alveolar macrophages in vitro. Toxicol Appl Pharmacol 1974;28:253–263.
107. Tipton IH, Shafer JJ. Statistical analysis of lung trace element levels. Arch Environ Health 1964;8:58–67.
108. Rae T. The toxicity of metals used in orthopaedic prostheses: an experimental study using cultured human synovial fibroblasts. J Bone Joint Surg 1981;63B:435–440.
109. Rae T. The hemolytic action of particulate metals. J Pathol 1978;125:81–89.
110. Faulkner-Hudson TG. Vanadium Toxicity and Biologic Significance. Amsterdam: Elsevier, 1964:76.
111. Lewis CE. Biologic effects of vanadium. II: The signs and symptoms of occupational vanadium exposure. AMA Arch Ind Health 1959;19:497–503.
112. Rae T. A study on the effects of particulate metals of orthopaedic interest on murine macrophages in vitro. J Bone Joint Surg 1975;57B:444–450.
113. Rae T. Biologic response to titanium and titanium aluminum vanadium alloy particles. I: Tissue culture studies. Biomaterials 1986;7:30–36.
114. Ducheyne T, et al. In vivo metal ion release from porous titanium fiber material. J Biomed Mater Res 1984;18:293–308.
115. Barbos M, Benvenuti A. Metallic debris arising from prosthetic abrasion: investigation of biodegradation of the materials and physiopathology of the bone. Ital J Orthop Traumatol 1983;9(3):377–86.
116. Cracchiolo A, Revell P. Metal concentration in synovial fluids of patients with prosthetic knee arthroplasty. Clin Orthop 1982;170:169–174.
117. Oonishi H, et al. Studies on corrosion of long retained metals in the living body. Acta Orthop Belg 1982;48:710–716.
118. Pazzaglia U, et al. Metal determination in organic fluids of patients with stainless steel hip arthroplasty. Acta Orthop Scand 1983;54:574–579.
119. Coleman, RF, Harrington J, Scales, JT. Concentration of wear products in hair, blood and urine after total hip replacement. Br Med J 1973;1:527–529.
120. Schniewind EO, Kasparek K, Ohnsorge J. Untersuchungen des Kontaktgewebes von Blount'schen Vitalliumklammern mit Hilfe der instrumentellen Neutronenaktivierungsanalyse. Z Orthop Grenzgeb 1975;113:209–216.
121. Evans EM, Freeman MAR, Miller AJ, Vernon-Roberts B. Metal sensitivity as a probable cause of bone necrosis and loosening of the prosthesis in total hip joint replacement. J Bone Joint Surg 1974;56B:626–642.
122. Jones DA, Lukas HK, O'Driscoll M, Price CH, Wibberley B. Cobalt toxicity after McKee hip arthroplasty. J Bone Joint Surg 1975;57B:289–296.
123. Dobbs HS, Minski MJ. Metal ion release after total hip replacement. Biomaterials 1980;1:193.
124. Abeln M. Spurenelemente im Serum nach Implantation von Kobalt-Chrom-Totalendoprothesen der Hufte—Untersuchungen mit Hilfe der Neutronenaktivierungsana-lyse. Thesis. Köln, 1977.
125. Mielke R, Henke G, Ehrenbrink H. Kobalt-und Chromkonzentrationen in der Synovialflussigkeit und ein Blutserum nach Implantation von Kneigelenkendo-prosthesen mit Hilfe der Neutronenaktivierungsanalyse. Z Orthop Grenzgeb 1981;119:767–768.
126. Michel R, et al. Trace elements burdening of human tissues due to corrosion of hip joint prostheses made of cobalt chromium alloys. Arch Orthop Trauma Surg 1984;103:85–95.
127. Bartolozzi A, Black J. Chromium concentrations in serum, blood clot and urine from patients following total hip arthroplasty. Biomaterials 1985;6:2.
128. Black J, Matin EC, Gelman H, Morris D. Serum concentrations of chromium cobalt and nickel after total hip replacement: a six months study. Biomaterials 1983;4:160.
129. McDougall A. Malignant tumour at site of bone plating. J Bone Joint Surg 1956;38B:709–713.
130. Delgado ER. Sarcoma following a surgically treated fractured tibia. Clin Orthop 1958;12:315–318.
131. Dube VE, Fisher DE. Haemangioepithelioma of the leg following metallic fixation of the tibia. Cancer 1972;30:1260–1266.

132. Taynton KJJ. Ewing's sarcoma at the site of a metal plate. Cancer 1980;45:413–415.
133. Dodion P, et al. Immunoblastic lymphoma at the site of an infected vitallium bone plate. Histopathology 1983;6:807–813.
134. Penman HG, Ring PA. Osteosarcoma in association with total hip replacement. J Bone Joint Surg 1984;66B:632–634.
135. Swan M. Malignant soft tissue tumor at the site of a total hip replacement. J Bone Joint Surg 1984;66B:629–631.
136. Bago-Granell J, et al. Malignant fibrous histiocytoma of bone at the site of a total hip arthroplasty. J Bone Joint Surg 1984;66B:38–40.
137. Lee H, et al. Malignant fibrous histiocytoma at site of metal implant. Cancer 1984;54:2286–2289.
138. Schottenfeld D, Haas JF. Carcinogens in the workplace. Cancer 1979;29:144.
139. Cancer facts and figures. Washington, DC: American Cancer Society, 1984.
140. Cancer incidence in Sweden. National Board of Health and Welfare. The Cancer Registry. Tryckindustri, Solna: 1983.
141. Cancer statistics regular series, MB1 #12, Office of Population and Census Surveys. London: Her Majesty's Printing Office, 1980.

■4■

Electrical Stimulation of Spinal Fusions

William J. Kane

Introduction

The ability of bone to respond to changes in the mechanical loads to which it is subjected led, in 1892, to the formulation of Wolff's law by the anatomist Julius Wolff. "The form of the bone being given, the bone elements place or displace themselves in the direction of the functional pressure, and increase or decrease their mass to reflect the amount of functional pressure." Bone not only alters its orientation in response to mechanical stress but also gains or loses substance.[1] Simply put, the internal architecture of bone is an expression of the external forces acting upon it. How this transduction of mechanical energy to a biological response occurs is imperfectly understood; it is hypothesized that through a negative feedback system the mechanical force effects a change in the crystalline systems of bone, and because bone is piezoelectric—which means that it generates an electric current when it is mechanically deformed—it was suggested that the electric signal was a component of the feedback loop.[2,3]

The loop can be pictured (Fig. 4.1) as mechanical energy being transduced to electrical energy, which in turn evokes a biological response that reacts against the mechanical force or energy. The exact nature of the source of the electric potential is still uncertain although there may be more than one source. Shamos and Lavine characterized the origin as the collagenous organic matrix of bone.[4,5] Becker et al.[6] believed the source to be a semiconductor rectification mechanism. Friedenberg and Brighton[7] described the chemical gradients of viable cells, and Anderson and Ericksson[8,9] considered the fluid to be streaming through the solid matrix. Lavine and Grodzinsky recently indicated that the "streaming potential mechanism appears to be the major contributor of mechanically generated potentials," based on the magnitude and time dependence of the potentials seen in fully wet bone. The electronegativity seen at a hard- or soft-tissue injury is not the result of the electromechanical activity of bone but "due to electrogenic pumps that are associated with living cells."[10] The elaboration of endogenous potentials led to many efforts to determine whether exogenous potentials could stimulate bone growth and healing. These trials encompassed direct, alternating, and pulsed currents, different current densities, varying electrode potential differences, electrodes of differing materials, and finally current sources that were totally implanted, totally external and some percutaneous. Other parameters studied included capacitive and inductive coupling, as well as time-varying magnetic fields and time-varying electrical fields. These basic studies, in turn, led to the clinical assessment of

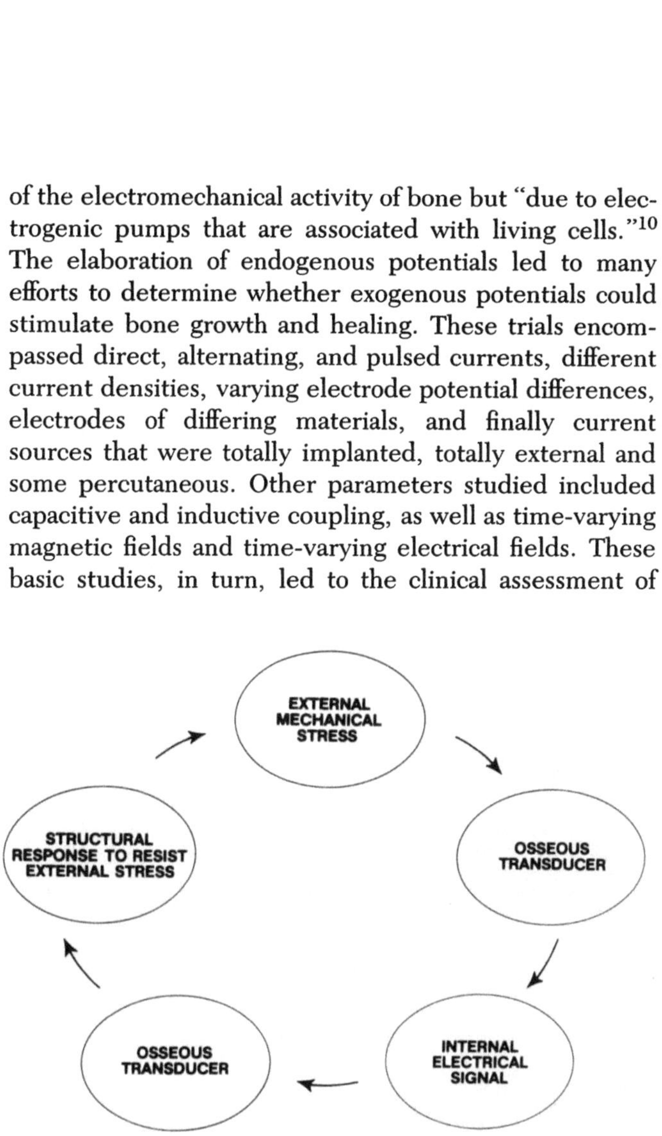

Figure 4.1. A hypothetical negative feedback loop demonstrates that external mechanical forces are transduced, or converted, into electrical signals, which in turn trigger a biological structural response that will resist the external forces. The exogenous electronic bone growth stimulator would enter the loop between the "Internal Electrical Signal" and the following "Osseous Transducer."

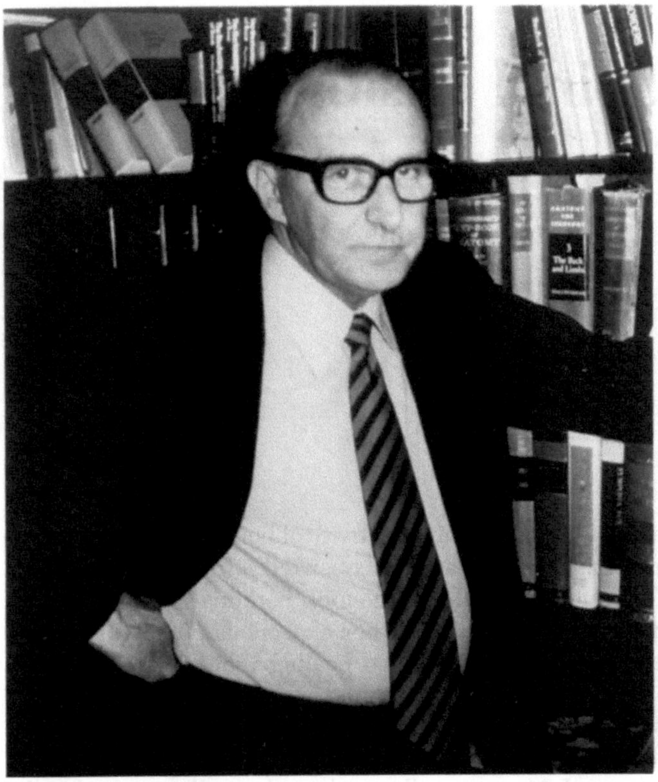

Figure 4.2. Allan F. Dwyer.

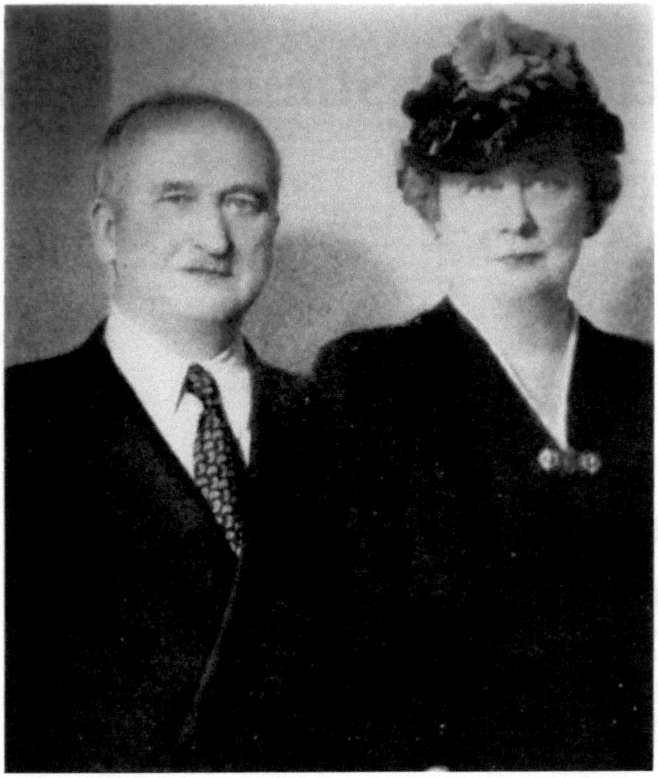

Figure 4.3 Fred H. Albee and Mrs. Albee. (Photograph courtesy of Hugo Kein.)

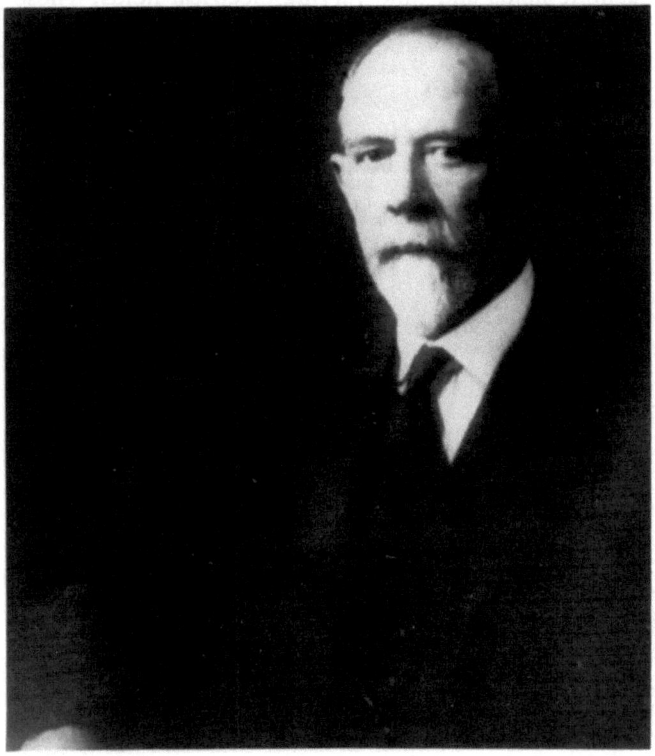

Figure 4.4 Russell A. Hibbs. (Photograph courtesy of Frank H. Bassett, III.)

electrical stimulation in facilitation of the healing of nonunions or delayed unions of the extremity long bones.[11]

Early Clinical Studies

Dwyer (Fig. 4.2) and Wickham, beginning in 1971, created a direct current device to stimulate bone healing in posterior spine fusions.[12] Seven decades earlier, Albee[13] (Fig. 4.3) and Hibbs[14] (Fig. 4.4) had almost simultaneously but independently reported on posterior spinal fusion for tuberculosis and other deformities of the spine. Over the ensuing years spinal fusions became commonplace especially in the lumbosacral region for pain, instability, and disease, in the thoracolumbar region for deformity, and in the cervicothoracolumbar regions for trauma and degeneration, but clinical success rates varied greatly according to anatomical region, etiological factors, and patient influences (age, compensation factors, etc.). It must be remembered that even with the achievement of a solid arthrodesis, a total cure in the clinical management of spinal pain, deformity, or disease is not assured. Clinicians dealing with patients with low back pain certainly recognize this; what they also recognize is that a solid arthrodesis is not always attained, nor is identifying a solid fusion an easy task.

A review of the fusion rates in lumbosacral fusions was presented at the International Society for the Study of the Lumbar Spine at Paris in 1981 by J. H. Evans et al. of Oswestry, England. They compiled 31 articles in which 3383 patients were assessed; the overall success rate was a reported 74% using varying types of lumbosacral fusions. Specifically, in regard to posterior or posterolateral fusions, Evans found 14 series encompassing 1705 patients with what was reported as a 79% success rate.[15] The word "reported" should be considered carefully because the ability to confirm the presence of a solid fusion is not the obverse of confirming a definite nonunion. Sacks, in 1965, stated "An accurate appraisal of successfully fused lumbar vertebrae can be made only by re-exploration of the fusion site."[16] Watkins echoed the same idea: "The only sure method of determining fusion in doubtful cases is by exploration."[17]

Because clear-cut pseudarthroses with motion amounted to 26% of the Evans compilation, the admonitions of Sacks and Watkins suggest an even higher percentage of failure if one were able to easily detect less obvious nonunions. Taking into account also the fact that these were the *published* series of lumbosacral fusions, one must wonder what the success rates would have been in those series that were not published either because of paucity of numbers or sparsity of success. The strong suspicion must be entertained that lumbosacral fusion rates in general are not as high as 74%, in the absence of internal instrumentation or other supplementations.

Dwyer and Wickham[12] were aware of the earlier work showing that direct current stimulation can induce or accelerate osteogenesis. They sought to mimic or enhance the zone of negativity by electrical stimulation to improve the reliability of operations for spinal fusion in the lumbosacral area. From February to September 1972, Dwyer performed 12 spinal fusions using a stimulator designed by Wickhan. The prototype stimulator had four titanium-tipped cathodes and one platinum-iridium-tipped anode, connected to the circuitry by 15-cm-long titanium leads insulated by silicone elastomer. (The very first anodic leads were of stainless steel, but were changed after four trials to platinum.) Each cathode carried 5 μA of current at loads that can vary from 0 to 100,000 Ω, and the battery capacity was sufficient to permit operation for 12 to 16 weeks. It is a tribute to Dwyer and Wickham that there have been no essential design modifications during 15 years of use, although the battery capacity has been increased to 24 to 26 weeks and the anodic lead has been eliminated, using the case of the battery as the ānode.

Dwyer, using a posterior approach, destroyed the facet joints and grafted a fibular strut to impart some stability. The cathodes were "inserted tightly into drill holes in the superior articular processes adjacent to the inferior articular processes of the vertebra above." The battery pack was placed deep to the deep fascia overlying the sacrospinalis and the anode was sutured to the sacral spine. Cancellous bone "was placed about each cathode." (Although bone graft is used to facilitate the fusion process about the facet points, it is reasonable but not proven that the cathode tips should be inserted into viable bone that would respond to the exogenous electrical signal. The graft bone could not respond to the exogenous signal until it had been colonized to the extent that it manifested some responsiveness to both exogenous and endogenous stimuli. This assumption has influenced the positioning of electrodes as described later under *Operative Technique*). Postoperative suction was used, as was an antibiotic regimen and a surgical corset. The stimulator was later removed on an inpatient basis from 5 to 16 weeks when, in most cases, the fusion area was completely exposed and macroscopically examined. (Dwyer, aside from the credit he must be given for the device and its clinical application, must also be acknowledged for his thoroughness in subjecting his patients to reoperation and exploration as was advocated by Sacks and Watkins.)[16,17] The bone appeared to form over an area 1 cm in radius around each cathode. In a number of instances the stimulator battery pack was removed and the electrode wires freed by a firm pulling motion without a complete exposure of the fusion.

Of 12 patients, only 1 was known to have a nonunion caused by a radiographically demonstrable anodic electrode failure due to corrosion. (Two other cases may possibly have had failure of the early fusion with fracture of the soft new bone. No other details were offered.) Dwyer and Wickham acknowledged the consequences of "inadvertent damage to the silicone insulation" on the early stainless steel leads. Tissue necrosis was found at reoperation about anodal sites where the silicone insulation had broken, leading to anodic destruction of the stainless steel lead. This problem disappeared with conversion of the stainless steel lead to titanium and with the use of thicker silicone insulation.

In a subsequent paper, Dwyer[18] noted that current flow in tissues is a flow of ions and that the chloride ion gives up its charge at the anode; it will attack stainless steel, forming ferric chlorides, nickel chlorides, and chromium chlorides, which are toxic and cause tissue destruction. Platinum, iridium, and titanium are free of this defect; oxidative products do not insulate the lead thus reducing current flow to ineffective levels.

Dwyer also indicated that he has used a different configuration (two cathodes and three anodes) "for anterior fusions." Seven single-level anterior fusions were performed and seven fused; five multiple-level anterior fusions were performed, and four were characterized as successful fusions and one the other "almost certainly successful."

Of considerable interest are the suggestions made by Dwyer that if he had used "a massive amount of cancellous graft the incidence of pseudarthrosis could have been lessened because although the bone would still have been immature at the time of battery removal, there would have been more of it to share the load," and, "I am also fairly sure that it would be better to use a battery with a longer life. All battery life is uncertain but our present batteries (1975) will last 3 months. I think a 6 to 12 month battery would assure much more chance of success."[18] In this article Dwyer candidly noted 7 certain failures of 47.

In addition to the 12 anterior fusions noted above, there were 35 posterior fusions but no certain failures of 13 single-level fusions, two certain failures and three probable failures of 13 two-level, fusions and five certain failures of 9 triple- level or greater fusions.

Experimental Data

In an editorial comment in a symposium on electrical current stimulation in spinal fusion, the editor, Mooney (Fig. 4.5), related an experimental series of five dogs in which posterior spinal fusions were done.[19]

"In each dog a posterior facet fusion was accomplished in the standard manner. Also, in each dog two electrical stimulators were used: each had four cathodes, one of which was placed at each of the eight facet joints operated upon. The engineers had tested the implants, and for each animal only one of the two was active. The other was a dummy. They appeared identical and thus the identity of the "live" one was unknown to the surgeon. Two months after surgery the animals were sacrificed and evaluated visually, radiographically, mechanically, and histologically. In the 40 joints operated upon (five animals, eight facets per animal), no difference could be distinguished between the 20 joints influenced by direct electrical stimulation and the 20 that served as controls. The appearance and mechanical testing were similar in each group. To the best of our understanding, we tried to reproduce the placement of cathodes and anodes as suggested by Dwyer, but it is quite possible that our animal placement was not the same as in the clinical studies he has reported."[19]

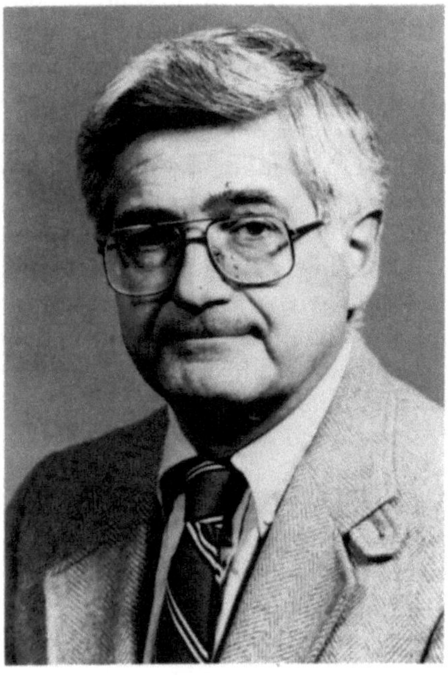

Figure 4.5 Vert Mooney.

I have included verbatim the methodology and results of Mooney's series because this set of experiments performed as a double-blind series and then judged by nonbiased evaluators certainly influenced the acceptance of the concept of electrical stimulation of spinal fusions.

Mooney himself in correspondence dated July 20, 1981 indicated: "As you recognize, this was not a very scientific study and did not deserve to be published. In that it has the opportunity of presenting some potentially negative information regarding the efficacy of electrical stimulation in lumbar fusions, it would be inappropriate for this information to be promulgated on such flimsy evidence."[20]

Numerous questions arise from this series which, except for the editorial aside, was never published. It is not known whether all 40 paired joints—stimulated and nonstimulated—fused, did not fuse, or simply some fused and some did not, but always as a pair independent of electrical stimulation. Can we decide whether stimulation is deleterious or helpful? If it is deleterious, can the dog overcome such an inference? Does it appear that stimulation is beneficial but we cannot recognize it because these dogs fused all treated joints independent of electrical stimulation? If electrical stimulation does have a beneficial effect, would it not be possible that the facet fusing (because it was stimulated) assisted in the attainment of fusion on the nonstimulated contralateral facet? Perhaps the active stimulator cathodes were not matched side by side in the same motion segment with the dummy cathodes; if so, then up to 20 paired nonstimulated facet joints all fused, in the absence of electrical stimulation but in the face of a foreign body, that is, the dummy cathode; this again indicates a high rate of fusion in the canine posterior facet when subjected to a "standard " fusion technique. It appears that this protocol simply does not allow the effect of electrical stimulation to manifest itself; if a protocol were developed that provided the opportunity for a failure of fusion, then the effect of the stimulation might be assessed.

Kahanovitz and coworkers[21] repeated Mooney's series using electromagnetic pulsing. They found that postoperative electromagnetic pulsing in adult dogs subjected to posterior spinal fusions showed "an unparalleled early osteogenic response in the stimulated group, but by 9–12 weeks, there did not appear to be any significant difference" in either group "as both were solidly fused by 12 weeks." This was essentially the finding of Mooney, that is, the dog fuses his posterior spine with speed and efficiency.

Nerubay et al.[22] performed two-level posterior spine fusions on 1-month-old pigs, half of which were stimulated at all four facets and half of which were not, since the battery pack was rendered inactive. At 1 month, 10 animals were sacrificed and no statistical difference was noted between the six stimulated pigs and the four nonstimulated pigs using histological and radiographic scoring. By 2 months, however, there was a significant increase of the fusion score in the active stimulator group ($p = .037$ using the Fisher's exact test for 2×2 tables). Comparing the total study groups, the results showed a statistically significant increase of fusion in the 2-month-old group ($p < .01$).

Kahanovitz and Arnoczky[23] performed one-level fusions at L1–L2 and at L4–L5 in large adult mongrel dogs. The facet joints were excised removing all cartilage and subchondral bone in the posterior two-thirds of the joints. Local spinous processes were used as bone graft, and a hole was drilled across both facets and the interposed bone graft at each level. The hole was filled with a cathodic electrode tip. An active bone growth stimulator was used in six animals and a dummy was used in six others. No other efforts at achieving a fusion, i.e. decortication of the other posterior elements or additional grafting, were involved in this series. The results with this protocol were markedly different from earlier research efforts of Mooney[19] and Kahanovitz.[21] There did not appear to be any appreciable radiographic or histological evidence of bony fusion in the 2-, 4-, or 6-week specimens in either the stimulated or control groups. At 12 weeks, all stimulated facet joints showed consistent radiographic and histological evidence of solid bony fusion. In contrast, the control or unstimulated facet joints showed no radiographic or histological evidence of bony fusion at 12 weeks. The authors noted the small sample size but also insisted "there can be little controversy over the distinctly different but consistent findings."

Later Clinical Studies

Dwyer et al.[24] reported on the early usage of the stimulator at the annual meeting of the Scoliosis Research Society in 1973. In 1980 at the annual meeting of the American Academy of Orthopaedic Surgeons, a report on 10 patients followed to fusion or failure was presented by Kane et al.[25] Of the 10 patients, 8 had previous surgery (an average of two previous procedures per patient) and 7 were involved in either workmen's compensation or personal injury litigation. Nine of the 10 fused, and 8 of 10 attained good (2) or excellent (6) results in terms of pain relief.

In a number of patients, pain relief was dramatic and virtually immediate, suggesting the possibility of an effect similar to that of a TENS (Transcutaneous Electrical Nerve Stimulation) unit, although a placebo effect cannot be ruled out. In attempting to salvage a small group of multiply operated patients with chronic low back problems, significant difficulties in designing a double-blind study arose. Recognizing these limitations, however, the authors were encouraged that the electronic bone growth stimulator enhanced lumbosacral fusions by stimulating local bone deposition.

Two years later in 1982, a series of 84 patients with a follow-up of at least 12 months was presented to the American Academy of Orthopaedic Surgeons by Kane et al.[26] Two patients are not included in the study, 1 because of loss to follow-up and the second because the stimulator was removed approximately 10 days postoperatively because of unexplained patient complaints of increased pain following implantation.

The follow-up and determination of solidity were performed by the operating surgeon, utilizing his own criteria of success whether that included plain films, tomograms, stress films, computer-assisted tomography (CAT) scan, or radioisotopic bone scans. This reliance on the operating surgeon for the definition of success or failure is a recognized shortcoming but is a failing common to the literature surveyed as well as to a specific comparison group that was also studied.

In the 82 patients, the success rate for the fusion was 91.5%. Although the data indicate a high rate of fusion for these patients, rhetorical questions were raised by the authors as to (1) whether or not this success rate might have been expected if the operations on this group of patients had been done without the use of electrical implants; (2) whether this group of patients was representative of patients undergoing this type of surgery in regard to such characteristics as age, sex, and the like, and (3) whether there were any characteristics in this group of patients which made them unique in the sense that one could not generalize the results in this group of patients to the general population of patients who are candidates for this type of surgery.

The review of lumbosacral fusions by Evans et al.[15] of Oswestry, England, presented at the International Society for the Study of the Lumbar Spine at Paris in 1981, has already been noted; in 31 papers, 3383 patients appeared to have an overall success rate of 74%. Because of the concern that this retrospective literature survey might not reflect the then-current spine fusion surgery results, a current survey of lumbosacral fusions at the major teaching hospitals of two university medical schools, South Carolina and Northwestern, was performed; 159 such patients were identified.

The comparison group and the implant group were then analyzed, and it was found that the implant group was representative of the general population of patients who are candidates for lumbosacral fusions in regards to such variables as age and sex, but not with regard to numbers of previous surgeries of the percentage of previous attempted fusions (Table 4.1). With respect to previous surgery the stimulator group had previous surgery 80.5% of the time as compared with 27.6% in the comparison group. In the 84 implant patients, there were 154 *previous* low back operations for an average of 1.83 per patient. The percentage having pseudarthrosis was 56.1% in the stimulator group as compared with 19.5% in the comparison group. The differences between the two series in regard to rates of prior surgery and pseudarthrosis were highly significant statistically ($p < .001$), which suggested that in regard to these two variables, the stimulator patients were not representative of the general population of patients who underwent this type of surgery.

However, the important questions were whether or not the higher success rate observed in the stimulator group could be attributed to the stated differences in these two variables and whether the history of previous surgery or the presence of a pseudarthrosis increases the probability of success in those patients in which the stimulator was implanted. Dyer, a statistician, determined that to the extent that previous failed surgery increases the probability of failure and to the extent that the implant series had a much higher proportion of patients with previous failed surgery, the failure rate expected in the stimulator series should have been higher than in the comparison group. In fact, the reverse was true; the fusion rate was 91.5% in the implant group versus 80.5% for the comparison group. In the implant group of 46 with pseudarthrosis, 42 achieved a successful fusion for a success rate of 91.3%.

At the same meeting in 1982, Brooks and Macy[27] reported on 13 patients undergoing L3 to sacrum or longer one-sided Watkins fusions using the stimulator. Of 13 patients, 9 attained good (5) or excellent (4) results, and 4 were rated poor although only 3 of the 43 levels did not fuse.

Table 4.1 Comparison of stimulated group and a nonstimulated comparison group[25] (Reprinted with permission of author and publisher.)

Parameter	Stimulated	Non stimulated[a]
Number	82	159
Mean age (yr)	41.2	40.0
Under 40 yr (%)	49	46
Males (%)	54	62
Previous Surgery (%)	81	28
Pseudarthrosis (%)	56	20
Success:		
Overall	75/82 (92%)	128/159 (81%)
Pseudarthrosis	42/46 (91%)	NA[b]

[a] Comparison group from northwestern South Carolina.
[b] NA, not available.

In 1984, Nerubay and Katznelson[28] reported on five spinal fusions for spondylolisthesis using the stimulator inserted into a strut-graft spanning L4 and S1 after removing the loose fragment. A Harrington distraction bar was inserted from L3 to S1. The patients were all in the second decade, and in 10 weeks the five patients "had good, solid fusion, judged clinically and radiographically." A year follow-up confirmed persistent good results.

While a true double-blind study was and is impossible because microammeters, are readily available that can reveal whether a unit is functioning or not and because most of these patients have litigation or compensation issues that generally preclude their participation in such studies, nevertheless a prospective randomized controlled trial series was begun using only "difficult patients." "Difficult patients" were defined as patients who had either one or more previous failed fusions, a grade II or worse spondylolisthesis, a multiple-level fusion, or a high-risk factor such as obesity. These patients were randomized by protocol as to whether they received a stimulator or not. The fusion rates of the two groups were assessed radiographically by the operating surgeon and by an independent radiologist at least 18 months postoperatively. Films included flexion-extension or side-bending and plain films, and in some instances the presence or absence of motion was determined by reoperation. The radiographs were reviewed by one of two independent radiologists without prior knowledge of the results as assessed by the investigator. This review confirmed a lack of bias in the investigator's assessment of fusion. Seven investigators in five different states had 63 patients; each operator had to have at least 4 patients in the study, at least 2 with a functioning stimulator and at least 2 without. Three patients were lost to follow-up, and in 1 the fusion attempt was discontinued. Statistical review confirmed the comparability of the groups (see Table 4.2). Success, defined as radiographic fusion, was achieved in 15 of 28 control patients (54%) compared with 25 of 31 treatment patients (81%). This result is statistically significant. ($p = .026$, one-tailed Fischer's exact test.) Results according to entry criteria and according to levels fused showed in each instance the superiority of stimulation (Tables 4.3 and 4.4).[29,30]

Concurrent with the randomized controlled trial, a nonrandomized study was conducted by a different group of clinical investigators. The protocol for the nonrandom study was identical to the random trial protocol, except that all patients received stimulation rather than being randomized into treatment and control categories. Results at 12 months post surgery were available on 116 patients

Table 4.2 Comparison of a stimulated group of "difficult patients" and a nonstimulated group of "difficult patients"[28] (Reprinted with permission of author and publisher.)

Parameter	Stimulated	Control
Number	31	28
Mean age (yr)	39.8	39.8
Under 40 yr (%)	49%	50%
Males (%)	68%	77%
Pseudarthrosis	35%	35%
Success:		
Overall	25/31 (81%)	16/28 (54%)
Pseudarthrosis	9/11 (82%)	4/10 (40%)

Table 4.3. Results by entry criteria[28] (Reprinted with permission of author and publisher.)

Criterion	Stimulated	Control
Previous failed fusion	82% (9/11)	40% (4/10)
Spondylolisthesis	100% (2/2)	83% (5/6)
Two or more levels fused	73% (11/15)	50% (6/12)
Other high risk factor	89% (8/9)	75% (6/8)

Table 4.4 Results by Levels Fused[28] (Reprinted with permission of author and publisher.)

Levels	Stimulated	Control
One	88% (14/16)	63% (10/16)
Two or more	73% (11/15)	42% (5/12)

by December 1984. Of 54 females and 62 males, the mean age was 45 years the median age 43 years, and the range 16 to 69 years. There were 29 patients (25%) with a previous failed fusion, including 6 patients with more than one previous failure.

At 12 months post surgery, successful fusion was achieved in 108 of 116 patients (93%). Of 62 males, 59 (95%) were assessed to have radiographic union, compared to 49 of 54 (91%) females. The over-50 age group had 43 of 43 successful fusions (100%). In the subgroup recognized as the highest risk, the previous failed fusion group, success was seen in 26 of 30 patients (87%).

The data were further analyzed to determine whether or not there was an increased risk of infection associated with this type of implantable bone growth stimulator. Out of all of the patients enrolled in both the random and nonrandom trials, only 1 of 466 patients (0.2%) was reported to have an infection.[31]

Operative Indications

Selection of patients will obviously depend on each surgeon's individual assessment and selection criteria; however, the following is offered as a general background for indications for use of the electrical bone growth stimulator. At the present time it is my opinion that the electrical bone growth stimulator (Fig. 4.6) for lumbosacral fusions is clearly indicated in those situations in which the risk of nonunion is, in general, higher than for typical lumbosacral fusions. More specifically, this includes patients with one or more previous surgical procedures, either with or without attempts at previous lumbosacral fusion, patients who have had tissue loss either as a result of tumor or previous surgery, and patients with symptomatic and progressive spondylolistheses.

Additionally, occasions will arise when primary lumbosacral fusions, either for lumbosacral instability secondary to degenerative disease or lumbosacral instability secondary to a spondylolysis, may, because of other factors, warrant the use of the electrical bone growth stimulator. Gradually, as more experience and information in the use of this device is acquired, its indications will be more clearly defined. I know of no specific contraindications to its use in the adult lumbosacral fusion.

Operative Technique[32]

The patient is positioned either in a prone position with pads under the iliac crests or in a modified knee-chest position. A midline incision is made from the spinous process above the intended fusion site to the spinous process of S1. By means of wide, long-handled periosteal elevators in conjunction with sharp dissection by scalpel, subperiosteal dissection of the musculature overlying the spinous processes, the laminae and the apophyseal joints, and the transverse processes is performed. Extreme care should be utilized to prevent fracture of the transverse

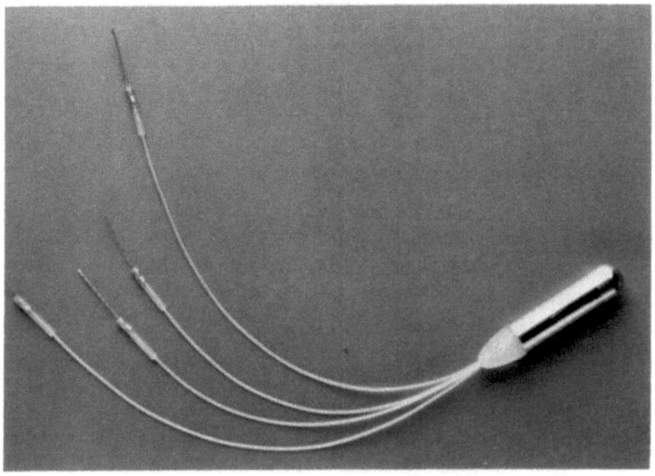

Figure 4.6 Totally implantable electrical bone growth stimulator consists of four cathodes, each delivering 5 μA, and the metallic case of the battery pack, which serves as anode. Electrical leads are insulated with nonconductive polymer.

processes as they are exposed and are denuded of soft tissue with a sharp, periosteal elevator or a chisel.

A self-retaining retractor should then be positioned lateral to the transverse process to facilitate further soft tissue dissection along the gutter lateral to the articular processes. If an L4-S1 fusion is to be achieved, the dissection should be completed to a point where the transverse processes of L4, L5, and the sacral ala are clearly and easily visualized. Up to this point it is suggested that the dissection be carried out one side at a time to reduce the pressure

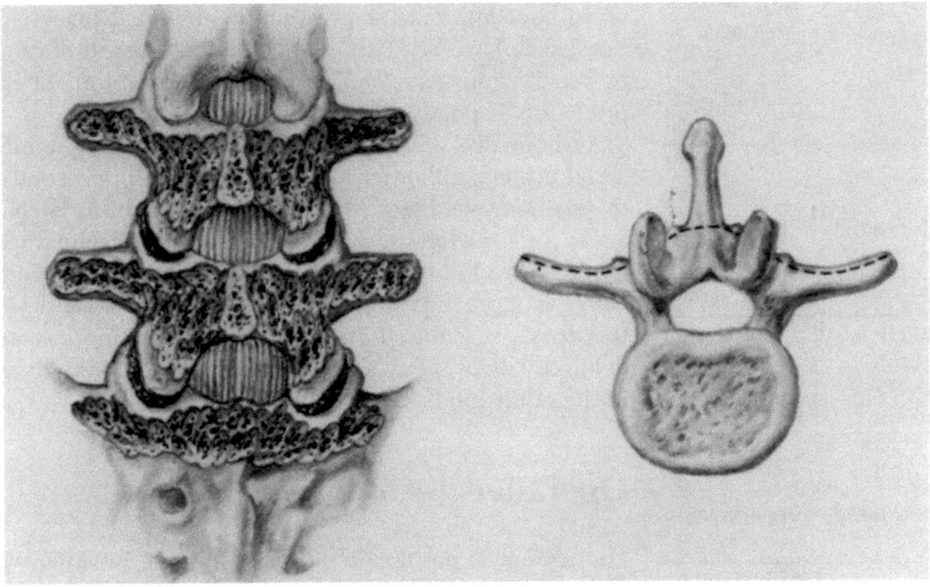

A

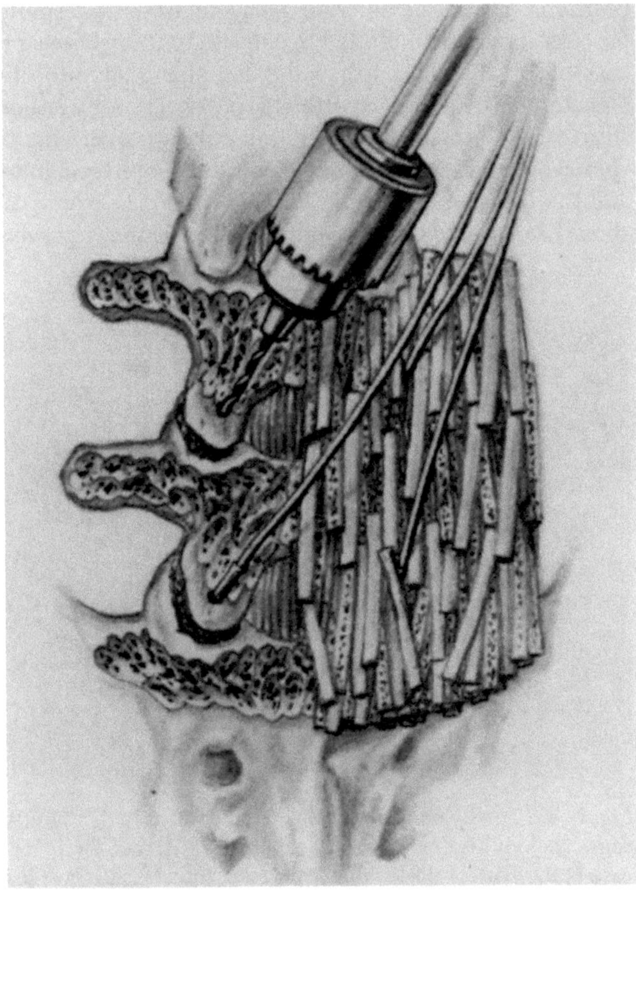

B

Figure 4.7 **A.** Posteroanterior view shows facet block grafts in place and decortication of posterior elements, lateral gutters, and transverse processes. Cross-sectional view (right) shows extent of decortication from transverse process tip to contralateral transverse process tip. **B.** Facet block complex, consisting of facets of adjacent vertebrae and intervening bone block, is then drilled with 1/16-in. bit (upper left facet complex); cathode is inserted through inferior facet of superior vertebra (lower left facet complex). Cathode tip may be bent back upon itself to prevent dislodgement. Cortical cancellous strips from the iliac overlay the decorticated posterior elements, lateral gutters, and transverse processes (right side of spine).

along the retractor, which has been located lateral to the tip of the transverse process. A similar dissection is carried out subsequently on the contralateral side.

Autogenous iliac bone graft of the corticocancellous variety can be obtained through the same midline incision of the skin when subcutaneous tissues are undermined laterally and caudally from its inferior portion. This allows the bone graft to be obtained from the posterior superior iliac spine region and its environs both inferiorly and superolaterally.

When subperiosteal exposure of the posterior elements and the transverse processes has been obtained, the facet joints are stripped of their joint capsules and the articular cartilage on both sides of the joint are removed by either a sharp dissection with a 1-cm-wide chisel, a needle-nosed rongeur, or a high-speed dental burr. The dissection is carried out beyond the cartilaginous surface to the cancellous bone (past the subchondral cortical bone). Care should again be exercised that the articular processes not be fractured at this point. A corticocancellous graft slightly larger in all dimensions than the denuded facet joint is then selected and snugly fitted into place by means of a bone punch. The resulting facet joint fusion (Fig. 4.7) should be quite stable and firm at the conclusion of the tamping after the method of Moe.[33]

Essential to the lumbosacral fusion is the creation of a large bed of bleeding bone by means of fish-scaling of the cortical bone in the area to be fused. This will include the transection of the spinous processes and decortication of the laminae as well as decortication of the transverse processes and the sacral ala. The decortication is not easily done after positioning of the cathodes and consequently should be performed previously, although this process of creating a bleeding bed of bone makes visualization somewhat more difficult for the positioning of the cathodes. This latter difficulty, however, is less troublesome than the difficulty of doing the decortication after the cathodes have been positioned. Before implantation of the generator, it is *imperative* that hemostasis via electrosurgical equipment be completed; electrocautery should never be used after implantation of a stimulator, as it may short out the internal circuits of the device.

To confirm the electrical activity of the stimulators, I have been in the habit of routinely testing each implant before its insertion in the patient. I do this by affixing the sterile hemostats of an appropriately designed amperage meter to the anode and one cathode and having the circulating nurse touch the amperage meter leads to the hemostats (Fig. 4.8). After testing has been accomplished, the hemostats that have been contaminated by the meter leads are removed by the circulating nurse and resterilized if necessary.

The resulting facet block complex consisting of the superior and inferior facets of adjacent vertebrae and the intervening bone block are then drilled with a 1/16-in.-diameter drill bit that is approximately the same diameter as the diameter of the tip of the cathode. The cathode is then inserted into the drill hole from medial to lateral through the inferior articulating process of the superior vertebra, the bone graft, and the superior articulating facet of the lower vertebra. To prevent dislodgement of the cathode, a portion of the tip of the cathode may be bent back on

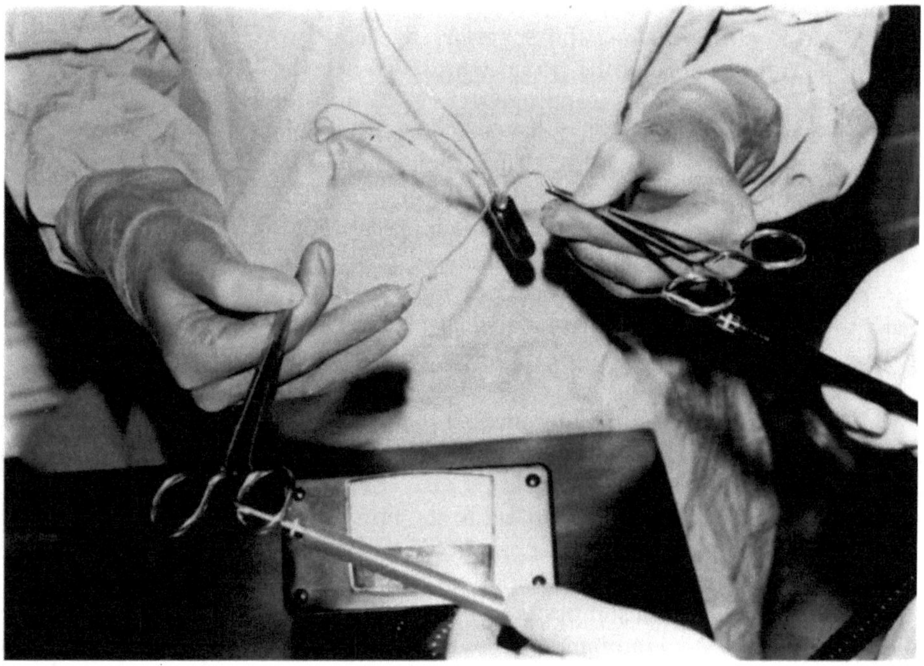

Figure 4.8. Leads of microammeter are touched to sterile hemostats that are in contact with anode and cathode of the stimulator; microammeter will read 20 μA (4 cathodes × 5 μA per cathode = 20 microamps). Hemostats are removed to be resterilized.

itself to form a barb, or a bit of bone graft may be tamped into the drill hole to hold the cathode in place. If placement of the cathodes would be more effective in the transverse process, this is an alternative placement site.

Pseudarthrosis Repair

For the patient with an identified pseudarthrosis, many of the same steps are undertaken; however, rather than concentrating on the facet joint fusion, which may be impossible, it is necessary to identify, debride, and decorticate the pseudarthrosis site. If the pseudarthrosis is large and easily identified, all the fibrous pseudarthrosis tissue should be removed using a sharp curette and/or needle-nosed rongeurs, cutting back to bleeding cancellous bone.

The identification of small pseudarthroses is facilitated by exerting pressure with a large, blunt periosteal elevator or other instrument along the course of the fusion mass. Motion will be detected at the pseudarthrosis site. It is necessary, when the pseudarthroses are difficult to identify, to begin a cautious decortication of a strip measuring approximately 5 to 10 mm wide from the superior to the inferior portion of the fusion site. This should be done on both sides of the midline. The shallow area of decortication will usually lead to identification of the inconspicuous pseudarthrosis.

The pseudarthrosis should be packed with cancellous graft. The final graft material may consist of corticocancellous strips with the cancellous portions placed into the pseudarthrosis site from the superior to the inferior margins of the fusion mass.

With respect to the placement of the cathodes along the pseudarthrosis, the cathodes should be positioned so that two cathodes are along the superior edge and two are on the inferior edge of the pseudarthrosis. When the sites have been selected, an appropriately sized drill bit (1/16 in.) is used to make four holes as close as possible to the rim of the pseudarthrosis. These holes should be within 5 mm of the rim because the field of osteogenic influence of the cathode transverses a cylindrical radius of approximately 5 to 8 mm. As mentioned previously, the cathode tip may be bent back on itself to form a barb to prevent dislodgement, or a small piece of bone graft may be driven snugly into the drill hole with the cathode.

Before closure, the titanium-encased battery pack, which also serves as the anode, is located just beneath the dorsal fascia in a tunnel created by a dissecting finger along the paramedian region cephalad to the fusion area. Alternately, the generator/anode can be placed in soft tissue above the iliac crest. It is important to ensure that the generator/anode is in soft tissue and not against bone. Additionally, the generator/anode should be positioned 8 to 10 cm from the cathodes.

The use of spinal instrumentation or metallic fixation devices has not been necessary in conjunction with the electrical bone growth stimulator, but if such a combination were to be used, every effort must be made to keep the leads from coming into contact with the metallic device, as this would cause the electrical impulse to dissipate along the metallic device and reduce the effectiveness of the bone growth stimulator.

Closure is accomplished in the usual fashion with interrupted suture of the layers. Drains or suction tubing are not ordinarily used at the site of the lumbosacral fusion and electrical bone growth stimulator, but if bleeding is profuse the surgeon should not hesitate to carefully insert a suction tube that could then be attached to intermittent suction. Similarly, suction-drainage of the iliac bone graft site will depend upon bleeding present at the time of closure. Drains or suction tubes are removed ordinarily at approximately 48 hours if the recovered blood has decreased to a level of approximately 30 cc per 8-hour time period.

Postoperative Regimen

Prophylactic antibiotic coverage is provided by the use of intravenous cefazolin sodium for 72 hours starting just before surgery. If an antibiotic sensitivity to this medication is anticipated, an alternative drug is selected.

Postoperatively, the patients are managed in a fashion comparable to the surgeon's usual postoperative program for a lumbosacral fusion. In my regimen, I use a lumbosacral chairback brace that is fitted approximately 3 to 5 days after surgery and then utilized continuously for 3 months, even during sleeping. It is removed only for bathing.

During the second 3 months, the brace is used continuously except during the sleeping hours; finally, during the third 3-month period, the brace is used for all activities except quiet at-home activities.

Generator Removal

At approximately 26 weeks, the patient is brought to the outpatient surgery area. Under sterile technique with local anesthetic and in conjunction with a recent anteroposterior film of the lumbar region, the generator is removed; no special effort is made to remove the cathode leads as their retention has proved to be routinely innocuous.

Satisfactory results are obtained following this technique. To date, there have been no reactions to the implant and no problems with the current generated either with respect to the central nervous system or the adjacent viscera. There have been no reports of spinal stenosis occurring at the site of electrical stimulation nor any reports of oncogenesis. The Food and Drug Administration has approved the totally implantable direct-current bone growth stimulator as "a spinal fusion adjunct to increase the probability of fusion success."[34] The totally implantable nature of this device precludes patient compliance from being a relevant factor in its utility.

Another method of presenting electrical and/or electromagnetic energy to the lumbar spine has been through the use of pulsing electromagnetic field (PEMF) devices, which are affixed over the lumbosacral spine for 8 to 10 hours[34,35]. Simmons studied 13 male patients suffering from failed posterior lumbar interbody fusions (PLIFs) with an average time of 40 months since the last surgical fusion attempts.[35] The devices promoted a significant increase in bone formation in 85% (11 of 13) of the patient pool and achieved body-to-body fusion throughout the intervertebral space in 77% (10 of 13) during the treatment period. The advantages of the system is that the treatment required no hospitalization, reduced morbidity, and avoided surgical risks. Brodsky reported his series managed in a similar fashion to Simmons as showing a 36% success rate in patients with pseudarthrosis after earlier attempts at lumbar spine fusions.[36]

Summary

A number of clinical trials have been made during the past 15 years. The original Dwyer series showed success in 40 of 47 patients (85%). The 1981 study showed 75 of 82 stimulated patients fused or 92%, compared with 128 of 159 controls or 81%. A further nonrandom study in 116 patients showed a 91% success rate. Finally, a randomized prospective control trial in "difficult patients" randomizing for all variables, including investigator differences, showed 25 of 31 stimulated patients fused (81%), compared with 15 of 28 controls (54%). These clinical trials, with the previously presented animal data and the extensive literature relating to the osteogenic nature of direct current, support the safety and efficacy of this device in spinal fusions.

The implantable stimulator is a supplement to a standard lumbosacral fusion or a pseudarthrosis repair and not a substitute for it. The stimulator does not accelerate fusion but is used to promote a higher percentage of fusion. It appears to be successful in that role when the need for supplementation of a fusion is present. Further studies are awaited with respect to the early work on the PEMF device.*

---

* No benefits in any form have been or will be received by the author from a commercial party related directly or indirectly to the subject of this chapter.

References

1. Wolff J. Das Gesetz der Transformation der Knochen. Berlin: Hirschwold, 1892.
2. Yasuda I. Piezoelectricity of living bone. J Kyoto Pref Univ Med 1953;53:325–328.
3. Fukada E, Yasuda I. On the piezoelectric effect of bone. J Physiol Soc Jpn 1957;12:1158–1162.
4. Shamos MH, Lavine LS. Physical bases for bioelectric effects in mineralized tissues. Clin Orthop 1964;35:177–188.
5. Shamos MH, Lavine LS, Shamos MI. Piezoelectric effect in bone. Nature (London) 1963;197:81.
6. Becker R, Bassett CAL, Bachman CH. Bioelectric factors controlling bone structure. In: Frost HM, ed. Bone Biodynamics. Boston: Little, Brown, 1964:209–244.
7. Friedenberg ZB, Brighton CT. Bioelectric potentials in bone. J Bone Joint Surg 1966;48A:915–923.
8. Anderson JC, Eriksson C. Electrical properties of wet collagen. Nature (London) 1968;218:166–168.
9. Anderson JC, Eriksson C. Piezoelectric properties of dry and wet bone. Nature (London) 1970;227:491–492.
10. Lavine LS, Grodzinsky AJ. Electrical stimulation of repair of bone. J Bone Joint Surg 1987;69A:626–630.
11. Lavine LS, Lustrin I. Shamos MH, Rinaldi RA, Liboff AR. Electric enhancement of bone healing. Science 1972;175:1118–1121.
12. Dwyer AF, Wickham GG. Direct current stimulation in spinal fusion. Med J Aust 1974;1:73–75.
13. Albee FH. Transplantation of a portion of the tibia into the spine for Pott's disease: a preliminary report. JAMA 1911;57:885–887.
14. Hibbs RA. An operation for progressive spinal deformities. NY Med J 1911;93:1013–1015.
15. Evans JH, Gilmore KL, O'Brien JP. How does fusion relieve low back pain. Orthop Trans 1982;6:32.
16. Sacks S. Anterior interbody fusion of the lumbar spine. J Bone Joint Surg 1965;47B:211.
17. Watkins MB. Posterolateral fusion in pseudarthrosis and posterior element defects of the lumbosacral spine. Clin Orthop 1964;35:80–86.
18. Dwyer AF. The use of electrical current stimulation in spinal fusion. In: Mooney V, ed. Symposium on the lumbar spine. Orthop Clin North Am 1975;6:265–273.
19. Mooney V. Editorial comment on the use of electrical current stimulation in spinal fusion. In: Mooney V, ed. Symposium on the lumbar spine. Orthop Clin North Am 1975;6:273.
20. Mooney V. Unpublished correspondence with WJ Kane, 1981.
21. Kahanovitz N, Arnoczky SP, Hulse D, Shires PK. The effect of postoperative electromagnetic pulsing on canine posterior spinal fusions. Spine 1984;9:273–279.
22. Nerubay J, Marganit B, Bubis JJ, Tadmor A, Katznelson A. Stimulation of bone formation by electrical current on spinal fusion. Spine 1986;11:167–169.
23. Kahanovitz N, Arnoczky SP. The efficacy of direct current electrical stimulation to enhance canine posterior spinal fusions. Presented at the North American Spine Society Annual Meeting, Banff Springs, Alberta, Canada, June 27, 1987.
24. Dwyer, AF, Yau AC, Jeffcoat KW. Use of direct current in spine fusion. J Bone Joint Surg 1982;56A:442.

25. Kane WJ, Bell WF, Porter IS. Supplementary electronic bone growth stimulation in lumbosacral fusions. Orthop Trans 1980;4:307–308.

26. Kane WJ, Lunceford EM, Dyer AR. An analysis of the utility of implantable bone growth stimulation in lumbosacral fusions. Orthop Trans 1982;6:464.

27. Brooks MO, Macy JR. One-sided long lumbar spine fusions with an implantable bone growth stimulator. Presented at American Academy of Orthopaedic Surgeons, New Orleans, Louisiana, 1982.

28. Nerubay J, Katznelson A. Clinical evaluation of an electrical current stimulator in spinal fusions. Int Orthop 1984;8:237–242.

29. Kane WJ. A prospective randomized assessment of the efficacy of electrical bone growth stimulation of lumbosacral fusions. Presented at the North American Spine Society Annual Meeting, Banff Springs, Alberta, Canada, 1987.

30. Kane WJ. Direct current electrical bone growth stimulation for spinal fusion. Spine 1988;13:363–365.

31. Kane WJ. Electrical bone growth stimulation. Presented at 7th American Orthopaedic Association International Symposium, Chicago, Illinois.

32. Kane WJ. A technique for insertion of the totally implantable bone growth stimulator for lumbosacral fusion via a midline approach. Englewood, Colorado: BGS Medical Corp., 1981.

33. Moe JH. A critical analysis of methods of fusion for scoliosis: an evaluation in two-hundred and sixty-six patients. J Bone Joint Surg 1958;40A:529–554.

34. Food and Drug Administration. Summary of safety and effectiveness: Osteostim HS11 implantable bone growth stimulator. Silver Spring, Maryland: Office of Device Evaluation, 1987.

35. Simmons JW. Treatment of failed posterior lumbar interbody fusion (PLIF) of the spine with pulsing electromagnetic fields. Clin Orthop 1985;193:127–132.

36. Brodsky AE, Khalil MA. Preliminary report on the use of EBI pulsing electromagnetic field therapy for treatment of pseudarthrosis of lumbar spine fusion. Presented at North American Spine Society Annual Meeting, Banff Springs, Alberta, Canada June 27, 1987.

5

Biomechanical Principles of Spinal Correction

Ronney L. Ferguson, Benjamin L. Allen, Jr., and Allan F. Tencer

The spine can be deformed by congenital, developmental, or traumatic events. The production, correction, and stabilization of spine deformities conforms to certain mechanical principles.[1–4] These principles can be used in designing spinal implant systems, testing systems before their clinical use, evaluating failures, and devising methods of augmentation to prevent further failure, and aid basic decision-making processes. A comprehension of spinal biomechanics is therefore crucial to the treating physician.

The advent of spinal column testing has made it possible to test and apply known mechanical principles to the design of spinal implantation systems. Mechanical testing of spinal implants may reveal weaknesses and strengths in the systems,[5–22] and critical analysis of successes as well as failures has allowed the physician and engineer to produce more reliable and stable constructs for spinal internal fixation.

Integral to the understanding and design of spinal implants is a knowledge of the mechanical properties of the bony spine and its supporting soft tissues. Numerous studies delineating these characteristics have been published.* The load applied to the spine can be measured or calculated and a spinal implant selected or designed such that bone-implant failure should not occur within the defined tissue envelope.[32]

Modeling of the spine by mathematical concepts has allowed computer analysis to simulate its functions, failures, and performance with different spinal implants attached.[33,34] This capability will improve with further understanding of the load-bearing characteristics of the spine, bone-implant junction mechanics, and the mechanical capabilities of differing spinal implant designs. This technology will make it possible to further our understanding and improve the design of spinal treatment systems.

* 7,10,13,23–31.

Advances are lost, however, if the practicing physician has no understanding of the principles used in arriving at the final product. Many spinal variables such as the degree of osteopenia and the appropriate implant to use with a particular deformity must be evaluated by the physician and the technique of treatment adjusted to those findings. Thus, some understanding of mechanical principles and testing of the spine, the spinal soft-tissue envelope, and spinal fixation devices is necessary to adequately treat spinal pathology.

The Column Concept

If the spine is considered to act as a column, then certain mechanical concepts can be applied to it.* Column mechanics were initially mathematically described by Euler. This model assumes that all loads on the column are vertical and centered over the column. The ends of the column are variably fixed or allowed to rotate. The in vivo human spine may vary from the model because mobile disc spaces and facet joints are interspersed throughout the spinal column and the loading is often eccentric, causing a moment to load the spine. Even so, column concepts hold some validity in the in vivo state.

Column Failure

Column failure can be typified mathematically as short or long column failure. Short column stability is expressed as $P < YA$, where P is the compressive load, Y is the yield strength of the spinal elements, and A is the cross-sectional area. As long as P (compressive strength) stays within a certain limit, the column remains stable and does not fail. If compressive load increases or the spinal elements lose stability (osteopenia, tumor, infection, soft-

* 1,2,28a,b,35,36.

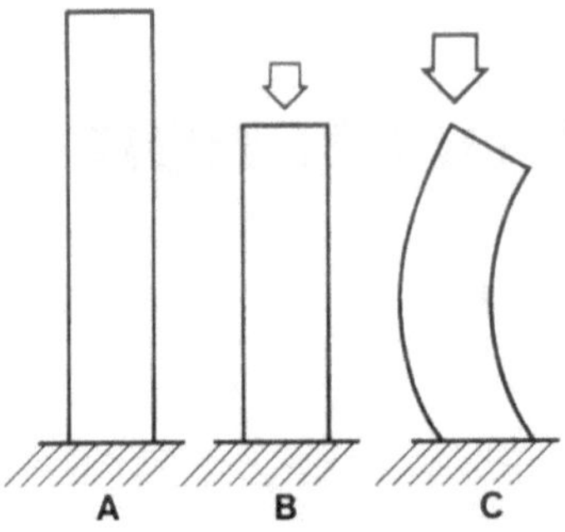

Fig 5.1

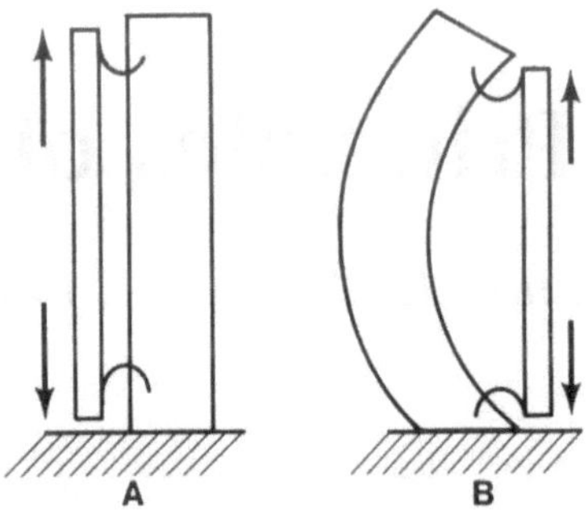

Fig 5.2

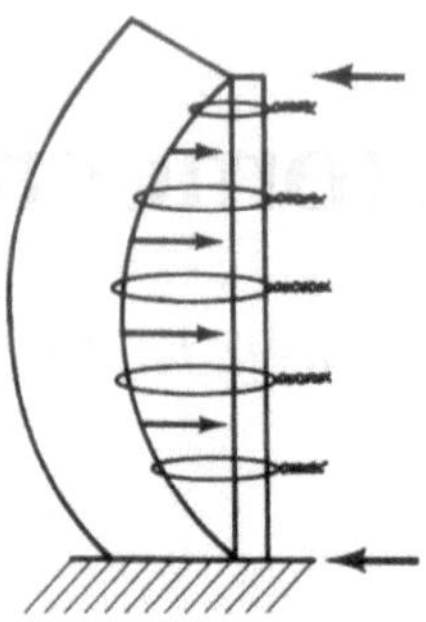

Fig 5.3

Figure 5.1. **A.** Column deforms with small loads (**B**) by shortening. **C.** As load increases, column bends. Enhanced bending occurs with taller columns, more slender columns, and columns with lower elastic modulus.

Figure 5.2. Axial loading can apply a distractive force to a shortened column (**A**) and thus lengthen it or (**B**) apply a moment to a bent column to straighten it.

Figure 5.3. Transverse loading of column will apply moment to correct bent column. This type of loading will not lengthen shortened column. Each loading point acts as three-point bend to correct bent column.

tissue degeneration), then the column may fail. This model is most applicable to traumatic deformities.[36]

Spinal deformities are more typified by long column stability. Long column stability is mathematically expressed as $P < K * EI/L^2$, where P is the compressive load, K is a constant representing degrees of freedom at the ends of the column, E is the column's modulus of elasticity (the mathematical ratio of stress to strain at any point in the elastic region of a material under test)[23], I is the area moment of inertia (a quantity that takes into account the cross-sectional area and distribution of material around an axis during bending)[23] and L is the length of the column. Unlike a short column with a load at one end, this column has the load distributed throughout; the weight at the top is very small by comparison. As the long column lengthens, as in a growing child, there is a greater tendency to deform. If the elasticity of the column increases, as might occur with certain collagen diseases known to predispose to scoliosis,[37] buckling of the column is more likely. These two correlations may have some relationship to the production of spinal deformity, at least in the mediolateral plane.[36]

When columns are loaded they initially deform by shortening. This occurs with small loads. Failure of the column does not occur, because removal of the load results in return of the column to its normal height. When the load increases to a critical loading value, the column also bends to accommodate the load (Fig. 5.1). If the load exceeds the yield strength of the column then failure of the column may occur (the column will not return to its original shape). This mechanical model correlates with spinal pathology seen in scoliotic, degenerative, and traumatic deformities of the spine.[2–4,36]

Column Correction

Two methods of correcting the deformed column exist. Axial loading may be used to either strengthen the shortened segment (Fig. 5.2A) or to create a moment to straighten a bent column (Fig. 5.2B): this involves a distractive or compressive force (or both) to correct a bent column.[1–4,35,36,49] The second method is to apply a transverse load to the center of the bent column, creating a moment in an effort to straighten the column[2,3,36] (Fig. 5.3): this will not lengthen a column that has shortened, but will straighten a bent column. The latter method represents bending correction. A combination of the two methods can also be used.[2,3,36]

A moment is equal to the product of the force applied and the length of the moment arm. A moment arm is the shortest perpendicular distance from the axis of rotation (the apex of the spinal deformity) to the force vector (the instrumentation applying the corrective force). The moment itself is the corrective load applied to the column multiplied by the moment arm. The magnitude of the moment can be directly affected by changing the length of its moment arm or by changing the direction or magnitude of the force applied to the moment arm. Thus, if a moment arm is becoming shorter, the force applied to the moment arm must be increased if the moment that is applied to the column is to remain constant. Because axial compressive devices (distraction or compression devices) (Fig. 5.4) and transverse corrective devices (segmental types of fixation) (Fig. 5.5) apply their corrective forces perpendicular to each other, their moment arms must also be perpendicular. Thus, theoretical differences in the correction that can be achieved exist. Almost all spinal instrumentations fit into one or the other of these categories or function with a combination of the two principles.

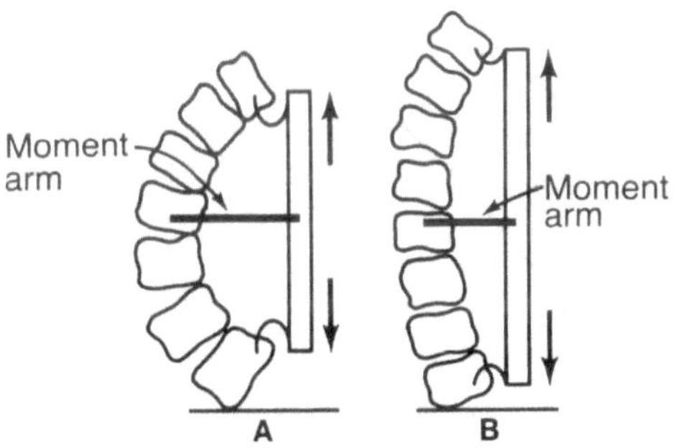

Fig 5.4

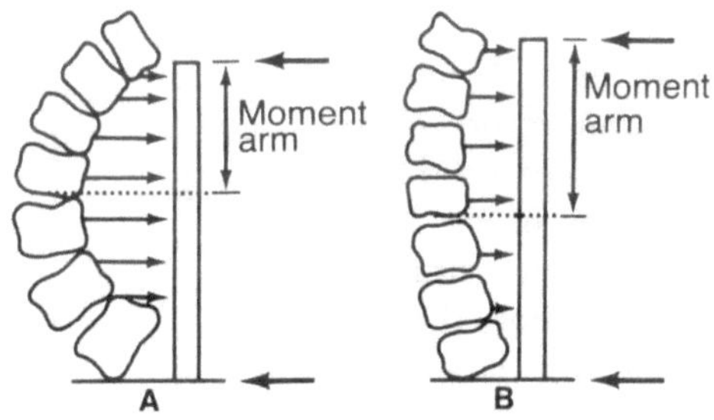

Fig 5.5

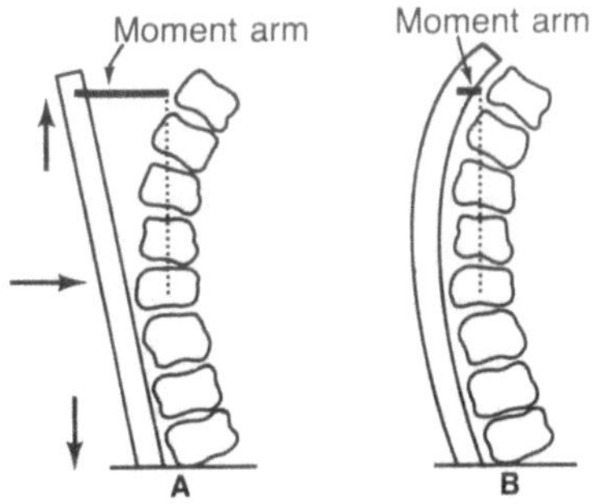

Fig 5.6

Figure 5.4. Axial loading. Corrective force is applied to long axis of spine. Moment arm is perpendicular to this and is measured from axis of apex of spine to axis of rod. The product of these is the moment that corrects the spinal deformity. **A.** In larger curvatures moment arm is longer, thus creating larger moment to correct spine per unit force applied to rod. **B.** As curvature of spine becomes smaller, so does moment arm, and consequently moment applied to correct spinal deformity lessens per unit force applied.

Figure 5.5. Transverse loading. Corrective force is applied perpendicular to long axis of spine. Thus, moment arm is measured from axis of apex of spine parallel to its long axis to end of load-applying device. **A.** In larger spinal curvatures, moment arm is smaller, thus creating smaller moment affecting correction on curved spine per unit force applied. **B.** As curvature lessens, moment arm lengthens, thus increasing moment applied to correct deformed spine per unit force.

Figure 5.6. **A.** Correction of kyphosis by axial loading device in distraction applies both axial force and transverse forces in manner of three-point bend. Thus, this is potentially a very powerful device for correcting kyphosis. Moment arm in this situation is measured from superior end of axis of rod to line drawn perpendicular to apex of axis of rotation of spine. **B.** If rod must be contoured to fit curve, then moment arm is decreased and resultant moment affecting straightening of deformity is thus lessened.

Axial Corrective Forces

Axial distractive forces applied to the concave side of a bent column result in a moment at both ends of the column and straightening of the column.[1–3,35,36] The moment arm is from the apex of the bent column to the point at which the axial loading (distractive) device interfaces with the column (see Fig. 5.4A): if the force is applied on the concave side (as in a scoliosis correction), the corrective moment is proportional to the angle of curvature of the spine;[3] the greater the angle of the bent column, the longer the moment arm[,] and the greater the moment per unit force applied to the column. As the angle of the column decreases, the force applied to straighten the column must increase dramatically because the moment arm is decreasing. Theoretically this type of system is best used to correct large angular deformities.[1] If axial distraction is applied to a 90° bend in a column, 70% of the distractive force is utilized by the moment in improving the curvature, whereas in a 45° bend only 35% of the distractive force is utilized by the moment for curve improvement.[36] All of the force is concentrated at the fixation sites. Increasing force at the bone-implant interface with a decreasing moment to correct the column bend may lead to failure of the implant.[30]

Axial distractive forces applied to the convex side of the column also create a transverse three-point bending force[4] (Fig. 5.6A): these two forces are complementary and can produce large moments. The moment arm in this axial distractive device is measured from the interface of the corrective device to a line perpendicular to the axis of rotation at the apex of the column's bend. If the instrument applying the axial distraction to the ends of the column is bent so that it conforms to the curve column, the moment arm is shortened and the force exerted is decreased (see Fig. 5.6B).

Transverse Corrective Forces

Unlike axial forces acting on a column, transverse forces applied to the concave side of the bent column create a longer moment arm as the curvature in the column becomes smaller (see Fig. 5.5). The correction occurs through a three-point bending mechanism. As each transverse fixation point is attached to the column, the next fixation point uses the previous point as one of its bending points in the three-point correction. If correction occurs within each fixation point, the moment arm lengthens with each fixation point to give a larger moment per unit force to correct the bent column. Transverse loading will not lengthen a shortened column, because the force is perpendicular to the long axis of the column and the moment arm lies in the direction of the axis of the column.

Transverse loading appears to be more efficient in correcting smaller degrees of curvature in a column.[2] This is true for the application of transverse forces to the convex side of the bent column. The moment arm in the convex placement of transverse fixation devices is measured from the ends of the bent column to the apex of the bend parallel to the column (just as in the concave situation in Fig. 5.6). As the column becomes straighter, the moment arm increases in length, thus allowing a larger moment to be applied to the bent column per unit of force applied.

White et al.[4] and Wenger et al.[2] have both calculated the degree of curvature at which axial and transverse forces are equally effective in producing a moment to correct a bent column. Assuming the columns have constant rigidity, White et al. determined this point to be 53° while Wenger et al. calculated it to be 44°. White et al. also showed a combination of axial and transverse forces to be the most efficient method of correcting the bending deformity of the column (Fig. 5.7).

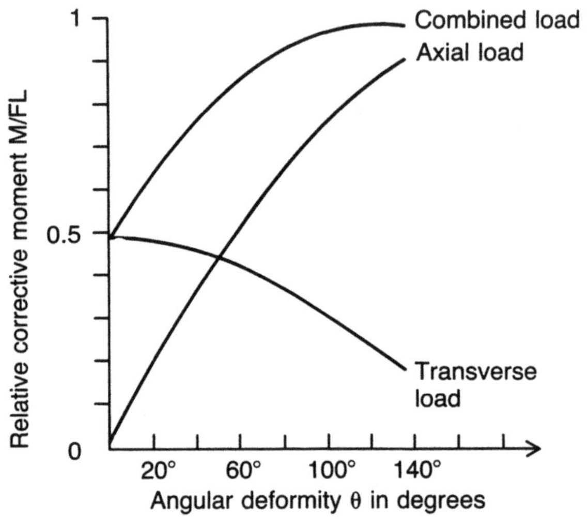

Figure 5.7. Graph demonstrates that as angle of curvature increases, axial loading device effectiveness improves and transverse loading device effectiveness decreases. Their axes cross at 53°, according to White and Panjabi. Note that devices that combine both methods of correcting column have higher efficacy than either of other two methods at any degree of curvature. (Reprinted with the permission of J.B. Lippincott, Co., as modified from White and Panjabi. The clinical biomechanics of scoliosis. Clin Orthop 1976;118:100–111.

Rotational Correction in the Transverse Plane

Axial correction moments have little to no effect on correcting axial rotation in the spinal column.[1] The force applied to the spine lies in a different plane than that which would be required to correct axial rotation.

Transverse instrumentations load the spine in the proper plane to produce derotation moments if the loading is on the concave side of the curve. In practice, however, instrumentations on the posterior aspect of the spine rarely produce enough of a moment to derotate the disc soft tissues.[2] Segmental anterior fixations may be more effective as they allow removal of the disc tissue before attempting correction.[38] Some residual rotation will always be present; Enneking[39] has shown that part of the rotational deformity is secondary to pedicular shortening on the concave side of the vertebrae in the scoliotic spine.

Instrumentations

The instrumentations that are presently available fall into either the axial loading type, the transverse loading type, or a combination of the two types. The instrumentations apply the forces to create the corrective moments that will straighten or lengthen the deformed spine.

Distraction Instrumentations

Distraction instrumentations load the spine axially. Examples of this type of instrumentation include Harrington distraction rod and hooks, the Jacobs' rods, Zielke instrumentation applied in distraction, Kostuik instrumentation, rod-screw-clamp (spinal fixator) applied with distraction, and the Milwaukee brace without pads.[1,32] The advantages of this system are that it has particular mechanical advantages in larger spinal curvatures (those above the 44° to 53° range).[2,3] It can lengthen a shortened segment of spine that is or is not bent. This may be very important in the management of spinal fractures with middle column failure.[7] There are several disadvantages of these instrumentations.[59b] As spinal curvatures become smaller, the amount of force applied to the bone–implant interface must be increased to maintain the corrective moment on the curvature. This places the system at jeopardy to fail especially when only two fixation sites are used. This is discussed in the section on bone–implant interface.

With axial loading of the spine, it is difficult to maintain sagittal curvatures especially when fixation is carried to the pelvis. Adjuncts such as Edwards sleeves or contouring the rods and using square hooks to prevent rotation of the rods have been proposed, but appear to have limited value in maintaining sagittal curvatures of the spine when axial distraction devices are used.[2] The Harrington distraction rod depends on intact ligamentous structures to distract against to maintain a load on the spine, which makes it very susceptible to loosening after creep occurs in the soft tissues. Nachemson[40] demonstrated that loads on the Harrington rod decrease to almost zero in the supine patient 2 weeks post instrumentation. This also makes this system a poor fixation system for use where all ligamentous stabilizers of the spine are disrupted by trauma.[7,41]

Axial distractive loading plus three-point bend loading are very efficient as a means of correcting kyphosis in either spinal deformities or trauma. The axial distraction is converted to a transverse force at the point of contact at the apex of the spine. This theoretical advantage holds true for short supple kyphoses that occur in conditions such as fractures. However, long rigid kyphotic deformities will usually require the rods to be bent to fit the spinal contour. This shortens the effective moment arm and thus makes the moment applied to the spine less effective in correcting the deformity.[4]

Compression Instrumentations

Compression instrumentations apply axial compression loading to the spine. When used on the convex side of a deformed spine, kyphosis, lordosis, and scoliosis can be corrected. Examples of this instrumentation include Gruca–Weiss springs, Harrington compression instrumentation, internal and external fixators of the spine, Edwards compression device, Dwyer instrumentation, and Zielke instrumentation applied in compression.

Compression instrumentation is most effective on larger curvatures, becoming less effective as the curvature is corrected. These systems have the advantage of using multiple fixation sites on the spine that can spread the load at the bone–implant interface, thus lessening the risk of failure of the bone or implant. The anterior spinal implants (Dwyer and Zielke devices) have the same axial compression mechanism for correcting the spine as the posteriorly placed Harrington compression devices. Anterior axial compressive spinal fixation devices can also correct transverse rotational deformities to some extent.[4]

Transverse Instrumentations

This type of instrumentation corrects the spine by segmentally applying forces perpendicular to the long axis of the spine. A three-point bending mechanism effects correction. Examples of this type of instrumentation include segmentally wired smooth rods with any of the reported configurations,[7,42–45] plate-and-screw fixation (Steffee, Luque, Roy-Camille, dynamic compression plate, slotted plate), rod-and-screw fixation, and cast or brace immobilization without lateral pads. These instrumentations are more effective in applying moments to small deformities of the spine. Theoretically, these instrumentations require little force to support a straight spine, making them good neutralization devices to fix nondeformed segments of the spine. Multiple fixation sites allow sharing of the loads applied to the laminae, pedicles, or spinous processes. Transverse instrumentations can be applied to the convex or concave side of the deformity with equal ease. Shortening in a column is not restored by this type of instrumentation so that it can not be expected to restore height to a traumatically shortened spinal motion segment.[7] When screws and fixed-hole plates or screws and rod clamp devices are used, lengthening of the spine can be maintained; smooth rods and wires will not maintain spinal length.[13] Sagittal curvatures can be maintained or produced with these instrumentations because the rod or plate can be contoured and then fixed to the spine.[2,46–48]

Combination Instrumentation

An instrumentation may use both axial and transverse loading principles to correct the spine. White et al.[3] (Fig. 5.7) demonstrated combination loading to be the most efficient means of accommodating the varying moment arm lengths of different deformed spinal geometries to produce an adequate correcting moment with minimum force. Examples of this type of instrumentation are the Cotrel–Dubousset instrumentation, Zielke system, segmentally wired Harrington distraction instrumentation, spinal fixators, distractive outriggers in combination with a fixed transverse loading device to support the correction gained with the axial loading device, and the Milwaukee brace with thoracic or lumbar pads. Instrumentations like the Cotrel–Dubousset system, certain of the spinal fixators, and the Zielke system have the potential to act as axial loading devices in both distraction and compression, as transverse loading devices, as a combination of both, or as neutralization systems. These systems have a very powerful potential for correction of spinal deformities. As the curvature of the spine is corrected and the axial loading moment becomes less effective, then the transverse component can be used to further straighten the deformed spine and at the same time provide load sharing with the axial corrective fixation device. This decreases the forces at the axially loaded end hooks.[3] The judicious use of the powerful mechanical advantage of the combined instrumentations should lead to fewer bone–implant interface failures.

Adjuncts to Spinal Instrumentation

Numerous methods of augmenting stability of spinal implants exist. These can be used when the bone is found to be severely osteopenic, when instrument fixation sites appear small, weak, or are absent, or when fixation by the instrumentation is suboptimal for whatever reason.

Wires

Wires may function as adjuncts to spinal fixation devices, as the primary fixation method to attach rods to the poste-

Table 5.1. Comparisons of ultimate strength and cycles to failure of 316L stainless steel (SS) wire and cable with MP35N wire and cables[a]

1.2-mm O.D.	UTS	Cycles to failure
Monofilament stainless steel	141 lb (625 N)	803
Monofilament MP35N	382 lb (1700 N)	1900
SS cable	147 lb (655 N)	5351 ± 397
MP35N cable #1	175 lb (780 N)	58683
MP35N cable #2	251 lb (1115 N)	64420 ± 8660

[a] From Georgette et al. The fatigue resistance of orthopaedic wire and cable systems. Proceedings of the Society of Biomaterials, 1984.

rior spinal elements or to connect adjacent posterior spinal elements to each other. The strength of the wire–bone interface depends on the strength of the tissue to which the wire attaches, the geometry of the wire–bone interface, and the material properties of the wire itself.* Geometry of the wire and bone are discussed in the section on bone–implant interface.

Material properties have proven important in preventing fatigue of wires. Different materials have differing elongation-to-failure characteristics, fatigue characteristics, and ultimate strengths. Various configurations of the same material may also display different loading properties. In Table 5.1 note that monofilament stainless steel wire and stainless steel cable have essentially the same ultimate strength yet very different fatigue strengths as measured by cycles to failure. Also note that metals of the same diameter may have very different strengths and fatigue characteristics. It must be pointed out that the stainless steel listed in this table is fully annealed. Incompletely annealed stainless steel has fewer cycles to failure for the same size and strength of material. Thus, multiple variables must be considered in choosing a particular wire for spinal implantation. Most prepackaged spinal fixation wires are fully annealed and made of either MP35N or 316L stainless steel with a diameter of 1.2 mm.

Methylmethacrylate

Methylmethacrylate can be used to augment other spinal instrumentations[52–58] or can be used as a primary fixation method.[59,60] Methylmethacrylate is not a glue but forms a mechanical interlock with the bony surface with which it comes into contact. Bone is 2.5 to 6 times stronger and about 10 times stiffer than methylmethacrylate and able to absorb more energy to failure.[61] If used as a primary means of fixation, reinforcement with a mesh or wires is usually required. Twisted wires embedded in methylmethacrylate significantly increase the tensile strength of the methylmethacrylate. The more strands of wire added to the construct, the more the tensile strength increases.[59,62] It may also be used as a spacer when bone has been removed and the healing potential of bone graft is limited.[53] Methylmethacrylate may be used to strengthen the bone–implant interface by promoting load sharing by a larger bony area.[63] It can be used to reinforce or repair areas where screws have pulled out of vertebral bodies or pedicles.[38,58]

Screws

Screw fixation of pedicles may be used as a primary fixation method for plates or rods[9,24,64–66] or as an adjunct to provide extra fixation sites for other methods of spinal fixation.[67,68] Screws may also be used for primary fixation across facet joints.[69,70] Pull-out testing of screws from vertebral pedicles has demonstrated several principles. Larger diameter screws with full thread designs appear to achieve better vertebral purchase.[24,71,72] Depth of purchase is also important. If the anterior cortex of the vertebral body is engaged, screws demonstrate greater pull-out strengths.[72] Depth of penetration of the screw into the cancellous vertebral body, although controversial, appears to correlate with increased pull-out strength.[24,72] Pull-out strength is increased if a screw fills the narrowest diameter of the pedicle.[72]

Cyclic loading studies have shown that deeper penetration into the vertebral body is correlated with the ability to withstand a greater number of cycles before loosening occurs.[72] Thus, the largest screw that will fit into the pedicle with the deepest depth of penetration will give the highest pull-out strength. Cross-linking of pedicle screws also improves screw pull-out strength[73] as does methylmethacrylate injected into osteopenic bone; methylmethacrylate injected into a screw hole from which a screw has pulled out will restore the pull-out strength to normal; and when injected into a screw hole under pressure will increase the pull-out strength up to twice normal. The larger the volume of methylmethacrylate injected, the greater the pull-out strength.[58]

Variation in pedicle size has been mentioned frequently.[24,31,72,74] Pedicles in the upper lumbar and lower thoracic spine may not accommodate 6.5-mm screws, and 4.5-mm screws may be too large for pedicles in the middle to upper thoracic spine.[31]

Transverse Couplers

Coupling rods with crossbars have two advantages. First, mechanical testing using both smooth rods and sublaminar wires and Cotrel–Dubousset instrumentation have demonstrated that torsional stiffness of the implant is improved with the crossbars. Second, minimal axial stiffening is also produced by the crossbars.[63,73,75,76] Theoretically, lateral

* 26,46,47,50,51,93.

bend stiffness should also improve by a factor of 3,[26] but this has not been tested experimentally.

Pelvic Fixation

Comparing pelvic fixation types and their relative efficiency is difficult. Although numerous techniques have been described,[42,65,77–81] few series of mechanical tests have been reported.[81,82] Axial loading methods (Harrington sacral hooks and sacral bars) appear to have significantly less load-bearing capacity than segmental types of fixation (Luque pelvic fixation, Galveston pelvic fixation, Asher pelvic fixation,[8b] pedicular screw pelvic fixation or rods or plates). Jacobs,[82] in a human cadaver study of pelvic fixation, found that while a flexion bending moment of 33.1 ± 6.7 N-m would pull out a conventional Harrington sacral bar from the pelvis, an 81.6 ± 16.8 N-m moment was required for failure using the Galveston L-rod technique of pelvic fixation. A study reported by Puno et al.,[81] measuring energy absorbed by several segmental pelvic fixation systems, demonstrated that the Steffee plate with two sacral screws was the stiffest construct and the Galveston technique of pelvic fixation was the least stiff. Methylmethacrylate has been shown to improve screw pull-out strengths in the sacrum[81] and has been used to augment loosened intralaminar pelvic fixation at revision.

Casting and Bracing

Casts and braces can act as both transverse loading devices, by applying loads directly to the skin over the spine or loading the rib cage, which subsequently loads the spine as in a thorocolumbar sacral orthosis (TLSO), or as axial loading devices, by distracting at the neck and chin as in the Milwaukee brace.[83] A combination of both principles is seen in the Milwaukee brace with lateral pads. Gaining control of the pelvis is necessary to stabilize the lumbosacral junction.[84] This is accomplished with molding of the brace or cast to the pelvis or incorporation of a thigh into the brace. External immobilization can be used as a primary fixation technique or as an adjunct to internal instrumentation. Nachemson and Elfstrom[40] implanted telemetrized Harrington distraction rods in patients with idiopathic scoliosis. These investigators compared forces on the rod with a Risser cast, a Milwaukee brace, and no support. They found the brace to be superior in terms of reducing the axial forces on the rod. They also found the brace to be effective even in the supine position. Nagel[85] tested five fresh human cadavers to determine range-of-motion measurements at the interspace of the first and second lumbar vertebrae after progressive disruption of the joint followed by internal and external stabilization; the Knight–Taylor brace was effective in limiting lateral motion, fair in limiting flexion-extension, and ineffective in preventing rotation. The three-point hyperextension brace was fairly effective for flexion-extension only. The body cast was effective in limiting all spinal motions.

Studies evaluating the immobilization potential of cervical orthoses found the Halo cast to give the best immobilization, followed by the Halo vest, four-poster braces, and soft-collar devices in that order.[49,86,87]

Bone–Implant Interface

No matter how large a moment is generated by an implant, or the ultimate strength and fatigue strengths of its components, if the bone–implant interface is unable to support the loads the corrective technique will fail.

Several approaches to improving load bearing at the bone–implant interface can be used. First, the load capacity limits of the interface need to be measured and not exceeded if possible. Second, mechanical means for decreasing bone–implant interface load can be used.

Waugh[30,89] has shown the thoracic laminae to be the weak points in the axial distractive hook systems. Distractive forces greater than 20 to 30 kiloponds (43.9–65.8 lb) may lead to failure of the thoracic lamina. A 20- to 30-kiloponds force was adequate to achieve 60 to 70% correction of a spinal deformity in a flexible curve. Forces above 30 kiloponds often caused pullout of the upper hook. Thus, in spines where large forces may need to be applied to the axial distraction rod to gain a sufficient moment for correction, the upper hook may be in jeopardy of dislodging.

McNeice et al.[26] performed 111 posterior pull-out tests on eight human cadaver spines to delineate failure loads and modes of failure using sublaminar single and double wires, cables, and steel bands. They found that single 1.2-mm wires (316L SS) cut through the lamina in 43% (22 of 51) of tests. Even when the failure mode involved was vertebral arch fracture (57% of single-wire tests), the wire cut deeply into the lamina. The mean load capacity for single wires was 850 Newtons (190 lb), with a range from 600 to 1200 Newtons. Double strands of 1.2-mm wire cut through the lamina in 25% (6 of 24) of tests and produced fracture of the vertebral arch or body in 75% of tests. The mean load capacity for double wires was 1100 Newtons (250 lb) with a range from 600 to 1300 Newtons. These results are in accord with those of Wenger et al.,[22] who reported midthoracic lamina to fail at an average load of 1032 Newtons. Vertebral arch fracture usually occurred at the junction between the lamina and pedicle in McNeice's study. Steel bands 4.76 and 2.3 mm wide caused vertebral arch or body fracture 100% of the time, but did not significantly increase the mean load capacity. In various osteopenic specimens, the verte-

Table 5.2. Comparison of spinal implants

Author	Date	Purpose	Specimen	Spine model	Load	Yield strength	Ultimate strength	Displacement per load	Result as	Instrument	Rank order of measurements					Comment
											Axial	Flex	Ext	LB	Tor	
Pinzur et al.[16]	1979	Fracture	Fr human	Flexion-fracture	Four point	—	Y	—	Stiffness	HCI	—	1	—	—	—	
										HDR	—	2	—	—	—	
										Weiss	—	3	—	—	—	
McAfee et al.[13]	1985	Fracture	Fr human	Intact	Pre-Comp-Tor	—	Y	—	Energy absorption	HDR	—	—	—	—	—	No significant difference
										LRI	—	—	—	—	—	
			Fr & embalm human	Burst	Axial Comp	—	—	Y	Displacement	Burst	4	—	—	—	—	
										LRI	3	—	—	—	—	
										HDR	2	—	—	—	—	
										HDR + SSI	1	—	—	—	—	
			Fr human	Torsion fracture	Pre-Comp-Tor	Y	—	—	Stiffness	Tor-fx	—	—	—	—	4	
										HDR	—	—	—	—	3	
										HDR + SSI	—	—	—	—	2	
										LRI	—	—	—	—	1	
Purcell et al.[18]	1981	Fracture	Fr human	Post defect flexion	Flexion	—	Y	—	Failure-moment	Intact	—	2	—	—	—	36% failure moment increase of 3 + 2 over 2 + 2
										HDR 2 + 2	—	2	—	—	—	
										HDR 3 + 2	—	1	—	—	—	
Ferguson et al.[7]	1987	Fracture	Fr human	Anterior-posterior column defect	Flex, Ext, Lat. Bend, Torsion	—	—	Y	Stiffness	Intact	—	—	—	—	—	
										AP model	—	—	—	—	—	
										HDR + SSI	—	—	—	—	—	
										Vermont	—	—	—	—	—	
										Roy-cam	—	—	—	—	—	
										C-Rod	—	—	—	—	—	
										J-Rod	—	—	—	—	—	
				Anterior-posterior middle (APM) column defect		—	—	—		APM model	—	6	6	6	5	
										HDR + SSI	—	3	3	4	2	
										Vermont	—	5	4	5	3	
										Roy-Cam	—	1	1	1	1	
										C-Rod	—	4	2	2	3	
										J-Rod	—	2	5	3	4	
Jacobs et al.[10]	1982	Fracture	Fr human	Posterior ligaments anterior slice defect	Four point	—	Y	—	Energy absorption	HCR-lam	—	1	—	—	—	
										Roy-Cam	—	2	—	—	—	
										HCR-trans	—	3	—	—	—	
										HDR 3 + 3	—	4	—	—	—	
										Weiss	—	5	—	—	—	
				Anterior body defect	Four point	—	Y	—	Energy absorption	HDR 3 + 3	—	1	—	—	—	30% stronger than 2 + 2
										HDR 2 + 2	—	2	—	—	—	
										Bohler	—	3	—	—	—	
				Combined anterior + posterior defect	Four point	—	Y	—	Energy absorption	HDR 3 + 3	—	1	—	—	—	
										HDR 2 + 2	—	2	—	—	—	
Stauffer et al.[20]	1975	Fracture	Embalm human	Flexion-rotation fracture	Flexion + Rotation moment	—	Y	—	Strength	HCR 2 + 2	—	1	—	—	1	
										HDR 2 + 2	—	1	—	—	1	
										Weiss	—	2	—	—	2	
Wenger et al.[22]	1982	Deformity	Calf	Scoliosis	Flexion, Axial, Rotation	—	Y	—	Failure load	HDR	4	3	—	—	—	
										HDR + HCR + TR	1	2	—	—	—	
										HDR + SSI	2	1	—	—	—	
										LRI	3	1	—	—	—	

Laborde et al.[11]	1980	Fracture	Fr & embalm human	Three-point bend	Four point	—	Y	—	Stiffness	Intact	—	2	1	1	—	
										HCR 2 + 2	—	1	4	2	—	
										HDR 2 + 2	—	3	3	3	—	
										Mesh 1 + 1	—	4	2	4	—	
Ward et al.[21]	1985	Deformity	Swine	Intact	Axial + Torsion	—	—	Y	Stiffness	HDR	1	—	—	—	1	Testing after 1000 cycles in torsion
										LRI	2	—	—	—	1	
Mino et al.[14]	1985	Deformity	Calf	Intact	Torsion	—	—	Y	Stiffness	HDR	—	—	—	—	3(3)	Non parentheses—max torque
										HDR + sublam.	—	—	—	—	3(3)	Parentheses—partial toughness
Puno et al.[17,81]	1986	Scoliosis	Fr human	Scoliosis	Axial, Flex, Ext, LB, Tor			Y	Energy absorption	Intact	1	3	5	4	3	Axial values in N-m
										CD	1	1	1	1	1	
										HDR	3	3	3	2	4	All other values in N-m rad
										HDR + HCR	1	2	4	2	3	
										HDR + SSI	1	3	2	2	5	
										LRI	2	4	3	3	2	
		Fracture	Fr human	Without vertebra	As above	—	—	Y	Energy absorption	Intact	1	3	3	1	2	
										CD	4	4	2	3	1	
										HDR	2	2	1	2	2	
										LRI	3	1	1	1	3	
				With vertebra +/− strut	As above	—	—	Y	Energy absorption	CD-strut	1	1	1	1	1	
										CD-no strut	2	2	2	2	2	
										LRI-strut	3	Fail	—	—	—	
Herring et al.[9]	1987	Spondylolisthesis	Calf	Spondylolisthesis model	Axial, Flex, Tor	—	—	Y	Stiffness	Steffee plate	1	1	—	—	1	
										¼ slot	2	3	—	—	2	
										¼ smooth	3	2	—	—	3	
										3/16 slot	4	4	—	—	4	
										LRI	3	2	—	—	6	
										Intact	5	5	—	—	5	
Mann et al.[12]	1987	Anterior decompression	Fr human	Anterior decompression—strut	Flex, Ext., LB	—	—	Y	% stiff	Graft	—	2	3	5/4	—	R/L = lateral bend (LB)
										Kostuik	—	3	2	3/3	—	
										Kaneda	—	1	2	1/1	—	
										I-plate	—	1	1	4/3	—	
										Rev. I	—	1	1	2/2	—	
Munson et al.[15]	1984	Fracture	Calf	Two (2) cm defect	Instrom	—	—	Y	Strain	HDR	2	2	—	2	2	
										HDR + SSI	1	1	—	1	1	
Cool et al.[6]	1987	Rotational test	Swine	Pre torques cycled 20 and 30 degrees	Torque tester	—	—	Y	Torques	LRI	—	—	—	—	1	
										HDR	—	—	—	—	2	
Gepstein et al.[8a]	1987	Fracture	Fr human	Burst fracture	MTS	—	Y	—	Failure moment stiffness	HDR 3 + 2	—	4	—	—	—	
										HDR 3 + 2 SSI	—	3	—	—	—	
										CD 2 + 1	—	1	—	—	—	
										CD 1 + 1	—	1	—	—	—	
										Intact	—	2	—	—	—	
Ritterbusch[19] et al.	1987	Deformity	Calf	30 degrees kyphosis 1000 cycles pre & post	MTS	—	—	Y	Stiffness	LRI	3	—	—	—	3	
										Wisc	2	—	—	—	2	
										HDR	4	—	—	—	4	
										CD	1	—	—	—	1	
Bone et al.[5]	1987	Fracture	Fr human	Burst	MTS	—	—	Y	Stiffness	Zielke-slot	2	—	—	—	3	
										T-plate	3	—	—	—	2	
										Broad plate	1	—	—	—	1	
										Kostuik	2	—	—	—	4	

bral arch tended to fracture at relatively low loads regardless of the type of sublaminar fixation.

Drummond et al.[50] studied wire pullout through the base of the spinous processes of Holstein calves. They demonstrated that pullout through a button–wire interface with force directed perpendicular to the button required an average of 176 lb of force. If the load was applied parallel to the face of the button, 115 lb of force was required. Sublaminar pull-out tests averaged 187.5 to 225 lb of force to failure.

Pedicle screw testing was previously discussed in the section on augmentation of spinal fixation with screws. The failure load of the Dwyer screw in pullout in the vertebral body has been measured to be 45 kiloponds (98.7 lb). This value would depend on the quality of the bone present in the vertebral body.

In evaluating multiple factors affecting the strength of the lamina and vertebral body, Calhoun et al.[88] found a positive correlation of lamina pull-out strength, indentation strength of the vertebral body, and bone mineral content. Age was negatively correlated to bone strength and bone mineral content.

Several mechanical means of improving the load-bearing ability of the bone–implant interface in the spine exist. Loads applied to the bone–implant interface due to the force exerted by the corrective implant can be decreased by using multiple fixation sites, adding transverse fixation to axial devices by passing wires about distraction rods and lamina or adding extra hooks from distraction rods to lamina, augmenting hook fixation sites, vertebral bodies, or pedicles with methylmethacrylate, or adding transverse loading support in the form of casts or braces. Also increasing the size, strength, and fatigue characteristics of the implant may improve its endurance limit and prevent implant failure.[87,90] All these mechanical methods may fail in the face of severe osteopenia, in the absence of fixation sites because of congenital defect or surgical removal, or in a very small individual with fragile bones. In some cases casting with or without recumbency may be the only means of obtaining fixation of a deformed or traumatized spine.

Mechanical Testing of Spinal Implants

Numerous studies have examined the mechanical stability of various spinal instrumentations. The results of these studies are occasionally contradictory but usually agree on certain major strengths and weaknesses of the implants. Many of these studies compared strengths to different standards (normal spinal stiffnesses, yield strengths, ultimate strengths, strengths or stiffnesses of other instrumentations, strengths or stiffnesses of fracture models), used a variety of models (human, calf, swine, plastic), examined varying spinal defects in the models, and used different modes to report their results (energy absorption, stiffness, failure moment, mode of instrument failure). Interstudy comparisons thus are difficult.

Table 5.2 lists the studies used to compare the spinal implants. The results are given in rank order from the authors' data, and are not necessarily the units used by the author to report his data. Statistical significance of the ranks cannot be assured for all studies.

Harrington compression instrumentation works well with posteriorly destabilized spinal segment. Harrington distraction instrumentation and Weiss springs were consistently inferior in stabilizing this injury when compared to the compression instrumentation.

Axial loads placed on the spinal model were best stabilized by combination axial-transverse loading systems and plate-screw systems. Harrington distraction instrumentation segmentally wired, Cotrel–Dubousset instrumentation, Wisconsin instrumentation, Steffee plates, and Roy-Camille plates proved to be the most effective posterior axial loading devices. The smooth rod-wire constructs consistently had the poorest results when tested with axial loading. Bone et al.[5] carried out anterior spinal instrumentation testing that used axial loading of instrumentation. The results demonstrate the broad dynamic compression plate (DCP) to give the best axial load-bearing results in a burst fracture model.

With flexion injuries (anterior and posterior column defects with occasional middle column defects as well)[7,41,91,92] tested with a flexion load, Harrington distraction instrumentation segmentally wired, plate-screw constructs such as Roy-Camille plates and Steffee plates, and Cotrel–Dubousset instrumentation proved to be the highest ranked constructs. Ferguson et al.[7,29] noted increasing instability in segmentally wired Harrington distraction rods with increasingly unstable spinal injury models. Extension of Harrington distraction instrumentation from two to three lamina above a fracture model increased the failure moment and energy absorbed to failure by 36% and 30%, respectively, in flexion loading.[10,18] The Jacobs' rod and clamp device proved to be stiff in flexion and to maintain its stiffness with increasingly unstable fracture patterns.[7]

In extension and lateral bend loading, plate screw devices and combination fixation devices ranked best. Torsional tests demonstrated Harrington distraction rods to have very poor stability. Segmental wiring of the Harrington distraction rod improved its torsional stiffness characteristics.[15] Transverse coupling improved rotational stability in all devices where it was applied.[21,73,75] Cotrel–Dubousset instrumentation, plate-screw fixation devices, and C- or L-rods (especially if coupled) ranked consistently as the best rotational stabilizing devices.

Testing by Ashman et al.[90] to examine the endurance limit (a stress below which failure will not occur regardless of the number of cycles used to test the implant) of metal implants demonstrated that the Harrington distraction rod with its ratchet-shaft junction and the Cotrel–Dubousset rods with knurling of the rods cause significant increases in stress, of 1.3 and 3.0 fold, respectively, at the stress-risers in the rods. They are thus theoretically at risk for failure from fatigue if arthrodesis of the spine is not achieved. Johnston et al.[87] have reported the theoretical susceptibility of implant failure in long pelvic fusions in which 3/16-in. 316L stainless steel L-rod having a residual of 38° or more of scoliosis. He stated that means of improving the endurance limits of this instrumentation might include larger diameter stainless steel rods, rods made of metals with higher ultimate and fatigue strengths, external support of the trunk, or cross-links between rods.

It appears that the large amount of mechanical testing done on spinal implants supports White's concept that combination fixation devices as well as screw-plate devices provide the greatest stability in in vitro tests. However, many of these tests only evaluate one mode of failure of the implant, ignoring biological variables such as stress bypass of the instrumented segment, the effect of trunk and spinal muscle forces, and creep of soft tissue (except where cyclic studies were done), as well as the interplay of all these variables. Definite conclusions cannot be made. It is probable that no one instrumentation construct will give the best results for all deformities.

Summary

Whether deformities of the spine are caused by trauma, degeneration, tumor, or idiopathic, congenital, or neuromuscular causes, mechanical principles to correct sagittal and coronal plane deformities are available. These principles have been demonstrated to have validity in the spine. They should be considered whether one is designing instrumentation systems or selecting instrumentations to correct specific deformities. Of equal importance is an understanding of the bony and soft-tissue envelope to which these instrumentations will be attached. Irrespective of the mechanical strengths of an instrumentation, if the bone is extremely fragile, failure of the bone–implant interface may be assured. This is not a problem of implant design but rather a problem of surgical judgment. In the final analysis, this variable is the most important one of all those discussed.[91]

References

1. Schultz AB, Hirsch C. Mechanical analysis of Harrington rod correction of idiopathic scoliosis. J Bone Joint Surg 1973;55A:983–992.
2. Wenger DR, Carollo JJ, Wilkerson JA. Biomechanics of scoliosis correction by segmental spinal instrumentation. Spine 1982;7:260–264.
3. White AA, III, Panjabi MM. The clinical biomechanics of scoliosis. Clin Orthop 1976;118:100–111.
4. White AA, III, Panjabi MM, Thomas CL. The clinical biomechanics of kyphotic deformities. Clin Orthop 1977;128:8–17.
5. Bone LB, Ashman RB, Roach JW, Johnston CE, II. Mechanical comparison of anterior spine instrumentation in a burst fracture model. Orthop Trans 1987;11:87.
6. Cool TA, Nasca RJ, Bidez MW, Lemons JE. Cyclic torsional testing with force-motion analysis of SSI and Harrington rod instrumentation. Orthop Trans 1986;10:8.
7. Ferguson RL, Tencer AF, Woodard P, Allen BL, Jr. Biomechanical comparisons of spinal fracture models and the stabilizing effects of posterior instrumentations. Spine 1988;13:453–460.

8a. Gepstein R, Latta L, Shufflebarger HL. Cotrel–Dubousset instrumentation for lumbar burst fractures: a biomechanical study. Orthop Trans 1987;11:452.

8b. Asher MA, Strippgen WE. Anthropometric studies of the human sacrum relating to dorsal transsacral implant design. Clin Orthop 1986;203:58–62.

9. Herring JA, Ashman RB. Biomechanical testing of instruments for the fixation of spondylolisthesis. Orthop Trans 1987;11:98–99.
10. Jacobs RR, Nordwall A, Nachemson A. Reduction, stability and strength provided by internal fixation systems for thoracolumbar spinal injuries. Clin Orthop 1982;171:300.
11. Laborde JM, Bahniuk E, Bohlman HH, Samson B. Comparison of fixation of spinal fractures. Clin Orthop 1980;152:303–310.
12. Mann KA, Found EM, Yuan HA, Lubicky JP, Fredrickson BE. Biomechanical evaluation of the effectiveness of anterior spinal fixation systems. Orthop Trans 1987;11:378.
13. McAfee PC, Werner FW, Glisson RR. A biomechanical analysis of spinal instrumentation systems in thoracolumbar fractures: comparison of traditional Harrington distraction instrumentation with segmental spinal instrumentation. Spine 1985;10:204–217.
14. Mino DE, Stauffer ES, Davis PK, Hester J. Torsional loading of Harrington distraction rod instrumentation compared to segmental sublaminar and spinous process supplementation. Orthop Trans 1985;9:119.
15. Munson G, Satterlee C, Hammond S. Betten R, Gaines RW. Experimental evaluation of Harrington rod fixation supplemented with sublaminar wires in stabilizing thoracolumbar fracture-dislocations. Clin Orthop 1984;189:97.
16. Pinzur MS, Meyer PR, Lautenschlager EP, et al. Measurement of internal fixation device support in experimentally produced fractures of the dorsolumbar spine. Orthopaedics 1979;2:28–34.
17. Puno RM, Hartjen CA, von Fraunhofer JA, Holt RT, Johnson JR. Biomechanical analysis of the Cotrel–Dubousset spine instrumentation systems. Orthop Trans 1987;11:404.
18. Purcell GA, Markolf KL, Dawson EG. Twelfth thoracic-first lumbar vertebral mechanical stability of fractures after

Harrington rod instrumentation. J Bone Joint Surg 1981;63A:71–78.
19. Ritterbusch JF, Ashman RB, Roach JW, Johnston CE, II, Birch JG, Herring JA. Biomechanical comparisons of spinal instrumentation systems. Orthop Trans 1987;11:87.
20. Stauffer ES, Neil JL. Biomechanical analysis of structural stability of internal fixation in fractures of the thoracolumbar spine. Clin Orthop 1975;112:159–164.
21. Ward JJ, Nasca RJ, Lemons JE. Cyclic torsional testing of Harrington and Luque spinal implants. Orthop Trans 1985;9:118.
22. Wenger DR, Carollo JJ, Wilkerson JA, Wauters K, Herring JA. Laboratory testing of segmental spinal instrumentation versus traditional Harrington instrumentation for scoliosis treatment. Spine 1982;7:265–269.
23. Frankel VH, Nordin M. Basic biomechanics of the skeletal system. Philadelphia: Lea & Febiger, 1980.
24. Krag MH, Beynnon BD, Pope MH, Frymoyer JW, Haugh LD, Weaver DL. An internal fixator for posterior application to short segments of the thoracic, lumbar, or lumbosacral spine: design and testing. Clin Orthop 1986;203:75.
25. Lin HS, Liu YK, Adams KH. Mechanical response of the lumbar intervertebral joint under physiological (complex) loading. J Bone Joint Surg 1978;60A:41–55.
26. McNeice G. Biomechanics research of fracture fixation: application to the thoracolumbar spine. Report to the University of Texas Medical Branch, Galveston, Texas, 1983.
27. Roaf R. A study of the mechanics of spinal injuries. J Bone Joint Surg 1960;42B:810–823.
28a. Schultz A, Andersson G, Ortengren R, Haderspeck K, Nachemson A. Loads on the lumbar spine. J Bone Joint Surg 1982;64A:713–720.
28b. Ferguson RL, Allen BL, Jr. A mechanistic classification of thoracolumbar spine fractures. Clin Orthop 1984;189:77–88.
29. Self J, Tencer AF, Allen BL, Jr, Ferguson RL. Design of laminar attachment device for posterior spinal instrumentation. Spine 1989;(in press).
30. Waugh TR. Intravital measurements during instrumental correction of idiopathic scoliosis. Acta Orthop Scand (Suppl) 1966;93:1–87.
31. Zindrick MR, Wiltse LL, Doornik A, Widell EH, Knight GW, Pathwardhan A, Thomas JC. Analysis of the morphometric characteristics of the thoracolumbar pedicles. Orthop Trans 1987;11:98.
32. Jacobs RR, Schlaepfer F, Mathys R, et al. A new instrumentation system for fracture-dislocation of the dorsolumbar spine. Orthop Trans 1981;5:17–18.
33. Belytschko TB, Andriacchi TP, Schultz AB, Galante JO. Analog studies of forces in the human spine: computational techniques. J Biomech 1973;6:361–371.
34. Schultz AB, Belytschko TB, Andriacchi TP. Analog studies of forces in the human spine: mechanical properties and motion segment behavior. J Biomech 1973;6:373–383.
35. Dunn HK, Daniels AU. The mechanics of the surgical treatment of scoliosis. In: Black JA, Dubleton J, eds. Clinical Biomechanics: A Case History Approach. New York: Churchill Livingstone, 1981:335–358.
36. Ogilvie JW. Biomechanics. In: Moe's Textbook of Scoliosis and Other Spinal Deformities. Philadelphia: Saunders, 1987;7–23.
37. Bradford DS, Lonstein JE, Moe JH, Ogilvie JW, Winter RB. Moe's Textbook of Scoliosis and Other Spinal Deformities. Philadelphia: Saunders, 1987.
38. Dwyer AF. Experience of anterior correction of scoliosis. Clin Orthop 1973;93:191–206.
39. Enneking WF, Harrington P. Pathologic changes in scoliosis. J Bone Joint Surg 1969;51A:165–184.
40. Nachemson A, Elfstrom G. Intravital wireless telemetry of axial forces in Harrington distraction rods in patients with idiopathic scoliosis. J Bone Joint Surg 1971;53A:445–465.
41. McAfee PC, Yuan HA, Fredrickson BE, Lubicky JP. The value of computed tomography in thoracolumbar fractures. An analysis of 100 consecutive cases and a new classification. J Bone Joint Surg 1983;65A:461–473.
42. Allen BL, Jr, Ferguson RL. Basic considerations in pelvic fixation cases. In: Segmental Spinal Instrumentation. ER Luque, ed. Thorofare, New Jersey: Charles B. Slack, Inc., 1984:185–220.
43. Dove J, Chan R, Ali MS. Biomechanics of segmental spinal wiring. Orthop Trans 1986;10:7–8.
44. Flatley TJ, Derderian H. Closed loop instrumentation of the lumbar spine. Clin Orthop 1985;196:273–278.
45. Goel VK, Nye TA, Clark CR, Nishiyama K, Weinstein J. Evaluation of an internal fixation device using the Selspot system—an application to the Luque closed loop system. Orthop Trans 1986;10:541.
46. Allen BL, Jr. Segmental spinal instrumentation with L-rods. AAOS: Instructional Course Lectures, Vol. 32, St. Louis. Mosby, 1983:202–208.
47. Allen BL, Jr. Biomechanical considerations in L-rod instrumentation. 19th Meeting of SRS Society, September 1984.
48. Allen BL, Jr, Ferguson RL. The Galveston technique for L-rod instrumentation of the scoliotic spine. Spine 1982;7:276–284.
49. Kostuik JP. Indications for the use of the Halo immobilization. Clin Orthop 1981;154:46–50.
50. Drummond D, Guadagni J, Keene JS, Breed A, Narechania R. Interspinous process segmental spinal instrumentation. J Pediatr Orthop 1984;4:397–404.
51. Georgette FS, Sander TW, Oh I. The fatigue resistance of orthopaedic wire and cable systems. Proceedings of the 10th Annual Society for Biomaterials Washington, DC, p 146, 1984.
52. Bryan WJ, Inglis AE, Sculco TP, Ranawat CS, Methylmethacrylate stabilization for enhancement of posterior cervical arthrodesis in rheumatoid arthritis. J Bone Joint Surg 1982;64A:1045–1050.
53. Dunn EJ. The role of methylmethacrylate in the stabilization and replacement of tumors of the cervical spine. Spine 1977;2:15–24.
54. Dunn HK, Bolstad KE. Fixation of Dwyer screws for the treatment of scoliosis. J Bone Joint Surg 1977;59A:54–56.
55. Herron LD, Dawson EG. Methylmethacrylate as an adjunct in spinal instrumentation. J Bone Joint Surg 1977;59A:866–868.
56. Lange DR. The mechanical bonding of methylmethacrylate to cancellous bone. J Bone Joint Surg 1979;61A:254–256.

57. Wang GJ, Reger SI, Shao ZH, Morton CL, Stamp WG. Comparative strength of anterior spinal fixation with bone graft or polymethylmethacrylate. Clin Orthop 1984;188:303–308.
58. Zindrick MR, Patwardhan A, Lorenz M. The effect of methylmethacrylate augmentation upon pedicle screw fixation in the spine. Orthop Trans 1986;10:540.
59. Hansebout RR, Blomquist GA, Jr. Acrylic spinal fusion. J Neurosurg 1980;53:606–612.
60. McAfee PC, Bohlman HH. Complications following Harrington instrumentation for fractures of the thoracolumbar spine. J Bone Joint Surg 1985;67A:672–686.
61. Crowninshield R, Pope MH, Hoaglund FT. A comparison of the tensile properties of bone and polymethylmethacrylate. J Bone Joint Surg [Am] 1974;56A:865.
62. Taitsman JP, Saha S. Tensile strength of wire-reinforced bone cement and twisted stainless steel wire. J Bone Joint Surg 1977;59A:419–425.
63. Johnston CE, II, Ashman RB, Corin JD. Mechanical effects of cross-linking rods in Cotrel–Dubousset instrumentation. Orthop Trans 1987;11:96.
64. Akbarnia BA, Merenda JT, Keppler L, Gaines R, Lorenz M. Surgical treatment of fractures and fracture dislocations of the thoracolumbar and lumbar spine using pedicular screws and plate fixation. Orthop Trans 1987;11:228.
65. Reed S, Wagner T. Preliminary report on lumbosacral fusion with pedicle screws and Steffee plates. Orthop Trans 1987;11:99–100.
66. Steffee AD. Complete reduction of grade IV spondylolisthesis using segmental spine plates and transpedicular screws. Orthop Trans 1987;11:228.
67. Luque E. Indications for SSI sublaminar intrapeduncular. Orthop Trans 1987;11:501.
68. Luque ER. Transpedicular segmental correction and fixation. Orthop Trans 1986;10:5.
69. Andrew TA, Brooks S, Piggott H. Long-term follow-up evaluation of screw-and-graft fusion of the lumbar spine. Clin Orthop 1986;203:113–119.
70. Kornblatt MD, Casey MP, Jacobs RR. Internal fixation in-lumbosacral spine fusion. Clin Orthop 1986;203:141–150.
71. Liu YK, Njus GO, Singerman R. Improvement of the mechanical properties of pedicle screws used in spinal internal fixation. Orthop Trans 1986;10:540.
72. Zindrick MR, Wiltse LL, Holland WR, Widell EH, Thomas JC, Spencer CW. A biomechanical study of intrapedicular screw fixation in the lumbosacral spine. Clin Orthop 1986;203:99–112.
73. Kling TF, Jr, Vanderby R, Jr, Belloli DM, Thomsen EL. Cross-linked pedicle screw fixation in the same vertebral body: a biomechanical study. Orthop Trans 1987;11:98.
74. Highland TR, Chan DPK. The pedicle of the spinal column: its anatomy and application in spinal surgery. Orthop Trans 1986;10:4.
75. Asher M, Carson W, Heinig C, Strippgen W, Lark R, Arendt M, Hartley M. A modular spinal rod linkage system to provide rotational stability. Orthop Trans 1987;11:124.
76. Moseley C, Mosca V, Lawton L, Koreska J. Improved stability in segmental instrumentation of neuromuscular scoliosis. Orthop Trans 1986;10:5.
77. Dubousset J, Guillaumat M, Cotrel Y. Correction and fusion to the sacrum of pelvic obliquity with CD instrumentation in children and adults. Orthop Trans 1987;11:96.
78. Edwards CC. A new method for direct sacral fixation: rationale and clinical results. Orthop Trans 1986;10:541.
79. Edwards CC. Spinal screw fixation of the lumbar and sacral spine: Early results treating the first 50 cases. Orthop Trans 1987;11:99.
80. McCarthy RE, Dunn HK. Pelvic fixation around the sacral ala with the Luque system. Orthop Trans 1987;11:88.
81. Puno RM, Bechtold JE, Byrd JA, Winter RB, Ogilvie JW, Bradford DS. Biomechanical analysis of five techniques of fixation for the lumbosacral junction. Orthop Trans 1987;11:86.
82. Jacobs RR. Personal communication, 1982.
83. Galante J, Schultz A, Dewald RL, Ray RD. Forces acting in the Milwaukee brace on patients undergoing treatment for idiopathic scoliosis. J Bone Joint Surg 1970;52A:498–506.
84. Lumsden RM, Morris JM. An in vivo study of axial rotation and immobilization at the lumbosacral junction. J Bone Joint Surg 1968;50A:1591–1602.
85. Nagel DA, Koogle TA, Piziali RI, Perkash I. Stability of the upper lumbar spine following progressive disruptions and the application of individual internal and external fixation devices. J Bone Joint Surg 1981;63A:62–70.
86. Johnson RH, Hart DL, Simmons EF, Ramsby GR, Southwick WO. Cervical orthoses. J Bone Joint Surg 1977;59A:332–339.
87. Johnston CE, Ashman RB, Sherman MC. Mechanical consequences of rod contouring and residual scoliosis in sublaminar pelvic SSI. Orthop Trans 1986;10:5–6.
88. Calhoun J, McNeice G, Allen BL, Jr, Ferguson RL, Meek-Chilton J. An analysis of variables affecting segmental spinal instrumentation. Orthop Trans 1985;9:538.
89. Waugh TR. The biomechanical basis for the utilization of methylmethacrylate in the treatment of scoliosis. J Bone Joint Surg 1971;53A:194–195.
90. Ashman RB, Birch JG, Bone LB, Corin JD, Herring JA, Johnston CE, II, Ritterbush JF, Roach JW. Mechanical testing of spinal instrumentation. Clin Orthop 1988;227:113–125.
91. Denis F. The three-column spine and its significance in the classification of acute thoracolumbar spinal injuries. Spine 1983;8:817–831.
92. Holdsworth F. Review article: fractures, dislocations, and fracture dislocations of the spine. J Bone Joint Surg 1970;52A:1534.
93. Winter RB, Lonstein JE, Vanden Brink K, Anderson MB. Harrington rod with sublaminar wires in the treatment of adolescent idiopathic scoliosis. A study of sagittal plane correction. Orthop Trans, 1987; 11:89.

II

Indications for Spinal Fusion

6

Assessing Spinal Instability or Indications for Spinal Fusion

John W. Frymoyer and Leon J. Grobler

Every year 10 million Americans have acute low back pain; only 286,000 (0.04%) require an operation, of which approximately one-fourth (70,000) are spinal fusions.[1] In the United States, 2% of the adult population have had a previous lumbar spinal operation, and it is probable there are 500,000 to 1,000,000 living adults who have had a lumbar spinal fusion.[2] These figures remind us spinal fusion is but a small part of the treatment for most low back disorders, and is usually indicated for the restoration of stability.

The Evolution of Spinal Stabilization and Fusion Techniques

The history of spinal fusion includes developments in concepts of mechanical spinal stabilization and biological spinal arthrodesis.

The earliest reported attempts to mechanically stabilize a spine were reported by Lange (1886) in Germany[3] and Hadra (1887) of Galveston, Texas.[4] More than 20 years elapsed before spinal arthrodesis was performed by Albee[5] and Hibbs[6] as a treatment for spinal tuberculosis. The subsequent developments have been directed to refinements of the metallurgical and biomechanical characteristics of stabilization devices, combined with an increased knowledge of the biology of graft materials and graft substitutes, and the optimal techniques for the placement of these bone grafts. From this accumulated knowledge it has been learned that long-term stability requires biological fusion, regardless of the devices used for spinal stabilization.

At the same time, our knowledge of what constitutes spinal stability and instability continues to be refined in light of improved clinical, radiographic, and biomechanical knowledge.

Assessing Spinal Stability

Hippocrates appears to have been the first person to have recognized the general problem of spinal instability when he wrote, "When a gibbosity seizes a person, it occasions a crisis in the then existing disease." Undoubtedly, he was describing spinal tuberculosis. Today an unstable spine is defined as a condition in which normally tolerated spinal movements and forces lead to abnormal displacements or deformities which places neurological structures at risk.[7] This definition is clinically applicable to spinal trauma, infectious processes, neoplasms, and spondylolisthesis, but continues to be less certain when applied to degenerative spinal conditions.

Determinants of Spinal Stability

The building block of the spine is the functional spinal unit (FSU) consisting of two vertebrae, the intervening disc, the facet joints, and the connecting spinal ligaments (supraspinous, interspinous, longitudinal ligaments, and ligamentum flavum). The vertebral column as an aggregate of functional spinal units requires muscles and their fascial envelopes for ultimate stabilization.

The elements of the FSU each contribute somewhat differently to spinal stability as a function of the applied loads and motions. Although it is convenient to think of motions as occurring in three isolated planes (flexion/extension, lateral bend, and rotation), spinal kinematics are far more complex. White and Panjabi[8] showed spinal movements are coupled, which means that primary or intentional movements in one plane are invariably accompanied by secondary or unintentional movements in another plane. Moreover, movements are not simply rotational about the three axes of the spine, but are also translational (Fig. 6.1).

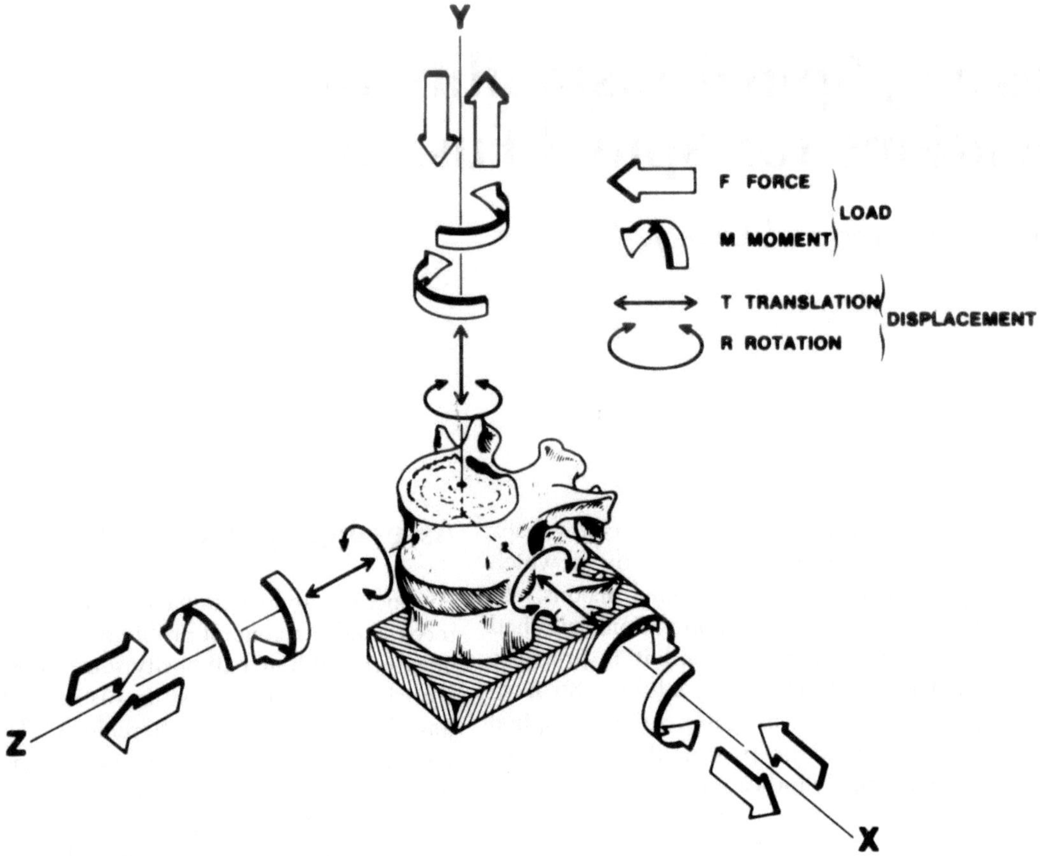

Figure 6.1. Rotation and translation occur about the three mutually perpendicular axes of the spinal motion segment, i.e., X, Y, and Z. (Reprinted from White and Panjabi[8] with the permission of the authors and publisher.)

The location of the axis changes with motion,[9] termed the instantaneous axis of rotation. Biomechanical studies in vitro[10] and in vivo[11] have established that the instant center in normal spinal specimens is located at the junction of the middle and posterior thirds of the disc. This instant center of rotation follows a fairly predictable course in the normal FSU.

Coupled behavior means that forces applied to a spine under normal physiological conditions will produce complex resultant stresses and strains. The "pure" loads experienced by the spine include compression, torsion, tension, and shear.

Compression Loading

Under compression loading the major elements affected are the vertebral bodies and discs. In the laboratory, compressive loads result in radial bulging of the discs, increases in the intradiscal pressures, and deformations of the vertebral endplates. If these forces are continued to failure, the endplates, rather than the disc, are disrupted.[12] Trabecular fractures in the region of the endplate are commonly observed in anatomical specimens and may cause some cases of back pain. The radiographic correlates of the compressive load-bearing portion of the FSU are the anterior and middle columns as defined by McAfee et al.[13] Under normal circumstances, the lumbar facet joints contribute no more than 25% to the compressive load-bearing capacities of the FSU.[14]

Torsional Loading

Torsional loading of the FSU produces stresses on both discs, the adjacent vertebral endplates, facets, and ligaments. Farfan's important studies have shown torsional loads in the lumbar spine are resisted 60% by the facet joints and 30% by the annulus and disc.[10] If torsion is applied to specimens without posterior elements, disruption of the fibers occurs primarily in the posterolateral corner of the disc. If the posterior elements of the FSU are intact, the torsional loads are resisted primarily by the facets up to the point of failure. The loads are then shifted to the posterior ligamentous complex, which fails if torsional forces are continued. These events correspond to failures of the posterior column.

Tension Loading

Tension loads are common in the posterior ligaments when the spine is flexed, particularly if there is an associated torsional component to that movement. The role of the posterior ligamentous complex as a tension-resisting component in fracture biomechanics is discussed later.

Shear Loading

Virtually every force applied to the spine results in a shear component. Thus, the applications of a compression load to a lordotic spinal segment will result in a shear load. Hutton and associates[15] evaluated the role of shear to the production of both spondylolysis and disc herniation. Their studies demonstrated that in lumbar flexion and extension the resultant shear loads are resisted by the neural arch. If motions are continued to failure, failures in the neural arch are produced and correspond to spondylolysis. If the loading conditions are repetitively applied through compression (with resultant shear), the disc may disrupt.

Role of Supportive Structures

The spine clearly is dependent on its supporting muscle/fascial envelopes. If an intact cadaveric spine, devoid of its muscles, is tested under compression, the specimen buckles at loads of less than 4 kg.[16] This behavior is not surprising to clinicians experienced in the management of paralytical curvatures of the spine. The musculature of an intact human spine has been likened to the stays on a sailboat. Electromyographic studies show, for a normal stance, that the electrically active muscles are the iliopsoas, but that the paraspinal muscles become active as soon as motion is initiated. In forward flexion the paraspinal muscles are electrically active until 60° to 70° of forward flexion is reached, at which point they become inactive. This observation has been interpreted to mean that the fully flexed spine is "hanging on its ligaments." Pressurization within the fascial envelope increases the effectiveness of muscle function, particularly in maintaining the erect spinal posture, whereas abdominal pressurization offsets only 5% of spinal compressive loads.

Assessing Spinal Instability

The preceding section detailed some attributes of the normal stable spine and how the various anatomical elements contribute to load bearing under different applied forces. Let us now examine the conditions that produce spinal instability and the indications for spinal stabilization and fusion procedures (Table 6.1).

Table 6.1 Spinal instabilities.

Fracture and fracture dislocations
Inflammatory lesions
Neoplasms
Spondylolisthesis
Degenerative disease

Fractures and Fracture Dislocations

Fractures and fracture dislocations, especially in the thoracolumbar area, have provided the greatest clinical information regarding spinal (in)stability. The primary objective in treating spinal fractures concerns, first, improving or preventing further anatomical displacement or deformities, and second, preventing the occurrence or progression of a preexisting neurological deficit. Both mechanical and neurological (nonmechanical) considerations should therefore be considered in deciding the correct approach in each case.

Defining spinal stability and therefore setting sound guidelines for treatment has been a major problem intriguing spinal surgeons during the past 30 years. Holdsworth[17] classified instability according to the fracture pattern observed on spinal radiographs, defining simple wedge fractures, burst fractures, and extension injuries as stable injuries, and shear fractures, rotational fracture/dislocations, and dislocations as unstable. He therefore divided the spine into two columns and believed that instability occurred after posterior complex disruption (Figs. 6.2A and 6.2B). More recent studies by Posner et al.[18] revealed that instability can only occur if both the posterior longitudinal ligament *and* the posterior annulus fibrosis are sectioned.

Aided by computed tomography (CT), McAfee[13] and Denis[19] advocated the usage of the three-column concept, thereby placing more emphasis on the role of the bony components, especially the middle column, in spinal sta-

A 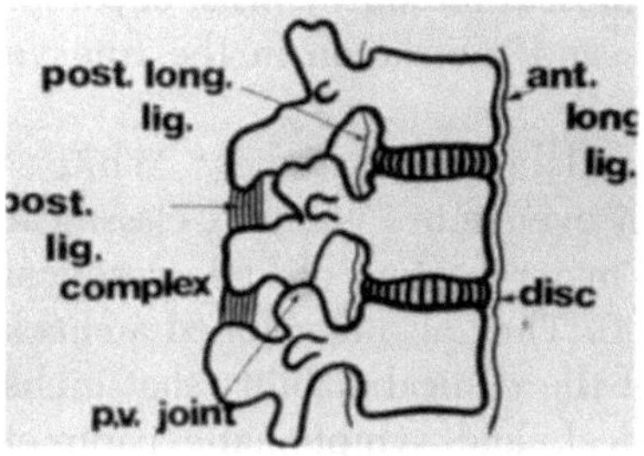

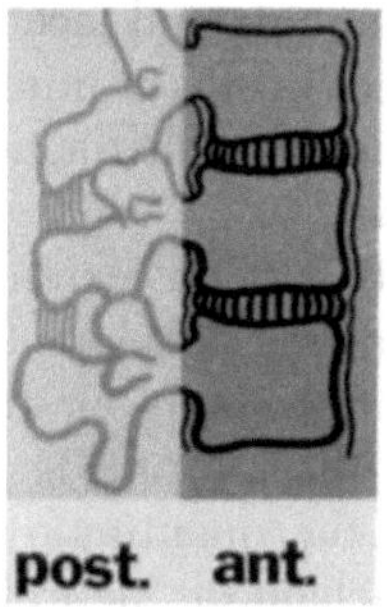 B

Figure 6.2. **A.** Anatomical structures are shown to more clearly demonstrate classification of spinal fractures. **B.** Holdsworth[17] initially classified spinal fractures by area of pathology (anterior or posterior) using posterior longitudinal ligament as reference point.

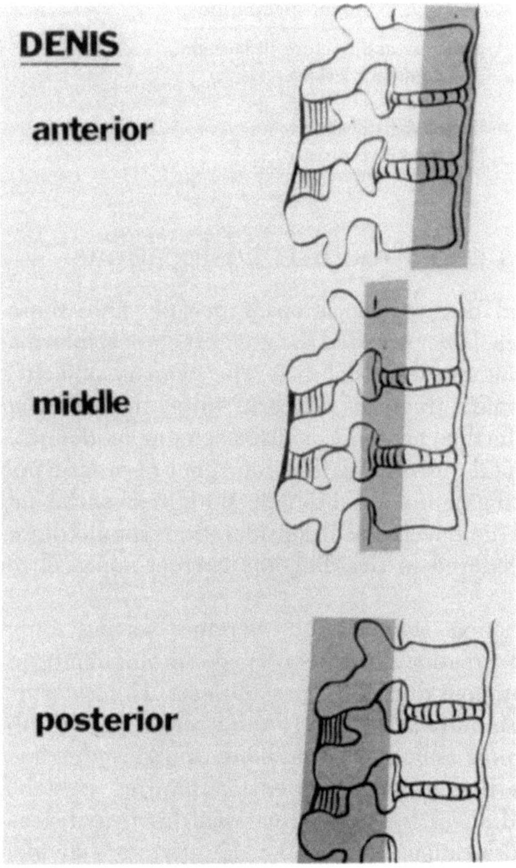

Figure 6.3. Denis,[19] following usage of computed tomography, emphasized importance of middle column and three-column concepts.

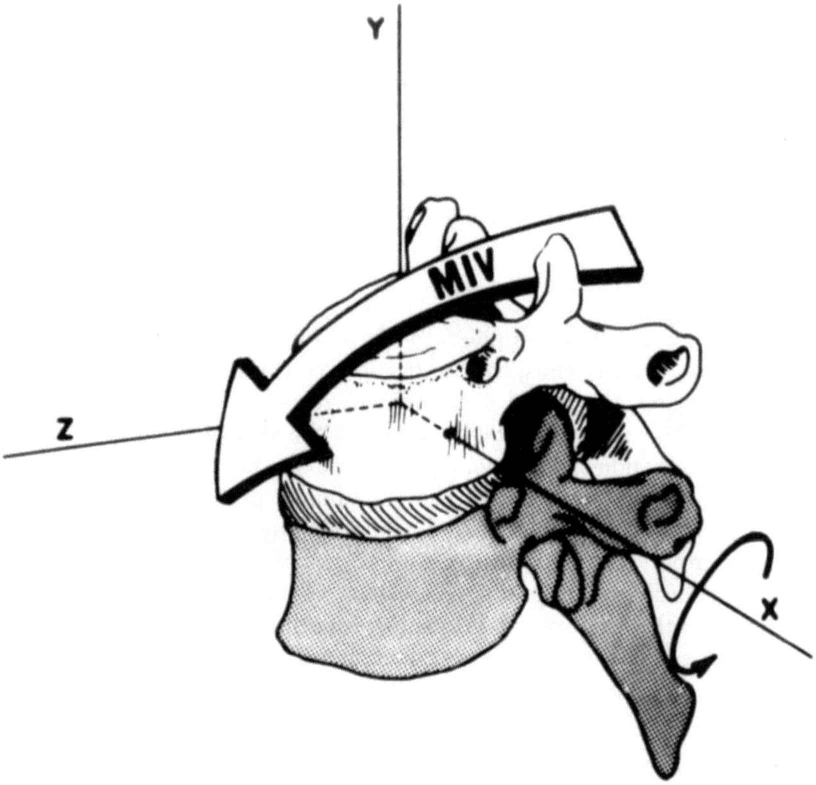

Figure 6.4. The major injury vector (MIV) according to White and Panjabi.[8] Bilateral facet dislocation in cervical spine is shown. Note that major force application is in translation along Z axis. Accompanying rotational component is depicted by *arrow* about X axis. (Reprinted from White and Panjabi[8] with the permission of authors and publisher.)

bility (Fig. 6.3). In this classification, the anterior column includes the anterior two-thirds of the vertebral body and disc, the middle column comprises the posterior one-third of the vertebral body, the annulus fibrosis, and the posterior longitudinal ligaments, and the posterior column includes the remaining posterior structures, including the ligaments and facet capsules. The authors suggested the mechanisms of injury most commonly consist of compression, axial distraction, and translation in the transverse plane.

Based on extensive laboratory studies, White and Panjabi[8] developed an even more complex classification that accounts for the major vectors of force responsible for the injury (Fig. 6.4). They also developed a checklist for the quantitation of the clinical stability that includes mechanical, neurological, and symptomatic parameters (Table 6.2).

Because mobility is of primary importance in the cervical spine, bony configuration is found to be less than optimal. Stability of the cervical spine depends on the susceptibility of the ligamentous structures to disruption in cervical injuries. Injured ligaments also tend not to heal as well as bone, thereby predisposing to long-term (chronic) instability.

Regarding the C1–C2 complex, the crucial stable structural component is the transverse ligament, and despite fractures of the ring of the atlas, stability prevails so long as the transverse ligament is intact. Following rupture of the transverse ligament, the C1 condyles drift apart,

Table 6.2 Checklist for instability in the lumbar (L1–L5) spine.

Element	Point value*
Cauda equina damage	3
Relative flexion sagittal plane translation >10% or extension sagittal plane translation >10%	2
Relative flexion sagittal plane rotation >0 degrees	2
Anterior elements destroyed	2
Posterior elements destroyed	2
Dangerous loading anticipated	1

* Total score of 5 indicates instability

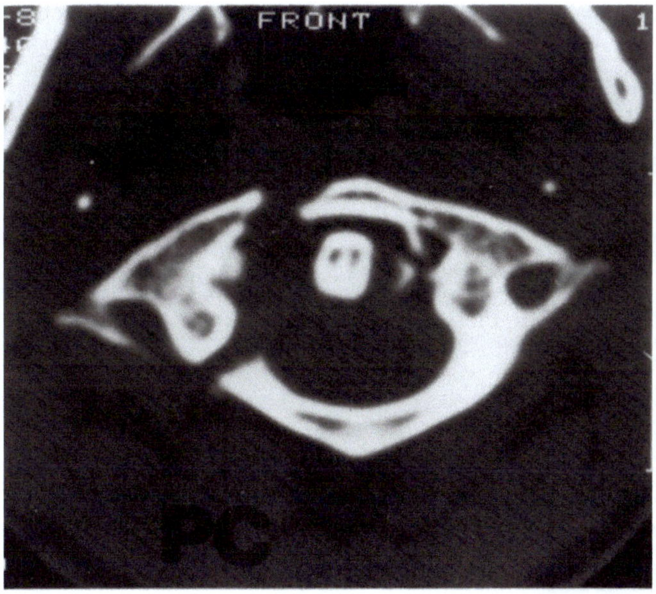

Figure 6.5. Computed tomography of bony C1 ring fracture and avulsion of transverse ligament insertion with resultant instability.

thereby creating an unstable situation; underlying neural damage may result (Fig. 6.5). Lateral displacement of more than 7 mm has been found to indicate an unstable C1 Jefferson fracture,[20] and decisive diagnosis of this situation is obtained by CT scan. It should also be emphasized that a fracture of the C1 ring may heal, but because of an undiagnosed transverse ligament rupture, chronic instability of C1–C2 may follow. This emphasizes the necessity of flexion/extension views after bony healing of C1 ring fractures.

Atlantoaxial instability is a classic example of ligamentous rupture leading to an unstable situation (Figs. 6.6A and 6.6B). Instability in trauma is present if the space between the dens and C1 arch exceeds 2 to 3 mm in the adult and 4 to 5 mm in children.[21]

Regarding C2 fractures (hangman's fracture), the crucial factor once again is a soft-tissue component, namely the presence or absence of C2–C3 disc disruption (Fig. 6.7), therefore necessitating careful flexion/extension views for diagnosis. The example illustrates the frequent necessity of judicious stress testing for instability in the cervical spine to diagnose the often-accompanying soft-tissue or ligamentous component. The important issue regarding stability in unilateral facet dislocation is the determination if it is a pure unilateral jumped facet or a unilateral facet fracture with or without subluxation. Rotational instability with resultant resubluxation is often found if an accompanying facet fracture is present (Figs. 6.8A and 6.8B). The clinical correlation of unstability occurs when unilateral facet dislocation is reduced very easily, which indicates it will tend to displace back to previous position just as easily. The value of the CT scan in cervical trauma in selected cases should also be emphasized.[22]

White and Panjabi[8] also classified cervical spine stability regarding horizontal displacement and angular motion. Horizontal displacement more than 3.5 mm and angular motion more than 11°, compared to adjoining spaces, are seen as signs of instability (Fig. 6.9). Herkowitz and Rothman[23] pointed out that initial normal radiographs can harbor an underlying unstable situation and emphasized the need for a high index of suspicion. After cervical

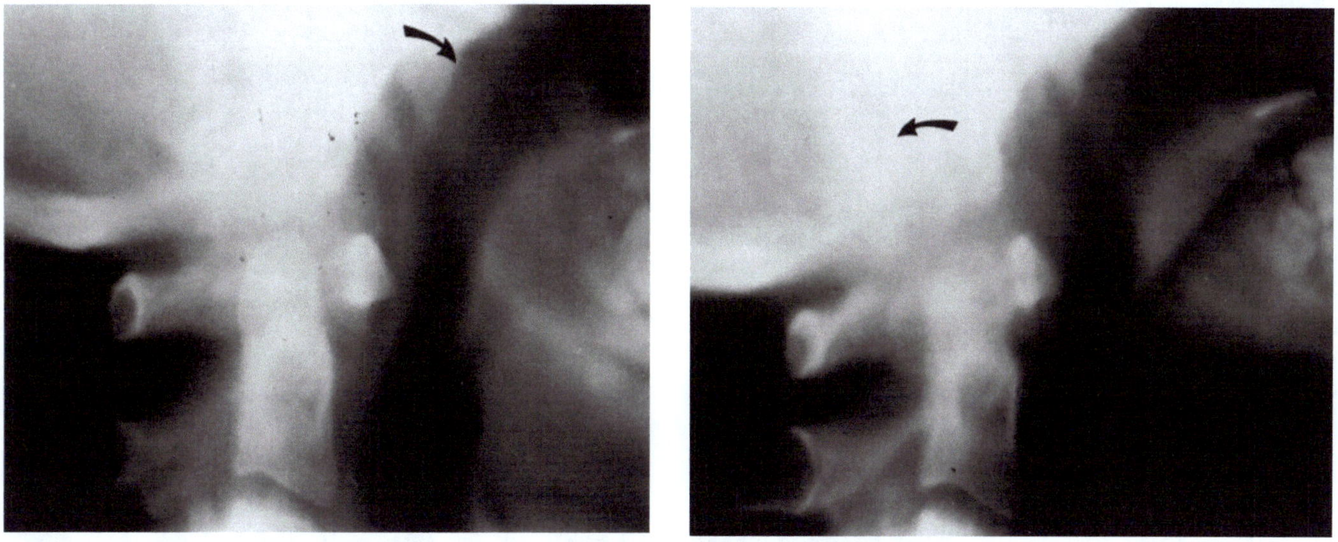

A B

Figure 6.6. Following transient loss of consciousness after motor vehicle accident, patient complained of minimal neck pain. Despite normal routine radiographs, flexion (**A**)/extension (**B**) views revealed increased A.D.I. (atlanto-dens-interspace) (*arrows*).

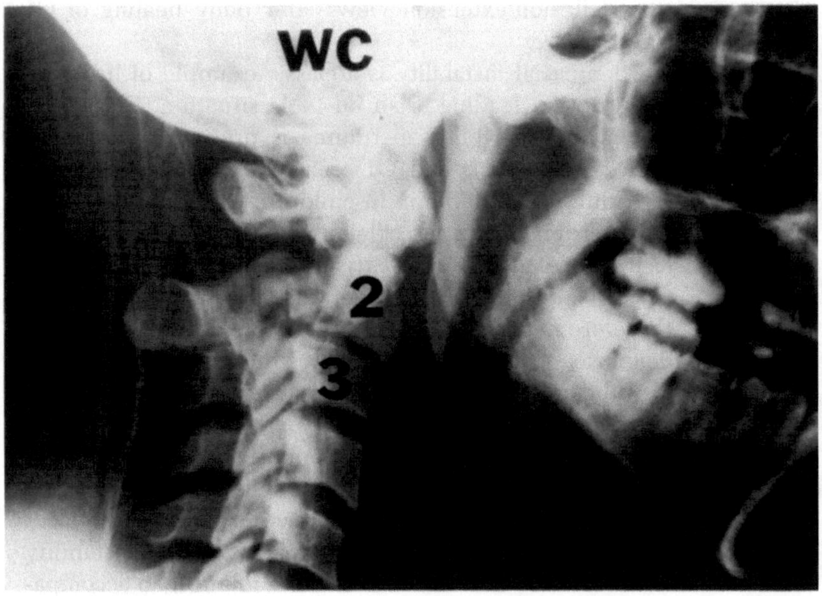

Figure 6.7. Hangman's fracture of C2 vertebra with translation C2–C3 caused by disc disruption and therefore potentially unstable.

Figure 6.8. **A** and **B.** Young adult presenting with neck and arm pain and C3–C4 subluxation (**A**). Reconstruction of computed tomography views in parasagittal view clearly outlines unilateral fracture of C3 inferior facet. On "unraveled" view (**B**), pathology is seen more clearly.

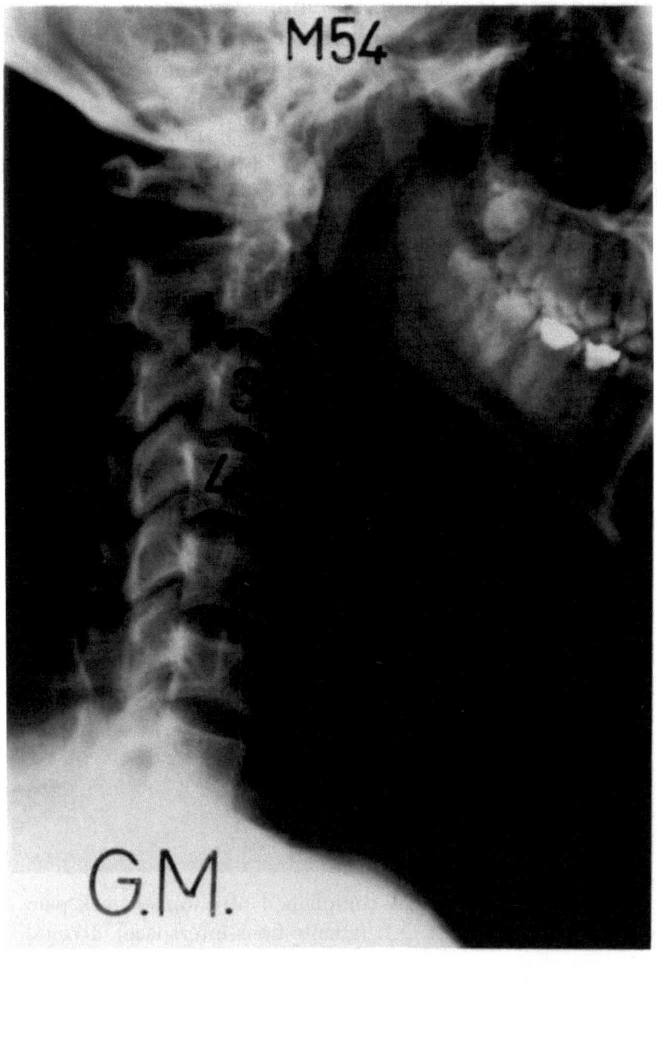

A

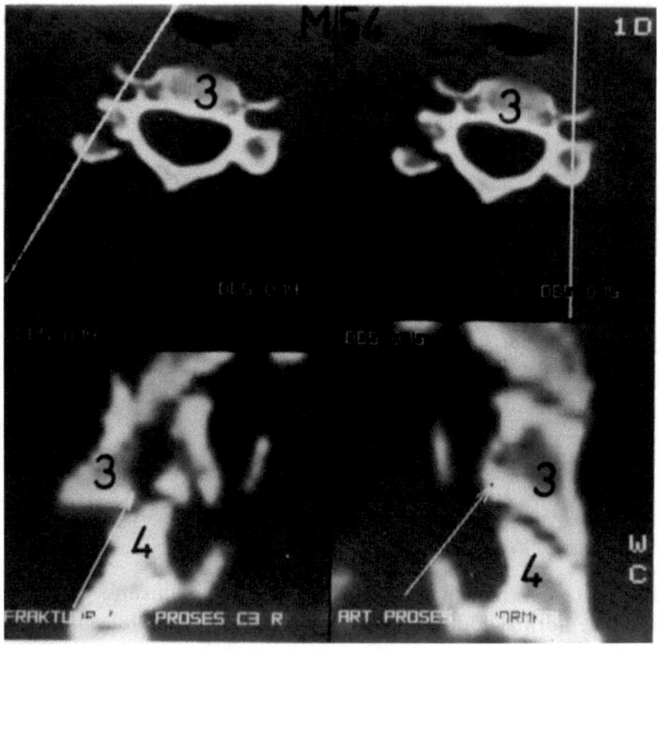

B

trauma, any signs of translation or indication of soft-tissue injury should indicate the need for thorough radiographic evaluation (Figs. 6.10A and 6.10B). This is especially important in high-risk groups, for example, head injuries, alcohol-related conditions, and multiple injuries. Even after no apparent injury is found on clinical grounds, follow-up evaluation 2 to 3 weeks later should include dynamic flexion/extension views to exclude ligamentous rupture that may have been masked by muscle spasm because of soft-tissue injury (Figs. 6.11A and 6.11B). Gaines et al.[24] emphasized that not only should the anatomy of the injury be assessed, but also the patient's functional demands must be taken into consideration in decision making.

Whitesides[25] defined spinal stability as the situation in which the spinal column (bony and ligamentous) can withstand stress without a progressive deformity or further neurological damage, therefore again linking the mechanical and neurological aspects of spinal stability.

It therefore follows that it is important in classifying spinal instability to assess the presence and possible increase in deformity as well as the neurological deficit. We discuss instability further, relative to spinal fractures, using both the mechanical and neurological concepts.

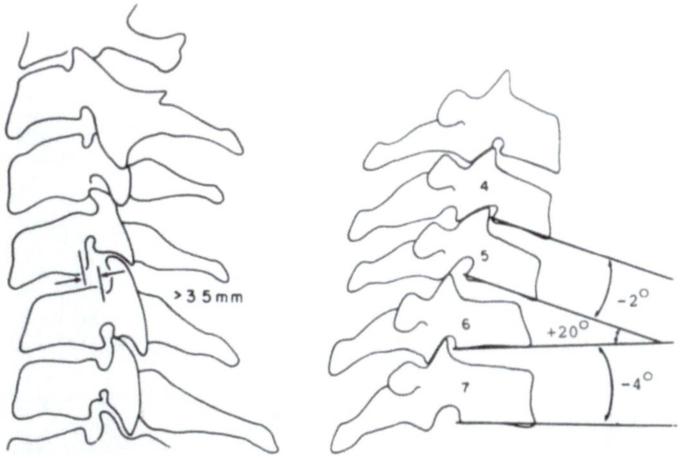

Figure 6.9. Criteria for cervical instability. [Reprinted from White and Panjabi[8] with permission of authors and publisher.]

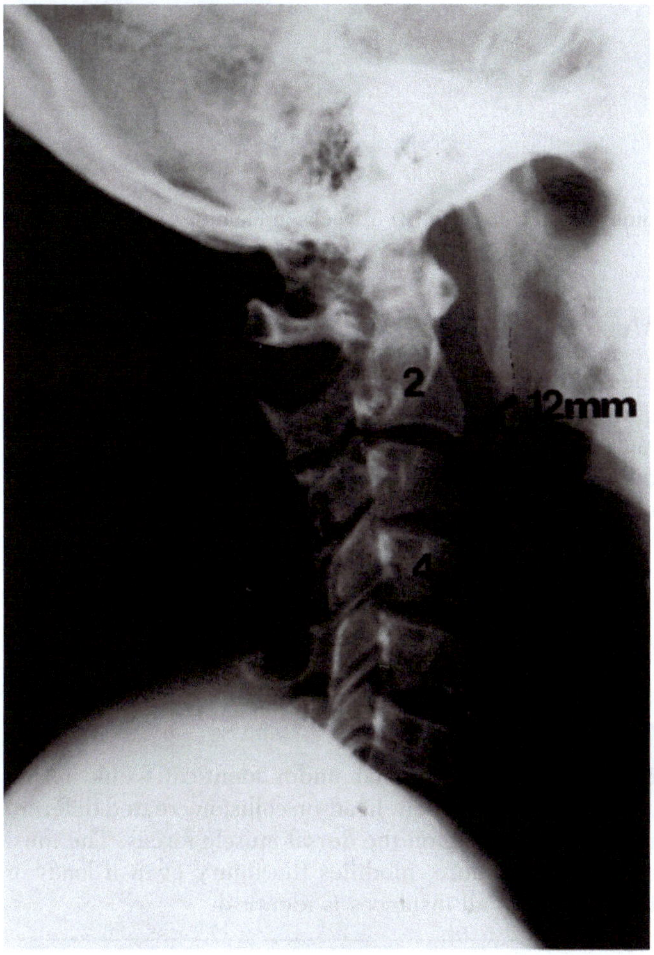

A

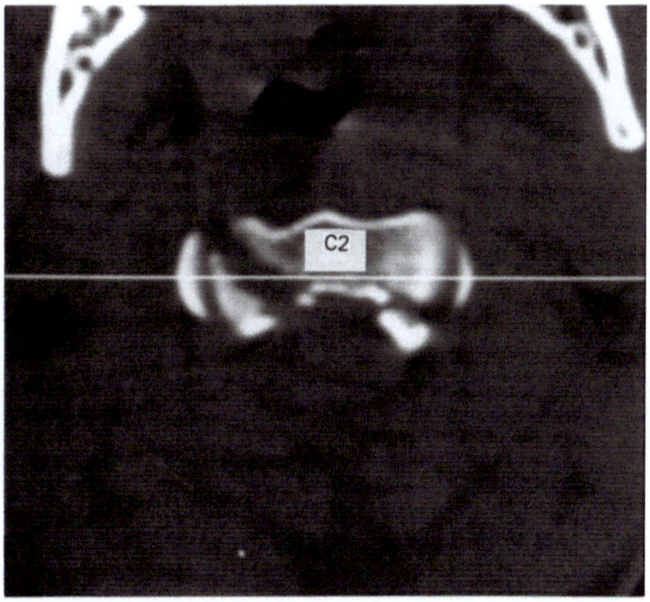

B

Figure 6.10. **A.** Apart from slight anterior displacement of C2, increased prevertebral space raised suspicion of underlying injury. Computed tomography (**B**) confirmed C2 body fracture. (Penning's normal values are C1 level, 10 mm; C2 level, 5 mm; C3 and 4 levels, 7 mm; from C5 downward, 20 mm.)

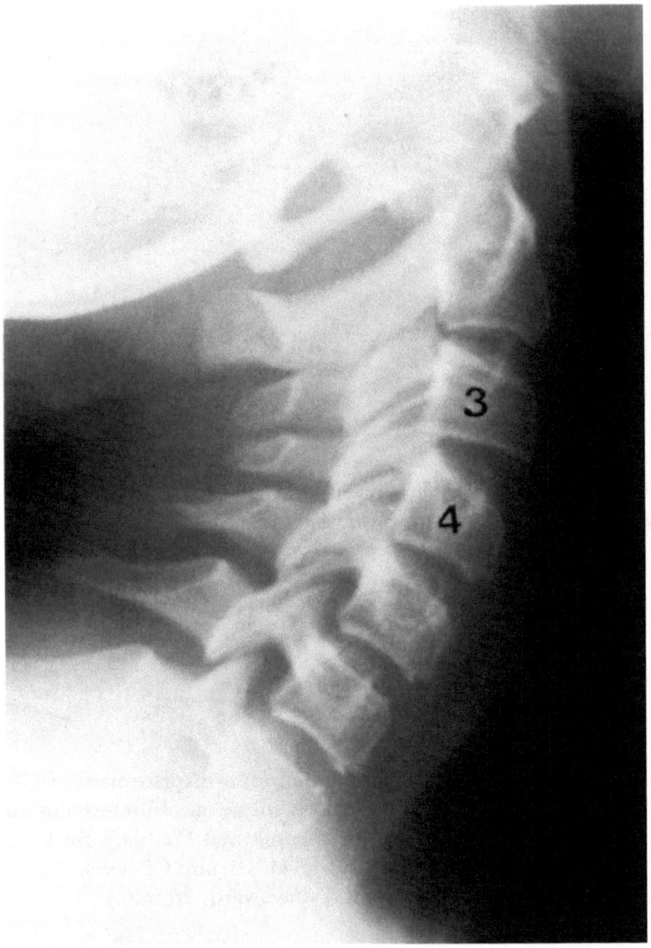

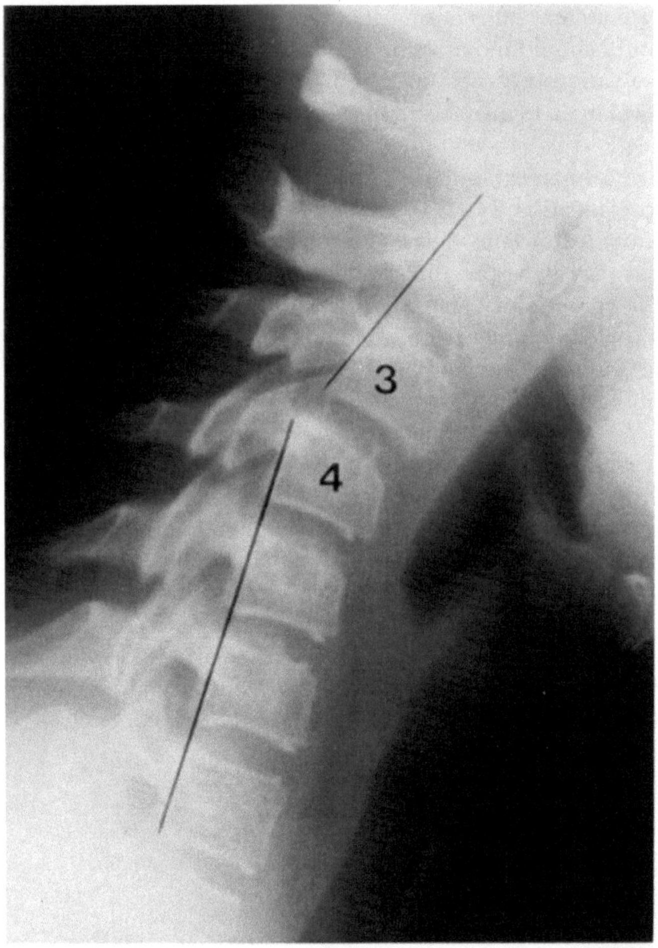

Figure 6.11 **A** and **B.** After initial "soft-tissue injury" of cervical spine (**A**), flexion view (**B**) 3 weeks after injury reveal posterior ligamentous rupture, confirmed at surgery.

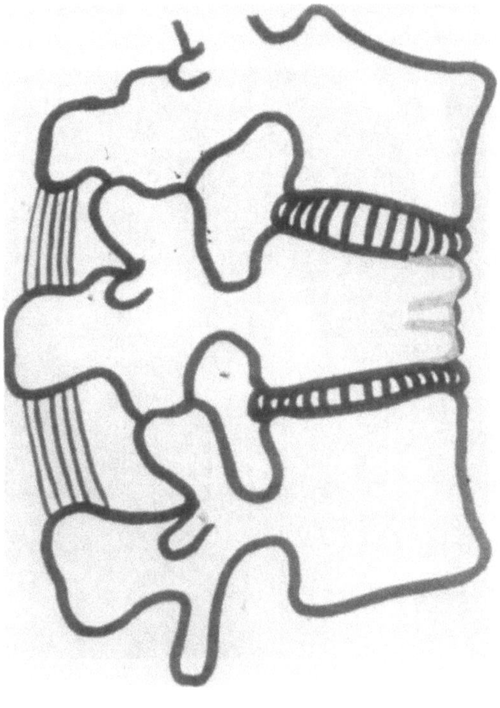

Mechanical Instability

Ideal (bio)mechanical management of spinal injuries requires a precise knowledge of the forces involved in creating the initial deformity and those resulting in the present displacement. Basically, three major deformities are most often encountered clinically:

- Compression loading
  - Flexion compression
  - Pure axial compression
- Flexion distraction
- Translation or shear loading.

Compression Loading

Krag et al.[26] showed that under identical trunk flexion and using a lap seat belt, head-on collision created different injuries depending on the dorsal muscle forces. The muscle force, therefore, modifies the injury even if loads or the loading in all instances is identical.

Figure 6.12. Diagram of typical compression fracture.

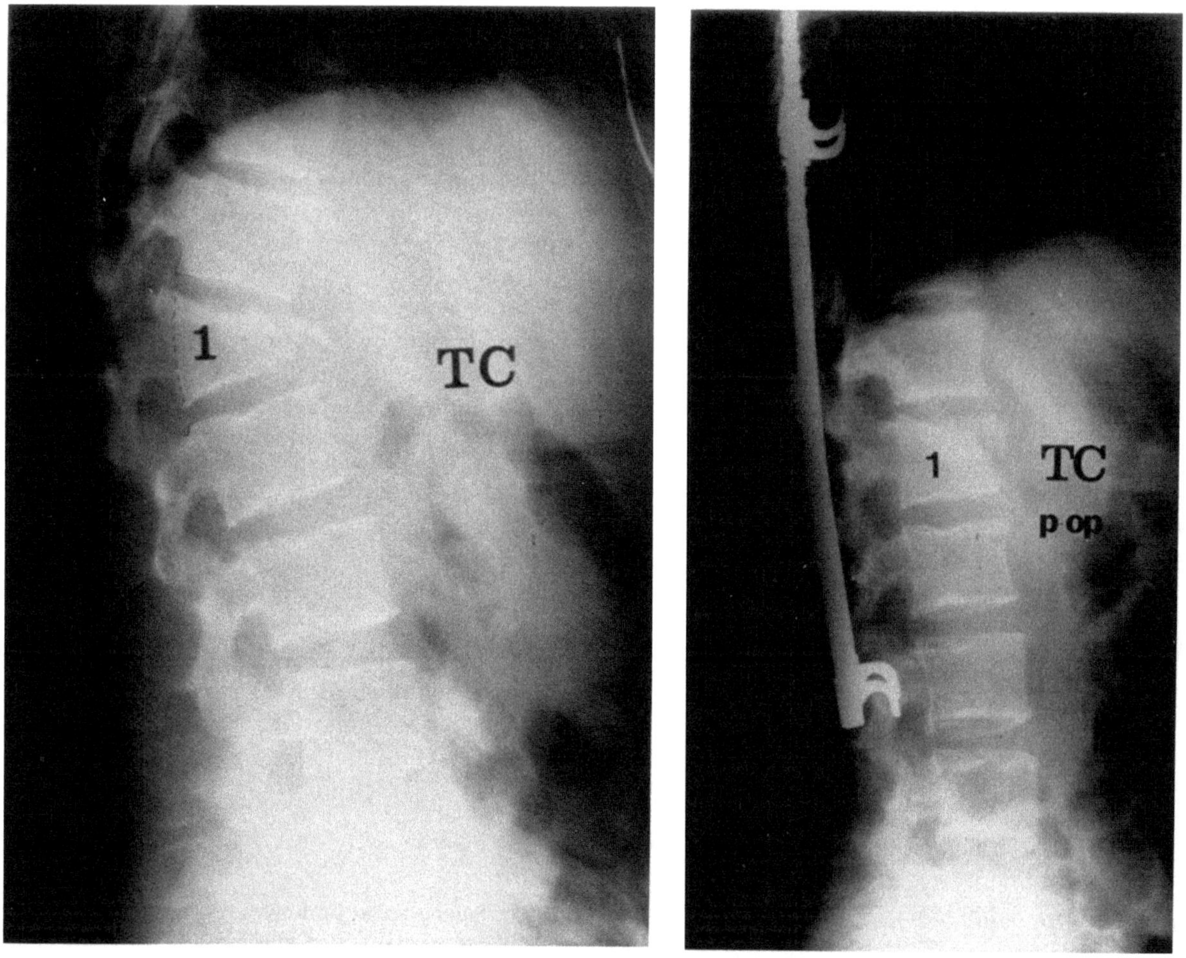

A B

Figure 6.13. **A.** This 30-year-old woman presented with definite local tenderness, palpable gap at T12–L1 junction, and neurological involvement. **B.** Realignment and stability obtained with Harrington rods and "fuse-short, rod-long" approach.

Flexion compression loading in its most simple form involves a flexion moment combined with axial compression, and the degree of deformity depends on the magnitude of the external forces. The mechanism of instability is based on a concept of anterior (compressive) weight-bearing column and a posterior tension-resisting column. One or both of these structures may be involved depending on the magnitude and direction of the force. The injury, on clinical grounds at least, is regarded as stable if: (a) the anterior bony column alone is involved; (b) not more than 50% of its anterior height is lost;[27] and (c) the posterior ligamentous complex remains intact (Fig. 6.12).

If the anterior column reveals loss of more than 50% of its anterior height, or involves, in addition, posterior ligamentous complex disruption, it is regarded as unstable (Figs. 6.13A and 6.13B). The precise evaluation of the posterior ligamentous complex (tension-resisting) is vital and should receive attention in both the clinical and radiological evaluation of these injuries. The diagnosis is obvious when local clinical assessment reveals posterior interspinous tenderness and a distinct palpable gap. Good supine static lateral radiographic evaluation, including tomography, may reveal definitive ligamentous rupture or avulsion fractures of the spinous process. In certain cases, carefully monitored flexion/extension radiographs may be considered, but seem to be less useful than in the cervical spine. Magnetic resonance imaging (MRI) may prove invaluable in the future. In the case of cervical as compared to thoracolumbar injuries, it is essential to realize the inadequacy of the bony components as a stability factor; potential ligamentous injuries should always be evaluated. Chronic instability in the sagittal plane results in progressive kyphotic deformity and may follow initial inadequate plain radiographs or flexion/extension radiographs or failure to perform carefully executed motion studies. However, flexion/extension radiographs should be avoided if a neurological deficit is present.

Pure Axial Compression

Axial compressive loads to failure will usually result in a burst fracture (Fig. 6.14), but what constitutes (in)stability

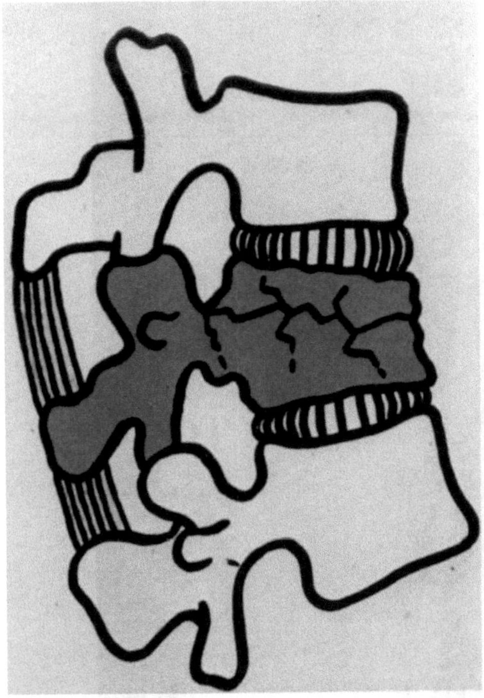

Figure 6.14. Diagram of typical burst fracture.

in this injury has not been totally resolved. McAfee[28] believed that instability in burst fractures resulted from posterior column disruption involving either soft-tissue or bony injury, and this followed an associated translatory, torsional, or lateral flexion movement. As the burst fracture combines both mechanical and neurological components of instability, a thorough assessment of both factors is essential in deciding on the merits for stabilization (Figs. 6.15A and 6.15B).

Therefore, the presence of a burst fracture previously considered stable by Holdsworth[17] could be highly unstable if concomitant posterior ligamentous disruption is present. The ability of the injured bony component (anterior and middle column) to withstand physiological stress must also be evaluated and, if needed, protected from load by appropriate surgical implant or eliminating the axial compressive loading if it is elected to treat the patient nonsurgically.

Axial compression in the cervical spine usually leads to a burst-type fracture in its most severe form, resulting in anterior compression of the spinal cord, and different degrees of neurological involvement follow. These cases frequently require anterior decompression and anterior interbody stabilization.

Figure 6.15. **A.** Radiographic findings in sagittal planes after motor vehicle accident and partial neurological deficit. **B.** Axial tomography shows involvement of middle column and posterior displacement of fragment. Decompression and stabilization procedure was performed.

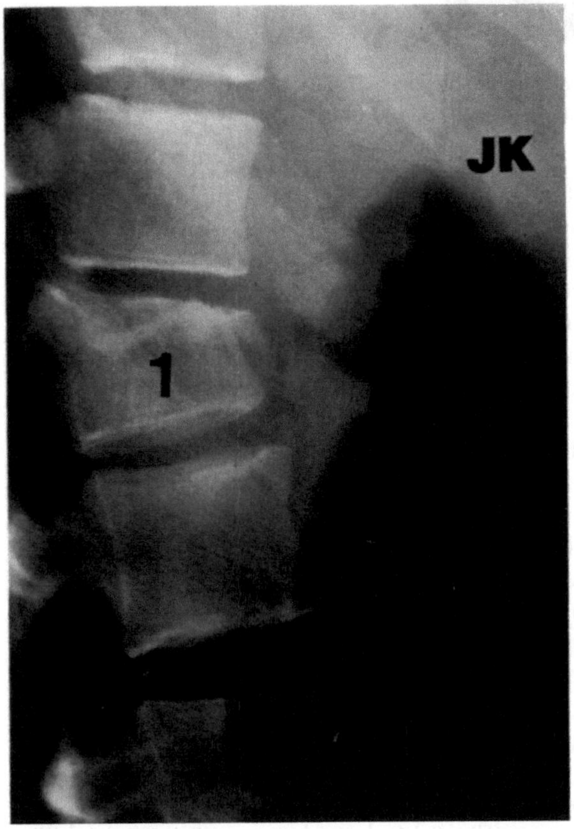

A

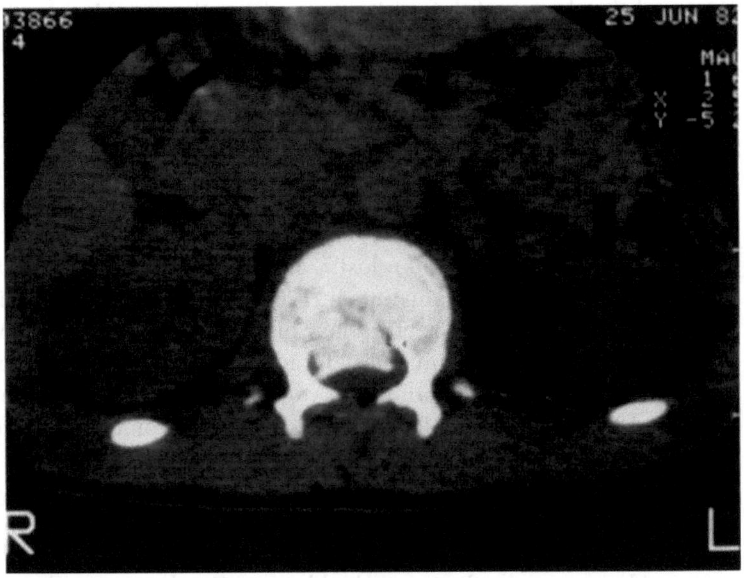

B

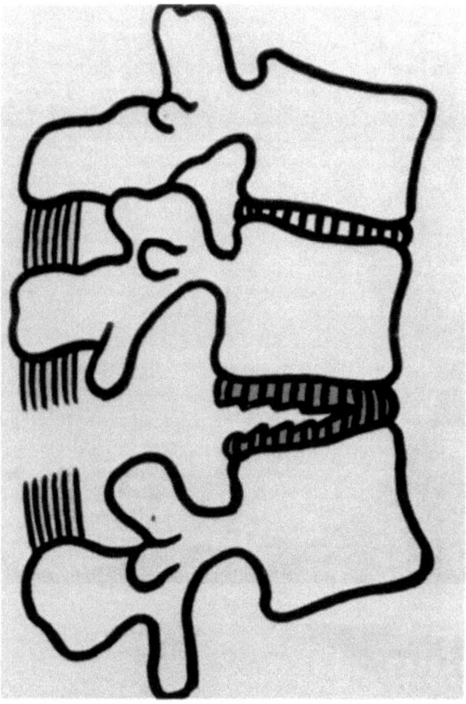

Figure 6.16. Diagram of typical flexion-distraction injury.

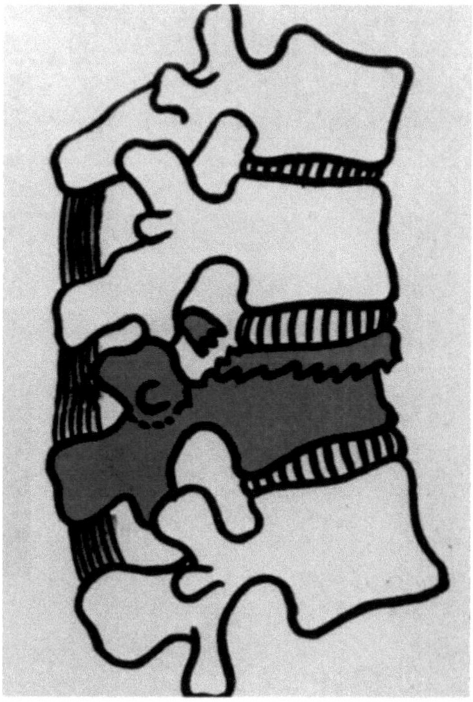

Figure 6.17. Diagram of fracture dislocation.

Flexion Distraction

This injury is only classified as being unstable if it also involves the middle column (Fig. 6.16). The relationship between the injury site loads and structural damage has been outlined by Pope et al.,[29] who emphasized that identical flexion producing moments at the thoracolumbar junction will result in various structural disruptions, determined by the weakest link in the chain. The central role played by the posterior ligamentous complex should be evaluated by thorough clinical and radiological evaluation. In view of the potential dangers of tension views in forward flexion, MRI may again be a diagnostic tool of future value in assessing stability.

Shear Translation or Shear Loading

Translatory displacement of more than 20% of the vertebrae indicates disruption of all three columns with resultant instability (Fig. 6.17). Reduction of a totally unstable injury may occur spontaneously, a point emphasized by McGuire[30] in his comparison of different methods in transferring patients. If a stabilization procedure is not done in these cases, the risk for further neurological compromise is obviously high.

More difficult than defining spinal instability with these injuries is determining its presence in a clinical situation. A clinical assessment, including a detailed history and a thorough physical examination, should be performed. Such analysis should include the history of load application and the presence or absence of neurological involvement, because these are the best predictors of instability. Potential unstable injuries are those in which the injuring forces are less severe (or less well understood), in which there is no neurological involvement, or in which stability is questionable. Detection of any neurological deficit, including a cystometrogram, is crucial in final decision making for correct management. In the presence of a partial or progressive neurological lesion, most surgeons seem to agree that surgery is indicated and final information regarding stability and methods to obtain it are decided at surgery.

Radiological assessment presents two major difficulties: the radiographs (1) available may reveal only the residual displacement, which could be the result of spontaneous reduction of a grossly displaced injury, and (2) ligamentous and other soft-tissue injuries cannot be detected on plain radiographs unless an avulsion injury of the spinous process is identified. An unstable complete posterior ligamentous complex disruption may, therefore, be indistinguishable from an apparently stable lesion.

Controlled tests by application of physiological stress may well aid in defining abnormal motion. Dynamic controlled radiography, that is, flexion/extension roentgenograms or stress testing, may be extremely useful in diagnosing and quantifying abnormal motion, especially in the cervical spine. White's stretch test[8] is another means of assessing instability, further adding to the database in deciding on the preferred treatment.

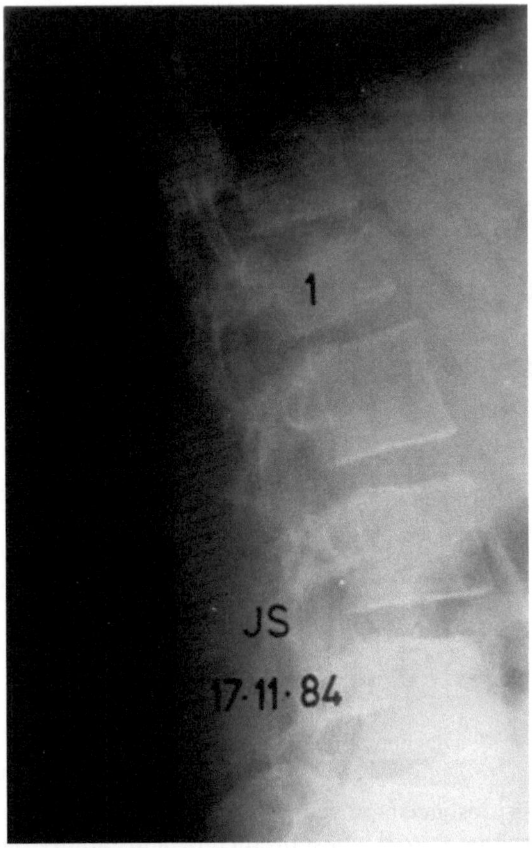

A

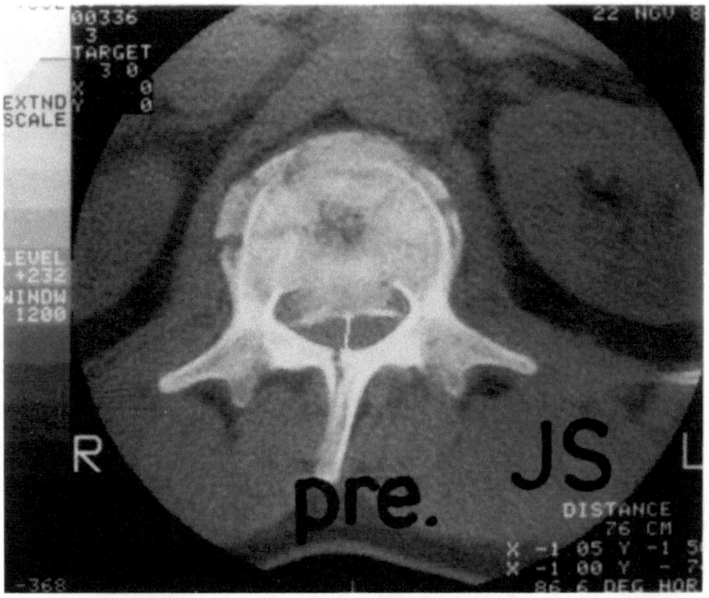

B

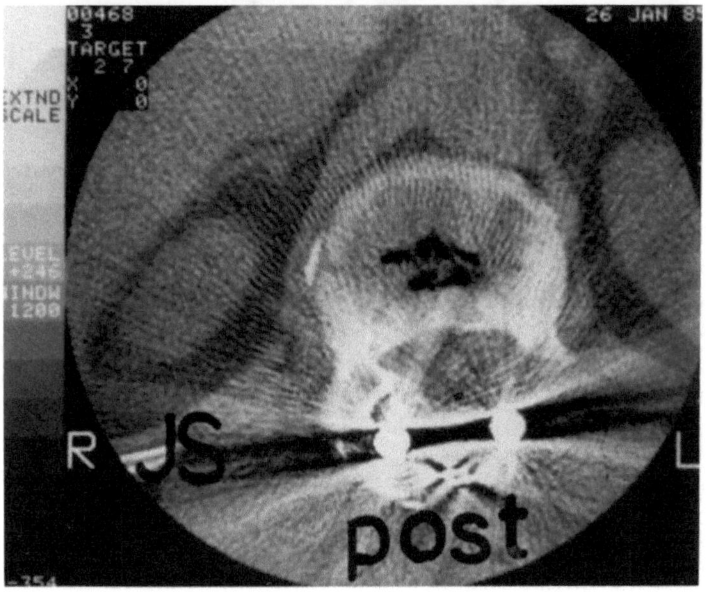

D

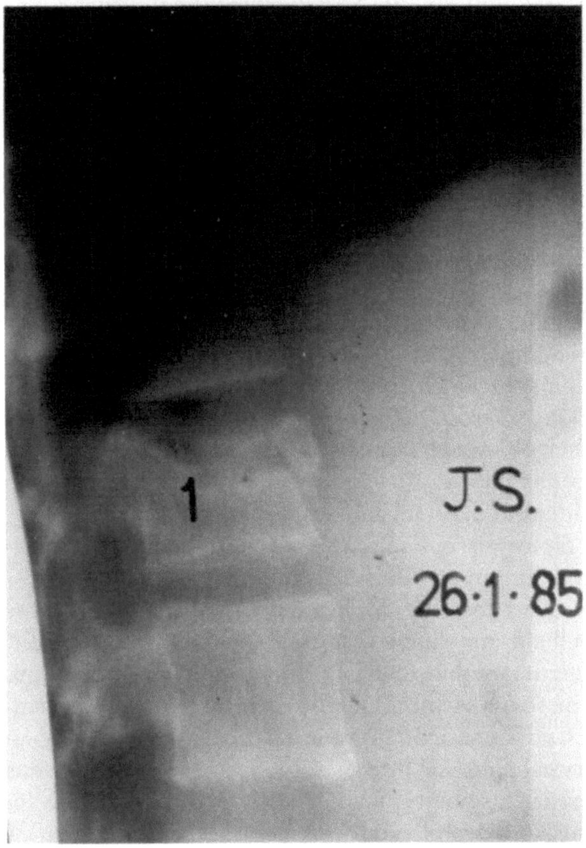

C

Figure 6.18. **A** and **B** 28-year-old engineer sustained L1 burst fracture with cord compression and partial neurological deficit. Posterolateral decompression via pediculectomy was followed by Harrington rod stabilization. **C** and **D.** Postoperative views show reduction and decompression.

Neurological Instability

Most investigators think that the mere presence of a partial or progressive neurological lesion signifies an unstable condition and treat the lesion by spinal stabilization after careful decompression of the neurological elements. The major decision in these cases is the method of fixation to be used rather than determining the need for stabilization. These injuries can be stabilized by an anterior, posterior, or combined anterior/posterior approach (Figs. 6.18A through 6.18D).

In patients with neurological deficit, stabilization following decompression of the neurological elements is essential after progressive kyphosis to prevent further deterioration.

If disruption of the posterior ligamentous structures is present, great care should be taken if an anterior interbody fusion is selected as it results in a high percentage of cases in further instability.[31] Posterior interspinous fusion is the surgical procedure most often employed but, following rotational instability as in unilateral facet dislocation, it may be essential to do facet fixation by wiring, therefore eliminating rotational instability. This may also apply to the C1–C2 level when using two lateral wires instead of a central wiring procedure, therefore preventing rotational displacement.

Spinal Infections

Inflammatory Lesions

Osteomyelitis and disc space infections primarily involve the anterior and middle columns of the spine and loss of bony support may result in both mechanical and neurological compromise (Fig. 6.19). Posterior involvement from hematogenous spread is uncommon, although it may be observed in patients with penetrating injuries and as a postoperative complication. Patients at particular risk for hematogenous infection are drug addicts, diabetics, those who are immunosuppressed, and those who have had recent genitourinary surgery. Although acute infection may be acompanied by the classic signs of fever, 40% have a more indolent course, and delays in diagnosis are common. This indolent course is even more likely if the offending organism is *Myobacteria*. The most reliable clinical signs are unrelenting spinal pain, unrelieved or even accentuated by rest, and elevations of the sedimentation rate. Early in the course of illness, plain radiography and even radionucleotide imaging may be negative and therefore are not reliable signs. The earliest confirmatory sign other than a positive culture from the disc or bone is the gallium scan, which converts to a positive image in 7 to 10 days. The technetium bone scan takes longer to convert and may be normal up to 21 days. If a specific bacteriological diagnosis is made early in the course of the illness, antibiotic therapy is effective in at least 60% of patients and instability is not a problem. However, delays in diagnosis or inability to eradicate infection with antibiotics are common and instability may result.

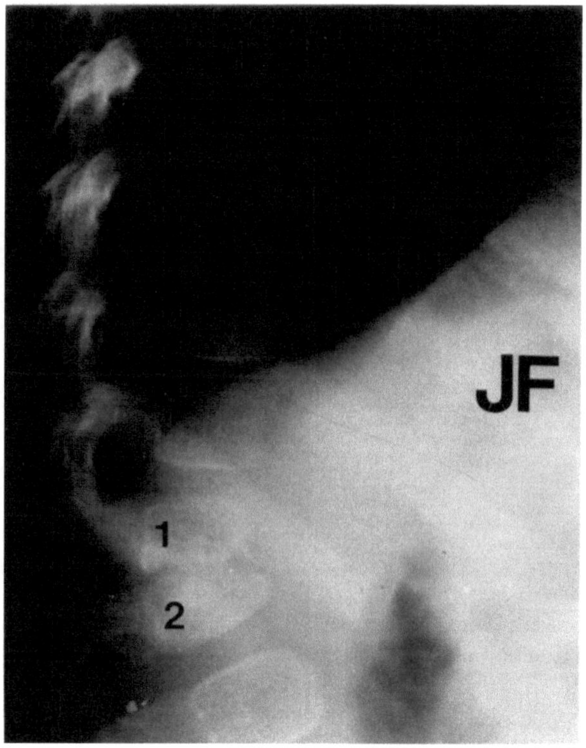

Figure 6.19. Typical radiographic appearance of tuberculous vertebral infection in young child with progressive kyphosis.

Three general reasons provide indications for surgical stabilization: (1) continuing evidence of infection manifested in systemic signs and elevated sedimentation rate when the patient is receiving adequate bactericidal antibiotic treatment specific to the organism; (2) progressive loss of anterior and middle columns, which commonly occurs when antibiotic treatment is providing ineffective control or there has been long delay in diagnosis; and (3) when infection is accompanied by increasing or new neurological signs or symptoms. Typically, postoperative infections, particularly after disc surgery, tend not to produce instability and usually result in spontaneous fusion.

Rheumatoid Arthritis

Rheumatoid arthritis is frequently associated with instability in the cervical spine, particularly at the occipital and C1–C2 level, but rarely affects the thoracic and lumbar spine. The mechanism is erosion of the supporting ligaments, and even adjacent odontoid in the case of C1–C2 (Fig. 6.20), and destabilization by involvement of the diarthrodial facet joints in the C2 through C7 levels. Patients with multiarticular, seropositive, nodular occurrence of cervical instability should be carefully evaluated,

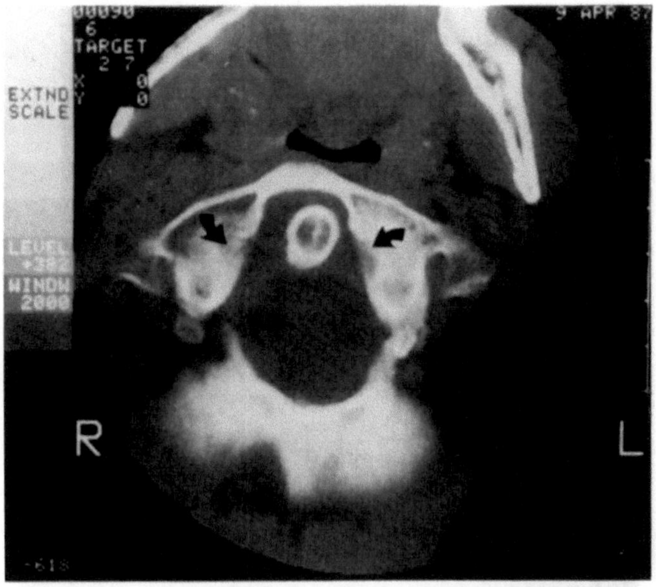

Figure 6.20. Localized erosion at sites of attachments of transverse ligament of C1–C2 articulation.

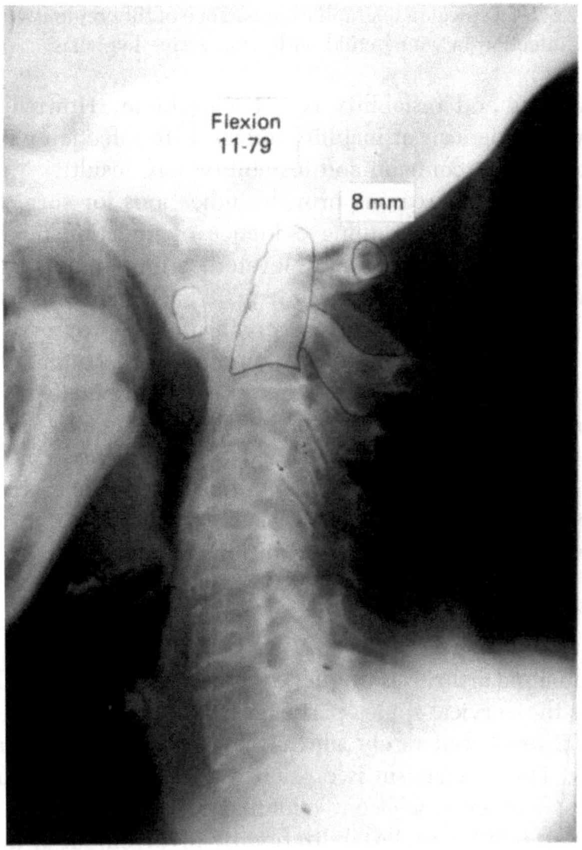

Figure 6.21. Patient suffering from long-standing rheumatoid arthritis and increased A.D.I. in absence of neurological findings.

particularly those who are undergoing surgical procedures that will require intubation. Radiographic indicators of instability are somewhat more controversial in rheumatoid disease than in trauma, as is the preferred management (Fig. 6.21). The mortality reported for surgical stabilization has been reported to be as high as 15%, and adequate stabilization may be difficult to achieve because of the associated osteoporosis. Thus, individual decisions are based on the overall health of the patient, the magnitude and progression of neurological involvement, and the patient's activity level. Prophylactic bracing is recommended in those patients who are not treated surgically.

Ankylosing Spondylitis

Patients with spinal ankylosis are at particular risk for unstable lesions, which may involve any level of the spinal column. These lesions may occur as the result of overt trauma or poorly advised spinal manipulation, or may be unrecognized by the patient presenting as a progressing kyphotic deformity. Historically, this last group of patients were presumed to have an inflammatory lesion, but Simmons[32] has provided convincing histological evidence for a traumatic basis. Unique to these patients is the complete involvement of all three columns and the difficulties in achieving adequate stabilization by conventional means (Figs. 6.22A and 6.22B).

Neoplasms

Most tumors involve the anterior elements, and the indications for surgical treatment are principally eradication of disease (Fig. 6.23). Primary mechanical instability is less commonly the problem, although surgical treatment may produce instability because of resection of the entire anterior and middle columns.

The corollary of the involvement in the anterior and middle columns is that posterior decompression, via a laminectomy, seldom results in adequate decompression. Furthermore, an unstable situation is furthered by removing remaining posterior structures leading to progressive anterior collapse and the potential increase of neurological deficit.

Metastatic tumors are quite common, with pathological evidence of vertebral spread identified in as many as 40% of patients with malignancies who have an autopsy, and usually involve the anterior and middle columns. The most common tumors with potential for vertebral metastatic spread are those of lung, breast, thyroid, and kidney. Pelvic neoplasms such as bowel, uterus, and bladder are less apt to metastasize to the vertebrae, but may directly extend into the lumbosacral spine. The indications for operation in both types of patients with metastatic and direct spread are a function of the tumor type and its

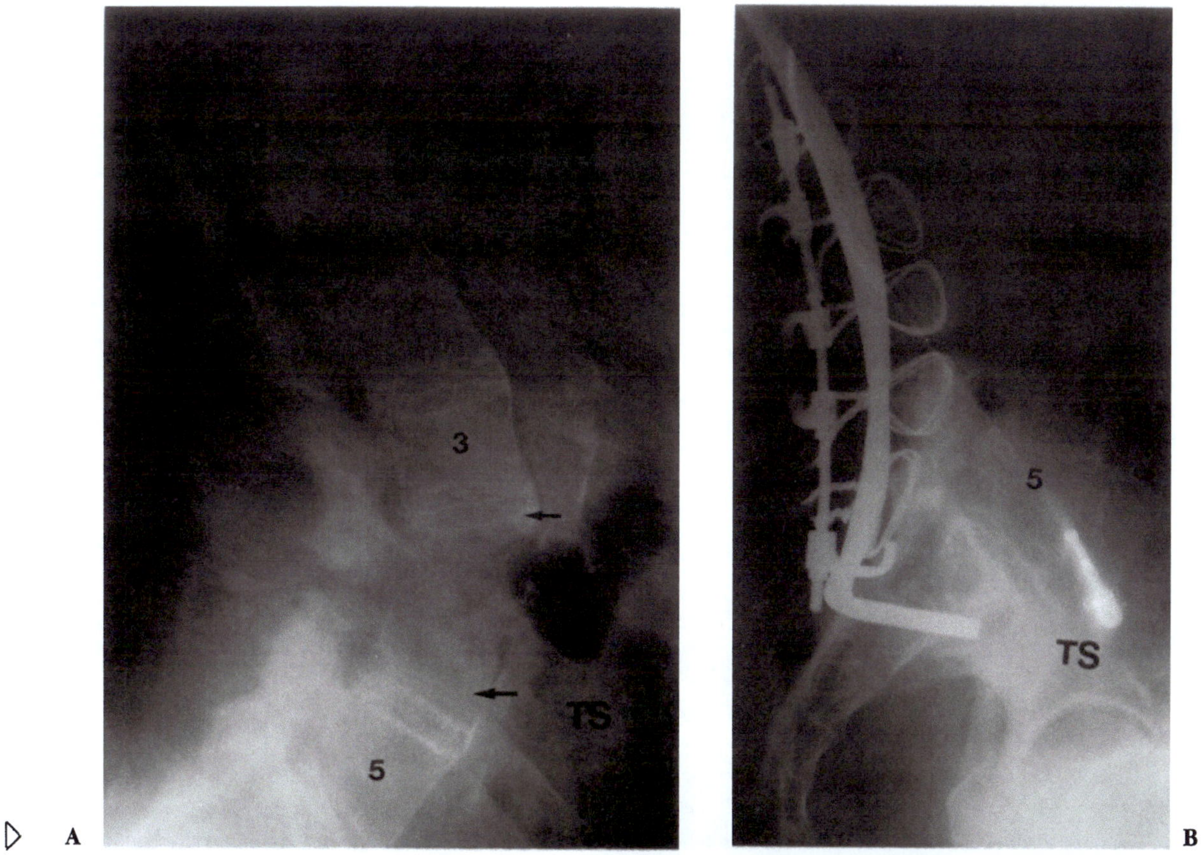

Figure 6.22. **A** and **B.** Because of spinal column rigidity, trauma often leads (**A**) to severe displacement (*arrow*) and necessitates unconventional fixation methods (**B**).

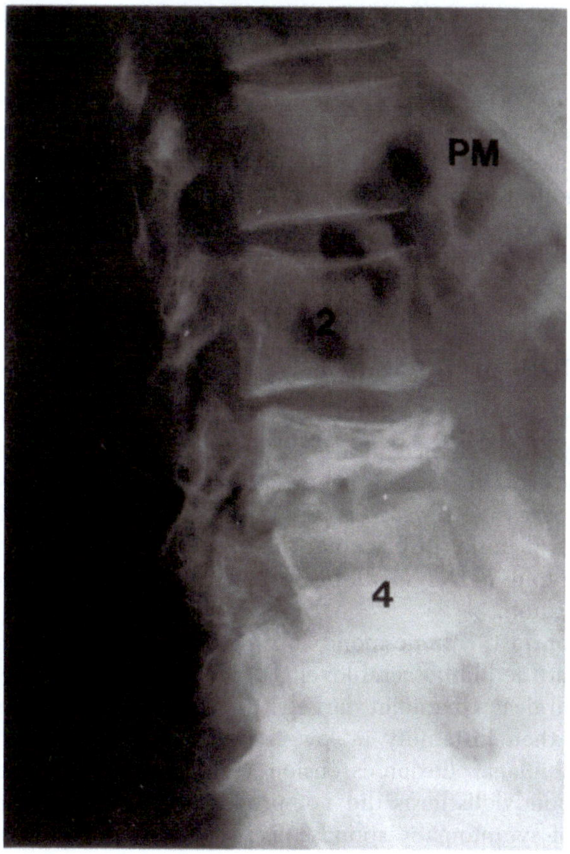

Figure 6.23. Complete loss of middle and anterior column stability from plasmacytoma in 52-year-old man.

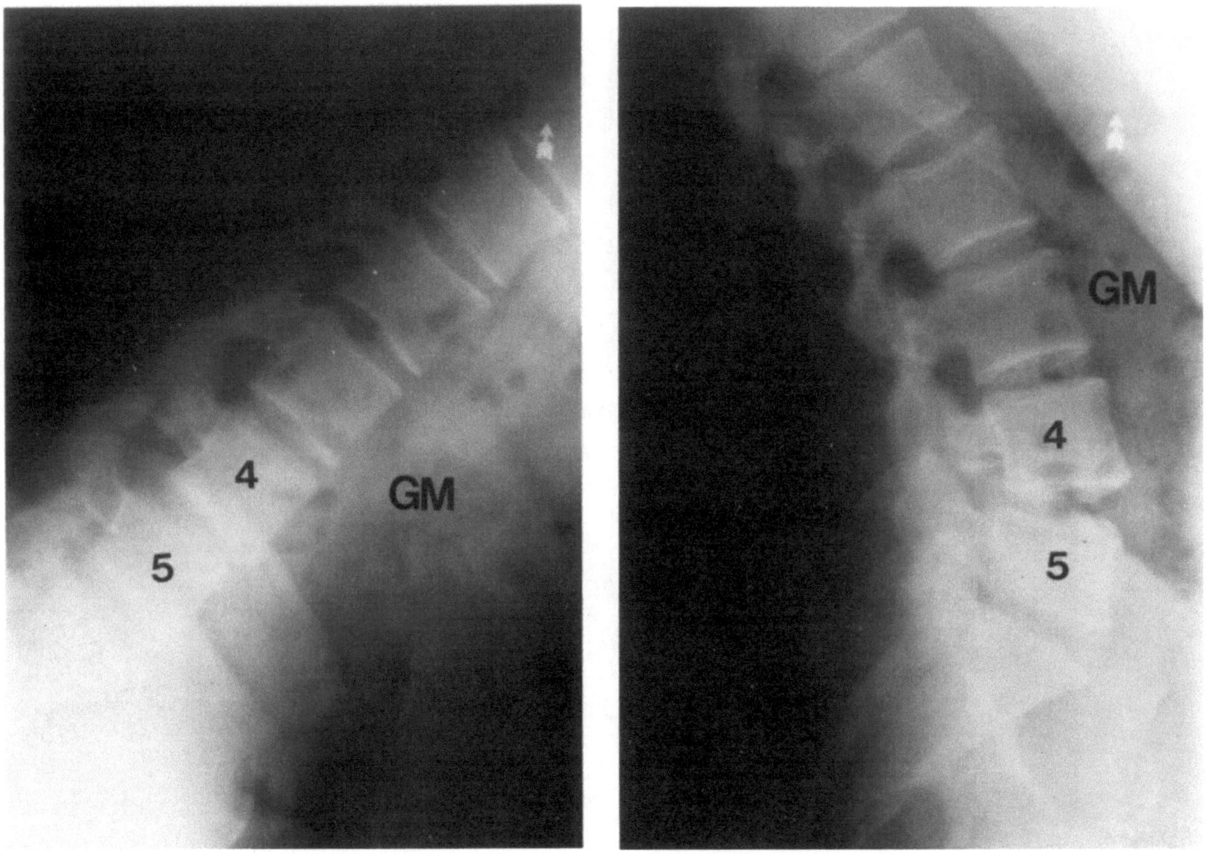

Figure 6.24. **A** and **B**. Flexion (**A**) extension (**B**) views in L4 isthmic lesion reveal increased translational and sagittal motion.

resistance or sensitivity to radiotherapy and chemotherapy, the expected life span of the patient, and the presence of mechanical instability or neurological involvement. The best indication is a patient with progressive deformity from anterior bone loss, pain, and impending neurological involvement, with a life expectancy of at least 3 to 6 months.

Spondylolisthesis

Most clinicians are well aware of the potential of dysplastic spondylolisthesis in children to progress, and no radiographic signs are known that predict a high risk of instability. Progressive slippage is reported to be as high as 50% of cases if initial displacement is more than 25%. Serial radiographs detect further slip and provide a basis for stabilization.

In contrast, isthmic spondylolisthesis in the adult population at the lumbosacral level is not a progressive lesion, and surgical treatment largely depends on symptoms rather than instability in low-grade lesions.[33] Pearcy,[34] using biplanar flexion/extension techniques, concluded that spondylolisthesis did not produce instability at the level of symptomatic spondylolisthesis. However, Lowe et al.[35] did find increased instability in the flexion/extension plane in grade III and IV slips, which they proposed may result from long-standing elongation of the ligaments and disc. Instability with increased slip angle may also occur after the Gill procedure.

In contrast to the L5–S1 isthmic lesion, there are indications that an isthmic lesion at the L4–L5 level may progress to a stage of instability in the third and fourth decades, manifested by progressive slip and increasing symptoms.[36] Thus, fusion is more likely to be indicated for instability (Fig. 6.24A and 6.24B).

Degenerative Disease

Instabilities Associated with the Degenerative Process

The classification and treatment of instabilities produced by spinal degeneration remain controversial. In this discussion, we focus primarily on the lumbar spine, although the general issues are applicable to the cervical spine. Although the definition previously given for instability is applicable to spinal degeneration, the clinical symptoms and signs and the objective radiographic correlates remain

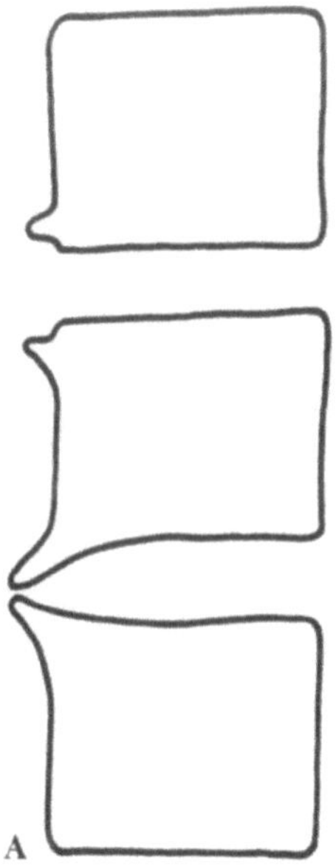

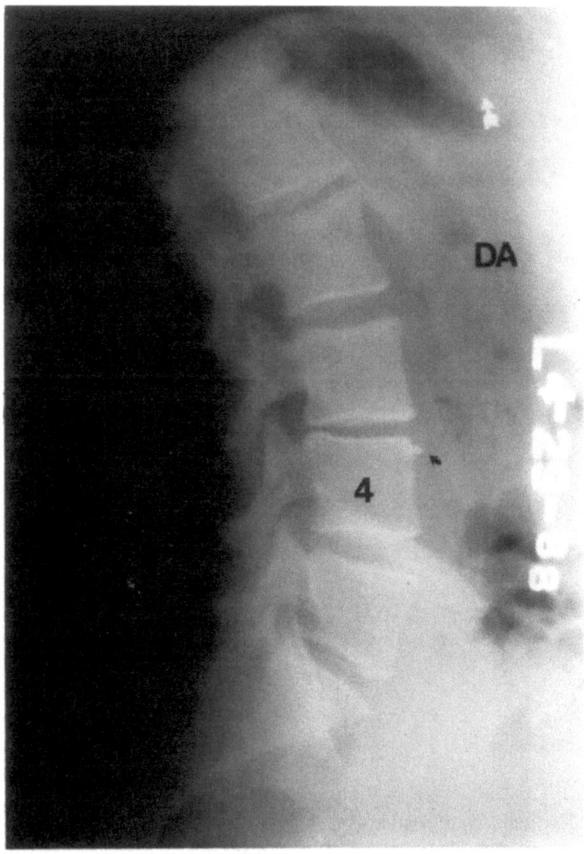

Figure 6.25. **A** and **B.** So-called traction spur, presumably caused by abnormal tension after transitional instability. This appearance is in contrast to more often encountered claw spurs.[68]

uncertain, yet "segmental instability" is the most common indication for lumbar spinal fusion.

In their original description of disc herniation, Mixter and Barr[37] proposed that the condition represents an unstable lesion of the lumbar spine and is best treated by decompression of the nerve root, accompanied by spinal fusion. This opinion dominated through much of the three decades since the 1930s.

Knutsson[38] in 1947 first identified "instability" in flexion/extension radiographs of patients with symptoms and signs suggestive of lumbar disc disease. He concluded that forward displacements of greater than 3 mm represent the earliest objective evidence of disc degeneration. Although Junghanns[39] had recognized forward slippage of the lumbar vertebra without defects in the pars interarticularis, Macnab's report of the clinical signs and symptoms that accompany these forward displacements focused greater attention on degenerative instability.[40] Macnab identified the condition to be most prevalent at the L4–L5 level and more common in females than males. Coincidentally, clinical and radiographic investigations furthered the broad concept of instability as a condition characterized by hypermobile lumbar motion segments, and abnormal translations during spinal flexion/extension, often accompanied by asymmetric disc space collapse. By 1957, Moran and King[41] had concluded instability accounted for at least one-quarter of the overall causation of low back pain. Macnab furthered the radiographic criteria to include traction spurs[42] (Figs. 6.25A and 6.25B), and proposed the biomechanical cause was abnormal tensions in the outer annular fibers produced by translational motions. In contrast, claw spurs resulted from physiological bulging of the disc under compressive loads. By 1970, degenerative spondylolisthesis and retrolisthesis were presumed to be identifiable by motion radiography and traction spurs before an actual deformity was obvious. At the same time, evidence had accumulated that disc herniation was not necessarily an unstable lesion, and fusion did not improve long-term results.[43]

In the past 15 years, biomechanical analysis has better defined lumbar spinal stability and instability. White and Panjabi in vitro[8] and others in vivo[11] have demonstrated coupled spinal motions, thus defining more completely the mechanical response of FSUs to externally applied loads. Farfan's studies directed attention to the important role of torsion as a major determinant of spinal degeneration.[10] His analysis of anatomical specimens provided compelling evidence that degenerative spondylo-

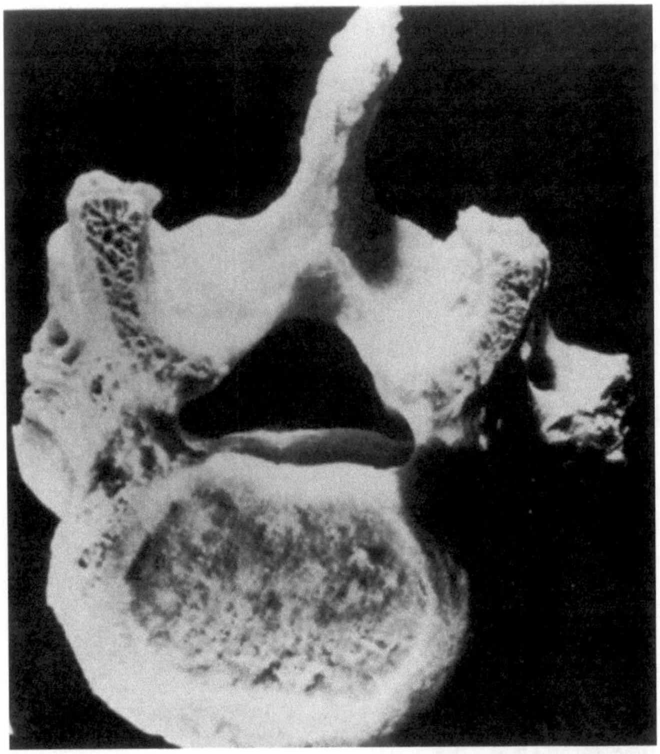

A

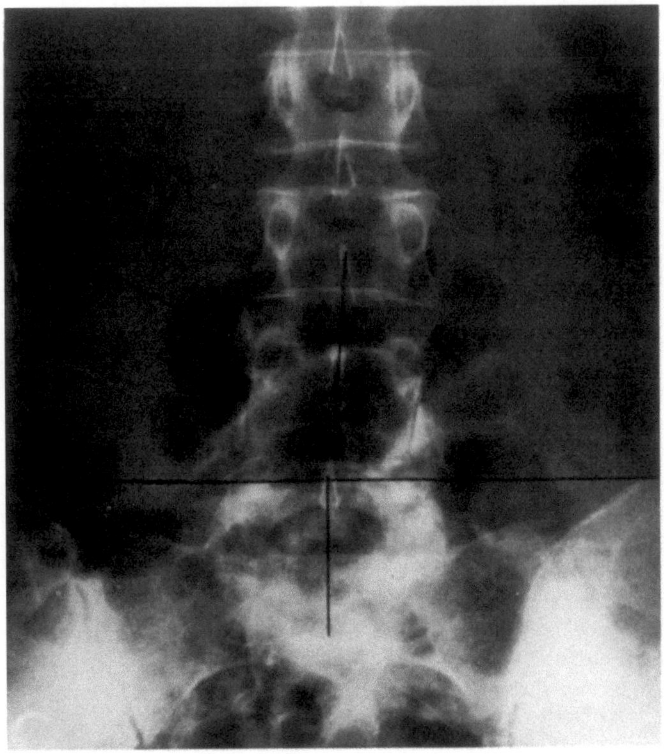

B

Figure 6.26. **A.** Axial view of anatomical specimen of degenerative spondylolisthesis demonstrates rotatory deformity to right encroaching on nerve root canal. (Reprinted from Farfan[10] with permission of author and publisher.) **B.** Disruption of spinous process line, which Farfan has proposed is yet another sign of axial rotational instability. (Reprinted from Farfan[10] with permission of author and publisher.)

listhesis is often accompanied by a torsional deformity (Figs. 6.26A and 6.26B).

Kirkaldy–Willis further conceptualized spinal degeneration as progressing in three sequential phases: dysfunction, instability, and stabilization.[44] In this pathological sequence, degeneration was more clearly delineated as involving both the disc and the two facets, that is, the "three-joint complex."

The dysfunctional phase is heralded by early acute episodes of low back pain, speculated to be produced by annular disruptions or early facet degeneration. In the unstable phase, the mechanical characteristics of the FSU are sufficiently disrupted that normally tolerated mechanical loads cause abnormal strains and result in symptoms. Kirkaldy-Willis and Farfan[45] defined instability as "the clinical status of the patients with back problems who, with the least provocation, step from the mildly symptomatic to the severe episode." They likened spinal instability to a "catastrophy fold" (Fig. 6.27A). This concept of spinal instability also seems implicit in Panjabi and Pope's illustration of stability and instability[46] (Fig. 6.27B).

In the final stabilization phase, healing is proposed to occur through biochemical changes in the disc, such as decreased water content, decreased proteoglycans, and increase in both the type and amount of collagen. The formation of spinal osteophytes produces a stiffer spinal motion segment. Symptoms at this stage may be minimal, or may be those of continuing low back pain, usually accompanied by neurological claudication. Deformities that are well recognized are degenerative spondylolisthesis and retrospondylolisthesis. In addition, it can be postulated "isolated disc resorption"[47] represents one possible endpoint of internal disc disruption. Crock[48] described isolated disc resorption as manifested by profound narrowing of the lumbar disc (usually less than 3 mm), accompanied by low back pain and, commonly, symptoms of lateral recess syndrome. In Crock's reported cases, isolated disc resorption most commonly was identified at the L5–S1 level.

As this concept of the three phases of degeneration has evolved, other load applications such as compression have been reevaluated in both laboratory and clinical settings. Hanson et al.[49] have shown that compressive overloads may produce endplate disruptions. Disruption of endplates may decrease the capacity of vertebral endplates to withstand further compressive loads, as well as permitting vascular ingrowth into the intervertebral disc, thus altering both its biological and mechanical behavior.

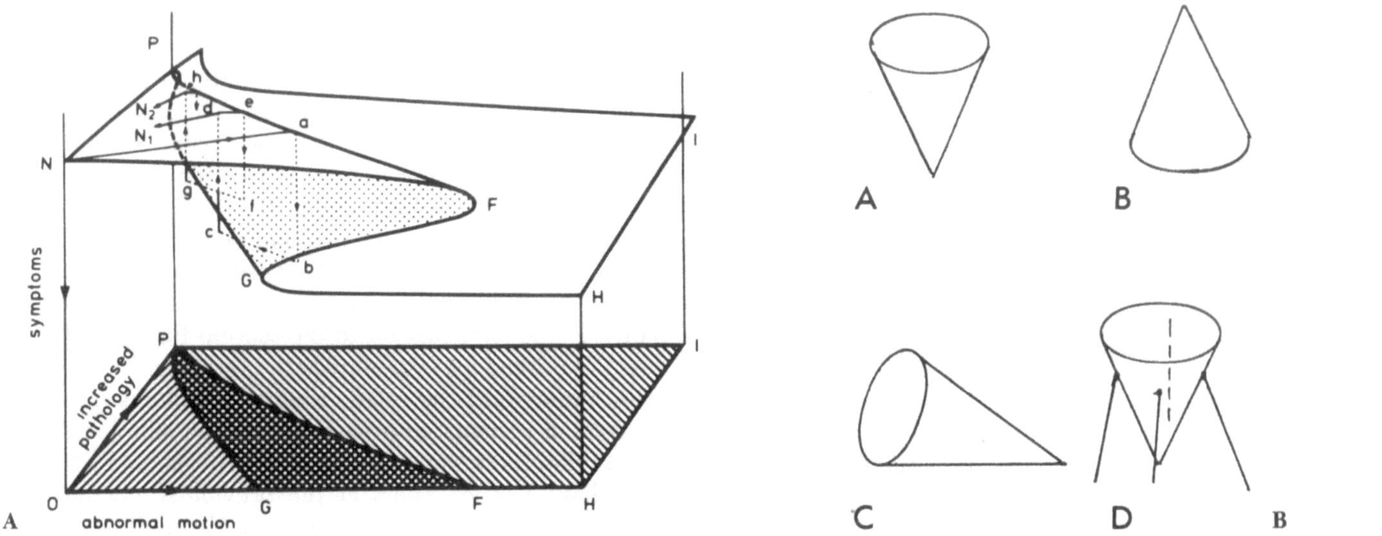

Figure 6.27. **A.** The catastrophy fold theory of segmental instability proposed by Kirkaldy-Willis and Farfan, graphically demonstrating that minimal changes in movement can be accompanied by catastrophic increase in symptoms. (Reprinted from Kirkaldy-Willis and Farfan[45] with permission of authors and publisher.) **B.** Mechanical conceptualization of instability proposed by Pope and Panjabi.[46] In Fig. 6.27A, cone is in unstable equilibrium; in Fig. 6.27B, it is in stable equilibrium. Condition of unstable equilibrium occurring in Fig. 6.27A can be converted to stabilized condition by addition of guide wires. This conceptualization emphasizes importance of muscles and ligaments to spinal stability.

The clinical syndrome that follows repetitive or acute compressive loads has been characterized by Crock as "internal disc disruption"[48] and is manifested by unrelenting back pain, systemic signs such as weight loss, normal spinal radiographs, and the reproduction of symptoms by discography.

Since about 1983, there have been further attempts to refine the definition of degenerative segmental instability in clinical radiographic and biomechanical terms. Abnormal motions have been reported to be palpable in unstable spinal segments, but convincing data are not yet available.[50] Attempts to measure spinal motion in vivo by three-dimensional techniques such as biplanar and stereometric radiographic techniques have not identified predictable patterns of instability.[51]

Sequential CT scans in different rotational positions, as well as application of spinal traction,[52] are newer methods reported to measure instability but have not yet been subjected to rigorous analysis. Historically, the relief of symptoms by spinal immobilization has been used to identify those patients who would respond to surgical stabilization. It is now evident that spinal braces do not predictably immobilize the lower lumbar spine, and in fact may increase spinal motions and stresses.[53] Immobilization is possible through cast application which includes one thigh. As an extreme, Olerud[54] has analyzed pain responses after the temporary placement of spinal fixators. Although the number of subjects was small, his studies suggest a positive response to rigid immobilization and predict a subsequent favorable outcome from spinal fusion. Obviously such an invasive procedure would require much greater analysis to be used as a diagnostic test.

Newer biomechanical studies have offered some potentially new insights. It has been postulated that "unstable" motions occur within the midrange of flexion/extension, or movements might be so subtle as to be unmeasurable by standard radiographic techniques. Gertzbein and colleagues[9] have carefully analyzed flexion/extension radiographs made at 10° increments in cadaveric specimens. They have shown the instant center of rotation in nondegenerative discs follows a fairly predictable pathway. In contrast, degenerative segments follow an erratic course (Fig. 6.28). However, they have not yet convincingly demonstrated that this radiographic method is applicable in the clinical setting.

Wilder[55] and others have also evaluated the behavior of spinal segments under physiological compressive loads, applied over multiple discrete areas. In nondegenerative discs, load displacement curves are quite predictable over a wide area of the disc as the load is shifted from the balance point toward the periphery. In some degenerative segments, a different mechanical behavior is observed. As the load application shifts from the balance point, small increments of changes are followed by sudden displacements of large magnitude. It is proposed that this mechanical behavior might represent an unstable motion segment. In the clinical setting, it could be postulated that similar displacements might occur, where small shifts in load lead to abnormal, and theoretically painful, alterations of stresses within the annulus.

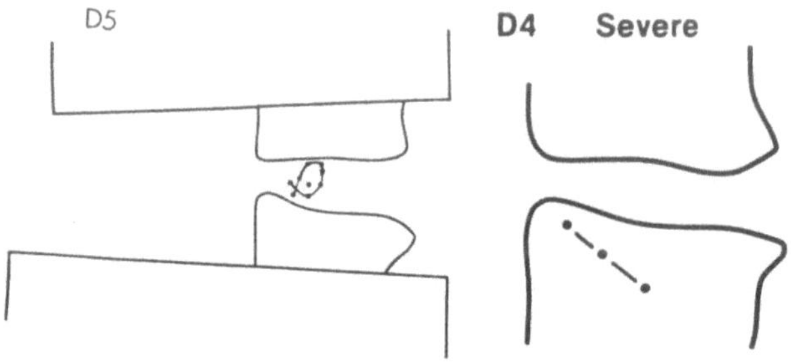

Figure 6.28. Gertzbein and associates[9] have studied movement of the centrode of motion between normal and degenerating vertebrae. Note relatively symmetrical course of nondegenerative segment and locus of motion at posterior middle one-third of disc. In contrast, under conditions of degeneration, the centrode length is longer and often not located in its more usual anatomical position. (Reprinted from Gertzbein et al.[9] with permission of authors and publisher.)

It should be apparent from the preceding discussion that degenerative instability remains elusive with respect to its diagnostic criteria. However, as the degenerative process progresses from the unstable to the stabilized phase, an evolving deformity represents a method that might provide classification of the unstable phase. It was this general consideration that led Frymoyer and Selby[56] to identify syndromes by radiographic criteria, which they argued would lead to a rational choice for fusion techniques. However, an analysis of epidemiological and clinical studies, radiographic data, and animal model experiments suggests major problems still remain in their definition, as well as its application to the clinical setting.

First, epidemiological studies show a significant prevalence of degenerative spondylolisthesis in the aging population.[57] Although this radiologic finding predicts an increased risk for low back symptoms, there are many subjects who have never had low back pain. Kirkaldy-Willis and Farfan[45] emphasize it is the combination of symptoms and radiographic findings that leads to the diagnosis of instability. Second, clinical and radiographic studies of patients who have had lumbar surgery reveal conditions that could be called unstable. For example, 20% of patients who have had L4 to the sacrum fusions fulfill Knutsson's criteria for instability at the next mobile level, yet this finding bears no relationship to symptoms. Similarly, 20% of patients who have undergone simple disc excision fulfill those same radiographic criteria, and additionally have traction spurs at the previously operated level.[58] Most typically, these radiographic findings are observed in females who have undergone L4–L5 disc excision, but the radiographic signs poorly predict the presence of symptoms. Third, recent radiographic studies, which have combined both flexion/extension films and biplanar techniques, have failed to demonstrate predictable patterns of instability.[59]

Last, animal experiments that attempt to reproduce instability have produced conflicting results. Sullivan and Farfan[60] tested a model of torsional instability by removing the facet joints on contralateral sides above and below the disc space in rabbits. Radiographic and unspecified pathological analysis suggested the disc space underwent accelerated degeneration. Cauchoix reproduced their experiment and reported acceleration of the degenerative process by histological criteria.[61] In our laboratories, we

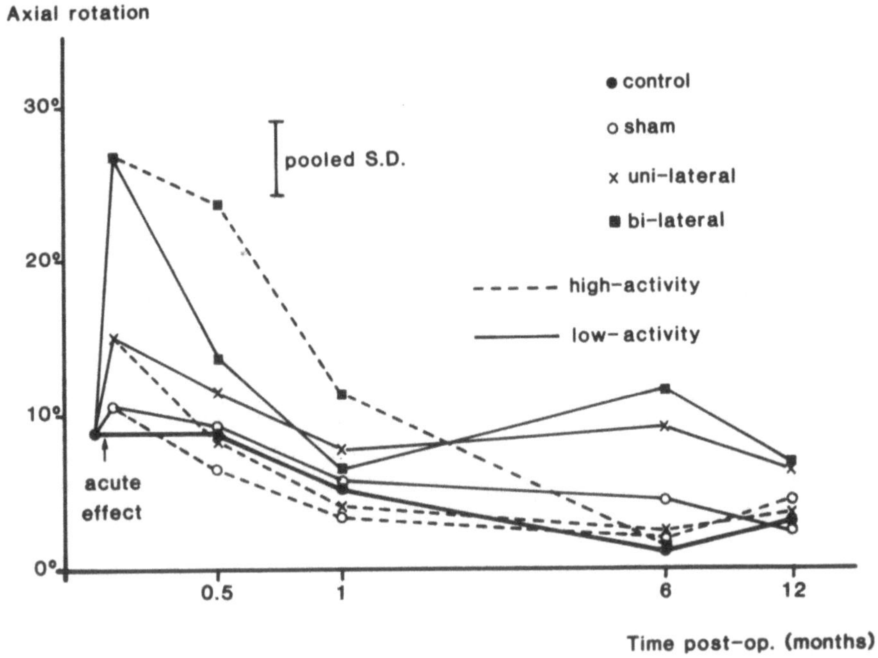

Figure 6.29. Experimental data from rabbits undergoing sham, unilateral, and bilateral facetectomies. Allowable range of axial rotation is given for each of time intervals, postoperatively, comparing groups of animals. Note initial instability is followed by trend toward restoration of stability; this progresses more rapidly in high-activity than in low-activity levels. (Reprinted from Stokes et al.[69])

have replicated the Farfan–Sullivan model, as well as tested a second model in which both facet joints are removed at the same level. The force displacement data (Fig. 6.29) demonstrate an initial instability followed by a progressive trend toward restabilization. The parallel biochemical studies, as well as histological analysis, fail to demonstrate convincing evidence of degeneration. Additional experiments compared high- to low-activity level animals and showed a trend toward more rapid resolution of the initial mechanical instability in the high-activity-level animals. The differences among the three studies might be explained by genetic differences, but our results suggest healing mechanisms may dominate in the evolution of unstable spinal conditions.

How then can we utilize the accumulated knowledge of instability to arrive at a scientific analysis of our patients with low back pain? The short answer is that in many instances we do not have the technology to do this in a rigorous, scientific manner. However, a more rational approach can be based on the following clinical principles: It is axiomatic that successful outcomes of surgical interventions in the lumbar spine correlate highly with the degree of concordance between clinical symptoms, clinical signs, and objective imaging studies. Thus, one can derive the general statement that a progressing deformity accompanied by signs and symptoms, particularly if they affect nerve roots, represent the best method of diagnosis. Moreover, there is ample evidence that spinal fusions performed for the complaint of low back pain have a predictably poor outcome; if there is uncertainty in diagnosis, surgery is more likely to fail.

The classification given in Table 6.3 represents a further application of the scheme proposed by Frymoyer and Shelby.[56] This operational approach is currently used in our hospital, but we emphasize that the scientific basis for this classification remains unproven, particularly for the objective confirmation of the "unstable phase."

Table 6.3 Classification of criteria for spinal fusion.

Primary degenerative instabilities	Fixed deformity
Translational	Degenerative spondylolisthesis
Retrolisthetic	Fixed retrolisthesis
Torsional	Degenerative spondylolisthesis
? Disc disruption	? Isolated disc resorption
Degenerative scoliosis	Fixed scoliotic deformity, at either single or multiple levels
Secondary instabilities (postsurgical)	
Post disc excision: Subclassified as translational, retrolisthetic, torsional, disc disruption, and scoliotic	
Post decompression: Either an increase of deformity, e.g., increased forward translation of a degenerative spondylolisthesis following decompression, or an acquired deformity subclassified as translational retrolisthetic, rotational, scoliotic	
Post fusion: Instability above or below fusion at the first mobile segment subclassified as for the postdecompression category	
Pseudarthrosis	

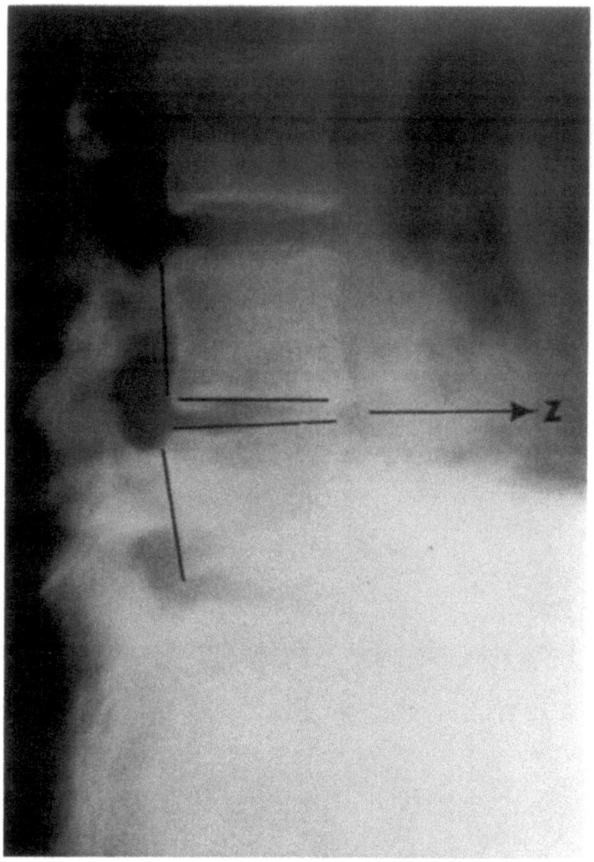

Figure 6.30. Increasing episodes of low back pain included symptoms suggesting L5 nerve root entrapment. On forward flexion, displacement in Z axis occurs between L4 and L5, representing early degenerative spondylolisthesis in its unstable phase.

1. *Transitional:* Our indication for spinal fusion is the patient who demonstrates forward displacements on plain, standing spinal radiographs, who has persistent or recurrent low back pain accompanied often by claudication, the disc space is still relatively preserved, there is minimal evidence of physiological stabilization by bridging osteophytes, and flexion/extension radiographs demonstrate motion greater than 8°. This definition fulfills the criteria for the early stage of degenerative spondylolisthesis. Less certain is the patient without an apparent deformity in plain radiographs who has persisting back pain with variable neurological symptoms. In these instances, flexion/extension radiographs demonstrating forward displacements greater than 4 mm, accompanied by traction spurs, and the relief of symptoms by facet blocks may represent a relative indication for spinal fusion (Fig. 6.30).

Although Goldner[62] has proposed anterior interbody fusion to be the operation of choice in these cases, the common need for posterior decompression has led us to conclude that transverse process fusion is most applicable. Internal fixation by Luque rods, Knodt rods, and the

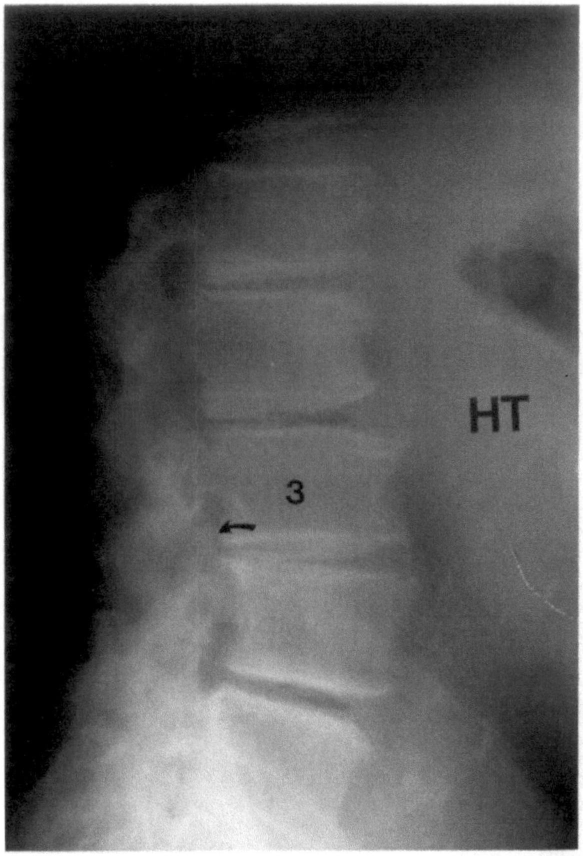

Figure 6.31. Male patient has increasing episodes of low back pain from multilevel degenerative disc disease. His major current symptoms are L4 nerve root irritation (*arrow*). Note posterior displacement of L3 on L4 on extension (retrospondylolisthesis).

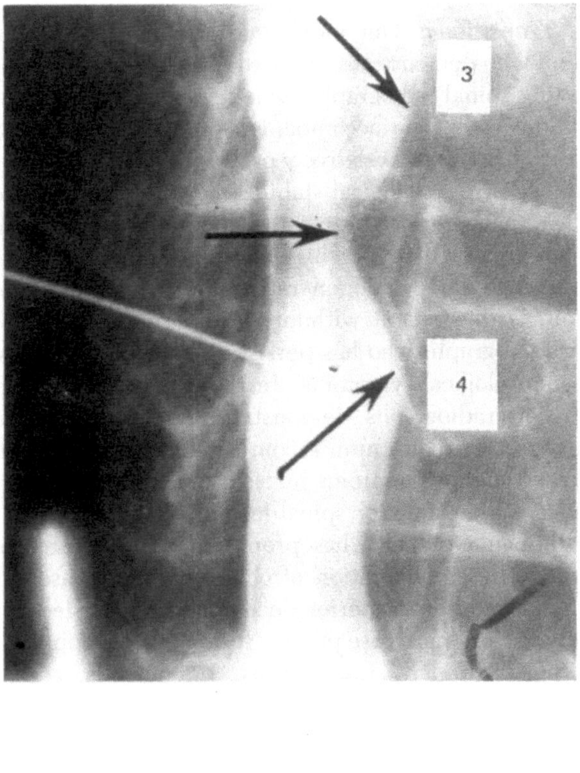

Kaneda device have been proposed as suitable methods, but the biomechanical advantage of pedicle fixation, particularly in osteoporotic bone, indicate these devices are most likely to be the reliable means of securing initial spinal stabilization.

2. *Retrolisthetic:* The indications here are basically the same as those previously given for translational instabilities; namely, the deformity is identifiable on plain spinal radiographs, the deformity increases and decreases during flexion/extension lateral films, and the patient has evidence of lateral recess symptoms, which may be intermittent or constant. Because adequate decompression of this condition may often require a sacrifice of more than one-third of the articular facets, this alone may serve as a sound biomechanical indication for fusion. A relative indication is the absence of deformity on lateral spinal radiographs with the demonstration of angulatory collapse of the disc space and retrolisthetic translations on flexion/extension radiographs and relief by facet blocks (Fig. 6.31). Reduction of the deformity is theoretically best provided by a distracting device such as the Knodt rod, but we now believe pedicle fixation is a more desirable method of stabilization.

3. *Torsional:* Our current inability to accurately diagnose a torsional deformity makes this diagnosis less certain, yet the biomechanical and anatomical data are persuasive. Because it is difficult to differentiate a torsional deformity from the more classically described translational deformity, indications are currently identical to those described previously. Radiographic signs, which may be suggestive, include malalignment of the spinous process at the affected level, as well as an unusual pedicle-to-pedicle defect seen on myelography as described by Farfan (Fig. 6.32). An additional "at-risk" sign is the position of the L4–L5 motion segment relative to the pelvis. Theoretically, the ideal fusion technique is an antitorsion fusion in which the facet on the side to which rotation is directed is first derotated toward the opposite side by a bone graft inserted into the joint. A smaller graft, which may be difficult to drive in because of the derotation that has been produced, is placed in the contralateral facet. We routinely supplement the facet fusion by transverse process fusion, although Farfan has indicated this may not be necessary in older patients. If the facets have been sacrificed, this technique is not applicable. Currently, alternative fixation devices, such as pedicle fixation systems which provide derotation, would seem a reasonable solution.

4. *Disc Disruption:* Crock's analysis of disc disruption suggests the most certain method of diagnosis is discography demonstrating disruption of the disc morphology,

Figure 6.32. Pedicle-to-pedicle defect (*arrows*) proposed by Farfan[45] as evidence of a rotational instability. (Reprinted from Frymoyer and Selby[56] with permission of publisher.)

sometimes with dissection of the dye along the posterior longitudinal ligaments, and the reproductions of the patient's symptoms[48] (Fig. 6.33). Some credence for this diagnostic method is the experimental finding of increased amounts of the neurotransmitter substance P in the dorsal root ganglion of animals after a discogram.[63] Additionally, anatomical dissections demonstrate nociceptor nerve endings in the peripheral fibers of the annulus, which could be activated during distention of the disc. Because the pathology is thought to involve primarily the anterior and middle columns, anterior interbody fusion has been the reported operation of choice. However, some surgeons have reported a lower-than-desirable rate of fusion with this technique, and there has been a reevaluation of the combined anteroposterior fusion (360°), either as a staged or single-operative intervention. This latter method has yet to be rigorously analyzed to determine its effectiveness. Resorption of the posterior fusion mass has been identified in a high percentage of cases, suggesting there may be either adverse biomechanical or physiological sequelae to this approach.[64]

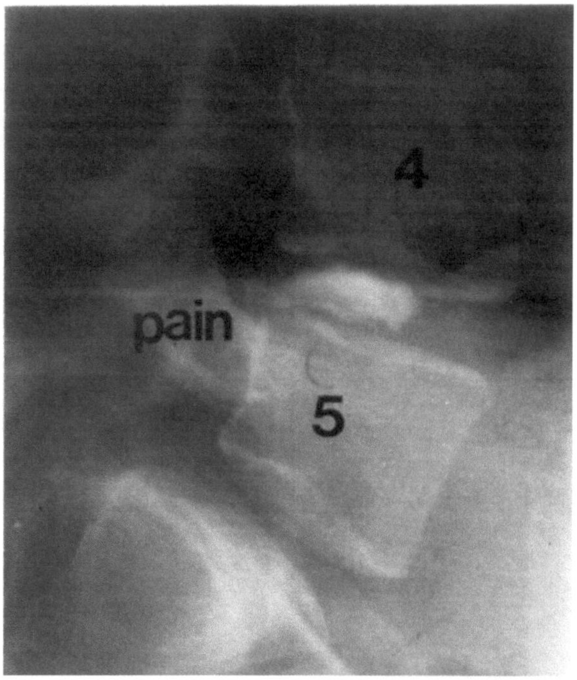

Figure 6.33. Discogram demonstrates posterior extrusion of dye with distention posterior along body of L5. Discography accurately reproduced this patient's symptoms, subsequently relieved by anterior interbody fusion.

5. *Degenerative Scoliosis:* The best demonstration of instability in degenerative scoliosis is progression of the curve over time in standing anterior/posterior radiographs, particularly when the patient has increasing symptoms of spinal stenosis or intractable back pain. In some patients, the deformity may be quite focal because of asymmetric collapse of the disc space (Fig. 6.34). Additional criteria are translations on lateral bending films. A significant rotational deformity accompanies many of these curves, and some of the single-level scoliotic deformities may represent a variant of the torsional deformity. The stabilization devices most effective are pedicle systems that have sufficient flexibility to conform to the curvature when it extends over multiple levels. The posterior Zielke or Wiltse devices currently best meet their objectives.

Secondary Instabilities

Post Disc Excision

The demonstration of abnormal translations on flexion/extension radiographs is found with sufficient frequency in asymptomatic, postoperative patients to make its usefulness suspect as a reliable radiographic sign. Clearly the best indication is increasing deformity over time, either as a translational, retrolisthetic, or torsional deformity. In our series of patients with failed low back surgery, instability was suspected and treated in 3%.[67] Choice of

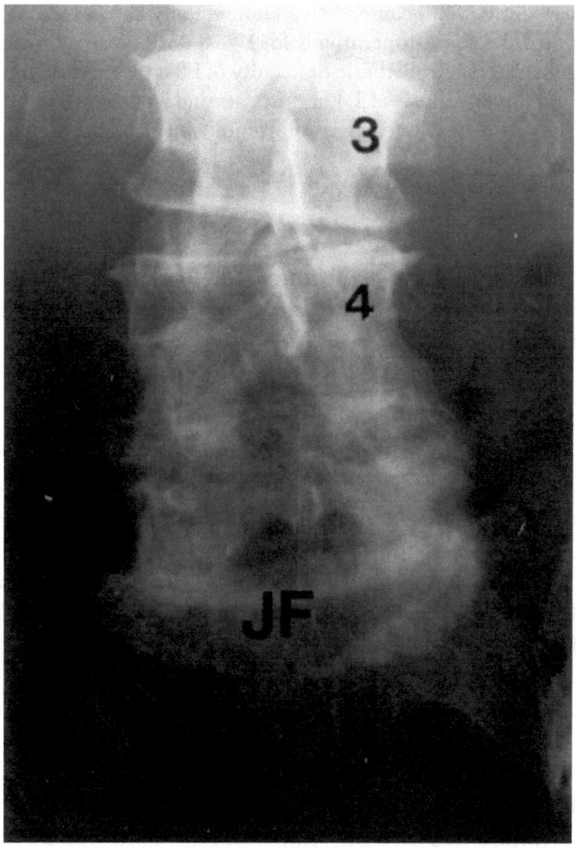

Figure 6.34. Patient with prior surgery with discitis at L4–L5 now presents with L4 nerve root symptoms. Note marked segmental collapse at L3–L4 level, consistent with instability. Progression of deformity occurred during period of 4 years.

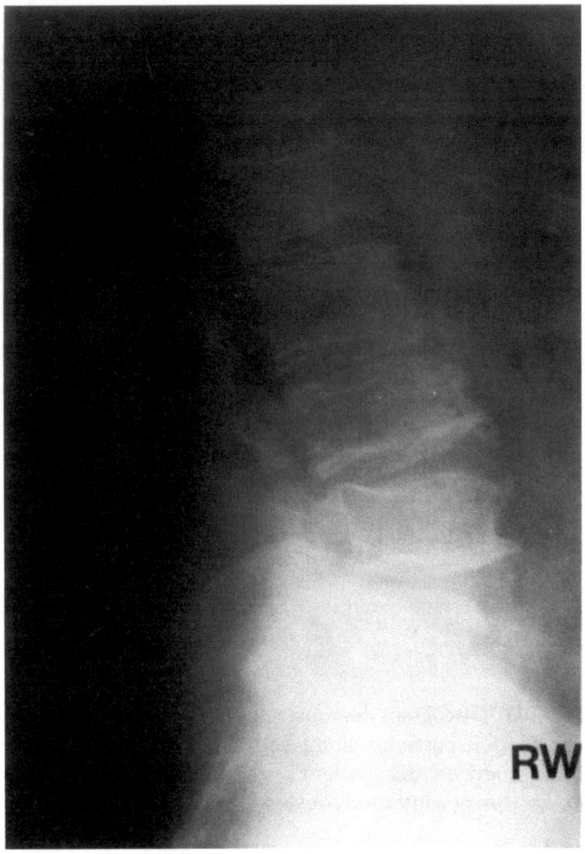

Figure 6.35. This 56-year-old male with multilevel spinal stenosis underwent wide decompressive laminectomy at L3–L4 and L4–L5. He did well postoperatively for 1 year until these radiographs demonstrated retrolisthetic deformity of L3 on L4 and degenerative spondylolisthesis at L4 and L5, secondary to complete facetectomy as necessitated by requirements of decompression.

fusion would seem logically to depend on the type of deformity, using the same criteria as described for primary instabilities.

Post Decompression

Two types of deformity are identified. The first is an accentuation of the preexistent deformity following decompression, most commonly identified in degenerative spondylolisthesis. This is most apt to occur when the indications for spinal fusion given previously are present at the time of the initial operation. It may also occur after sacrifice of facets for decompression in retrolisthetic deformities. A second type of deformity most commonly follows multilevel decompressions in degenerative spinal stenosis or scoliosis. In these instances, a variety of unstable patterns may be identified at different spinal levels (Fig. 6.35). Before the advent of pedicle fixation correction of such deformities was virtually impossible, but newer devices, such as Steffee plates and posterior Zielke instrumentation, have proven particularly useful. When osteoporosis is present, methylmethacrylate has been shown to increase the pull-out strength of the pedicle screw and is indicated. Johnson[65] found that the cervical facet joints account for 40% of spinal stability and, therefore, it is essential to preserve these joints when doing posterior decompressions. Wide laminectomies alone are often well tolerated, but may lead to instability if the facet joints are also included. Even in cases where the facet joints are preserved, progressive deformity may occur as time goes by.

Post Spinal Fusion

Instability Above a Fusion. It has been shown in laboratory and clinical studies that fusions from L4 to the sacrum produce abnormal stresses at the next mobile spinal level. However, the demonstration of "Knutsson's sign" is not reliable because it is a common finding in asymptomatic patients.[58] The most common pattern observed is a progressive degenerative spondylolisthesis, accompanied by signs and symptoms of acquired spinal stenosis.[66] If a patient is developing intractable low back pain, Knutsson's sign is present, and temporary relief follows facet block. This may serve as a relative indication for fusion, particularly if the symptoms can be reproduced by discography. Although fusion may be done anteriorly or posteriorly, a short pedicle fixation device, such as the Vermont Fixator, may provide more certain fusion in this situation.

Pseudarthrosis. The determination that pseudarthrosis is causing symptoms is difficult because many patients with this finding are asymptomatic. Clinical and radiographic signs that may be helpful, but are equivocally diagnostic, are (1) relief of symptoms following local anesthetic injection into the defect; (2) reproduction of symptoms by discography; (3) an easily visible defect on plain radiographs accompanied by forward motion greater than 4° in flexion/extension radiographs; and (4) a recurrent disc protrusion with unequivocal radiculopathy. We have delayed repair of pseudarthroses identified 6 months postoperatively, and waited for a minimum of 1 year before considering refusion because patients may improve during that interval. The 50% success rate that follows refusion and a solid arthrodesis suggests the need for caution in these patients.[67] Currently, we advocate anterior interbody fusion, with or without posterior fusion and instrumentation, or simply posterior fusion with pedicle fixation as solutions to this problem.

References

1. Rutkow IM. Orthopaedic operations in the United States, 1979 through 1983. J Bone Joint Surg 1986;68A:716–719.
2. Frymoyer JW, Pope MH, Clements JH, Wilder DG, MacPherson B, Ashikaga T. Risk factors in low-back pain: an

epidemiological survey. J Bone Joint Surg 1983;65A:213–218.
3. Lange F. Support of the spondylolitic spine by means of buried steel bars attached to the vertebrae. J Orthop Surg [Am] 1910;8:344.
4. Hadra BE: Wiring of the spinous processes in Pott's disease. Trans Orthop Assoc 1981;4:206.
5. Albee FH. Transplantation of a portion of the tibia into spine for Pott's disease. JAMA 1911;57:885.
6. Hibbs RH. An operation for progressive spinal deformities. NY J Med 1911;93:1013.
7. Frymoyer JW, Krag MH. Spinal stability and instability. In: The Unstable Spine. New York: Grune and Stratton, 1986.
8. White AA, Panjabi MM. Clinical Biomechanics of the Spine. Philadelphia: Lippincott, 1978.
9. Gertzbein SD, Seligman J, Holtby R, Chan KH, Kapasouri A, Tile M, Cruickshank B. Centrode patterns and segmental instability in degenerative disc disease. Spine 1985; 10(3):257–261.
10. Farfan HF. Mechanical Disorders of the Low Back. Philadelphia: Lea & Febiger, 1973.
11. Stokes IAF, Wilder DG, Frymoyer JW, Pope MH. Assessment of patients with low back pain by biplanar radiographic measurement of intervertebral motion. Spine 1981;6:233.
12. Perey O. Fracture of the vertebral end-plate in the lumbar spine: an experimental investigation. Acta Orthop Scand (Suppl) 1957;25.
13. McAfee PC, Yuan HA, Fredrickson GE, Lubicky JP. The value of computed tomography in thoracolumbar fractures. J Bone Joint Surg 1983;64A:461.
14. Lorenz M, Patwardhan A, Vanderby R. Load-bearing characteristics of lumbar facets in normal and surgically altered spinal segments. Spine 1983;8:122.
15. Hutton WC, Stott JRR, Cyron BM. Is spondylolysis a fatigue fracture? Spine 1977;2:202.
16. Lucas DB, Bresler B. Stability of the ligamentous spine. Biomech Lab Report #40. San Francisco: University of California.
17. Holdsworth FW. Fractures, dislocations and fracture dislocations of the spine. J Bone Joint Surg 1963; 45B:6.
18. Posner I, White AA, Edwards WT, et al. A biomechanical analysis of the clinical stability of the lumbar and lumbosacral spine. Spine 1982;7:374–389.
19. Denis F. The three-column spine and its significance in the classification of acute thoraco-lumbar spinal injuries. Spine 1983;8:817.
20. Fielding JW, Cochran GVB, Lawsing JF III, Hohl M. Tears of the transverse ligament of the atlas. A clinical and biomechanical study. J Bone Joint Surg 1974;56A:1683–1691.
21. Penning L. Obtaining and interpreting plain films in cervical spine injury. In: The Cervical Spine, pp. 62–95. The Cervical Spine Research Society. Philadelphia: Lippincott, 1983.
22. Binet EF. Cervical spine tomography in trauma. Spine 1977;2:163.
23. Herkowitz HN, Rothman RH. Subacute instability of the cervical spine. Spine 1984;9:348–357.
24. Gaines RW, Humphries WG. A plea for judgment in management of thoraco-lumbar fractures and fracture dislocations. Clin Orthop 1984;189:36–42.
25. Whitesides TE. Traumatic kyphosis of the thoracolumbar spine. Clin Orthop 1977;128:78.
26. Krag MH, Pope MH, Wilder DG. Mechanisms of spine trauma and features of spinal fixation methods. Part I, Mechanisms of injury. In: Ghista D, ed. Spinal Cord Injury Medical Engineering. Springfield, Illinois: CC Thomas, 1986.
27. Whitesides JR, Shah SGA. On the management of unstable fractures of the thoracolumbar spine. Spine 1976;1:99.
28 McAfee PC, Yuan HA, Lasada NA. The unstable burst fracture. Spine 1982;7:365.
29. Pope MH, Krag MH, Wilder DG. Mechanisms of spine trauma and features of spinal fixation methods. Part II, Fixation methods. In: Ghista D, ed. Spinal Cord Injury Medical Engineering. Springfield, Illinois: CC Thomas, 1986.
30. McGuire RA, Neville S, Green BA, Watts C. Spinal instability and the log-rolling maneuver. J Trauma 1987;27(5):525–531.
31. Bailey SI, Bell D. Failures of anterior bone grafting of injured cervical spine. J Bone Joint Surg 1977;59B:509.
32. Simmons EH. Kyphotic deformity of the spine in ankylosing spondylitis. Clin Orthop 1977;128:65–77.
33. Fredrickson BE, Baker D, McHolick WJ, Yuan HA, Lubicky JP. The natural history of spondylolysis and spondylolisthesis. J Bone Joint Surg 1984;66A:699–707.
34. Pearcy M, Shepherd J. Is there instability in spondylolisthesis? Spine 1985;10(2):175–177.
35. Lowe RW, Hayes TD, Kaye J, Bagg RJ, Luekens CA. Standing roentgenograms in spondylolisthesis. Clin Orthop 1976;117:80–84.
36. Frymoyer JW, Wiltse L, Grobler LJ. Unpublished data.
37. Mixter WJ, Barr JS. Rupture of the intervertebral disc with involvement of the spinal canal. N Engl J Med 1934;211:210–215.
38. Knutsson F. The instability associated with disc degeneration in the lumbar spine. Acta Radiol 25:593
39. Junghanns H. Spondylolisthesen ohne Spalt im Zwischengelenkstück. Archiv für orthopädische und Unfall-Chirurgie 1930;29:118–127.
40. Macnab I. Spondylolisthesis with an intact neural arch—the so-called pseudo-spondylolisthesis. J Bone Joint Surg 1950;32B:325.
41. Moran FP, King T. Primary instability of lumbar vertebrae as a common cause of low back pain. J Bone Joint Surg 1957;39B:6–22.
42. Macnab I. Backache. Baltimore: Williams & Wilkins, 1977.
43. Frymoyer JW, Hanley E, Howe J, Kuhlmann D, Matteri R. Disc excision and spine fusion in the management of lumbar disc disease: a minimum ten-year followup. Spine 1978;3:1–6.
44. Kirkaldy-Willis WH. Presidential symposium on instability of the lumbar spine. Introduction. Spine 1985;10(3):254.
45. Kirkaldy-Willis WH, Farfan HF. Instability of the lumbar spine. Clin Orthop 1982;165:110.
46. Pope MH, Panjabi M. Biomechanical definitions of spinal instability. Spine 1985;10(3):255–256.
47. Crock HV. Isolated lumbar disk resorption as a cause of nerve root canal stenosis. Clin Orthop 1976;115:109–115.
48. Crock HV. Internal disc disruption: a challenge to disc prolapse fifty years on. Spine 1986;11:650–653.
49. Hansson T, Roose B. Microcalluses of the trabeculae in

lumbar vertebrae and their relation to the bone mineral content. Spine 1981;6:375–380.
50. Paris SV. Physical signs of instability. Spine 1985;10(3):277–279.
51. Stokes IAF, Wilder DG, Frymoyer JW, Pope MH. Assessment of patients with low back pain by biplanar radiographic measurement of intervertebral motion. Spine 1981;6:233.
52. Friberg O. Lumbar instability: A dynamic approach by traction—compression radiography. Spine 1987;12(2):119–129.
53. Nachemson A, Schultz A, Andersson G. Mechanical effectiveness studies of lumbar spine orthoses. Scand J Rehabil Med 1983;15(Suppl 9:139–149).
54. Olerud S. External fixation as a stabilizer in connection with anterior fusions in the lower lumbar spine. 12th International Conference on Hoffmann External Fixation. Bavaria, West Germany: Garmisch-Partenkirchen/Murnae, 1986.
55. Wilder DG. On loading of the human lumbar intervertebral motion segment. PhD Dissertation, Civil and Mechanical Engineering Dept., University of Vermont. Ann Arbor: University Microfilms International, 1986.
56. Frymoyer JW, Selby DK. Segmental instability: rationale for treatment. Spine 1985;10:280–286.
57. Valkenburg HA, Haanen HCM. The epidemiology of low back pain, pp. 9–22. In: Symposium on idiopathic low back pain. St. Louis: Mosby, 1982.
58. Frymoyer JW, Hanley EN, Howe J, Kuhlmann D, Matteri RE. A comparison of radiographic findings in fusion and nonfusion patients ten or more years following lumbar disc surgery. Spine 1979;4:435–440.
59. Stokes IAF, Frymoyer JW, Lunn RA. Segmental motion and segmental instability. Orthop Trans 1986;10:517–518 (abstr).
60. Sullivan JD, Farfan HF, Kahn DS. Pathologic changes with intervertebral joint rotational instability in the rabbit. Can J Surg 1971;14:71–79.
61. Cauchoix J, Yaacoubi, E, Romero CG, Heripret G. An experimental model of lumbar degenerated disc in rabbits. In: Proceedings of the International Society for the Study of the Lumbar Spine, annual meeting, Montreal, Quebec, Canada, 1984.
62. Goldner JL. The role of spine fusion: Question 6. Spine 1981; 6:293.
63. Claverie G, Weinstein J. The pain of discography. Presented at the International Society for the Study of the Lumbar Spine, Miami, Florida, 1988
64. Gill K, O'Brien J. Resorption of the lateral bone graft used in the simultaneous combined anterior and posterior lumbar fusion procedure. A radiographic observation in a review of 38 patients. Presented at the International Society for the Study of the Lumbar Spine, Dallas, Texas, 1986.
65. Johnson RM, Owen JR, Panjabi MM, Friedlander GE, Southwick WO. Biomechanical stability of the cervical spine using a human cadaver model. Orthop Trans J Bone Joint Surg 1980;4:42.
66. Brodsky AE. Post-laminectomy and post-fusion stenosis of the lumbar spine. Clin Orthop 1976;115:130–139.
67. Frymoyer JW, Hanley E, Howe J, Kuhlmann D, Matteri R. Disc excision and spine fusion in the management of lumbar disc disease: a minimum ten-year followup. Spine 1978; 3:1–6.
68. Macnab I. The traction spur. An indicator of segmental instability. J Bone Joint Surg 1971;53A:663–670.
69. Stokes IAF, Counts DC, Frymoyer JW. Experimental instability in the rabbit lumbar spine. Spine 1989; 14(1): 68–72.

III

Anatomy and Surgical Approaches

■7■

Anatomy and Surgical Approaches of the Spine

Howard B. Cotler and Michael G. Kaldis

Embryological Development of the Spine

In the second week of intrauterine development, the notochord arises from complex migration and invagination of cells within the primitive streak. The ectoderm over the notochord gives rise to the neural plate of the neuroectoderm. This then forms the neural groove and subsequently the neural tube, which dilates cephalad to form the encephalon and caudad to form the spinal cord. The neuroectoderm differentiates into three layers; the central ependymal, an intermediate mantle, and a peripheral marginal layer, which form the ependymal lining of the central cord of the spinal cord, the gray matter, and white matter, respectively. Dura mater or the pachymeninx apparently develops as a condensation from surrounding mesoderm, while the arachnoid and pia mater or leptomeninges probably develop from the ectodermal neural crest cells.

Somites arising from the paraxial mesoderm develop in a craniocaudal direction on or about the third week. The somites then divide, at the end of the fourth week, into three cell colonies (Fig. 7.1) that develop into dermis and subcutaneous tissue, musculature, and vertebrae, or the dermotome, myotome, or sclerotome, respectively. Remnants of the degenerated notochord develop in the intervertebral disc to become the nucleus pulposus. The mesenchymal vertebrae arising from the somite develop areas of chondrification forming the vertebral body, pedicle, and transverse processes. Enchondral ossification in prenatal and postnatal development eventually give rise to the bony vertebrae.

Anatomy of the Spinal Cord

The spinal cord extends from the base of the skull and usually ends at the L1–L2 intervertebral disc.[1,2,3] According to McCotter,[4] the average cord length is 45 cm in males and 42 cm in females. In this study, termination of the cord varied from T12 to L2 with 77% at the L1–L2 intervertebral disc.

In general, the cord is wider in the lateral diameter than in the anteroposterior plane. The intumescentia cervicalis and lumbalis[5] are enlargements of the spinal cord at the cervical and lumbar level. The cervical enlargement averages 13.2 by 7.2 mm; the thoracic enlargement is 8 by 6.5 mm; and the lumbosacral swelling averages 9.6 by 8 mm. Spinal canal diameters, as determined by Aeby,[6] are 24.5 by 14.7 mm in the cervical region; in the thoracic region, 17.2 by 16.8 mm; and in the lumbar region, 23.4 by 17.4 mm.

The spinal nerve roots include 8 cervical, 12 thoracic, 5 lumbar, 5 sacral, and 1 coccygeal. The dorsal and ventral roots form the spinal nerve which, with the spinal ganglion, lies in the intervertebral foramen. These roots vary in length and direction according to their respective cervical, thoracic, or lumbar levels. Dorsal and ventral rami form distal to the intervertebral foramina. The cauda equina is made up of the roots caudal to the conus medullaris. The conus is then continued as the filum terminale. The filum is surrounded by dura to its terminal attachment on the dorsal coccyx.

In cross section, the outer contour of the spinal cord is formed by the following: posterior median sulcus, posterior median septum, posterolateral sulcus, posterior intermediate sulcus, anterior median fissure, and anterolateral sulcus. The spinal cord is generally divided into the peripheral white and the central gray matter (Fig. 7.2). The gray matter contains anterior and posterior columns as the anterior and posterior horns, respectively. The posterior columns receive impulses via the dorsal nerve roots, whereas the anterior columns receive impulses from the dorsal roots and the central nervous system, which give final input into voluntary muscle control. The preganglionic sympathetic neurons are within the lateral gray matter of all thoracic and the first and second lumbar

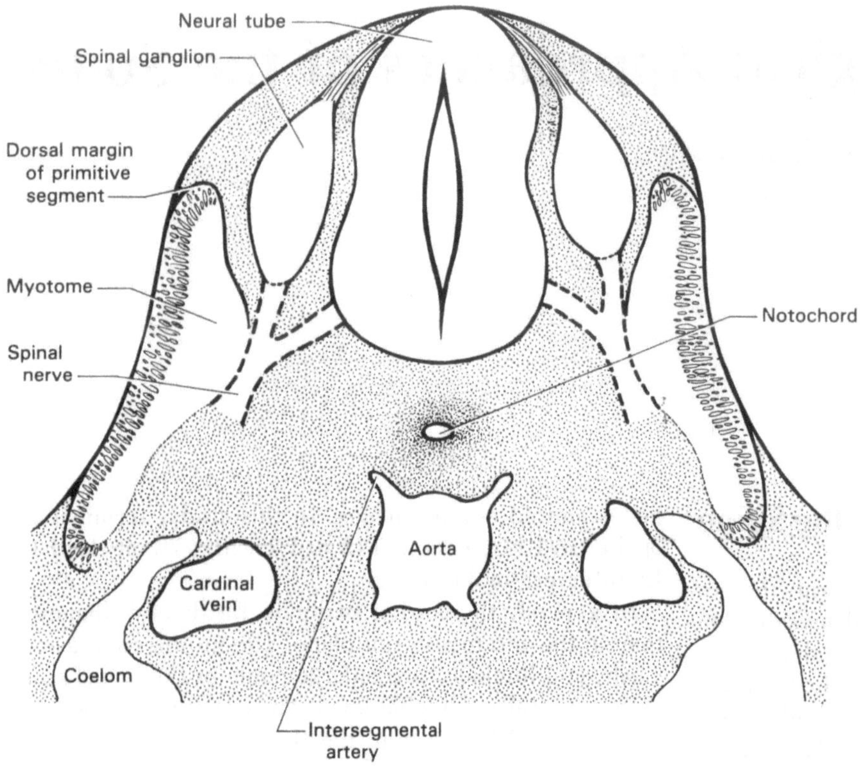

Figure 7.1. Development of the spine. Four-week embryo demonstrates result of somite division.

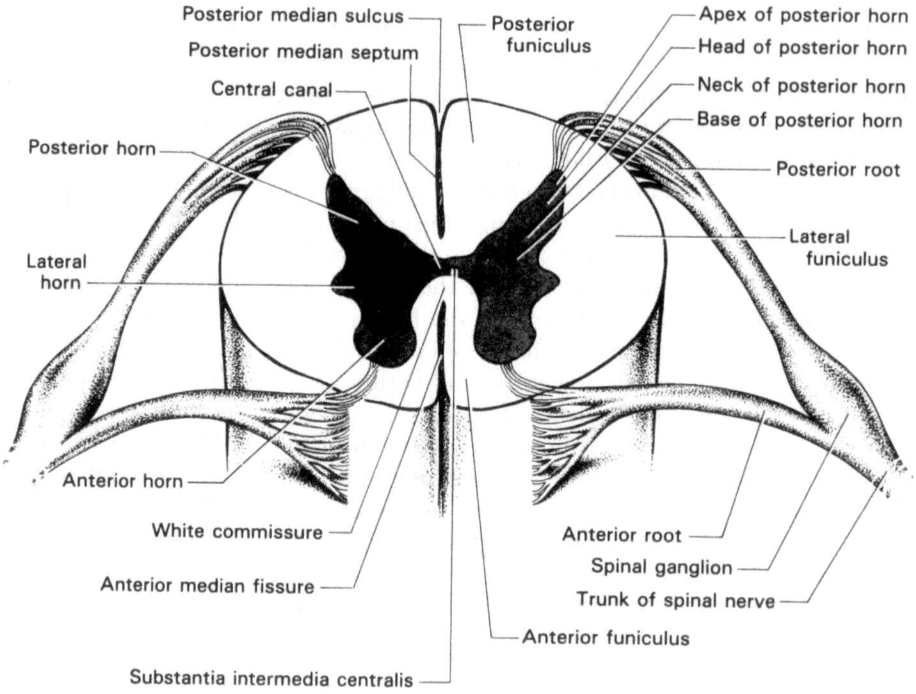

Figure 7.2. Cross section of spinal cord.

segments of the cord. The posterior horn, or somatosensory zone, receives and forwards impulses entering the spinal cord via posterior nerve roots. Between the posterior and anterior horns is the intermediate gray matter, containing the visceromotor and viscerosensory zones that provide visceral function. The anterior or somatomotor horn receives impulses from higher centers, the dorsal roots, and contains the median nuclei to axial muscles, lateral nuclei to shoulder and pelvic girdle, and central column to the diaphragm and pelvic muscles.

The white matter of the cord consists of the posterior, lateral, and anterior funiculi. The two posterior funiculi, gracilis and cuneatus, contain afferent fibers from cells of the dorsal root ganglion that are primarily for proprioception, pressure, and discriminative touch. The lateral funiculi contain ascending and descending tracts. The most important is the lateral spinothalamic tract, which carries pain and temperature sensation as it crosses anterior to the central canal and then ascends in the anterolateral portion of the lateral spinal cord. The lateral corticospinal tract decussates at the pyramid of the medulla and descends for voluntary muscle control. The innermost fibers of this tract supply cervical muscles, and fibers corresponding to the thoracic, lumbar, and sacral region that occur laterally in the cord. The anterior funiculus contains the anterior spinothalamic, ventral corticospinal, and spinotectal tracts. The spinothalamic tract crosses and ascends for light touch sensation; the ventral corticospinal tract descends and serves to control muscle contraction and tone; and spinotectal tract ascends with afferent impulses from the viscera.

The spinal meninges include the dura mater, arachnoid, and pia mater. They provide protection and nourishment to the spinal cord. The dura mater is the outermost layer extending from the foramen magnum where it is continuous with the intracranial dura to the sacral level surrounding the filum terminale. Superficial to this layer is the epidural space, and deep to it is the subdural space. The next deeper layer is the arachnoid membrane, which surrounds the subarachnoid space containing the cerebrospinal fluid (CSF). The CSF is produced by the choroid plexuses in the brain; its volume is estimated to be about 135 ml (75–150 ml), of which 55 ml is in the subarachnoid space. Approximately 300 ml of CSF is produced daily.[7] The pia mater is the innermost layer and intimately lines the neural structures. The spinal cord is stabilized by paired denticulate ligaments from the lateral columns that are continuous with the pia and extend to the dura. These are attached to the entire length of the spinal cord, originating between the dorsal and ventral roots.

Termination of the dural sac is variable between S1 and S4, according to studies performed by Lanier[8] and Louis.[3,9] This termination is primarily at S1 and S2. The dura and arachnoid join at or just distal to the dorsal root ganglia to obliterate the epidural space. Arachnoid

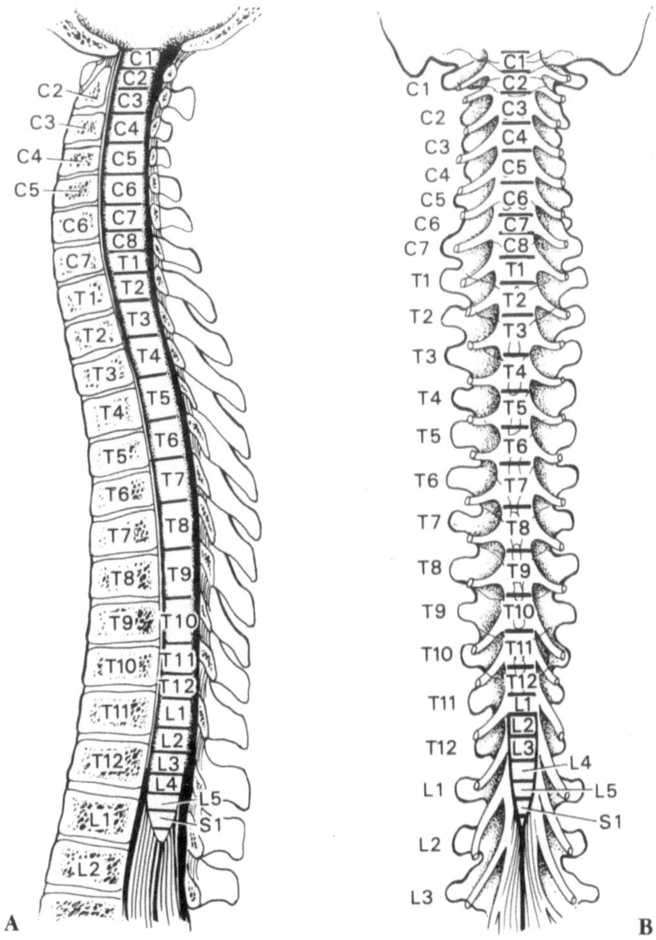

Figure 7.3. Vertebromedullary topography on (**A**) median sagittal section of spine and (**B**) viewed from posterior aspect of spine.

trabeculae within the subarachnoid space are between the arachnoid membrane and pia mater. The subarachnoid space terminates at the same level as the dura and is widest at the lumbar cistern.

The vertebromedullary topography varies somewhat according to the termination of the cord, which is usually at the L1–L2 disc space. Each medullary segment is a myelomere that gives rise to a spinal nerve root (Fig. 7.3).

The topography of the spinal nerve roots is determined by the segment of origin and passage through the dura and intervertebral foramen. Exiting of the nerve root varies with level of dural termination. With termination of the dura at S1 (approximately 43%),[3] the cervical roots emerge below the corresponding disc, except C8, which emerges at the C7–T1 disc space. Thoracic roots exit above the corresponding disc, yet the lower thoracic nerve roots exit half a vertebra above the disc. The lumbar root exits at the corresponding vertebral body.

With respect to the intervertebral foramina, nerve root

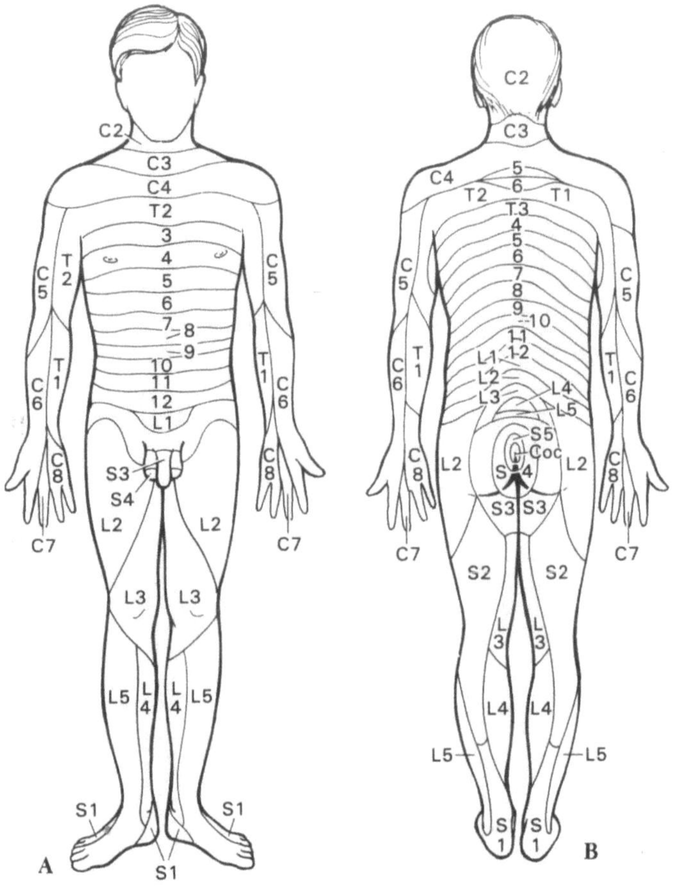

Figure 7.4. Sensory dermatomes.[66] **A.** Front view. **B.** Back view.

passage becomes more oblique in the caudal direction. At the cervical level, the nerve roots are almost transverse as they progress through their corresponding intervertebral foramina and occupy three-fourths of the foramina. In the thoracic region, the root passes just inferior to the superior pedicle of the foramina, occupying one-fifth of the space.[3] The lumbar spinal roots take a more diagonal course to occupy one-third of the foramina.[3]

The dermotomal (open sensory) and myotomal (open motor) distribution is important in the diagnosis of spinal pathology. The spinal nerve dermotomes are depicted in Fig. 7.4. More important dominant nerve root innervation of muscles is listed in Table 7.1)[10]

Vascular Supply of the Spinal Cord

The arterial supply of the spinal cord arises from the anterior spinal artery, lying in the anterior median fissure, and the two posterior spinal arteries, running along the posterolateral sulci. The anterior spinal artery arises from the vertebral artery whereas the posterior spinal arteries arise either from the inferior cerebellar artery or the vertebral artery. Radicular branches of the spinal arteries are quite variable in size and distribution, as shown by Hassler[11] and Turnbull.[12] The largest radicular arteries appear to be in the lower cervical and thoracolumbar regions. The first large radicular artery to the cervical cord (artery of the cervical enlargement of Lazorthes)[13,14] usually originates from the deep cervical artery, accompanies the C6 spinal nerve root, and supplies the cervical enlargement (intumescentia cervicalis). The largest radicular artery accompanies the ventral root between the T7 and L4 levels (more often on the left side) supplies the intumescentia lumbalis, and has been named the arteria radicularis anterior magnus, artery of Adamkiewicz,[13] or artery of the inferior enlargement of Lazorthes.[14,15]

Table 7.1. Dominant nerve root innervation of key muscles[10]

C4	Diaphragm
C5	Deltoid and/or biceps
C6	Wrist extensors
C7	Triceps
C8	Flexor profundus
T1	Hand intrinsics
T2–L1	Sensory level
L2	Iliopsoas
L3	Quadriceps
L4	Tibialis anterior
L5	Extensor hallucis longus
S1	Gastrocnemius
S2–S5	Sensory level

Contrary to the popular classical opinion[16] regarding the tenuous arterial blood supply of the spinal cord (especially the thoracic cord), many independent researchers (e.g., Lazorthes and Gouaze[17,18]; Crock and Yoshizawa[19]; Louis[20]) have provided a more realistic assessment of the spinal blood supply. Their studies show the presence of metametric radiculomedullary spinal arteries accompanying each spinal nerve to the spinal cord and demonstrate a rich anastomotic network of spinal arteries.

The anterior spinal artery and its branches appear to supply the anterior and intermediate gray matter, base of the posterior gray column, and anterior and lateral funiculis.[21] The posterior spinal artery and its branches supply the posterior funiculis, most of the posterior gray columns, and superficial lateral funiculis[21] (Fig. 7.5).

The two veins of the spinal cord are located in the anterior median fissure and the posterior median sulcus of the spinal cord. The spinal venous circulation drains primarily into the azygos system and joins directly into the venae cava.

Innervation of the Spine

The nerve supply of the spine arises from the dorsal rami of the spinal nerves, meningeal nerve, and sympathetic trunk (Fig. 7.6). The dorsal ramus branches at the facet joint capsule into the medial and lateral rami. The medial

Figure 7.5. Vasculature of spinal cord. **A.** Extrinsic and intrinsic vessels. **B.** Intrinsic vascular territories.

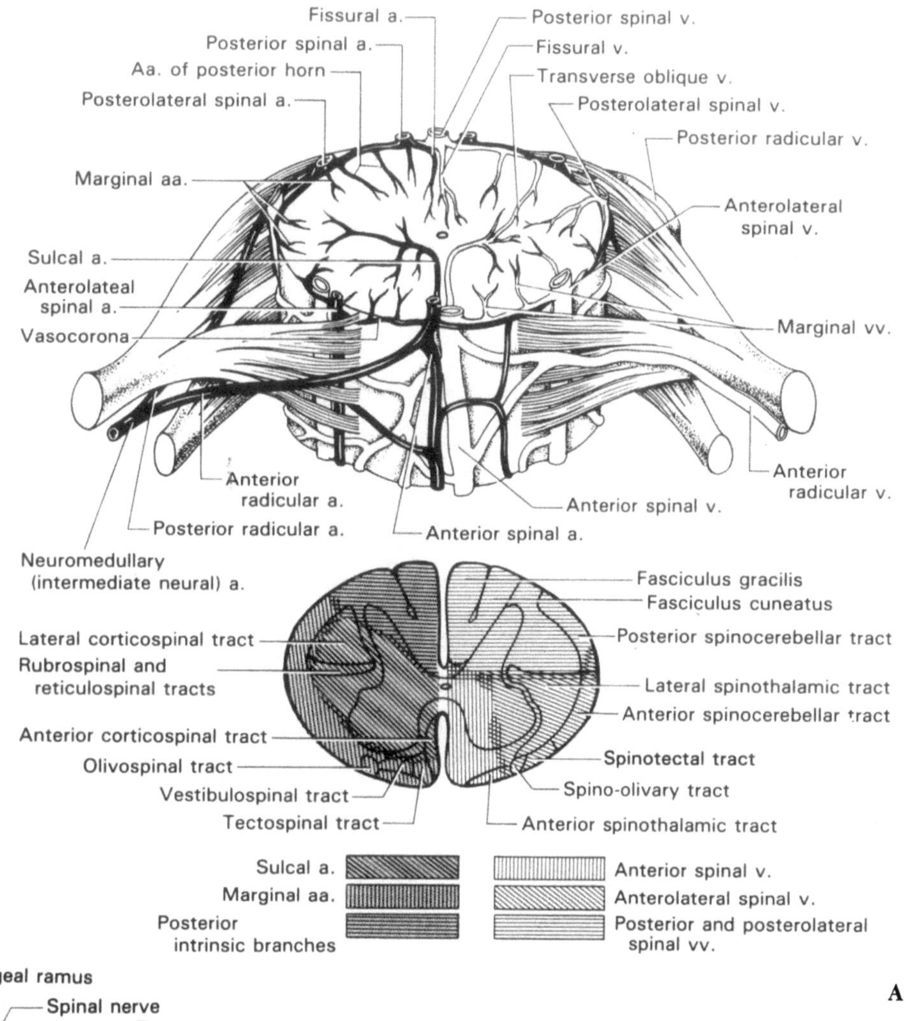

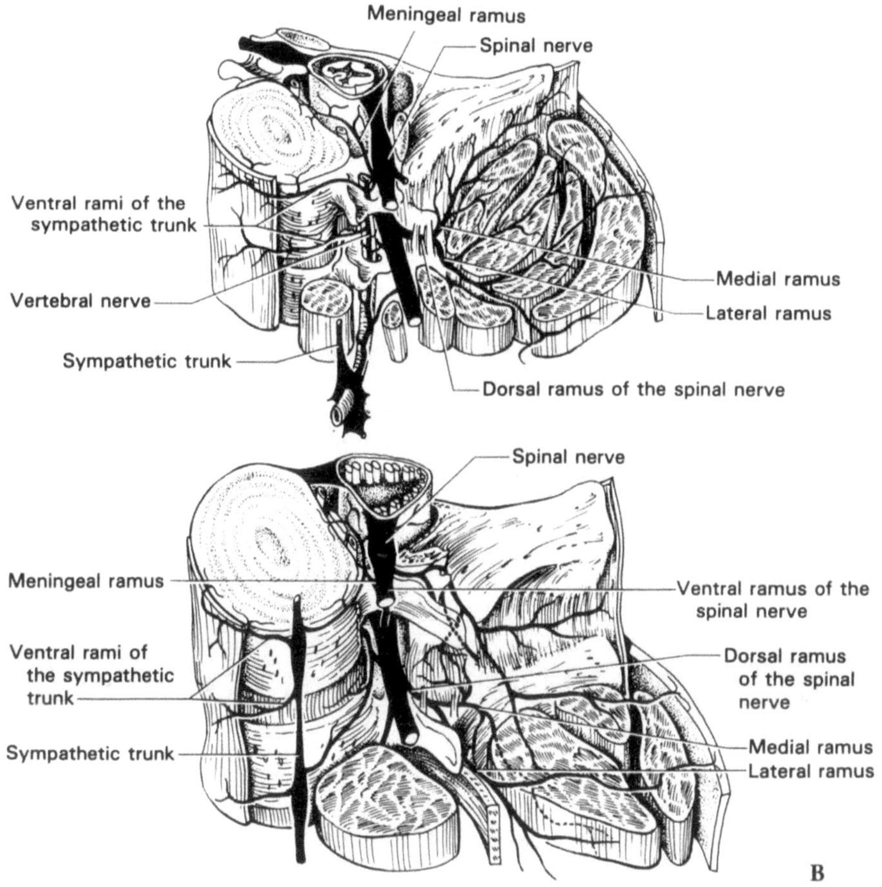

Figure 7.6. Intrinsic innervation of spine. **A.** The cervical spine. **B.** The lumbar spine.

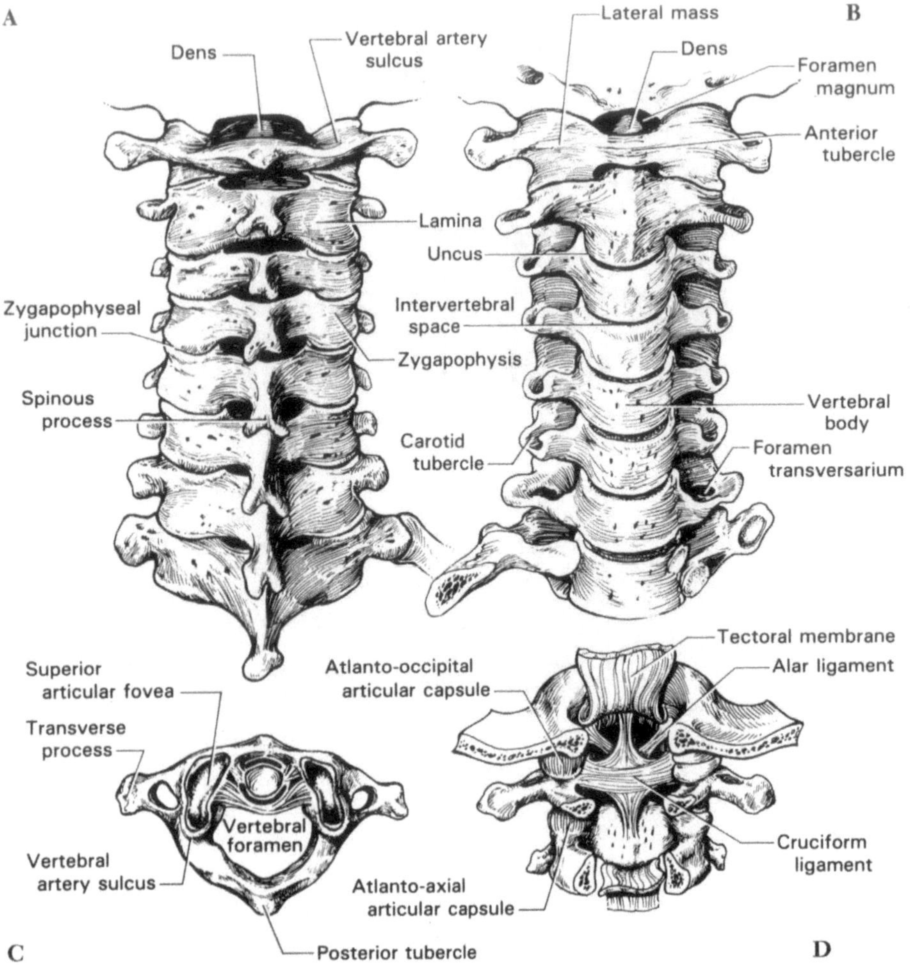

Figure 7.7. Bony morphology of cervical spine. **A.** Posterior aspect. **B.** Anterior aspect. C. Superior aspect of atlas. **D.** Posterior aspect of craniovertebral articulation.

ramus innervates the zygapophyseal joint, ligamentum flavum, interspinous ligaments, supraspinous ligaments, medial spinal muscles, and dorsal cutaneous region of the neck, trunk, and buttocks. The lateral ramus innervates the intertransverse ligaments and muscles, iliolumbar ligaments, sacroiliac joints, and the lateral part of the spinal muscles and dorsal skin.[22,23,24]

The meningeal or Luschka's sinuvertebral nerve has fibers from the spinal nerve and sympathetic trunk. It traverses superior to the intervertebral foramen and innervates the dura, posterior longitudinal ligament, superficial and posterior portion of the annulus fibrosis, peridural venous plexuses, and ligamentum flavum in the prearticular region. Fibers arising from the sympathetic trunk innervate the anterior longitudinal ligament and the superficial part of the annulus fibrosis.[3,25] To date, no author has documented nerve fibers in the nucleus pulposus or the deepest part of the annulus fibrosis.

Vertebral Bony Anatomy

The vertebral column is formed by 7 cervical, 12 thoracic, 5 lumbar, 5 fused sacral, and 5 fused coccygeal vertebrae. In general, the typical vertebra consists of the body, pedicle, lamina, transverse process, spinous process, and superior and inferior articular facets. The intervertebral disc is between each vertebral body from C2 to the sacrum. The vertebrae are formed from spongy bone with hyaline cartilage endplates.

Surgical Anatomy and Approaches to the Cervical Spine

Bony Morphology of the Cervical Spine (Fig. 7.7)

The cervical spine consists of seven vertebrae. The vertebral body is convex in the anterior posterior plane and concave superiorly. Each vertebra contains both a vertebral and transverse foramen. The costal process arises from the body whereas the transverse process lies at the lamina pedicle junction. The anterior and posterior tubercles, formed at the costal and transverse process, respectively, provide a sulcus for the spinal nerve. At the C6 level, the carotid tubercle, or Chassaignac's tubercle, is prominent and provides a good surgical landmark. The spinous processes are bifid from C2 to C6, whereas the atlas or C1 lacks a spinous process and C7 has a single spinous process.

The atlas or first cervical vertebra consists of an anterior and posterior arch with articular fovea cephalad and caudad. The atlantooccipital joint, formed by the articulation between the atlas and occipital condyles, is stabilized by a lateral ligament and posterior atlantooccipital membranes. The anterior arch of C1 provides articulation, with the dens supported by the transverse or cruciform ligament forming the atlantoaxial articulation. The tectorial membrane extends from the anterior foramen magnum to the posterior surface of the axis. The axial and alar ligaments join the foramen magnum and dens. The articular surfaces between the atlantooccipital and atlantoaxial articulations are horizontal, and without these strong ligamentous structures the articulation would be a very unstable configuration.

The axis or second cervical vertebra is composed of a much thicker lamina with a longer spinous process. The superior articular surface of the axis forms the atlantoaxial articulation with the inferior articular fovea of the atlas. The inferior articular process of the axis is similar to the remaining cervical vertebrae.

From C2 to T1, the zygapophyseal articulations form a shingled configuration inferiorly and posteriorly. The transverse processes contain the foramen tranversarium, which allows passage of the vertebral artery, veins, and nerve. The cervical vertebral canal varies in shape from oval in the upper portion to triangular in the lower portion. As in other regions of the spine, the canal is bound by the vertebral bodies and intervertebral discs anteriorly, and lamina and ligamentum flava posterolaterally. The anterior and posterior longitudinal, intertransverse, interspinous and supraspinous, and nuchae ligaments all add additional support to the cervical articulations.

Anatomical landmarks of the anterior neck that correspond to cervical spine level include the following: hard palate, arch of the atlas; inferior border of the mandible, C2/C3; hyoid bone, C3, thyroid cartilage, C4/C5; cricoid cartilage, C6; and carotid tubercle, C6. Using these consistent bony landmarks, anterolateral incisions may be planned for the exposure of the desired level (Fig. 7.8).

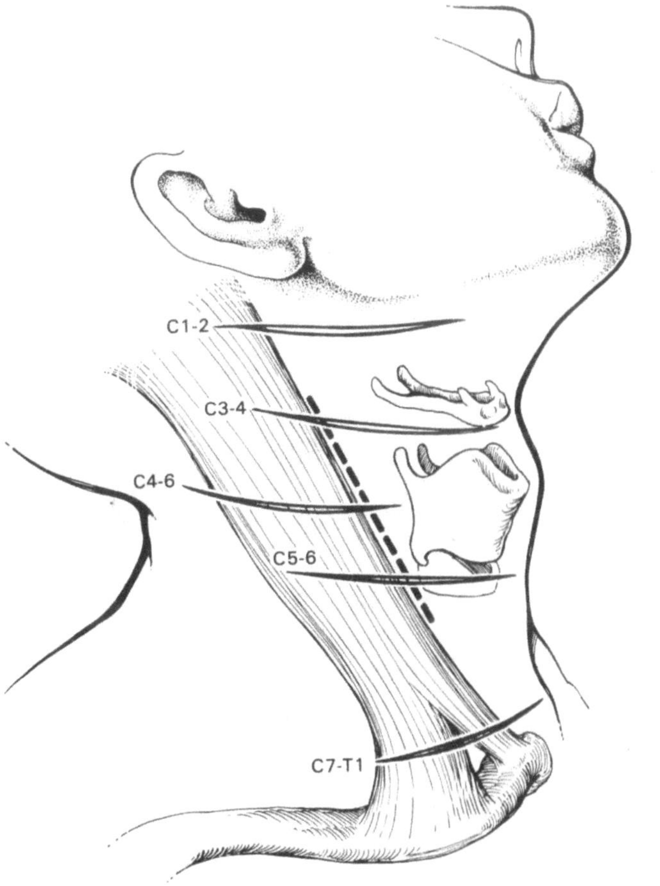

Figure 7.8. Topographical anatomy of cervical spine. Cosmetic transverse incision from anterior border of sternocleidomastoid to midline will allow adequate exposure of three vertebral bodies and two disc levels. Extensive vertical incision (*dotted line*) along anterior border of sternocleidomastoid allows longer exposures of cervical spine.

Cervical Myology

The most superficial posterior paracervical layer is the trapezius, which originates from the superior nuchal line and all cervical spinous processes (Fig. 7.9). The intermediate layer consists of the splenius capitus, extending from the occipital bone to the spinous processes of C7 to T3. The deep layer consists of the semispinalis capitus and cervicis, longissimus capitus, and the levator scapulae. The semispinalis capitus is the most superficial, extending from its origin at the cervical transverse processes to insertion in the occipital bone. The semispinalis cervicis originates in the upper thoracic transverse processes and inserts into the cervical inner spinous region. The longissimus capitus and levator scapulae are located at the level of the neuroforamen. Muscles around C1 and C2 (nuchal region) include the rectus capitus major (C2 spinous process to occipital bone), rectus capitis minor (C1 to occipital bone), obliques capitis inferior (spinous process of C2 to transverse process of C1), and obliques capitis superior (tubercle of C1 to occipital bone) (Fig. 7.10).

In the upper anterior cervical spine, the craniovertebral junction is surrounded by the buccal region anteriorly and the vertebral canal superiorly. The buccal cavity allows

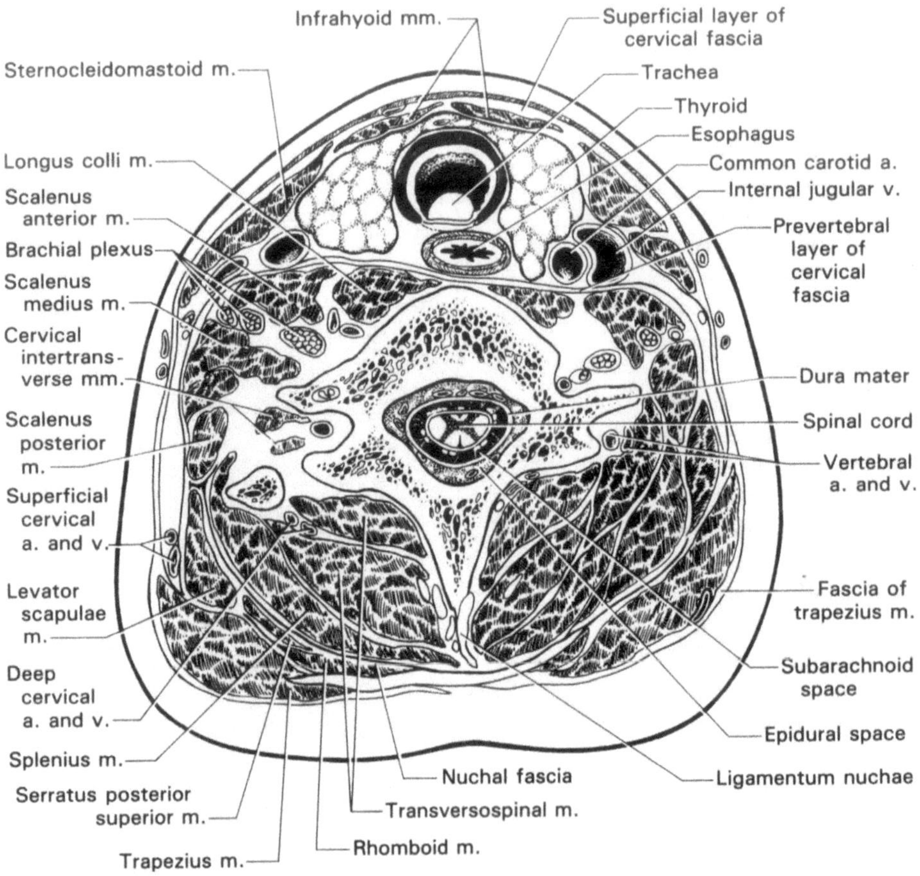

Figure 7.9. Cross section of neck at C_6.

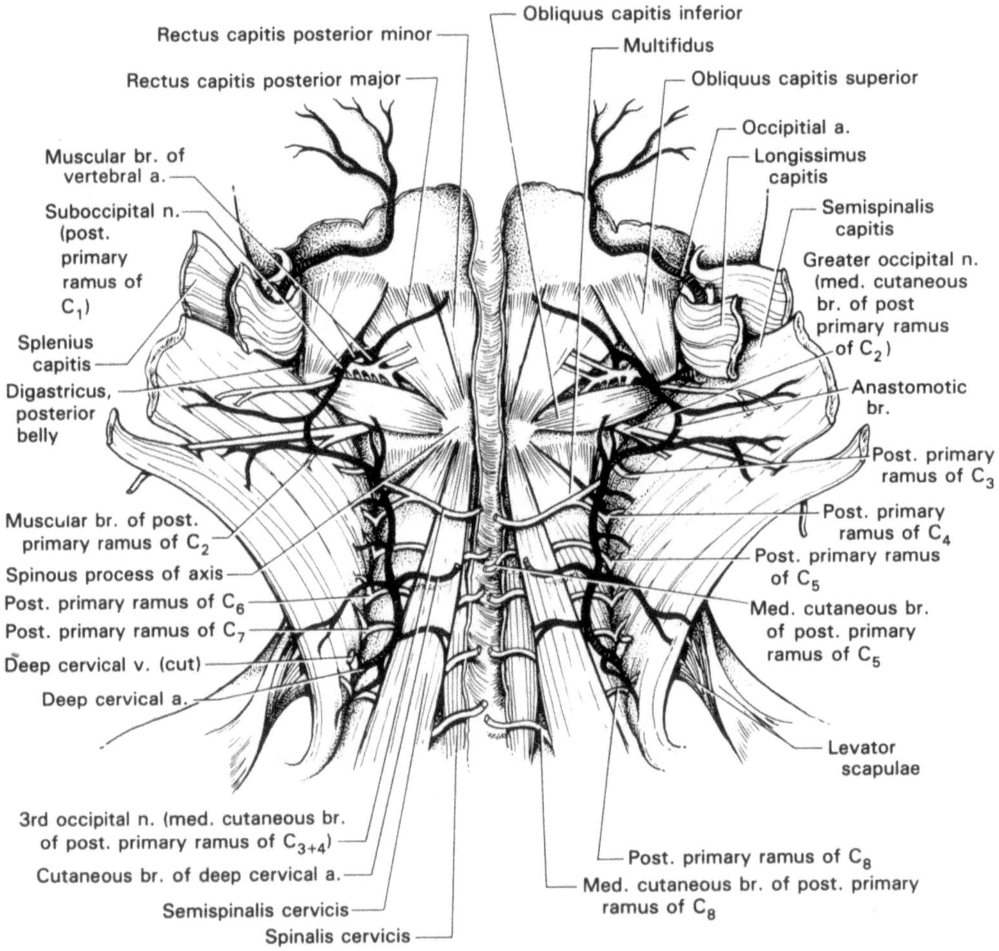

Figure 7.10. Nuchal region.

Figure 7.11. Cervical myology.

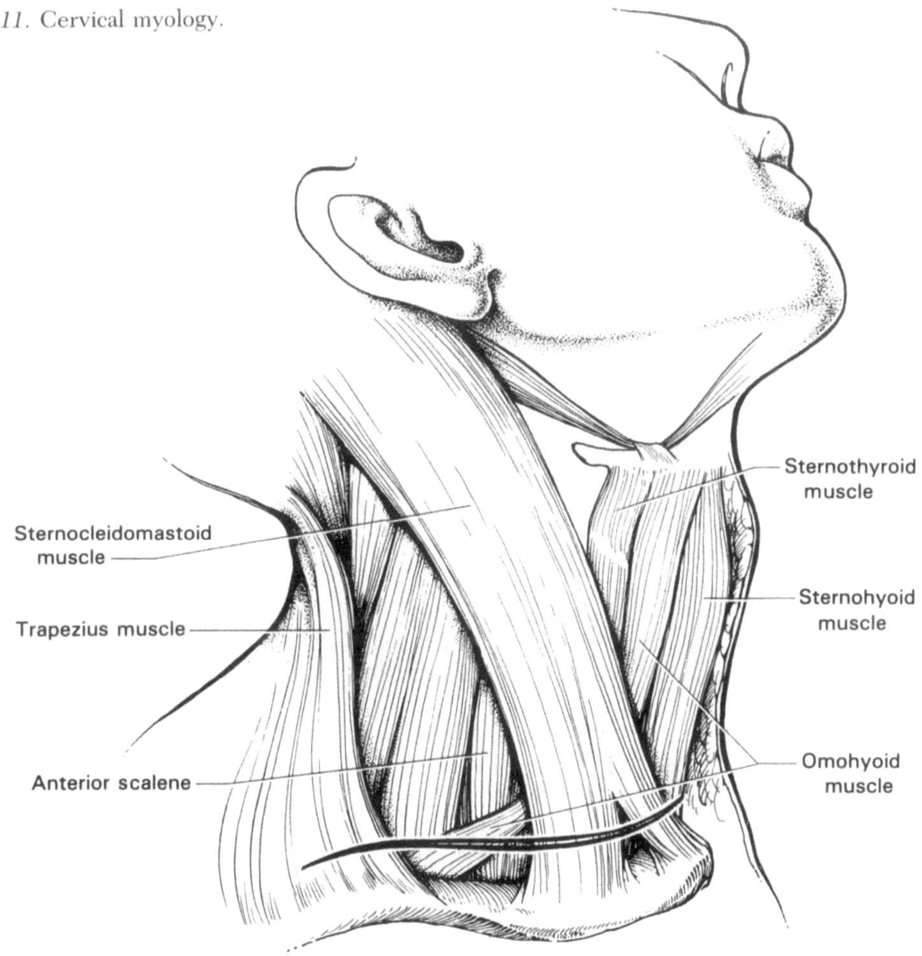

access to the atlas, axis, and upper half of C3. At this level, the pharynx and prevertebral muscles (rectus capitus, anterior and lateralis longus colli, and longus capitus) overlie the cervical spine.

The anterior anatomy of the neck can be divided into layers and triangles (Fig. 7.11). The most superficial layer deep to the skin in the subcutaneous tissue is the platysma muscle. Its fibers extend from the mandible to the clavicle. The superficial cervical fascia deep to the platysma surrounds the neck and envelops the sternocleidomastoid and trapezius muscles. Deep to this fascial layer are the anterior and posterior cervical triangles. The boundaries of the anterior triangle are the sternocleidomastoid, inferior mandibular margin, and median line of the neck. It is further subdivided into the submandibular triangle (bordered inferiorly by the digastric muscle), the submental triangle (bounded by the body of the hyoid bone and the anterior belly of the digastric muscle on each side), the carotid triangle (bordered by the superior belly of the omohyoid muscle, digastric muscle, and sternocleidomastoid muscle), and muscular triangle (bounded by the superior border of the omohyoid, the anterior border of the sternocleidomastoid, and the anterior median line of the neck). The posterior triangle is delineated by the trapezius muscle, the sternocleidomastoid muscle, and the middle third of the clavicle.

The pretracheal fascia surrounds the strap muscles and is continuous with the carotid sheath at its lateral margin. The strap muscles in the infrahyoid region include the sternohyoid, the omohyoid, thyrohyoid, cricothyroid, and sternothyroid muscles. The digastric and stylohyoid muscles in the suprahyoid region. The prevertebral fascia is the deepest layer and envelops the scalenus and longus colli muscles. Deep to the prevertebral fascia is the anterior longitudinal ligament of the cervical spine.

Neurovascular Structures of the Cervical Spine

The vascular structures of the posterior cervical spine include the vertebral arteries, occipital artery and vein, cervicalis profundo and ascendens, descending scapular artery, posterior jugular vein, and azygos cervical vein.

The vertebral artery is the first branch off the subclavian artery and ascends through the foramen transversarium of the sixth cervical vertebra. At the atlantooccipital joint, the vertebral artery lies posterior and enters the vertebral

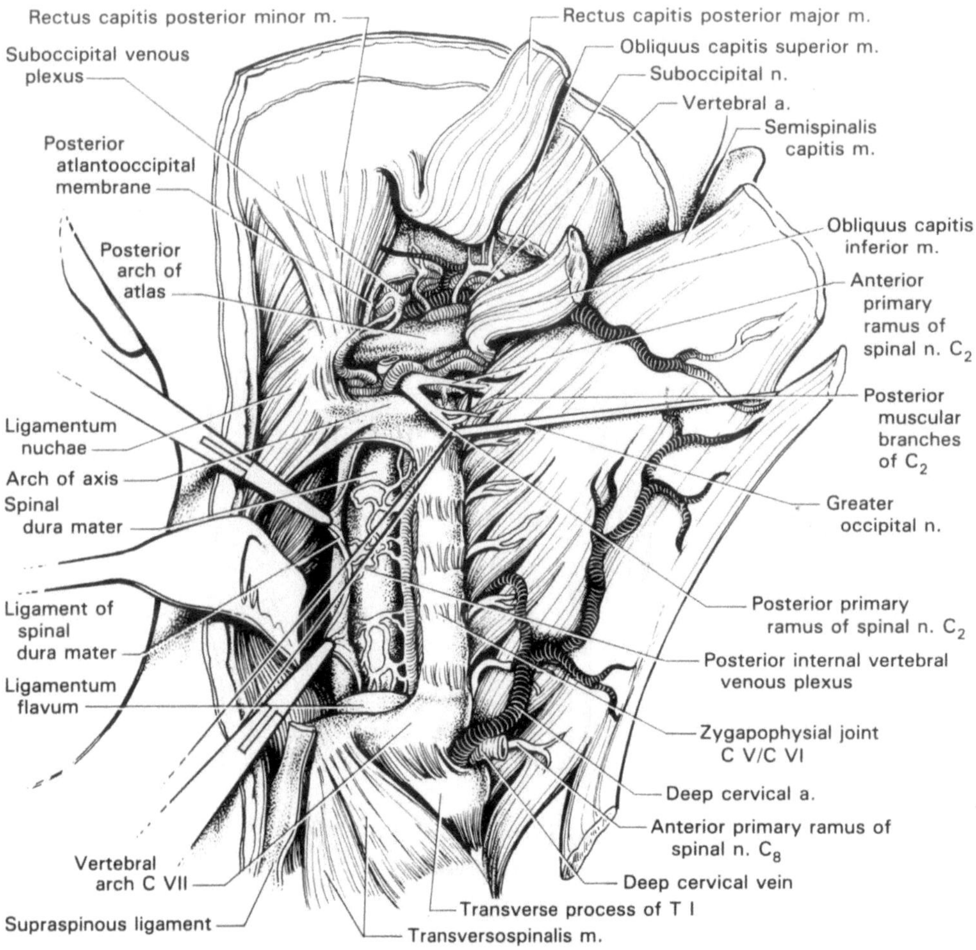

Figure 7.12. Suboccipital region and cervical spinal canal.

canal at the superior margin of the atlas. The occipital artery arises from the external carotid and ascends between the lateral tubercle of the atlas and mastoid. The cervical artery ascends along the posterior articulations of the cervical vertebrae. The major veins include the posterior jugular, descending along the cervical laminae, and the cervical azygos vein, descending along the spinous processes.

The neural structures of the posterior cervical spine exit intervertebral foramen with the exceptions of the C1 and C2 nerves. The C1 or the suboccipital nerve exits at the level of the C1 vertebra and innervates muscles of the suboccipital triangle, which include the obliques capitus inferior and superior and the rectus major. The C2 or greater occipital nerve exits inferior to the obliques capitus inferior muscle to ascend through the semispinalis capitus (Fig. 7.12). The remaining cervical nerves exit the intervertebral foramen and pass lateral to the posterior articular masses.

Neurovascular anatomy in the anterior cervical region can be subdivided into structures found in the anterior and posterior triangles (Fig. 7.13). In the posterior triangle, the external jugular vein crosses the sternocleidomastoid muscle and descends into the fascia to drain into the brachiocephalic vein. The great auricular nerve extends along the sternomastoid with the external jugular vein. The accessory nerve innervates the sternocleidomastoid and trapezius muscles. Other motor nerves, which are named by the muscles they innervate, are deep to the fascia of the posterior triangle and innervate the levator scapula, rhomboids, and serratus anterior. The transverse cervical artery, arising from the thyrocervical trunk or the second branch of the subclavian artery, transverses the base of the posterior triangle across the brachial plexus. More anterior to the sternocleidomastoid lies the internal jugular vein, along with the phrenic nerve that is deep to the fascia.

Medial to the internal jugular vein in the anterior triangle is the common carotid artery with its internal and external branches. The superior thyroid artery, the first branch from the external carotid artery, passes deep to the sternothyroid muscle supplying the thyroid gland. The lingual artery, the second branch of the external carotid artery, passes deep to the digastric and stylohyoid muscles.

Major neural structures in the anterior triangle are the vagus nerve, ansa cervicalis, hypoglossal nerve, and supe-

Figure 7.13. Neurovascular anatomy in anterior cervical region.

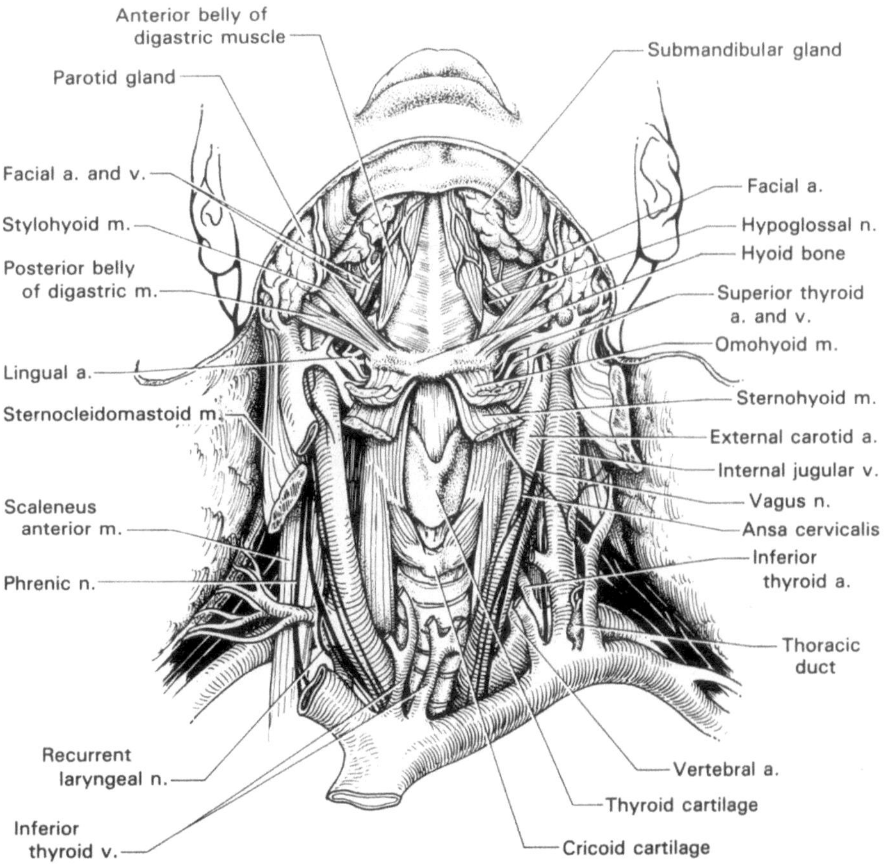

rior laryngeal nerve. The vagus nerve lies between the carotid artery and internal jugular vein, giving off the recurrent laryngeal nerve supplying the larynx and a major branch to the heart. The superior laryngeal nerve, also arising from the vagus, gives sensory input to the larynx and base of the tongue and somatic fibers to the cricothyroid muscle and lower esophageal constrictor (cricopharyngeus muscle). The hypoglossal nerve passes superior to the greater horn of the hyoid bone to supply extrinsic muscles of the tongue. The ansa cervicalis arises from the hypoglossal nerve and traverses superficial to the carotid arteries to supply the infrahyoid muscles.

Major structures at the base of the anterior neck include the sympathetic chain and thoracic duct. The sympathetic chain is posterior to the common carotid artery outside the sheath. It traverses the prevertebral fascia forming the superior cervical ganglion (C1), the middle cervical ganglion (C6) just anterior to the inferior thyroid artery, the vertebral ganglion (C7) adjacent to the thoracic duct, and the cervicothoracic (stellate) ganglion (T1), which is posterior to the vertebral artery. The thoracic duct lies posterior to the esophagus and drains into the left subclavian vein.

Surgical Approaches to the Cervical Spine (Fig. 7.14)

Transoral Approach to the Cervical Spine

The transoral approach to C1 and C2 has been described by various authors[26,27,28] (Fig. 7.15). This approach may be indicated for infections or tumors involving the anterior aspect of C1 or C2.

The transoral approach begins with the neck in hyperextension under endotracheal anesthesia via tracheostomy. A gag is placed in the mouth. The uvula and soft palate is reflected on itself and sutured. The incision is extended approximately 5 cm beginning 1 cm below the anterior tubercle of the atlas. The dissection is carried down to bone and the soft tissues are elevated away from the midline. Stay sutures are then placed. This allows exposure to the lateral masses of the atlas and axis. It is important to note that the incision should not be extended too low to avoid difficulty with closure. In addition, exposure beyond the lateral masses risks injury to the vertebral vessels. The closure is usually done with absorbable suture, and should include the anterior longitudinal ligament, buccopharyngeal fascia, constrictor muscles, and pharyngeal mucosa.

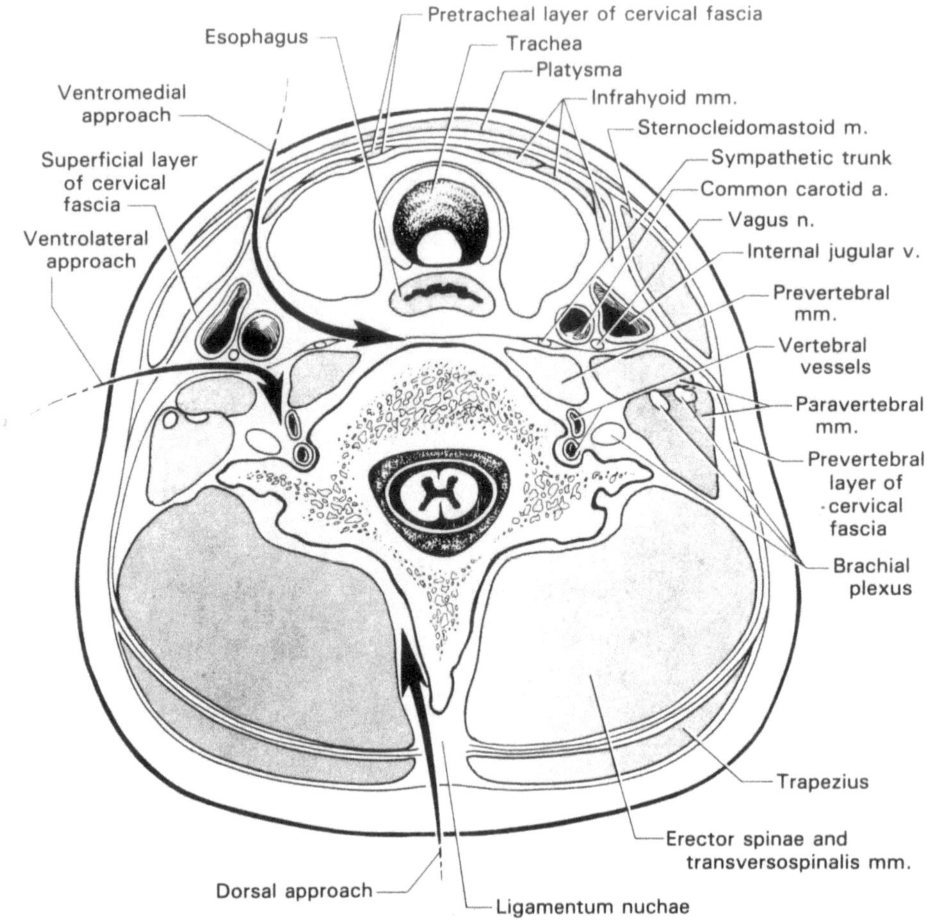

Figure 7.14. Surgical approaches to cervical spine.

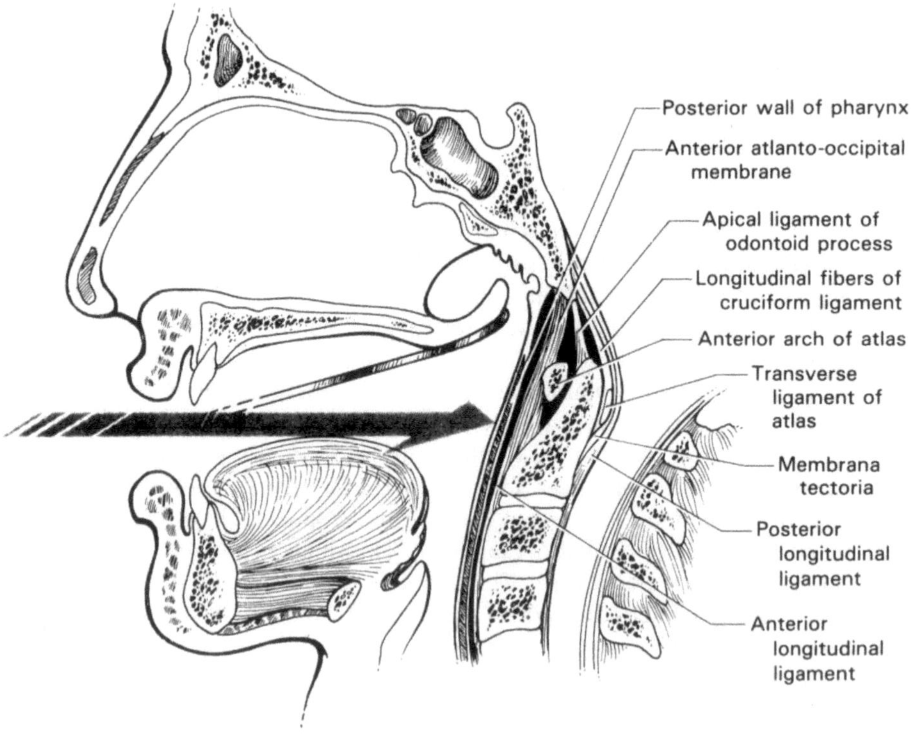

Figure 7.15. Transoral approach to cervical spine.

Figure 7.16. Anterior medial approach to cervical spine.

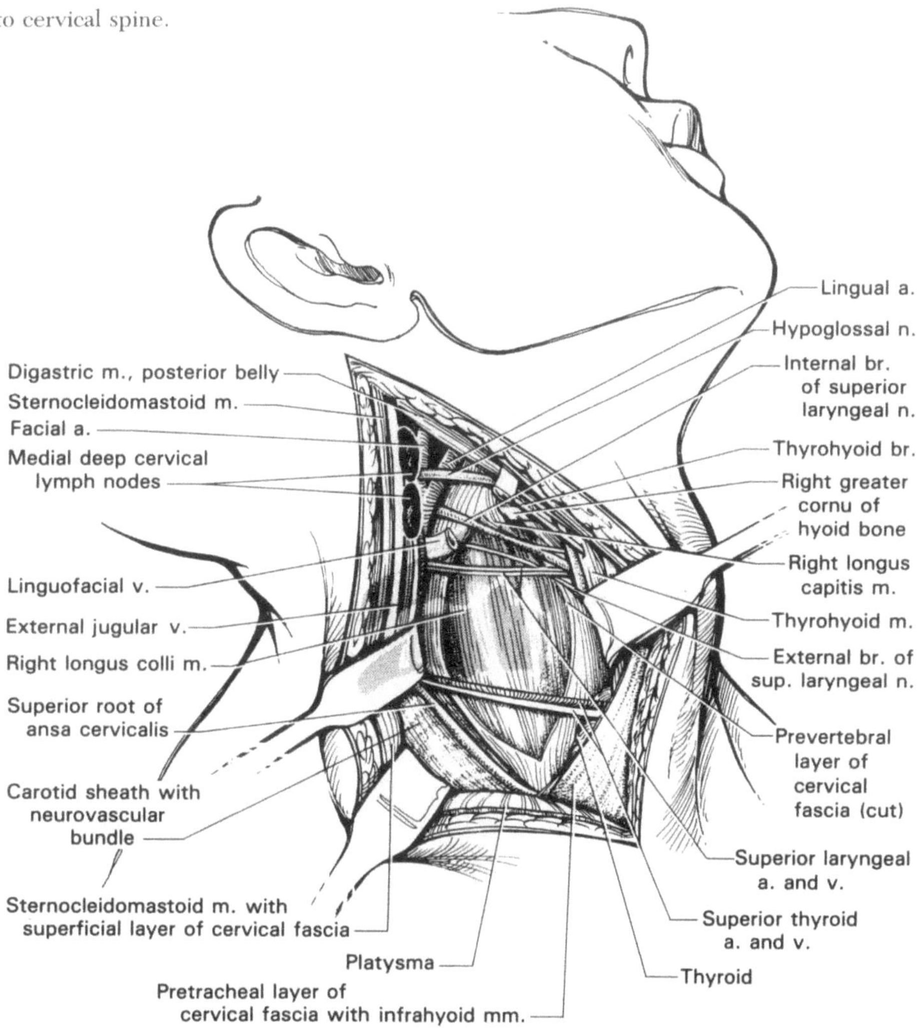

Possible complications with the transoral approach include infection, nasal-toned voice, injury to vertebral vessels, and injury to the internal carotid if stay sutures are placed too deep in the pharyngeal wall.

Anterior Medial Approach to the Cervical Spine

The anterior medial approach allows exposure of the upper and midcervical spine (Fig. 7.16). Numerous authors, including Southwick and Robinson,[26] Bailey and Badgley,[29] and Riley[30] have described this approach, which has been used for excision of herniated disc(s), interbody fusion(s), tumors, osteomyelitis, fractures, and other midcervical pathology.

The technique is described with a transverse or longitudinal skin excision. Bailey and Badgley prefer a right-sided approach and exposure of the recurrent laryngeal nerve as it crosses the neck at the level of the seventh cervical vertebra. Southwick and Robinson recommend the left-sided approach as the nerve lies in the tracheoesophageal groove and does not need to be exposed. If the transverse incision is chosen, the incision is made in the skin crease in the midline across the sternocleidomastoid muscle. The longitudinal incision extends from two finger breadths below the mastoid process along the anterior sternocleidomastoid border to the sternum. The platysma is split along its fibers, and the superficial fascia is incised along the anterior border of the sternocleidomastoid muscle.

By approaching the spine anterior to the sternocleidomastoid, any level between C1 and T2 may be exposed. This allows exposure of the carotid sheath and its contents, which are retracted laterally, as is the sternocleidomastoid muscle. The omohyoid muscle may be retracted or transected for better exposure. The carotid tubercle serves as a landmark for the C6 level. The middle thyroid vein superficial to the middle cervical fascia is ligated. The esophagus, trachea, and thyroid gland are retracted medially to further expose prevertebral fascia and underlying longus colli muscle. The inferior thyroid artery and vein at the C6–C7 level are retracted for more distal exposure, and the superior thyroid artery and vein and superior

Figure 7.17. Carotid triangle.

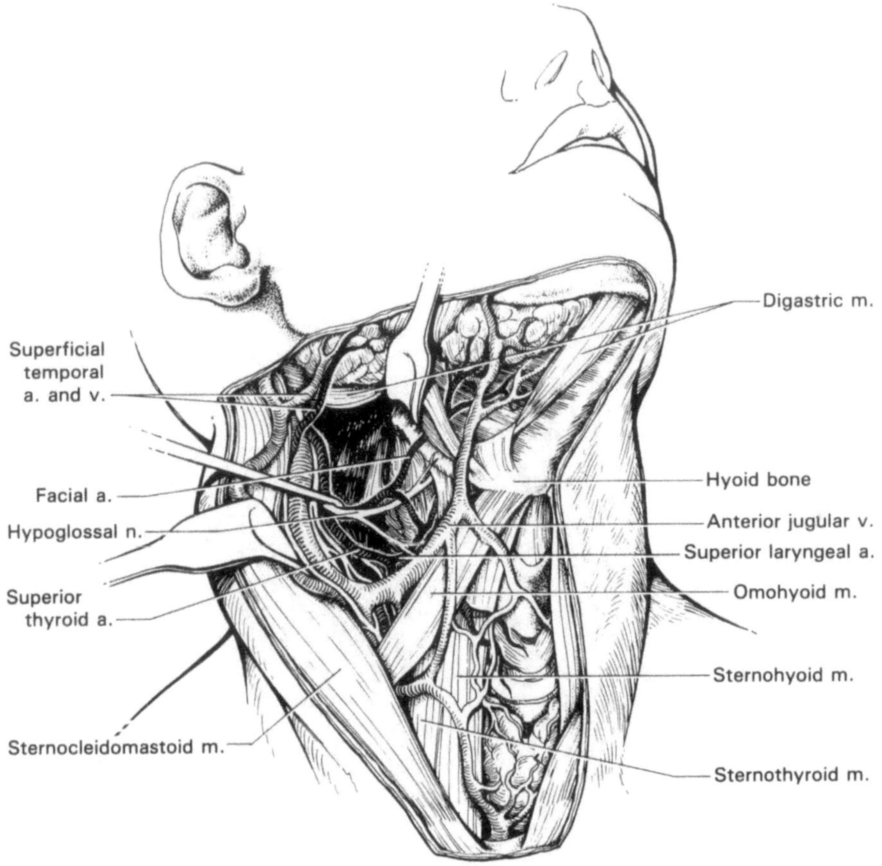

laryngeal nerve at C3–C4 level are retracted for cephalad exposure. The prevertebral fascia and longus colli muscle are split and elevated to expose the anterior longitudinal ligament and underlying vertebral body and intervertebral disc.

Potential complications in this approach include esophageal perforation, Horner's syndrome secondary to sympathetic chain damage, thyroid vessel damage, postoperative hoarseness caused by injury to the superior or recurrent laryngeal nerve, and vertebral artery perforation.

Anteromedial Approach to C1–C2–C3

The anteromedial approach to the upper cervical spine has been described by De Andrade and Macnab[31] in its use for occipital cervical fusion. The procedure is indicated for patients who have an unstable spine and cannot undergo a posterior fusion because of previous laminectomy. although this approach is limited by the complex anatomy, it may be used in drainage of infection and anterior fusion.

The surgical approach is usually made on the right or left side by a transverse skin incision made one-finger breadth below the mandible extending posteriorly to the mastoid process. The platysma is incised the length of the incision to expose the carotid triangle (Fig. 7.17). This triangle is bounded superiorly by the posterior belly of the digastric muscle, posteriorly by the sternocleidomastoid, and inferiorly by the omohyoid muscle. It should be noted that branches of the ansa cervicalis (greater auricular nerve and anterior cervical nerve) cross the proximal portion of the sternocleidomastoid muscle and should be spared. Important neurovascular structure in this carotid triangle include the hypoglossal nerve, lingual artery, facial artery, superior thyroid artery, and carotid artery. These structures pass from lateral to medial within the middle cervical fascia.

The dissection is carried out bluntly to expose the plane between the carotid sheath and its contents laterally and the strap muscles medially. Further exposure allows identification of the hypoglossal nerve, which lies superficial to the lingual and facial arteries. The hypoglossal nerve is retracted cephalad and the lingual and facial arteries may be ligated. The superior thyroid artery, branching off the external carotid artery, and the superior thyroid vein are retracted caudad. The superior laryngeal nerve is also retracted caudad. Blunt dissection is continued in the retropharyngeal space to the prevertebral fascia and longus colli muscle, which is elevated to expose the atlantoaxial joint, and, more cephalad, the basiocciput. The wound closure should not include deep sutures, but only those in the platysma and skin.

This approach is potentially fraught with multiple complications. The complications in the original report noted temporary hoarseness and permanent inability to shout

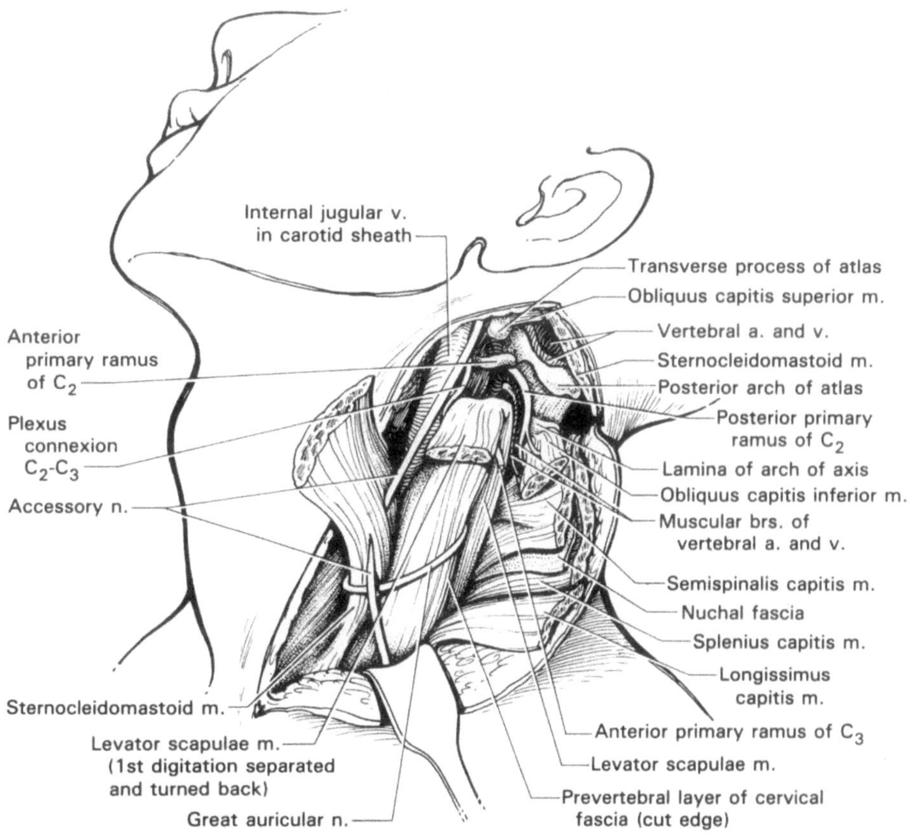

Figure 7.18. Anterolateral approach to atlas (C1) and axis (C2).

or sing high notes in all patients, probably because of recurrent laryngeal nerve injury.

Anterolateral Approach to the Upper Cervical Spine, C1–C2–C3

The anterolateral approach to the upper cervical spine was described by Whitesides and Kelly[32] and Whitesides and McDonald.[33] This approach was similar to that described by Henry[34] for exposure of the vertebral artery.

Whitesides described the anterolateral approach for C1 and C2 fusion in a patient with progressive kyphosis whose head could not be extended nor rotated because of a previous posterior cervical fusion. This approach has also been used for post traumatic instability, os odontoideum, rheumatoid arthritis and tumors of the upper cervical spine.

In preparing for the approach, the patient is supine with the head in skeletal traction. A curvilinear transverse skin incision is made from the mastoid process along the anterior sternocleidomastoid border. The greater auricular nerve and other cutaneous sensory nerves may be retracted or sacrificed if necessary. The sternocleidomastoid and splenius capitus muscle is detached from the mastoid process leaving a fascial edge for later repair (Fig. 7.18). This allows exposure of the major structures exiting the jugular foramen, which include the spinal accessory nerve (cranial nerve XI), vagus nerve (cranial nerve X), glossopharyngeal nerve (cranial nerve IX), and hypoglossal nerve (cranial nerve XII) (Fig. 7.19). The spinal (XI) accessory nerve courses laterally to enter the sternocleidomastoid muscle two finger breadths inferior to the mastoid process. The facial nerve exits the stylomastoid foramen between the mastoid and styloid process. Bony landmarks comparable in the vicinity are the transverse processes of C1 and C2 and the anterior tubercle of C2. Careful dissection of the spinal accessory nerve allows further retraction of the sternocleidomastoid muscle laterally. The carotid sheath, internal jugular vein, hypoglossal nerve, and vagus nerve are retracted medially. Blunt dissection in the retropharyngeal space allows exposure of the prevertebral fascia and anterior longitudinal ligament, which are incised in the midline for the exposure of C1, C2, and C3. Wound closure should be done over a drain in separate layers for the platysma, subcutaneous tissue, and skin.

Like the anteromedial approach, problems with retropharyngeal edema and subsequent airway obstruction can be avoided by tracheostomy. Other complications may include vascular or neural injury, although the incidence of infection is much less than with the transoral approach.

Lateral Approach to the Cervical Spine (Verbiest)

Verbiest[35,36] described his experience with the lateral approach to the cervical spine. Indications included bony

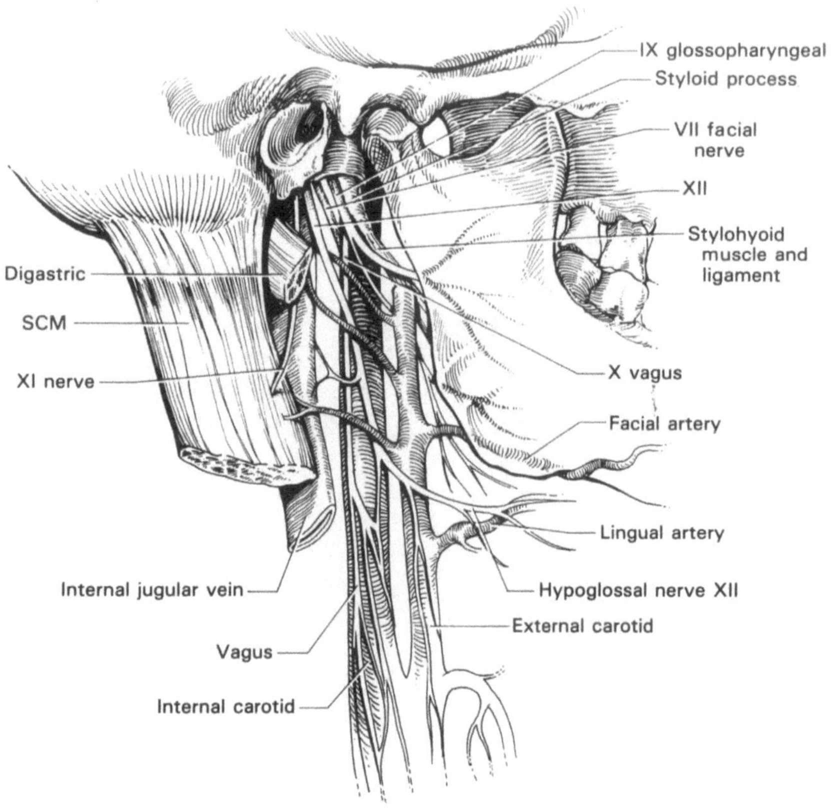

Figure 7.19. Jugular foramen.

spur, nerve root or vertebral body compression, lateral disc herniation, traction brachial plexopathy, and traumatic deformities of the cervical spine. The primary advantage of the lateral approach is that it allows visualization of the cervical nerve root.

A transverse or longitudinal skin incision is used, depending on the number of cervical levels of exposure desired. To expose C3, C4, and C5, the transverse incision is extended from the cricoid cartilage to the anterior sternocleidomastoid border. This incision may be made more caudad for exposure of C6 and C7. The longitudinal incision along the anterior sternocleidomastoid border allows exposure of multiple levels (Fig. 7.20).

The platysma is split the length of the incision. The superficial fascia surrounding the sternocleidomastoid muscle is incised to expose the anterior border. The interval between the sternocleidomastoid muscle and the strap muscles is then developed. The carotid sheath and its contents are palpated and retracted laterally with the sternocleidomastoid. The middle cervical fascia is bluntly dissected to further develop the interval and allows retraction of the strap muscles, esophagus, and trachea medially. The longus colli and longus capitus muscles are exposed by incising the prevertebral fascia in a longitudinal fashion. The sympathetic chain is anterior to the transverse process and is either in the posterior carotid sheath or between the sheath and longus colli in connective tissue. The anterior tubercle of the transverse process and the costotransverse lamellae of the cervical vertebra to be exposed are palpated. The costotransverse lamella is a small nubbin of bone that connects the anterior tubercle to the vertebral body and covers the foramen transversarium that houses the vertebral artery. The vertebral artery medially and cervical nerve root laterally are then exposed by excision of the corresponding costotransverse lamella and anterior tubercle. This excision is done after stripping the longus colli muscle and longus capitus muscle attachments laterally from the anterior tubercle. Bleeding may be noted if there is interruption of the venous plexus surrounding the vertebral artery. This may be controlled by local pressure.

Possible complications from this approach are injury to neural or vascular structures and, as this is a technically demanding procedure, it is rarely indicated.

Lateral Approach to the Cervical Spine (Hodgson)

Hodgson[3] described a lateral approach to C3 through C7 for tuberculosis. Hodgson and associates advocated this approach, which avoids the thyroid vessel, vagus nerve, and superior laryngeal nerve. Because of the manner in which the cervical spine is exposed, Hodgson thought that injury to the cervical cord was less likely using this exposure.

An oblique incision is made on the right side of the neck in the skin crease (Fig. 7.21). This is done inferior to the hyoid bone, and the platysma is split the length of the incision. The posterior third of the sternocleidomas-

Figure 7.20. Lateral approach (Verbiest) to cervical spine.

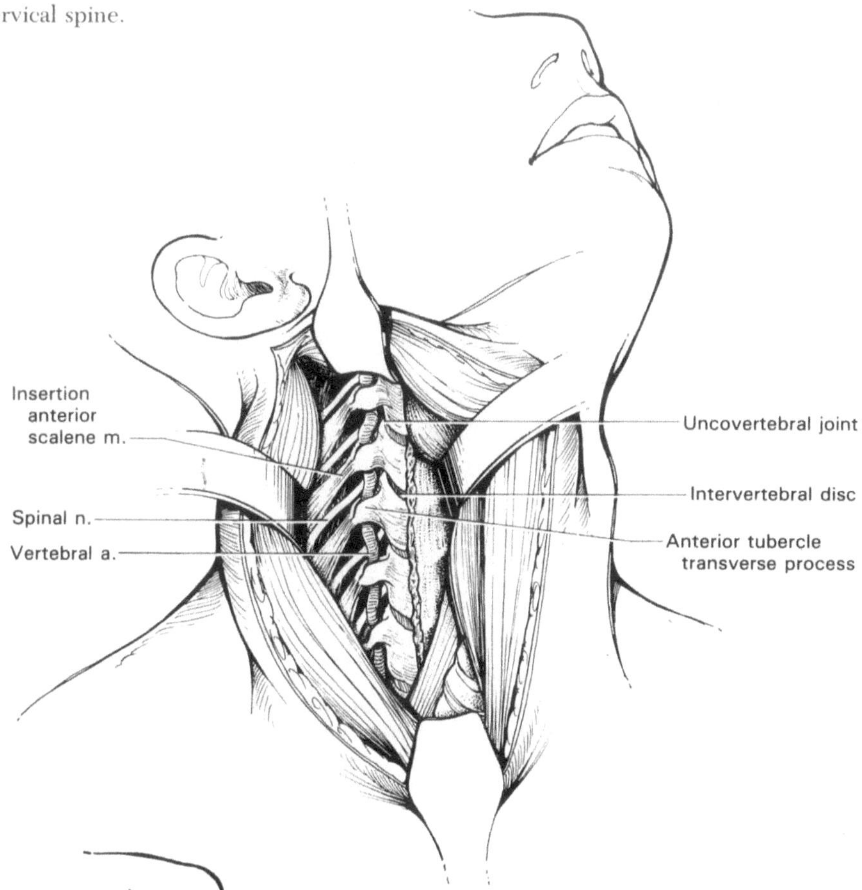

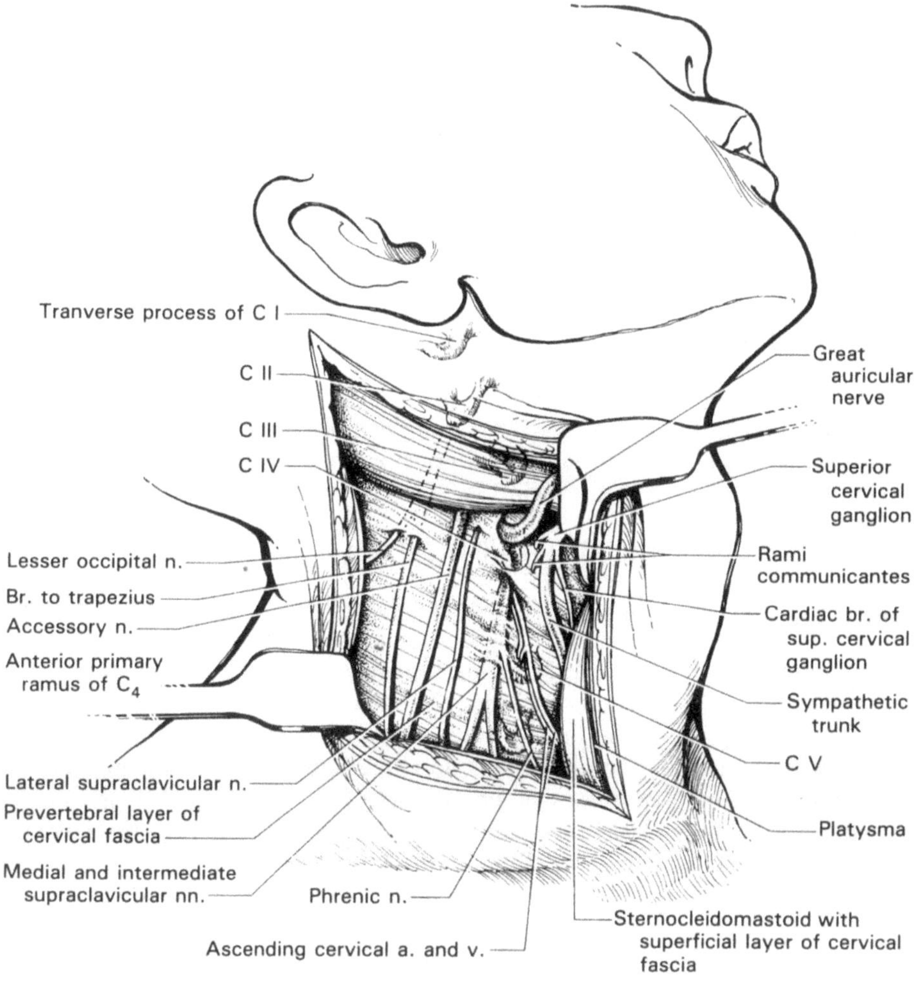

Figure 7.21. Lateral approach (Hodgson) to cervical spine.

toid muscle may be incised to enhance exposure. The external jugular vein is divided if necessary.

The dissection is carried through the posterior triangle fat pad posterior to the carotid sheath and its contents. The cervical sympathetic chain along the prevertebral soft tissue is identified. The carotid sheath, the musculovisceral structures, and the sternocleidomastoid are retracted anteriorly to allow exposure of the spine. The prevertebral fascia and longus colli muscle incised in the midline and the desired cervical level is exposed.

Complications resulting from this approach are similar to those resulting from any other anterior cervical approaches.

Posterior Approach to the Cervical Spine

The midline posterior approach to the cervical spine may be indicated for decompression or stabilization in various pathological conditions. The patient is placed in the prone position with the head in skeletal traction or some other holding device. A midline skin incision is made using the prominent spinous processes of C2, C7, and T1 as bony landmarks. A localizing roentgenogram may be taken as indicated.

The dissection is carried through the subcutaneous tissue and the ligamentum nuchae is incised along the spinous processes. The paraspinous muscles are stripped subperiosteally using the Cobb elevator and/or electrocautery as indicated. The dissection is carried laterally along the lamina, facet joints, and transverse processes if needed. Great care must be taken during the dissection to limit the exposure so a "creeping fusion" will not occur. Also, the articular capsules must not be violated if the level is not to be included in the fused segment. Bleeding may be encountered from segmental arteries between the transverse processes and adjacent facet joints. The vertebral arteries are well protected in the foramen transversarium, although they may be inadvertently injured if pathological bony destruction is present. The indicated surgical procedure is carried out and the wound is closed in layers. Complications resulting from this approach are rare, but bleeding and infection can occur.

Posterior Approach to the Atlas and Axis

The patient is placed in the prone position with the head in traction or some other type of holding device as indicated. A midline skin excision is made from the occiput to the spinous process of C3. The dissection is carried through the subcutaneous tissue and the ligamentum nuchae is incised. Hemostasis is obtained with electrocautery. The paraspinous muscles are elevated subperiosteally along the posterior tubercle of C1 the spinous process of C2 and the base of the skull with the Cobb elevator and/or electrocautery as needed. The dissection is carried away from the midline along the lamina to allow for further exposure of C1 and C2. Caution should be exercised at the atlantooccipital membrane and the groove of C1 where the vertebral artery can be damaged. The indicated surgical procedure may then be carried out, followed by a layered closure.

Thoracic Spine

Bony Morphology of the Thoracic Spine

The thoracic spine, as previously mentioned, contains 12 thoracic vertebra. Those at the midthoracic level have the characteristic features of a thoracic vertebra. The spinous processes are oriented in a vertical shingled fashion. The spinal canal is triangular with nearly equal anterior, posterior, and transverse diameters, with the diameter increasing toward the cervical and lumbar level. The thoracic transverse processes of the upper 10 thoracic vertebrae articulate with the ribs at the anterolateral costal facet and the tubercle of the rib to form the costotransverse articulations (Fig. 7.22). The thoracic vertebral bodies are progressively larger in size from T1 to T12. The vertebral bodies of T1 through T8 have superior and inferior costofovae that articulate with the head of the ribs, whereas the remaining thoracic vertebral bodies have only a superior fovae.

The thoracic spine has variable kyphosis. Each lamina overlaps the more inferior lamina like shingles on a roof. The pedicles arise from the superior aspect of each vertebral body with the intervertebral foramina just inferior to the pedicle.

The following topographical relationship exists between the tip of the thoracic spinous process and thoracic vertebral body:[3]

T1 through T3: Upper half of vertebral body below
T4 through T6: Lower half of vertebral body below
T7 through T9: Upper half of vertebral body below
T10 through T12: Level of intervertebral space below.

Myology of the Thoracic Spine

The posterior muscles of the thoracic spine include superficial and deep extensor muscles. The superficial muscles (Fig. 7.23) include latissimus dorsi, rhomboideus, and serratus posterior. The deeper muscle layer is composed of the erector spinae muscles (Fig. 7.24).

The latissimus dorsi has some origin from the spinous processes of L5 through T6. The rhomboideus muscle arises from the spinous processes of C7 to the spinous processes of T4 and inserts into the scapula. The serratus posterior superior aponeurosis arises from spinous processes of C7 through T3 and inserts on the ribs 2 through 5. The serratus posterior inferior aponeurosis arises from

Figure 7.22. Bony morphology of thoracic spine. **A.** Posterior aspect. **B.** Anterior aspect. **C.** Lateral aspect of costovertebral articulation. **D.** Superior aspect of costovertebral articulation.

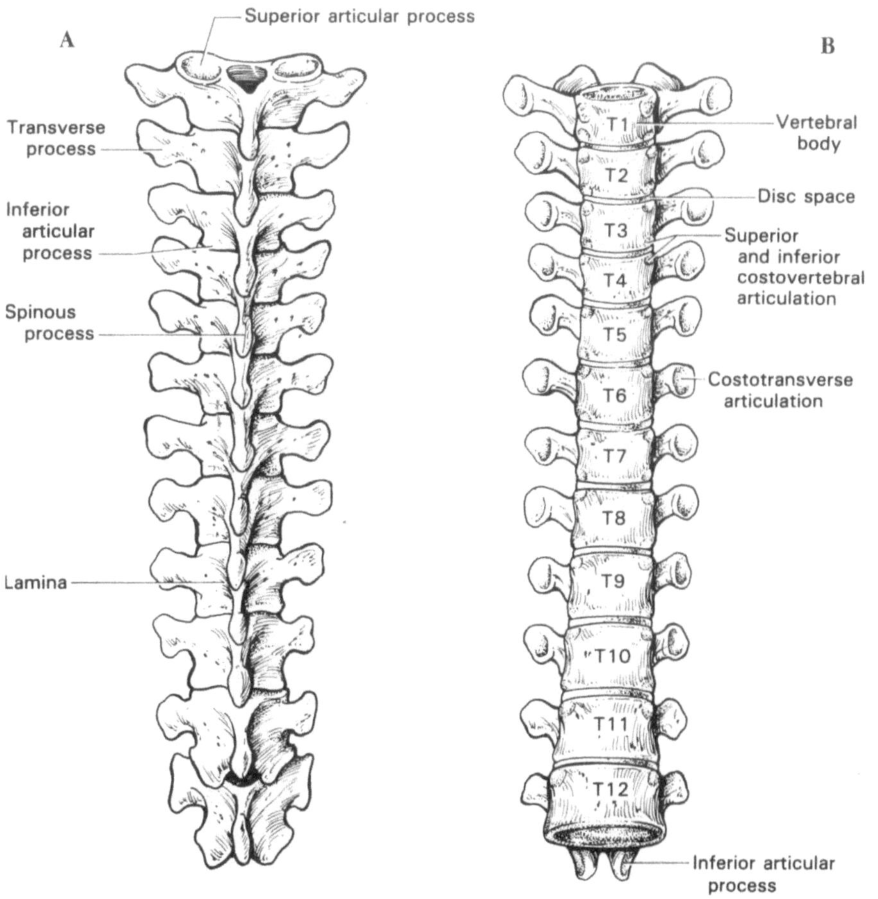

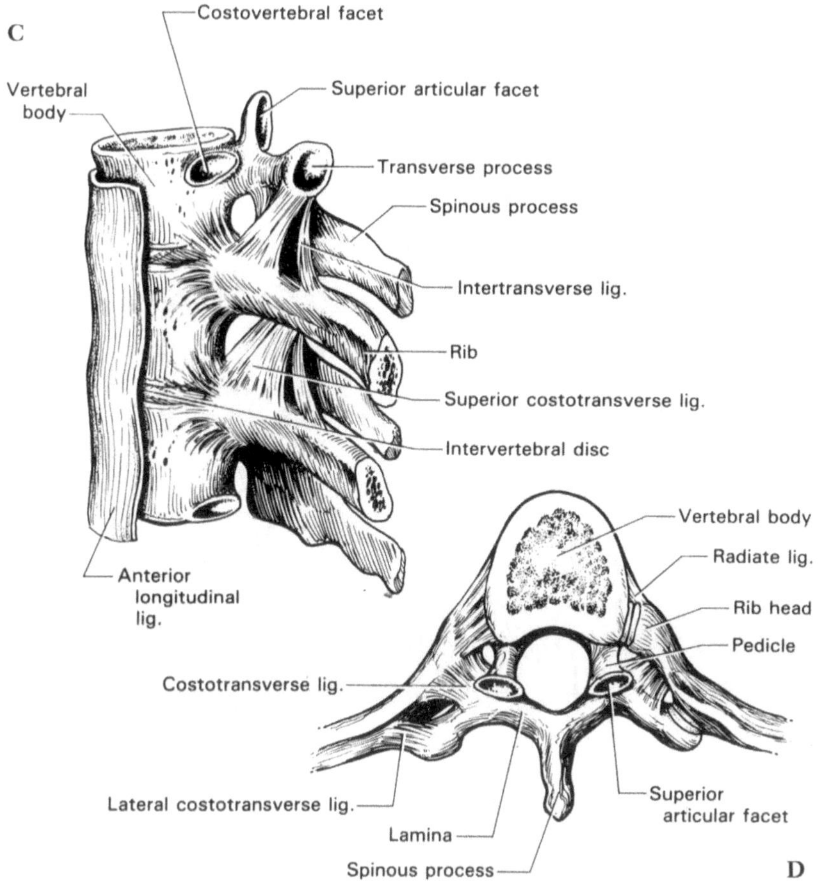

Figure 7.23. Superficial muscles of back.

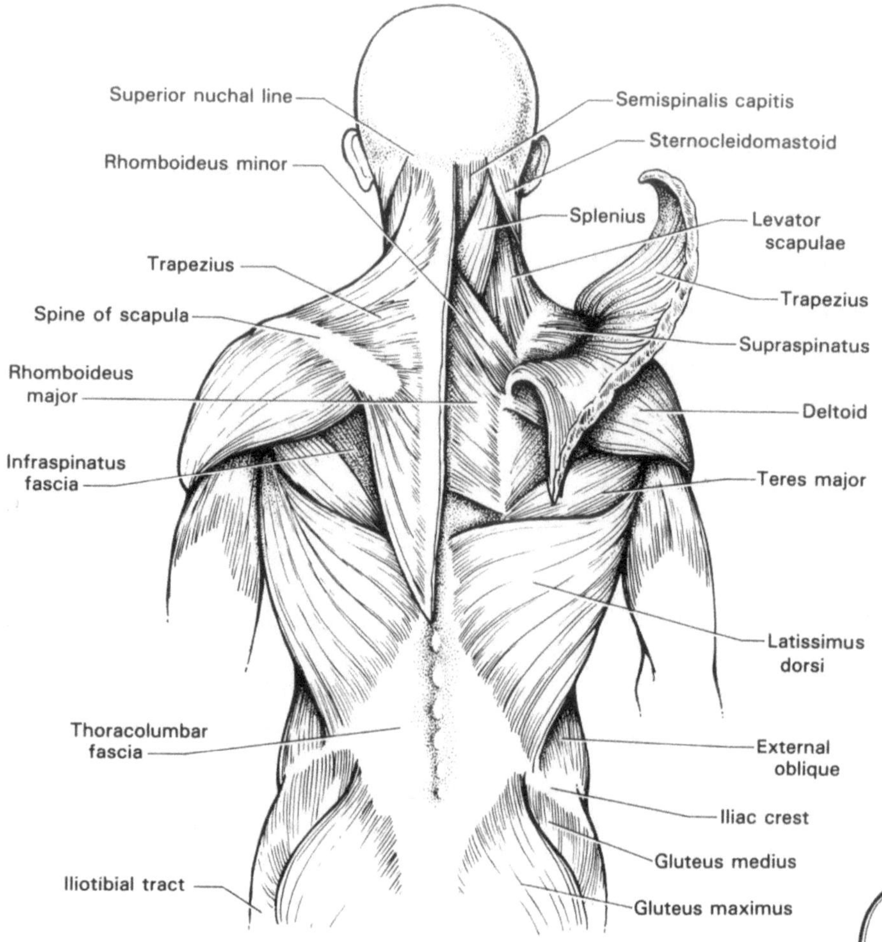

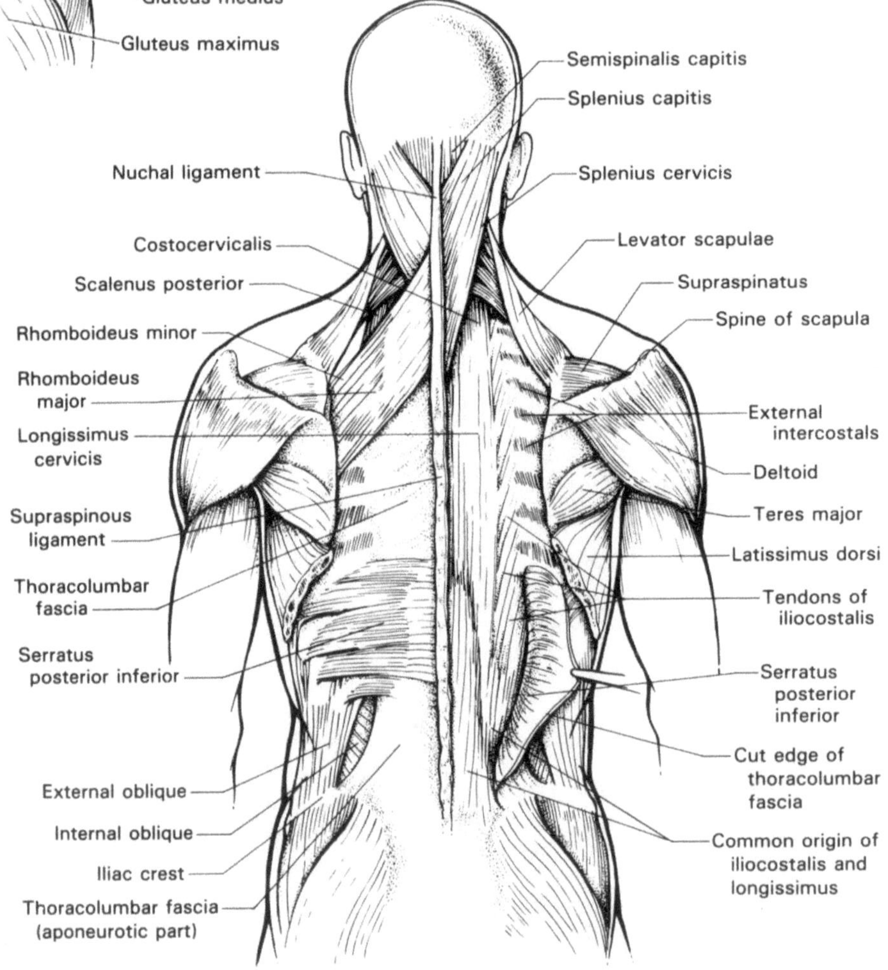

Figure 7.24. Deep muscle layers of back.

Figure 7.25 Cross section of chest wall at T6.

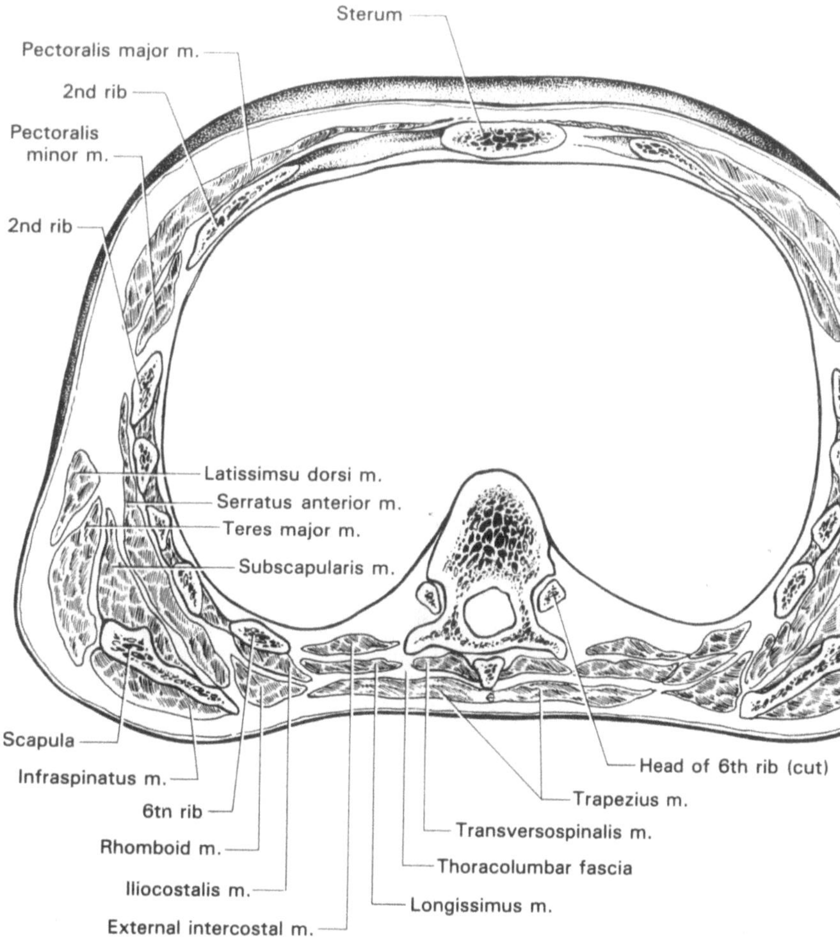

T11 through L2 spinous processes and inserts on ribs 9 through 12.

The erector spinae muscles of the thoracic region include the longissimus thoracis, spinalis thoracis, interspinalis thoracis, transversospinalis, and iliocostalis. Most of these muscles are innervated by the dorsal rami of the spinal nerves. The longissimus thoracis arises from the erector spinae mass and inserts on the transverse processes and ribs of T3 through T12. Medial to the longissimus is the spinalis thoracis, which originates from the spinous processes of T11 through L2 and inserts on spinous processes of the upper four to eight thoracic vertebrae. The interspinalis thoracis are less well developed than those found in the cervical region between the spinous processes. Transversospinalis muscles are found between the spinous processes and the transverse processes. The iliocostalis thoracis is the most lateral portion of the erector spinae muscles, arising from the lower six ribs and inserting into the upper six ribs.

Anatomy of the Thoracic Wall

The anterior thoracic wall includes the mammary layer, superficial muscle, and the intercostal layers. The mammary layer overlies the pectoralis muscles, encompasses the area from the third to the seventh rib. Deep to this is a superficial muscular layer that includes the pectoralis muscles, serratus anterior, and abdominal musculature (rectus abdominis and external oblique). The intercostal region is divided into the external intercostal muscle, fibrocellular layer, middle intercostal muscle, middle intermuscle cellular tissue, and internal intercostal muscles (Fig. 7.25). The neurovascular bundle lies uder the costal groove between the internal and middle intercostal muscles.

The lateral thoracic wall musculature is bounded by the latissimus dorsi posteriorly and pectoralis major anteriorly. The fibers of the serratus anterior interdigitate with the external oblique muscle fibers. The intercostal layers are similar to that described for the anterior thoracic wall.

In the posterior thoracic wall, the musculature deep to the skin and subcutaneous tissue includes three primary layers. The trapezius and latissimus dorsi are the most superficial. The rhomboid major and minor muscles and

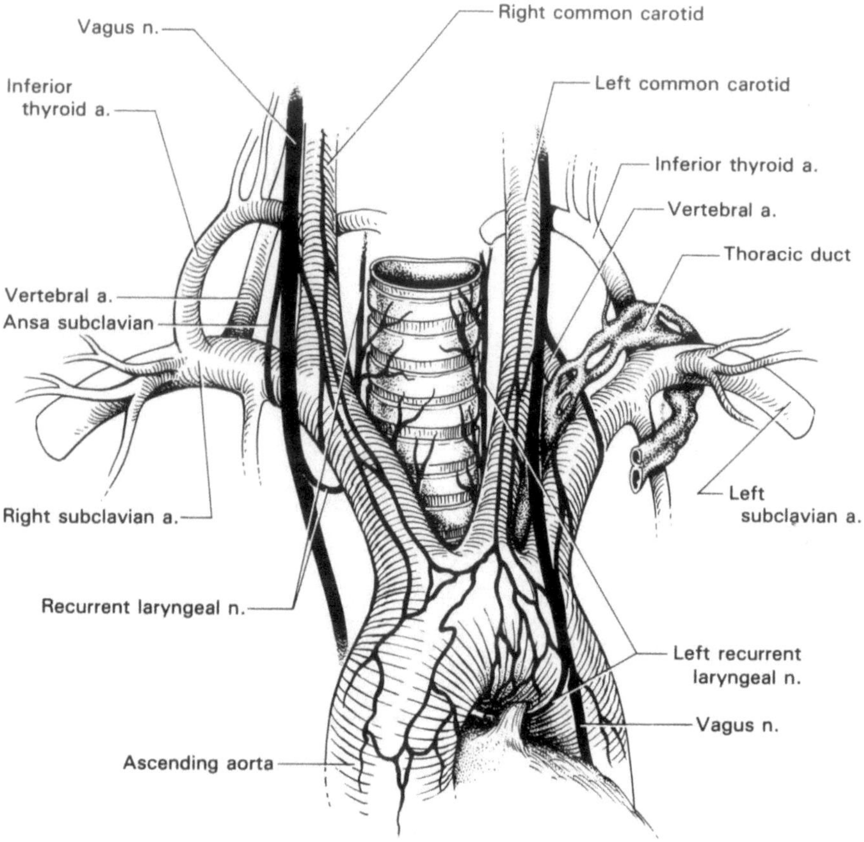

Figure 7.26. Nerurovascular structures of anterior cervicothoracic region.

the erector spinae muscles form the middle layer. The intercostal layers form the deep portion of the posterior thoracic wall.

Neurovascular Anatomy of the Thoracic Spine

The anterior cervicothoracic region has numerous important neural and vascular elements (Fig. 7.26). The aortic arch and the superior vena cava give off many branches in this region. The brachiocephalic trunk gives off the right common carotid and the right subcvlavian arteries, and on the left, these arteries arise from the aortic arch. The right and left subclavian veins and the right and left internal jugular veins drain into the right and left brachiocephalic trunks, respectively. The right and left internal thoracic arteries branch off the subclavian arteries and descend along the sternal margin.

The major neural structures in the region are the vagus, phrenic, and recurrent laryngeal nerves. The right vagus lies anterior to the right subclavian artery and gives off the right recurrent laryngeal nerve, which ascends adjacent to the trachea. The left vagus nerve descends along the left carotid artery. Anterior to the aortic arch, the left vagus nerve gives off the left recurrent laryngeal nerve at the ligamentum anteriosum. The phrenic nerves descend along the superior vena cava on the right and the aortic arch on the left.

In the upper thoracic prevertebral region, branches of the thyrocervical arterial trunk run toward the anterior vertebral bodies of T2 and T3. The costocervical trunk in the paravertebral region anastomose with the intercostal vessels. The intercostal veins drain into the azygos vein on the right and the hemiazygos vein on the left. The thoracic duct ascends along the left upper thoracic vertebral bodies and eventually drains into the left subclavian vein and brachiocephalic trunk.[38] The important neural structures in this area include the sympathetic trunk along the right anterior costal vertebral region and the intercostal nerves. The neurovascular structures of the anterior and lateral chest wall include the supraclavicular nerve, superficial cervical artery, and external thoracic artery anteriorly, and the thoracodorsal artery, subscapular artery, and long thoracic nerve laterally.

In the mediastinum, the major vascular structure on the right is the azygos vein, which lies anterolateral to the thoracic vertebral bodies from T4, at the azygos arch, to the T10–T11 level. The azygos vein drains into the superior vena cava. The vagus nerve descends along the esophagus at this level. On the left, the hemiazygos veins

Figure 7.27. Surgical approaches to thoracic spine.

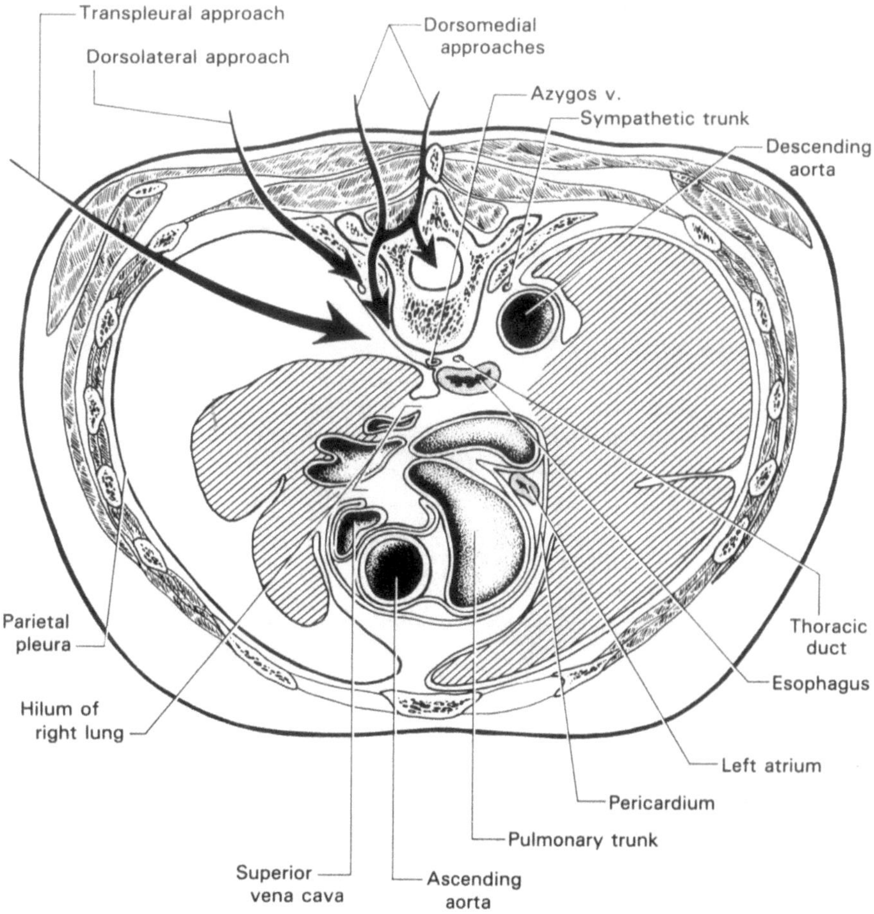

ascend and descend along the lateral thoracic vertebral bodies. The intercostal veins anastomose with the azygos system bilateral. At the T6–T7 level, the hemiazygos vein crosses anteriorly to anastomose with the azygos vein. The intercostal arteries arise from the aorta at this level.

Surgical Approaches to the Thoracic Spine

(Fig. 7.27)

Posterior and Posterolateral (Costotransversectomy) Approach to the Thoracic Spine

The posterior approach to the thoracic spine provides direct access to the posterior elements and may be indicated for biopsy, debridement, decompression, or fusion for various pathological conditions. The posterolateral (costotransversectomy) approach[39] provides direct access to the posterior elements and pedicles but limited exposure to anterior disc spaces and/or vertebral bodies. The posterolateral exposure is indicated for biopsy, drainage, limited debridement, limited decompression,and limited fusion when an extrapleural approach is needed.

With the patient in the prone position, a midline, posterior incision is made over the spinous processes of the thoracic spine. The thoracic fascia is divided in the midline, and the paraspinous musculature is elevated subperiosteally using the Cobb elevator or electrocautery to the facet joints. The dissection may be carried out laterally to expose the transverse processes or ribs as needed. After the procedure is performed, the wound is closed in layers.

A posterolateral (costotransversectomy) approach may be performed through a midline posterior or curved paramedian incision.[39] The trapezius muscle is cut in line with its fibers, and the paraspinal muscles are divided to expose the rib and costotransverse junction. The rib is subperiosteally exposed for 6 to 8 cm lateral to the midline and removed. All muscular attachments are elevated off the transverse process, and the transverse process is removed. The retropleural space is then exposed by blunt dissection. A layered closure is performed after the completion of the indicated procedure. The possible complications are injury to the dura, intercostal nerves or arteries, and pneumothorax.

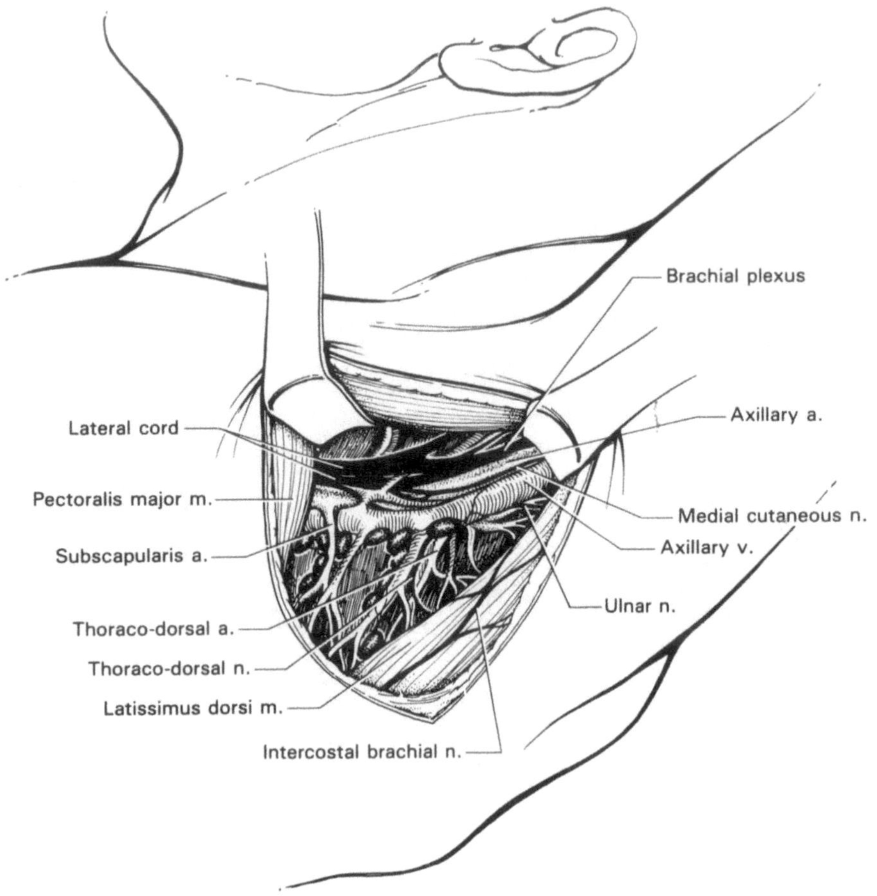

Figure 7.28. Transaxillary approach to thoracic spine.

Transaxillary Approach to the Upper Thoracic Spine

The transaxillary approach[40–44] (Fig. 7.28) allows exposure of the upper thoracic spine to the T1 vertebral body. It is used for females and thin males for indicated pathology, but cannot be used in patients with well-developed pectoralis major and latissimus dorsi muscles or when an extensive exposure is needed.

With the patient's arm abducted, a transverse skin incision is made along the axillary hairline. The dissection is carried through the subcutaneous tissue to expose the pectoralis major muscle, which is divided. The latissimus dorsi muscle is retracted posteriorly. The chest wall is exposed and the ribs are palpated. The intercostal brachial cutaneous nerve is sacrificed. The periosteum is elevated along the second or third rib and a segment is removed. The parietal pleura is incised and exposure is obtained with a rib spreader. The lung is retracted inferiorly and the parietal pleura is incised along the upper thoracic vertebral bodies. The intercostal vessels are ligated at the level being exposed. Complications for this procedure are as from any thoracotomy (hemothorax, pneumothorax, pleural hernia, etc.), numbness of the arm secondary to sacrifice of the intercostal brachial cutaneous nerve or intercostal brachial neuralgia, winging of the scapula if the long thoracic nerve is divided, and brachial plexus injury.

Split Sternal Approach to the Cervicothoracic Spine

The split sternal approach was described by Cauchoix and Binet,[45] Hodgson and Yau,[40] and Louis[3] (Fig. 7.29). Hodgson and Yau proposed a transverse skin incision made above the suprasternal notch and extended distally along the midsternum in a T-shape. Cauchoix and Binet, as well as Louis, preferred a cervical incision along the anterior left sternocleidomastoid. The procedure is indicated for extensive disease of the cervicothoracic junction. The sternohyoid and sternothyroid muscles are divided transversely in the suprasternal region. The xiphisternum is exposed and resected. Blunt finger dissection is used to free tissue from the posterior aspect of the sternum. Midsternotomy is then performed allowing exposure of the pleura. The pleura is stripped from the left of the thymus, which is then retracted to the right. The left brachiocephalic vein is ligated with or without later reanastomosis. The left inferior thyroid artery is then ligated. The dissection is carried between the left carotid artery and the

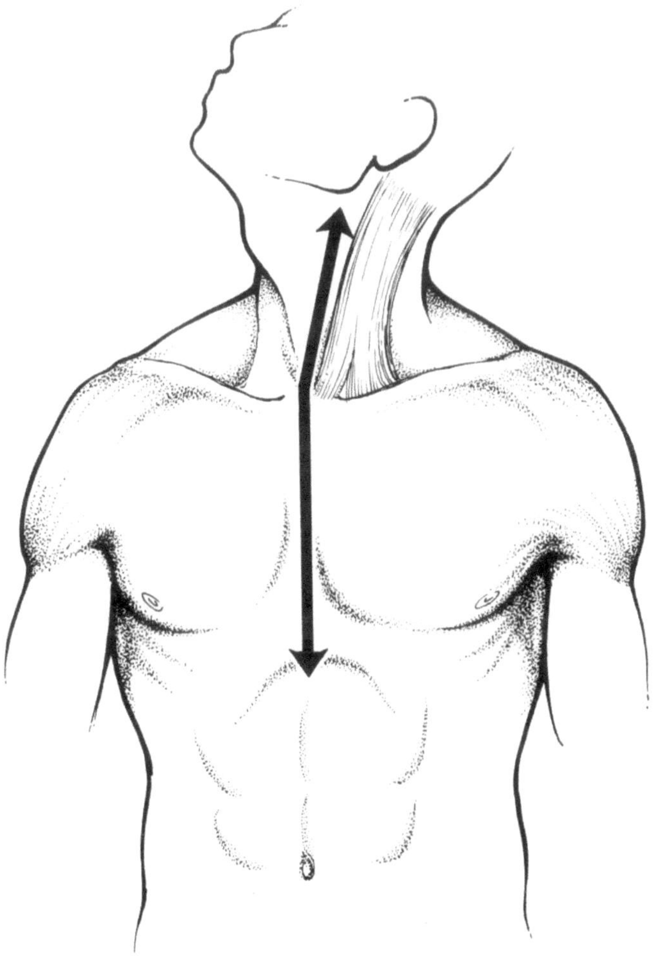

Figure 7.29. Split sternal approach to cervicothoracic spine.

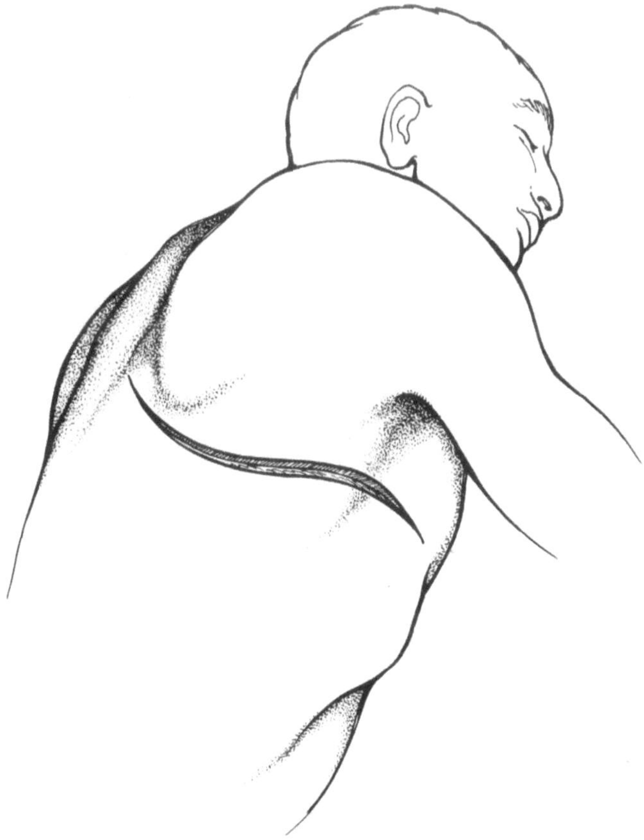

Figure 7.30. Transthoracic approach to upper thoracic spine.

right brachiocephalic trunk. The trachea, esophagus, and thyroid are retracted to the left. This interval allows exposure of C4 through T4. The anterior longitudinal ligament is incised to allow for exposure of the anterior vertebral bodies.

Complications from the split sternal procedure may be from the loosening of vascular sutures, pseudarthrosis of the sternum, swelling of the arm, pigeon chest deformity in children, and a high operative mortality (40%) in one series.[46]

Transthoracic Approach to the Upper Thoracic Spine

Thoracotomy at the level of the third rib allows exposure of C7 to T4 for indicated pathology.[40–42] The patient is placed in the lateral decubitis position with the right side of the patient up. When approaching the high thoracic spine, it is easier to mobilize or divide the azygos vein than to mobilize the firmly fixed aortic arch. Exposure of the lower thoracic or the thoracolumbar spine is better approached from the left side as it is easier to control and mobilize the aorta than the vena cava. The incision is made from the third costochondral junction along the caudal scapular border to the paraspinous region of T1 (Fig. 7.30). Underlying muscles (latissimus dorsi, rhomboid, trapezius, and serratus posterior) are incised carrying the dissection onto the rib. The periosteum is completely stripped from the third rib, which is then excised and used for bone graft later in the procedure. The rib bed is incised and the parietal and visceral pleurae is separated using finger dissection. The rib spreader is then placed to expose the thoracic contents. The lung is retracted carefully allowing visualization of the anterior costal veins, aorta, and cervicothoracic spine. The overlying parietal pleura is incised, and intercostal vessels are ligated or cauterized to expose the desired vertebral level. It is important to expose the intervertebral disc initially because this is the avascular plane. Complications from this approach are primarily pulmonary.[47]

Thoracotomy Approach to the Thoracic Spine

Exposure of the mid- and lower thoracic spine can be done through thoracotomy.[40,41,48–51] The rib to be excised

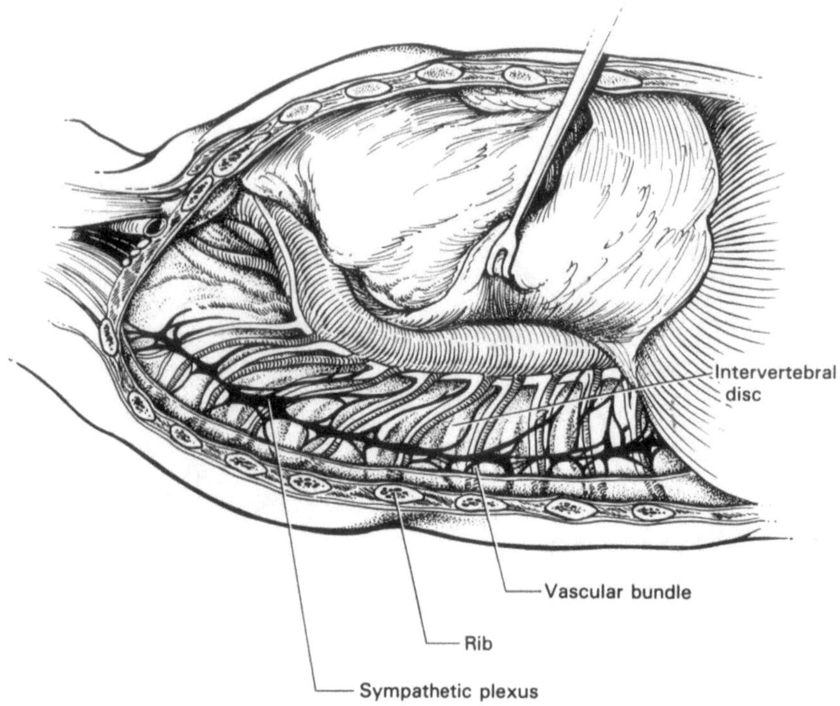

Figure 7.31. Transthoracic approach to midthoracic spine.

is usually two levels higher than the center of the vertebral lesion, which, in the midaxillary line, is opposite the kyphosis or center of the vertebral lesion.

The incision is made with the patient in the lateral decubitus position with right side down. It is extended from the sternocostal junction to the paraspinous region. The thoracic musculature is sharply incised or cut with electrocautery. The periosteum is incised and elevated circumferentially around the appropriate rib. The rib is excised, and the periosteum of the rib bed is incised. The rib spreader retractor is placed allowing exposure of the thoracic cavity. The lung is retracted medially. The parietal pleura overlying the aorta and spine is incised along the spine. An intercostal vein and artery cross each vertebral body (Fig. 7.31); therefore, the avascular intervertebral disc is exposed first. The segmental vessels are then ligated or cauterized for further exposure of the appropriate body and intervertebral space. Complications are as from any thoracotomy.

Approach to the Thoracolumbar Spine

Exposure of the T12–L1 vertebral level is carried out via thoracotomy over the tenth rib.* This allows exposure to the thoracic and abdominal cavity. The skin is incised from the posterior paraspinous region along the tenth rib, then extending anteriorly along the lateral border of the rectus abdominis muscle (Fig. 7.32). The dissection

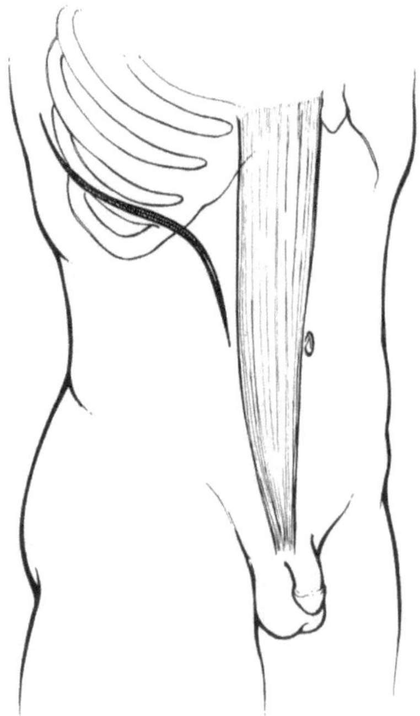

Figure 7.32. Thoracoabdominal approach via tenth rib.

is carried through the subcutaneous and muscular layers. The periosteum of the tenth rib is incised and elevated allowing resection of the rib. The pleura along the rib bed is incised. The costal cartilage is used as the landmark for retroperitoneal exposure and repair of the diaphragm. The peritoneum is bluntly dissected off the diaphragm

* 40,41,47,49,51.

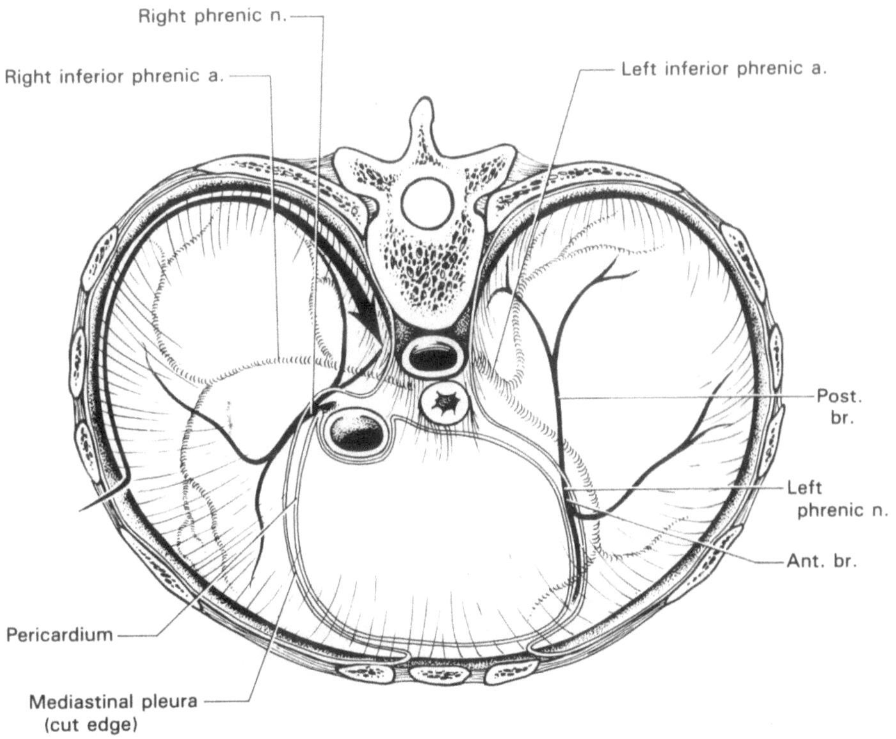

Figure 7.33. Division of diaphragm for exposure of thoracolumbar spine.

and vertebral column. The abdominal extension of the approach is then completed by incising the external oblique, internal oblique, and transversus abdominis muscles. The diaphragm is then incised along the costal margins circumferentially (Fig. 7.33). The diaphragmatic crus insertion on the anterolateral vertebral column is incised to allow exposure of the T12–L1 level. The psoas muscle is also detached for further exposure. The parietal pleura is incised at the thoracic level, and exposure of the vertebral column is completed after ligation or cauterization of the intercostal vessels. Complications are those as previously described for a thoracotomy with the addition of a possible diaphragmatic hernia.

Eleventh-Rib Surgical Approach to the Thoracolumbar Spine

The surgical approach to the thoracolumbar spine with resection of the eleventh rib is somewhat similar to previously described approaches.** A major difference is the dissection between the retroperitoneal and extrapleural plane (Fig. 7.34). Following resection of the eleventh rib, the costal cartilage is used as the primary landmark. The rib bed is incised and the parietal pleura is bluntly dissected off the endothoracic fascia and diaphragm, reflecting it cephalad. The diaphragm is then detached from its insertion to the twelfth rib and reflected cephalad. The peritoneum is then bluntly dissected from the diaphragm allowing retraction of the peritoneal contents anteriorly. The crus of the diaphragm and psoas muscles detach from the upper lumbar segments for further exposure of the vertebral column. Complications are as previously described for the tenth-rib approach.

** 40,41,48,49,52.

Lumbosacral Spine

Bone Morphology of the Lumbosacral Spine

The lumbosacral spine is a very mobile transitional portion of the spine that connects a firmly fixed pelvis to a relatively immobile thoracic spine. It may be divided into five lumbar vertebrae, sacrum, and coccyx. The lumbar vertebrae maintain a lordotic configuration. The interlaminar spaces are widest at the lumbar levels as compared to other spinal levels. As at other spinal levels, there is articulation between inferior and superior articular processes, but is vertically oriented. The isthmic region and the superior articular facet mark the origin of the transverse processes. The accessory articular processes are found at the isthmus transverse process junction. The lumbar vertebral bodies are supported by the intervertebral disc spaces, which are widest anteriorly. Each intervertebral foramen is bounded by the pedicle above and below, and the foramina have their greatest dimension in the lumbar region compared to other spinal levels. The pedicle is the key to all intracanal anatomy. The pedicle is located by interest-

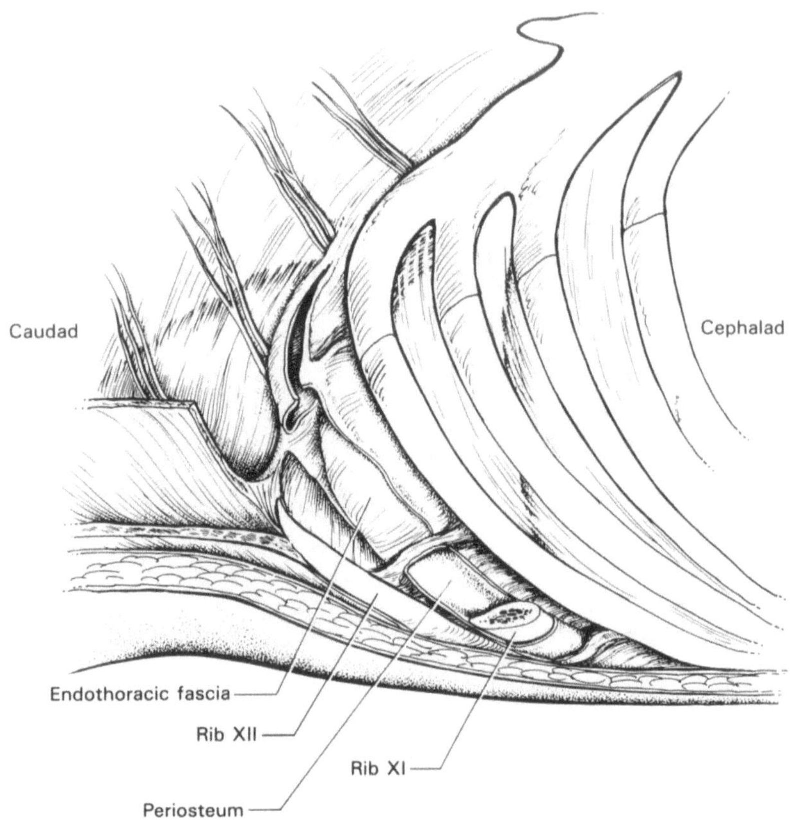

Figure 7.34. Thoracoabdominal approach via eleventh rib; retroperitoneal, extrapleural space is identified.

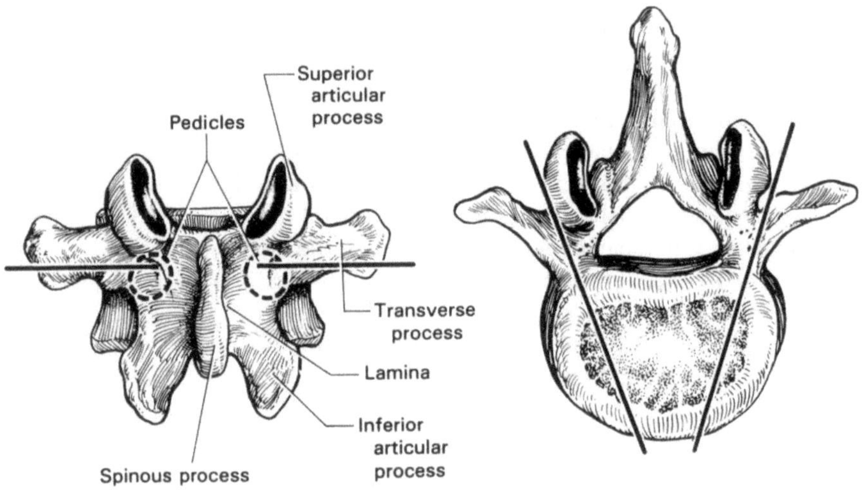

Figure 7.35. Locating the pedicle. **A.** Posterior landmarks. **B.** Axial view.

ing lines, one line being parallel to the midportion of the transverse process and one parallel to the lateral margin of the superior articular process. The pedicles subsequently converge at 20° toward the midline (Fig. 7.35). The spinous processes posteriorly correspond to their respective lumbar level anteriorly. The sacrum articulates with the fifth lumbar vertebrae at its superior articular process, but lacks interlaminar spaces and zygapophyseal articulations. The sacrum contains a midline sacral promontory, four paired sacral foramina at the lateral portion of the sacral grooves, with the sacral ala lying lateral to the foramina (Fig. 7.36). Laterally, the sacrum articulates with the ilium. The sacrum terminates into the fused coccygeal segment.

Ligamentous structures of the lumbar spine include many of those found at other spinal levels. Anterior and posterior longitudinal ligaments form the boundaries of the vertebral bodies (Fig. 7.37) and are loosely and firmly connected, respectively, to the annulus fibrosis. The ligamentum flavum is in the interlaminar region. Most posterior are the interspinous ligaments between each spinous process. The dorsal and ventral sacroiliac-iliac ligaments extend from the sacrum to the ilium with the dorsal being the stoutest. The iliolumbar ligaments extend from the

Figure 7.36. Tendons and muscles of lower end of spine.

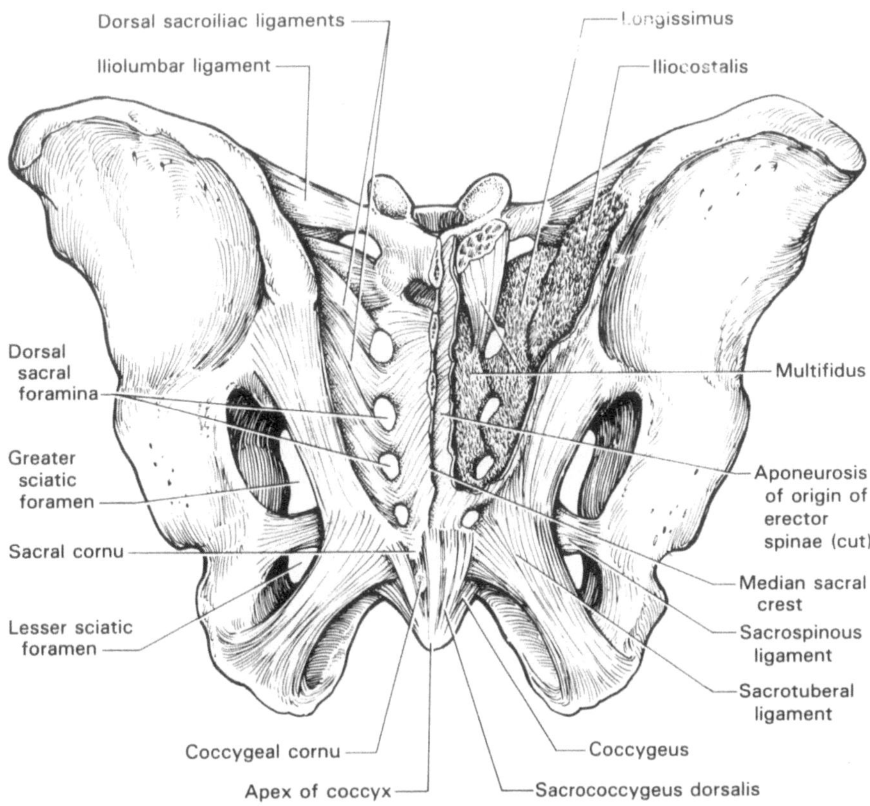

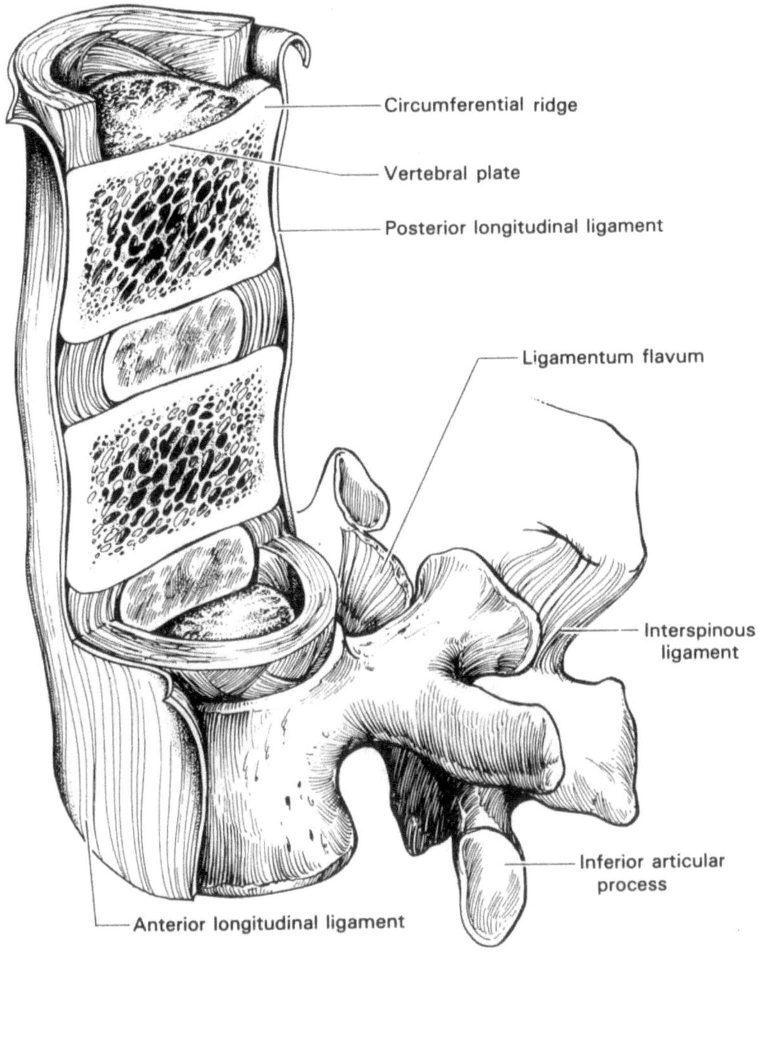

Figure 7.37. Ligamentous structures of lumbar spine.

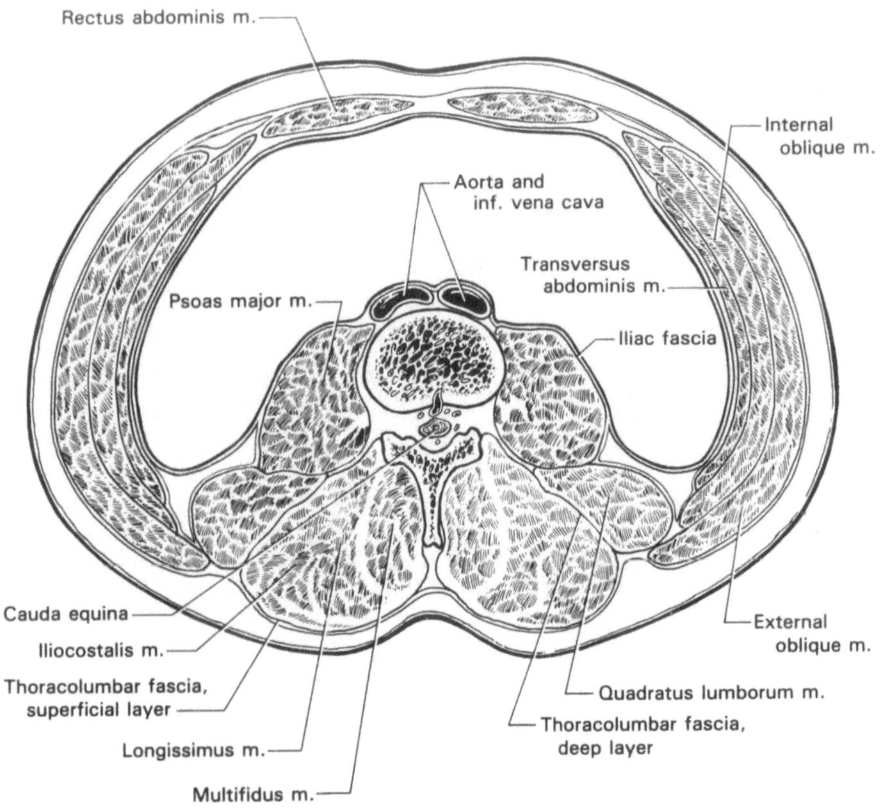

Figure 7.38. Cross section of body wall at L4 vertebral body.

transverse processes of L4 and L5 to the iliac crest. The sacroiliac-sciatic ligaments extend from the sacrum to the sciatic spine.

The zygapophyseal articulation of the lumbar region is formed by the superior facet supplying the anterolateral articulation and the inferior facet the posteromedial articulation. Each articulation is supported by a capsule, ligamentum flavum, and interspinous, supraspinous, and intertransverse ligaments.

Myology of the Lumbar Spine

As described for the posterior thoracic spine, muscles of the posterior lumbar spine include the erector spinae complex. These are the interspinalis lumborum, transversospinalis lumborum, longissimus lumborum, and iliocostalis lumborum.

Abdominal wall musculature is important in anterior approaches to the lumbar spine (Fig. 7.38). These include the external oblique, internal oblique, and transversus abdominis and rectus abdominis muscles. The external oblique muscle lies most superficial, arises from the lower ribs interdigitating with the serratus anterior and latissimus dorsi, and terminates in an aponeurosis which helps form the rectus sheath in the midline and extends to the inguinal ligament. The internal oblique muscle, deep to the external oblique, arises from the thoracolumbar fascia, iliac crest, and iliac fascia. The aponeurosis of the internal oblique forms the anterior and posterior rectus sheath in the midline. The transversus abdominis muscle is deep to the internal oblique horizontally oriented fibers. The upper fibers insert into the rectus sheath whereas the lower aponeurosis fuses with the internal oblique aponeurosis to form the posterior rectus sheath. The lowest portion of the transversus aponeurosis forms part of the anterior rectus sheath. The peritoneum forms the deepest layer of the abdominal wall surrounding the abdominal contents.

Neurovascular Anatomy of the Lumbosacral Spine

The retroperitoneal region adjacent to the lumbosacral spine contains major neural and vascular structures (Fig. 7.39). The iliohypogastric and ilioinguinal nerves descend along the psoas and quadratus lumborum muscles in the paravertebral region. The genitofemoral and lateral cutaneous nerves traverse the psoas muscle more caudad toward the iliac fossa. The sympathetic trunk and ganglia descend between the psoas and lumbosacral spine.

The prevertebral vasculature includes the aorta on the left and the inferior vena cava on the right. The aorta bifurcates at the L4–L5 intervertebral disc region into

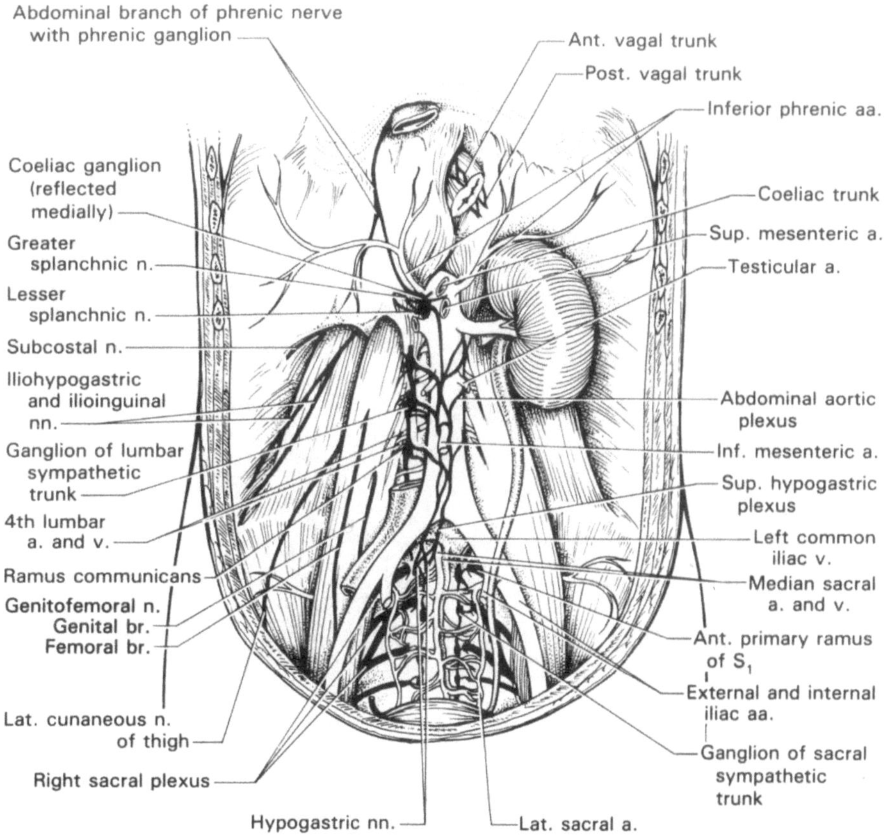

Figure 7.39. Lumbar prevertebral and presacral areas.

the common iliac arteries, which traverse obliquely at the L5 vertebral body. The major arteries of the lumbar region branch off the posterior aorta and descend along each lateral vertebral body to the intervertebral foramina. Adamkiewicz's artery usually passes at the L1–L2 intervertebral foramina supplying the lumbar swelling.

The inferior vena cava ascends from the common iliac veins at the L5 level. It lies posterior to the aorta along the anterior vertebral column. In most cases, each lumbar vein originates from the paravertebral musculature, anastomoses with lumbar and spinal plexus veins, and traverses along its corresponding vertebral body to the inferior vena cava.

Surgical Approaches to the Lumbosacral Spine (Fig. 7.40)

Anterior Retroperitoneal

The anterior retroperitoneal approach was previously described with the patient in the supine position to allow for opening of the disc space with placement of a bridge at the lumbosacral region.[40] The right lateral decubitus position is now preferred by most authors.[40,53] It decreases the need for retraction because the viscera falls away from the operative field. The left side is approached because the aorta is much more easily retracted off the spine, and the left iliac vessels are longer, allowing for retraction. Indications for this approach include intervertebral lumbar fusion in patients with failed posterior lumbar surgery, interbody fusion for degenerative disc disease, atypical low back pain and lower extremity discopathy, often with arthrosis and instability, failed fusion, spondylolysis and spondylolisthesis, infection, tumor, and trauma.

The skin incision in the retroperitoneal approach extends from the midaxillary line to the edge of the rectus sheath (Fig. 7.41). The level of incision is placed according to the intervertebral space to be exposed, between the twelfth rib and the iliac crest; above the umbilicus, for L2–L3 exposure; and at the umbilicus, for L3–L4 exposure. An incision is placed between the umbilicus and symphysis in the upper half for L4–L5 exposure and lower half for L5–S1 exposure.

After the incision has been made, electrocautery is used to divide the muscles of the abdominal wall in line with the incision. This includes the external oblique muscle, internal oblique muscle, and transversus abdominis muscle. The thin transversalis fascia is then carefully incised posteriorly to allow exposure of the extraperitoneal space. The peritoneum is bluntly dissected off the transversalis fascia and interposing retroperitoneal fat toward the midline rectus sheath. Any violation of the peritoneum should be repaired.

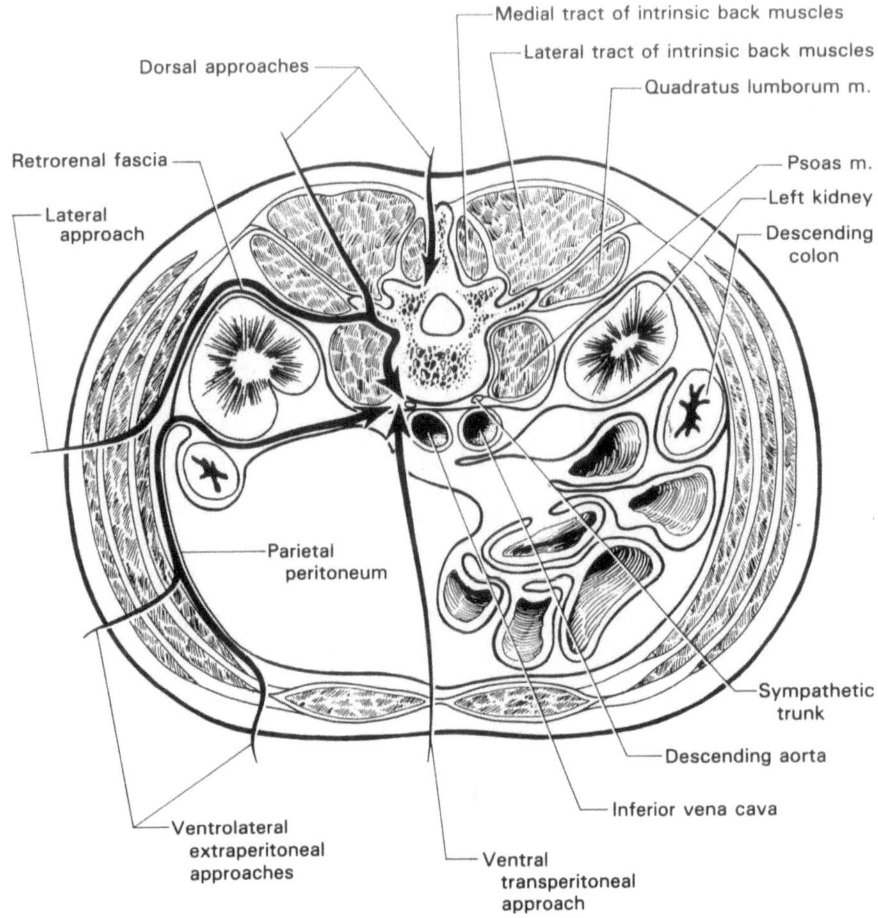

Figure 7.40. Surgical approaches to lumbosacral spine.

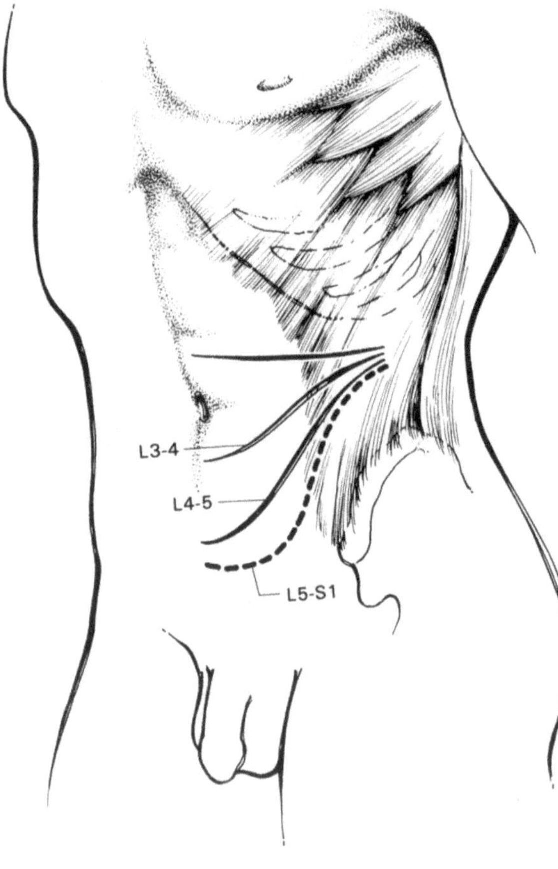

Figure 7.41. Anterior retroperitoneal approach to lumbosacral spine.

The dissection is carried down to the psoas muscle allowing retraction of the peritoneal contents medially. The ureter can be identified on the inferior surface of the peritoneal reflection. If there is any doubt as to the location of the ureter, either the suspected structure may be pinched to observe for peristalsis or a urological consultation obtained preoperatively for passage of ureteral catheters. The genitofemoral nerve lies on the surface of the psoas muscles, as previously described. The dissection is carried medial to the psoas for exposure of the aorta, sympathetic chain, and spine. The vertebral body and intervertebral space are palpated, and gentle blunt dissection is used to retract the aorta and vena cava off the spine. The dissection is carried cephalad toward the aortic bifurcation and caudally along the common iliac artery. Some sympathetic fibers over the vessels may be divided. Lumbar vessels along the vertebral bodies may be ligated and divided. More distal at the L4–L5 intervertebral level, the iliolumbar vein, which overlies the L5 vertebral body, is ligated. The common iliac vessels are further dissected from the spine at this level. It is important to note that there may be a wide variation in the venous anatomy at the lower lumbar spine; therefore, caution should be used.[54] On completion of the indicated lumbar spine procedure, retractors are removed and each muscle layer of the abdominal wall, followed by subcutaneous tissue and skin, is repaired. Complications may be from injury to neurovascular or urologic structures.[54,55]

Transperitoneal

The anterior transperitoneal approach to the lumbosacral spine was used early on for the treatment of spondylolisthesis[56–58] and tuberculosis.[41] Others have used it for L5–S1 interbody fusion, degenerative disc disease, and spondylolisthesis.[59,60] Knowledge of the anatomy of the abdominal cavity, as well as the previously described anatomy of the lumbar spine, is required for this approach.

The patient is placed in the supine position with some hyperextension of the lumbar spine to allow maximum opening of the intervertebral disc space. Slight trendelenberg of the operating room table will help maintain the large and small bowel in the upper abdomen.

The skin incision is made in the midline from the supraumbilical region to the pubic symphysis, or it may be made transverse in the infraumbilical region. In the midline incision, the rectus sheath is incised retracting the rectus abdominis muscle laterally. With the transverse incision, the rectus sheath is incised and the rectus muscle is transected. The peritoneum is carefully incised the length of the incision (Fig. 7.42). The large and small bowel is then retracted proximally to allow for exposure of the posterior peritoneum. The underlying great vessels and lumbosacral spine are palpated. Saline may be infused deep to the peritoneum to delineate the retroperitoneal space. The posterior peritoneum is incised in the midline from the sacrum to the aortic bifurcation. The iliac artery, iliac vein, and sympathetic plexus are identified. Avoid damage to the iliac vein, which overlies the L5–S1 intervertebral disk space, as injury will result in excessive postoperative swelling of the leg. Careful blunt dissection is used to retract the iliac vessels and superior hypogastric plexus from the left to right. The middle sacral artery and vein may require ligation. The anterior longitudinal ligaments may then be incised for further exposure of the disc or vertebral body.

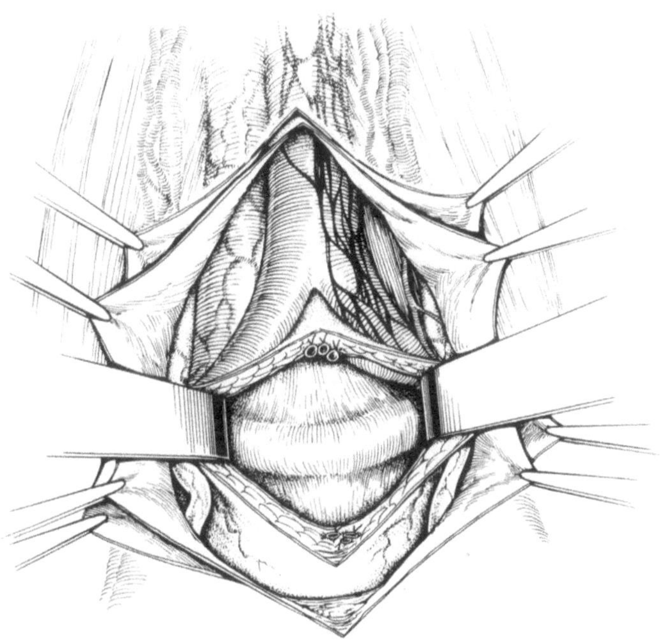

Figure 7.42. Transperitoneal approach for exposure of L5–S1 disc.

This approach may be extended cephalad for exposure of the L4–L5 or L3–L4 intervertebral disc space. This is carried out by extension of the posterior peritoneal incision over the iliac vessels and along the lateral border of the spine. Injury to major neurovascular structures is the most frequent complication.

Posterior Paraspinous

The paraspinal sacroiliac-spinalis muscles splitting approach to the lumbosacral spine, as described by Wiltse,[61,62] may be used for posterior lumbosacral fusions, spondylolisthesis, fusion, and/or decompression of the lumbosacral spine, and for correction of a pseudarthrosis of the lumbosacral spine. It allows for better exposure of the lateral structures of the lumbosacral region. In comparison to the paraspinal approach[63] which dissects lateral to the sacroiliac-spinalis muscle, this approach allows for easier laminectomy and nerve root decompression.

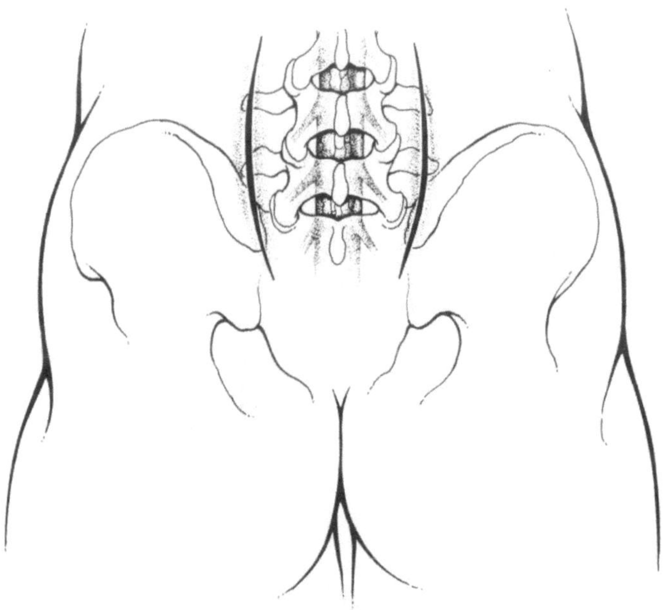

Figure 7.43. Bilateral posterior paraspinal approach to lumbosacral spine.

Two curved skin incisions are made over the paraspinous region just medial to the posterior superior iliac spines (Fig. 7.43). The cluneal nerves, which are about a handbreadth lateral to the posterior superior iliac spine, are avoided. The dissection is then extended through the lumbar fascia and bluntly through the sacroiliac-spinalis muscle. This allows exposure of the L5 lamina and transverse process, sacral ala, and L5–S1 facet joint. The dissection may be extended to higher lumbar levels as indicated. Muscle and fascial attachments are elevated off the lamina, transverse process, sacrum, and facet joints. Those levels not to be included in the fusion are left free of dissection. Laminectomy is carried out as needed. Posterior iliac bone graft may be harvested with the same approach.

Midline Posterior

The midline posterior approach[64–67] to the lumbosacral spine is well known to most spine surgeons. This approach may be used for lumbosacral fusion and degenerative disc disease, spinal stenosis, spondylolisthesis, and herniated nucleus pulposus of the lumbosacral spine. The skin incision is made over the midline spinous processes of the lumbar spine (Fig. 7.44). The dissection is carried down to the subcutaneous tissue. The lumbar fascia is incised the length of the incision of that portion of the spine to be exposed. The periosteum is incised along the spinous process with electrocautery or sharp dissection. The paraspinous muscles are elevated subperiosteally using the Cobb elevator or electrocautery along the spinous process of the lamina to the facet joints. This dissection is carried out as needed beyond the facet joints to expose the transverse process, which lies at the level of the facet joints.

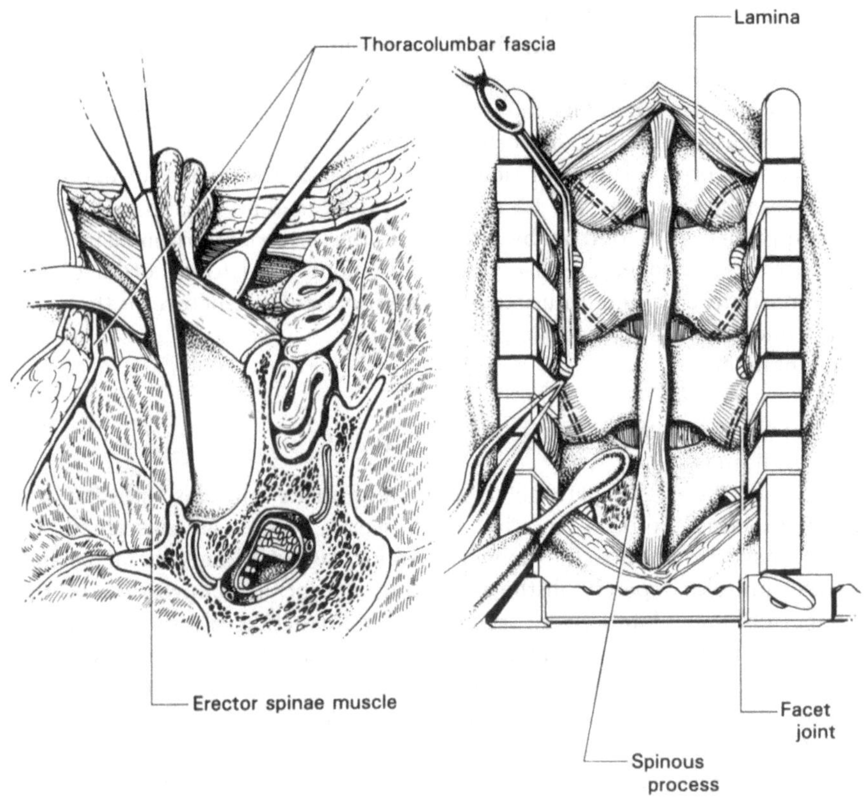

Figure 7.44. Midline posterior approach to lumbosacral spine. **A.** Dissection of paraspinal musculature with periosteal elevator. **C.** Exposure of posterior elements of spine.

After exposure is made, Taylor retractors or self-retaining retractors may be used. The indicated fusion or laminectomy is then performed. The wound is closed placing sutures in the deep fascia, subcutaneous tissue, and skin. Usually a drain is inserted prior to closure deep to the muscular fascia and possibly in the superficial fascia in the presence of dead space or excessive adipose tissue.

Summary

We have tried to provide a detailed description of the embryology of the spine, and of the anatomy of the spine including its bony morphology, myology, and neurovascular surrounding structures, both anteriorly and posteriorly. In addition to the detailed anatomical description of the spine, the neuroanatomy of the spinal cord has been presented. Only through the thorough understanding and knowledge of this complex spine anatomy can one proceed with the surgical approaches to the spine. The operating surgeon must realize that a careful soft-tissue dissection is important so that the fusion bed can be meticulously prepared and in the optimal condition for a solid arthrodesis.

Acknowledgment. A debt of gratitude is owed to Patricia Carlson, of The University of Texas/M.D. Anderson Cancer Center Medical Illustration and Graphic Design Department, for her brilliant illustrations.

References

1. Reimann AF, Onson BJ. Vertebral level of termination of the spinal cord with report of a case of sacral cord. Anat Rec 1944;88:127.
2. Hollinshead WH. Anatomy for Surgeons: The Back and Limbs, Vol. 3. 3rd Ed. Philadelphia: Harper and Row, 1982.
3. Louis R. Surgery of the Spine. Berlin: Springer-Verlag, 1983.
4. McCotter RE. Regarding the length and extent of human medulla spinalis. Anat Rec. 1916;10:559.
5. Elliot HC. Cross-sectional diameters and areas of the human spinal cord. Anat Rec 1945;93:287.
6. Aeby C. Die Altersverschiedenheiten der menschlichen Wirbelsäule. Arch Anat Physiol (Anat Abt) 1879:77.
7. Noback CR, Demarest RJ. The Human Nervous System. 2nd Ed. New York: McGraw-Hill, 1967:38.
8. Lanier RR, Jr. The presacral vertebrae of American white and Negro males. Am J Phys Anthropol 1939;25:341.
9. Louis R. Contribution a l'etude topographique des racines rachidiennes et de la moelle avec les lomes et les disques intervertebraux. Marseille: These, 1961.
10. American Spinal Injury Association (ASIA). Standards for neurological classification of spinal injury patients. Chicago: ASIA, 1987.
11. Hassler O. Blood supply to the human spinal cord. A microangiographic study. Arch Neurol 1966;15(3):302–307.
12. Turnbull IM, Brieg A, Hassler O. Blood supply of cervical cord in man. J Neurosurg 1966;24:951.
13. Adamkievicz A. Die Blutgefässe der menschlichen Rückenmarksoberfläche. Sitzungsber Akad Wissensch Wen Math Nat Klasse 1882;85:101.
14. Lazorthes G, Poulhes J, Bastide G, Roulleau J, Chanchalle AR. Recherches sur la vascularization arterielle de la moelle. Applications a la pathologic medullaire. Bull Acad Natl Med (Paris) 1957;41:464.
15. Cayaffa JJ. Anatomy and vascular supply of the spinal cord. In: Calenoff L, ed. Radiology of Spinal Cord Injury. St. Louis: Mosby, 1981.
16. Zeitlin H, Lichtenstein BW. Occlusion of the anterior spinal artery: clinicopathologic report of a case and a review of the literature. Arch Neurol Psychiatry 1936;36:96.
17. Lazorthes G, Gouaze A, Bastide G, Soutoul JH, Zadeth O, Santini JJ. La participation des arteres radicullares lombosacrees a la vascularization fonctuinnelle de renflement lombaire. C R Assoc Anat 1966;135:580.
18. Lazorthes G, Gouaze A, Zadek JO, Santini JJ, Lazorthes Y, Burdin P. Arterial vascularization of the spinal cord: recent studies of the anastomotic substitution pathways. J Neurosurg 1971;35:253.
19. Crock HW, Yoshizawa H. The Blood Supply of the Vertebral Column and Spinal Cord in Man. New York: Wien Springer, 1977.
20. Louis R. Topographie vertebromedullaire et vertebroradiculaire. Anat Clin 1978;1(1):73.
21. Herren RY, Alexander L. Sulcal and intrinsic blood vessels of human spinal cord. Arch Neural Psychiatry 1939;41:678.
22. Bogduk N, Long DM. The anatomy of the so-called articular nerves and their relationship to facet denervation in the treatment of low back pain. J Neurosurg 1979;51:172.
23. Bradley KC. The anatomy of back ache. Aust N Z J Surg 1974;44:227.
24. Yinchuan. Anatomical observations on lumbar nerve posterior rami. Clin Med J 1978;4(6):492.
25. Bogduk N. The innervation of the lumbar spine. Spine 1983;8(3):286.
26. Southwick WO, Robinson RA. Surgical approaches to the vertebral bodies in the cervical and lumbar regions. J Bone Joint Surg 1957;39A:631.
27. Fang HSY, Ong GB. Direct anterior approach to the upper cervical spine. J Bone Joint Surg 1962;44A:1588.
28. Apuzzo MLJ, Weiss MH, Heiden JS. Transoral exposure of the atlantoaxial region. Neurosurgery 1978;3(2):201.
29. Bailey RW, Badgley LE. Stabilization of the cervical spine by anterior fusion. J Bone Joint Surg 1960;42A:564.
30. Riley LH. Surgical approaches to the anterior structures of the cervical spine. Clin Orthop 1973;91:16.
31. DeAndrade JR, Macnab I. Anterior occipito-cervical fusion using an extrapharyngeal exposure. J Bone Joint Surg 1969;51A:1621.
32. Whitesides TE Jr, Kelly RP. Lateral approach to the upper cervical spine for anterior fusion. South Med J 1966;Aug:879.
33. Whitesides TE, Jr, McDonald AP. Lateral retropharyngeal approach to the upper cervical spine. Orthop Clin North Am 1978;9(4):1115.
34. Henry AK. Extensile Exposure. 2nd Ed. Z. Edinburgh: Churchill Livingstone, Edinburgh, 1973.
35. Verbiest H. Anterolateral operations for fractures and dislocations in the middle and lower parts of the cervical spine. J Bone Joint Surg 1969;51A(8):1489.

36. Verbiest H. A lateral approach to the cervical spine: Technique and indications. J Neurosurg 1968;28:191.
37. Hodgson AR. An approach to the cervical spine (C3–7). Clin Orthop 1965;39:129.
38. Probst-Proctor SL, Rinsky LA, Bleck EE. The cisterna chyli in orthopaedic surgery. Spine 1983;8(7):787.
39. Capener N. The evaluation of lateral rhachotomy. J Bone Joint Surg 1954;36B:173.
40. Hodgson AR, Yau ACMC. Anterior surgical approaches to the spine. In: Apley AG, ed. Recent Advances in Orthopaedics. Baltimore: Williams and Wilkins, 1964:289–323.
41. Kirkaldy-Willis WH, Allen PBR, Rostrup O, Willox GL. Surgical approaches to the anterior elements of the spine: Indications and technique. Can J Surg 1966;9:294.
42. Cotler HB, Cotler JM, Cohn HE, Israel HI, Gartland JJ. Intrathoracic chordoma presenting as a posterior superior mediastinal tumor. Spine 1983;8(7):781.
43. Honnart F. Vois D'abord en Chirurgie Orthopedique et Traumatolique. Paris: Masson, 1978.
44. Atkins HJB. Sympathectomy by the axillary approach. Lancet 1954;538.
45. Cauchoix J, Binet JP. Anterior surgical approaches to the spine. Ann R Coll Surg Engl 1957;21:237.
46. Hodgson AR, Stock FE, Fang HSY, Ong GB. Anterior spinal fusion—the operative approach and pathological findings in 412 patients with Pott's disease of the spine. Br J Surg 1960;48(208):172.
47. Cotler HB, Cotler JM, Stoloff A, Cohn HE, Jerrell BE, Martinez L, Northrup BE, Osterholm JL, Rosato FE. The use of autografts for vertebral body replacement of the thoracic and lumbar spine. Spine 1985;10(8):748.
48. Smith TK, Stallone RJ, Yee JM. The thoracic surgeon and anterior spinal surgery. J. Thorac Cardiovasc Surg 1979;77(6):925.
49. Bradford DS, Winter RB, Lonstein JE, Moe JH. Techniques of anterior spinal surgery for the management of kyphosis. Clin Orthop 1977;128:129.
50. Dwyer AF. Experience of anterior correction of scoliosis. Clin Orthop 1973;93:191.
51. Riseborough EJ. The anterior approach to the spine for correction of the axial skeleton. Clin Orthop 1973;93:207.
52. Mouat TB. The operative approach to the kidney of Bernard Frey. Br J Urol 1939;2.
53. Flynn JC, Hoque MA. Anterior fusion of the lumbar spine. J Bone Joint Surg 1979;61A:1143.
54. Harmon PH. A simplified surgical technic for anterior lumbar discectomy and fusion; avoidance of complications; anatomy of the retroperitoneal veins. Clin Orthop 1964;37:130.
55. Johnson RM, Mcguire EF. Urogenital complications of anterior approaches to the lumbar spine. Clin Orthop 1981;154:114.
56. Capener N. Spondylolisthesis. Br J Surg 1932;19:374.
57. Burns BH. An operation for spondylolisthesis. Lancet 1933;i:1233.
58. Mercer W. Spondylolisthesis. Edinb Med J NS 1936;43:545.
59. Freebody D, Bendall R, Taylor RD. Anterior transperitoneal lumbar fusion. J Bone Joint Surg 1971;53B:617.
60. Lane JD, Moore ES, Jr. Transperitoneal approach to the disc in the lumbar area. Ann Surg 1948;127:537.
61. Wiltse LL. The paraspinal sacrospinalis-splitting approach to the lumbar spine. Clin Orthop 1973;91:48.
62. Wiltse LL, Bateman JG, Hutchinson RH, Nelson WE. The paraspinal sacrospinalis-splitting approach to the lumbar spine. J Bone Joint Surg 1968;50A:919.
63. Watkins MB. Posterolateral fusion of the lumbar and lumbosacral spine. J Bone Joint Surg 1953;35A:1014.
64. Hoppenfield S, de Boer P. Surgical Exposures in Orthopaedics. Philadelphia: Lippincott, 1984.
65. Watkins RG. Posterior approach to the lumbar spine. In: RG Watkins, JS Collis, Jr, eds. Lumbar Discectomy and Laminectomy. Aspen: Rockville, 1987.
66. Austin GM. The spinal cord: basic aspects and surgical considerations. 2d Ed. Springfield, Illinois: Thomas, 1972:762.
67. Bauer R, Xerschbaumer K, Poisel S. Operative approaches. In: Sharon GS, trans. from Germ. Orthopaedic Surgery and Traumatology. New York: Thieme, 1988;2–89.

IV
Fusion Techniques

■8■

Fusion Techniques for Spinal Infections

Taylor K. Smith

Background

The earliest application of spinal fusion was for the treatment of spinal infections. It was found that tuberculosis and other infections that were thought to be tuberculous were often controlled by putting the involved spinal segment to rest by immobilization or arthrodesis. Before antibiotics, this principle extended also to other joints where plaster immobilization, extraarticular arthrodesis, and intraarticular arthrodesis were the mainstays of the treatment of joint infections.

Sayre,[1] in the latter half of the nineteenth century, popularized the ambulatory cast treatment of infections of the spine. His ability to reverse paraplegia and bring an infectious process to a quiescent state by immobilizing the spine with a body cast that was applied while the patient was suspended by his head and shoulders was truly a remarkable feat. Other forms of spinal immobilization such as plaster beds and elaborate orthotic devices were developed to arrest the movement of the spine and bring the disease under control. Hibbs[2] in 1912 described the first operative arthrodesis of the spine for tuberculosis. He accomplished spinal fusion by stripping the lamina, spinous processes, and articular processes of soft tissue, and then crushed the osseous structures together thus obtaining a fusion.

Albee,[3] also in 1912, described arthrodesis of the spine that was accomplished by splitting the spinous processes and inserting a bone graft taken from the tibia. It is remarkable that many spinal infections could be brought under control by accomplishing an arthrodesis before the advent of effective antibiotics. Arthrodesis of the spine remains an effective method of putting an infected segment of the spine to rest thus keeping the infectious disease under control and preventing the progression of deformity. Since the early part of the twentieth century, arthrodesis has also been used to maintain correction of a deformity caused by infection, and for arresting painful motion after destruction caused by infectious disease. The history of arthrodesis of the spine, therefore, is also the history of the treatment of spinal infections.

Diagnosis of Spinal Infections

Even in this day of modern technology, the diagnosis of a spinal infection is all too often delayed or missed.[3,4] In countries where tuberculosis is not a common occurrence, one rarely thinks of granulomatous disease or pyogenic disease as a cause of spine pain and deformity. Although certainly not common, tuberculosis and other granulomatous diseases still occur fairly often, especially in areas where emigrants from developing countries are constantly arriving. The emergence of human immunodeficiency virus diseases and the use of immunosuppression with organ transplantation and the treatment of rheumatological diseases opens the door for opportunistic infections that may involve the spine. Therefore, spinal infections should be on the list of differential diagnoses in every patient presenting with spine pain, deformity, or unexplained neurological involvement. The history is helpful if it places the patient in a high-risk category.

Pain is usually the most prominent early complaint of spinal infection, although certainly granulomatous diseases can progress quite extensively without much apparent pain. The onset of weakness and/or bowel and bladder control problems should alert one to early neurological complications of spinal infection. The historian should carefully search out other foci of infection such as symptoms related to the genitourinary tract, including hematuria and recent genitourinary instrumentation, cholecystitis, dental infections, or the more obvious pulmonary symptoms of active tuberculosis. The young child frequently will complain of pain in his buttocks or legs and

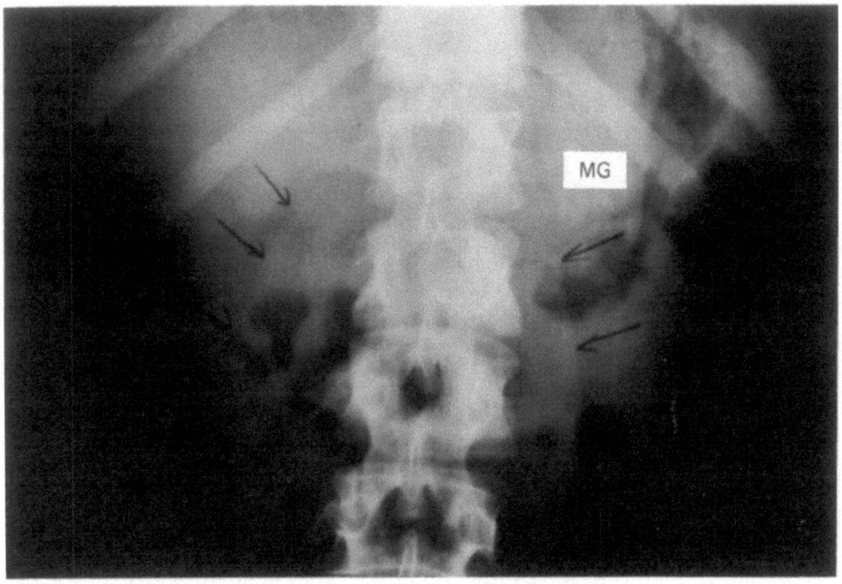

Figure 8.1 Psoas abscess (*arrows*) of spinal tuberculosis as seen on KUB radiograph.

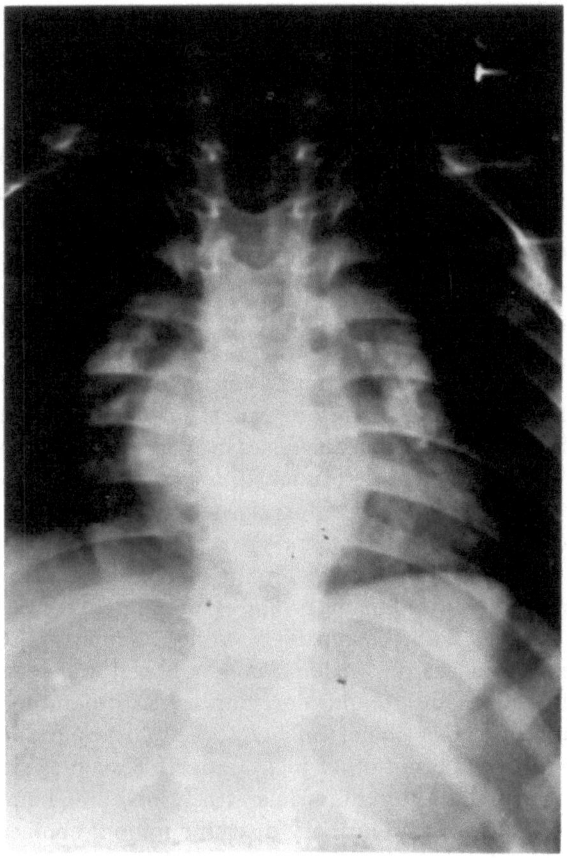

Figure 8.2. Paravertebral abscess seen behind cardiac shadow of patient with spinal tuberculosis.

frequently will simply refuse to walk when vertebral osteomyelitis or discitis becomes symptomatic.[5]

The physical findings of infection of the spine may be subtle, or they may be frankly obvious, as in a gibbous deformity or the development of a pointing psoas abscess in the groin or over the trochanteric areas. A poker spine and resistance to attempts at spinal flexion are frequently seen. A spinal infection leading to a psoas abscess may cause a hip flexion and abduction deformity caused by the abscess. Old evidence of spinal infection such as scars in the groin from previous spontaneously drained psoas abscesses should alert one that a superinfection with a contaminating organism may have occurred. Rarely, a spinal abscess in the thoracic area will evacuate into the lung and the sputum may produce sequestra along with the other pyogenic materials.

The laboratory evaluation of a patient with spinal infection should include the routine CBC and sedimentation rate studies. A chronic infection frequently will lead to anemia, but the white count may not be elevated. The sedimentation rate, however, is almost always elevated unless an anergic response has developed from overwhelming sepsis and poor nutrition. Skin tests should be ordered not only to rule out various organisms but to demonstrate the patient's immunocompetence. Plain radiographs will frequently localize the site of the infection, but sometimes in the early stages the plain films are not helpful. Careful attention to the soft-tissue shadows such as psoas abscesses (Fig. 8.1) and paravertebral abscesses (Fig. 8.2) in the thoracic area may focus attention on in-

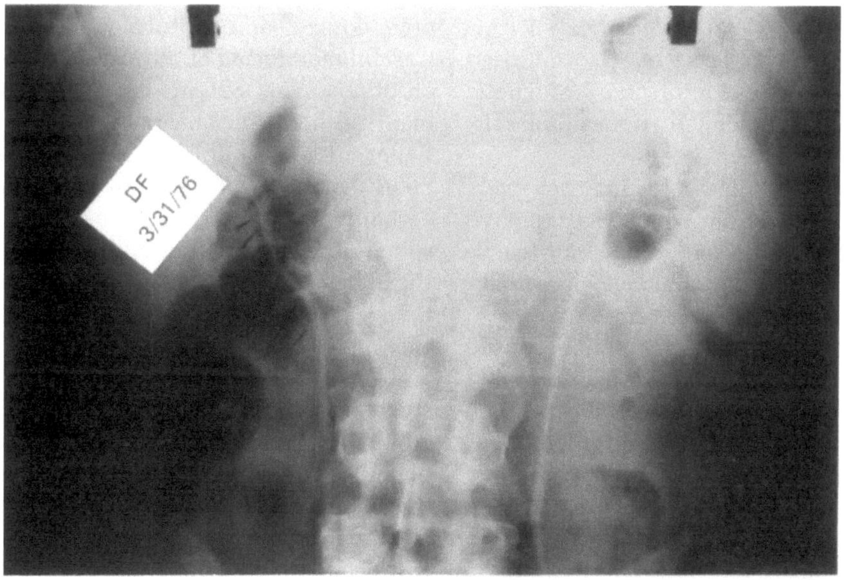

A

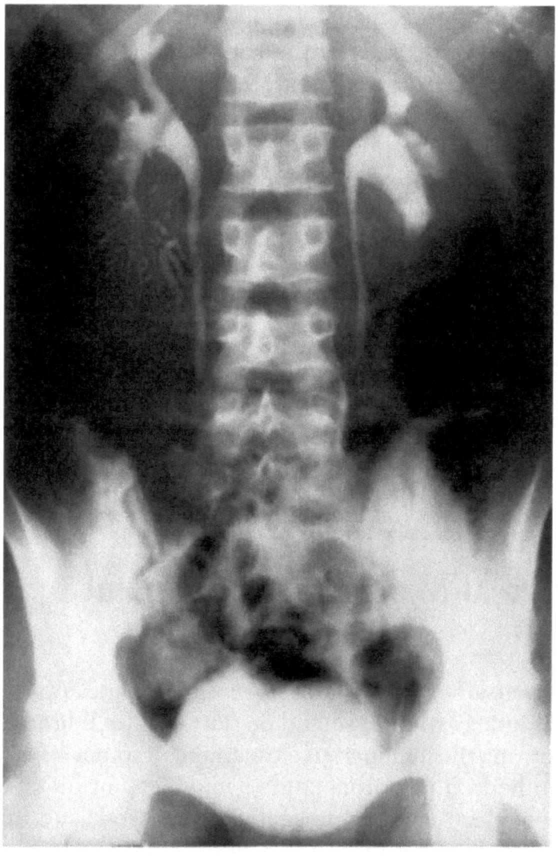

B

Figure 8.3. **A.** Intravenous pyelography shows ureteral displacement by psoas abscess. **B.** Renal tuberculosis with blunting of calyces.

volved vertebrae. Further definitive radiographic studies of the spine, including tomography and computerized tomography, should be used because the disease quite often is much more extensive than was originally apparent on the radiographs. Chest radiographic studies should be done on all patients suspected of having spinal infections, because active pulmonary disease may be present. An intravenous pyelogram (IVP) is an excellent screening study, because patients with granulomatous disease of the spine, especially tuberculosis, often have infection of the genitourinary tract. One can also see the displacement of the ureters by psoas abscesses; further, if retroperitoneal surgery is contemplated, the status of the kidneys and ureters should be determined before surgery

(Figs. 8.3A and 8.3B). Other selective studies such as an upper GI series or gallbladder series may be indicated if these areas are possible sources for infection. Magnetic resonance imaging (MRI) is helpful to determine soft-tissue and neurological involvement.

The definitive diagnosis of a spinal infection, however, depends on obtaining material from which the infective organism is grown. It therefore becomes necessary to culture the blood, the urine, and any drainage that might be present, and in many cases to perform a biopsy to obtain culture material from the spine itself and to rule out tumor.[6] If an operative procedure has been determined to be necessary to evacuate an abscess, perform an arthrodesis, or correct a spinal deformity such as kyphosis, the biopsy can be obtained at the time of the definitive surgical procedure. If, however, it is necessary to establish a bacteriological diagnosis before or rather than surgery, several options are available.

An open biopsy has the greatest morbidity, but it does provide for obtaining adequate samples of tissue and fluids. It is important to discuss with the pathology department and the bacteriology department the particular biopsy procedure and thus determine the correct handling of the biopsy material. Performing an open biopsy with no results is an unfortunate situation that occurs all too often. Indiscriminate use of antibiotics before biopsy is probably the greatest cause for obtaining a negative biopsy. Needle biopsies of abscesses or bone can be carried out with a variety of instruments. It is best to obtain a tissue sample if at all possible, because histological diagnosis as well as bacteriological diagnosis frequently can be established by an adequate piece of tissue or abscess wall. A computerized tomography-directed needle biopsy is an accurate technique for obtaining material from the designated site. Only a few areas, such as the midthoracic or the upper cervical area are inaccessible to needle biopsies.

Nonsurgical Management of Spinal Infection

When the causative organism has been identified, appropriate antibiotic treatment should be started. Much literature concerning the nonoperative treatment of spinal infections has relied on data from studies in which antibiotics we now consider relatively ineffectual were used, and in which control of antibiotic levels was poor. Now, infections in most cases can be adequately treated and controlled, and in many cases cured with appropriate antibiotics, rest, adequate nutrition, and close observation of the patient for response to the treatment.

There are a few specific indications for surgical intervention in the treatment of spinal infections, and if these are not met, a trial of adequate nonsurgical management should be attempted. Selection of the appropriate antibiotic, dosage, and route of administration is important. Careful monitoring of the systemic effects of the antibiotic on other organ systems is of course mandatory, because many of these substances are toxic to vital organ systems. Penetration of antibiotics into abscess cavities and other poorly vascularized areas is in most cases adequate, but certainly one cause of failure of medical management of spinal abscesses is the failure of the antibiotic to reach the infecting organism because of the presence of avascular tissue or sequestra that harbor the organism and rekindle the infection.

Rest of the spine is important for the management of spinal infection. This is best accomplished with bed rest. In the past, plaster beds or cast immobilization in recumbency was advocated. In most cases adequate bracing can be obtained with newer, lightweight materials, which are much more acceptable to the patient than a plaster cast. The length of immobilization with bed rest and casting or bracing is determined by the response of the patient to medical management. If the patient's pain, malaise, and fever resolve, if the patient develops an appetite and begins to gain weight, and if the patient's laboratory parameters such as white blood count and sedimentation rate begin to return to normal, these offer certain evidence that the spinal infection is coming under control. Radiographic confirmation of healing lags far behind the clinical course, and is not as reliable. On the other hand, progression of the disease as seen on radiographs and failure of the laboratory parameters to return to normal, along with persistent symptoms of pain, fever, and malaise, all indicate that the chosen medical treatment is ineffectual.

The patient's immunological status should be carefully monitored. The effect of nutrition on the host's ability to fight infection cannot be underestimated, and hyperalimentation, either enterically or parenterally, should be considered for all patients who show nutritional assessment parameters indicating protein and calorie malnutrition. The serum albumin and total lymphocyte counts have been shown to have a direct correlation with the patient's ability to fight infection and heal damaged tissue, and these two parameters can be easily monitored.[7,8]

It has been shown time and again that nonsurgical management of spinal infections, including tuberculosis, can be effective, but a considerable amount of time and resources must be expended to ensure a satisfactory outcome.[9,10]

Surgical Management of Spinal Infections

There are specific indications for operative intervention in the management of spinal infections. The recent onset of neurological deterioration is probably one of the most demanding indications for surgical intervention.[11] It is imperative that the surgical intervention not increase the instability of the spine or inadequately decompress the spinal canal contents when surgery is being performed for neurological deterioration. Other reasons for surgical intervention include the failure to respond to what is considered to be adequate nonsurgical management consisting of rest, antibiotics, nutritional support, and time. Unacceptable structural abnormalities such as kyphotic deformities, instability, or growth disturbances can also be indications for operative intervention.

Finally, a strong case can be made for operative intervention for spinal infection to hasten the patient's recovery even though the infection might adequately be controlled and rendered quiescent with months of antibiotic treatment, bed rest, and systemic support. Quite often the healing process can be markedly accelerated by evacuation of abscess material, sequestra, and avascular material, and by the creation of a spinal arthrodesis. Time and again we have seen how rapidly a patient's clinical course will change with the evacuation of an abscess, although the patient had been on antibiotics for a prolonged period before surgery. That is not to say that the patient would not have eventually recovered under the nonsurgical management, but it certainly appears that in many cases the surgical intervention hastens the patient's return to health. The goal of surgical intervention in the management of spinal infections should be to establish a diagnosis, adequately decompress any structures that might be compromised by the abscess or sequestra, establish drainage of the abscess if necessary, and to effect an arthrodesis of the spine to render the infection quiescent and in some cases to correct an unacceptable deformity.

Many of the fusion techniques discussed elsewhere in this book are not applicable in dealing with spinal infections because of the hazard of introducing hardware or polymethylmethacrylate into a focus of infection. It has been found, however, that bone grafting in the face of infection, after adequate debridement has been carried out and appropriate antibiotic treatment has been started, does not constitute an excessive risk to the patient. This holds true for both granulomatous and low-grade infections as well as the more virulent pyogenic infections. The key is adequate debridement, resection of bone back to good bleeding cancellous bone, firm fixation of bone grafts into a good cancellous bed, adequate postoperative immobilization, and the establishment of adeqnate antibiotic coverage (Figs. 8.4A–8.4E). The creation of instability by the evacuation of an abscess to decompress compromised neural tissue without the establishment of stability with the use of an arthrodesis only replaces one problem with another problem that may be more serious. In most cases, it is feasible as well as the better course of action to accomplish all these goals with one operative procedure.

Timing of Arthrodesis for Spinal Infections

If surgical intervention has been chosen, then the earlier the disease can be extirpated, the pathological organism determined, and the appropriate antibiotic coverage established, the better the chance of arresting the disease. The earlier that decompression of neurological structures and stabilization and immobilization of the involved segment with bone grafting and casting or bracing can be effected, the better the chance for recovery from neurological injury and deformity.[12]

The question of when to start appropriate antibiotic coverage often arises. If a definitive diagnosis has been established preoperatively by appropriate cultures, then preoperative antibiotics should be started. Abscesses in general facilitate dissection at surgery, and thus if surgery is necessary then it should be carried out before antibiotics can heal a lesion and create a scar that makes surgery more difficult.

As suggested, the nutritional status of the patient is of prime importance in the conquest of spinal infections. Surgery of a severely malnourished patient should be delayed, if at all possible, until the catabolic state has been addressed and perhaps reversed. This of course is not possible if neurological structures are compromised, but certainly the patient should be in optimal condition before surgery. Preoperative blood transfusions, intravenous hyperalimentation, and preoperative physical and respiratory therapy are of great benefit to these seriously ill patients.

Bone Grafting Techniques for Spinal Infections

In spite of the advances that have been made in allografting, autogenous bone graft material is still the best. It is preferred that the patient's own bone be used unless there is a contraindication or the defect is too great to fill with the patient's own bone. Cortical-cancellous grafts from the ilium are usually the grafts of choice (Figs. 8.5A and 8.5B). More cortical grafts such as fibular or tibial cortical grafts have the strength that is often necessary, but the lack of cancellous bone delays the revascularization of the graft and increases the chance for nonunion or late fracture of the graft. In the upper thoracic area ribs are readily accessible and make excellent graft material (Fig. 8.6). A combination of ribs and iliac crest frequently is used where a large defect must be bridged with a strong graft that will vascularize readily (Fig. 8.7). The graft should be placed into good beds of bleeding cancellous bone and should be surrounded by vascular soft tissues. Careful keying of the grafts into the bone above and below the fusion site, and adequate postoperative immobilization

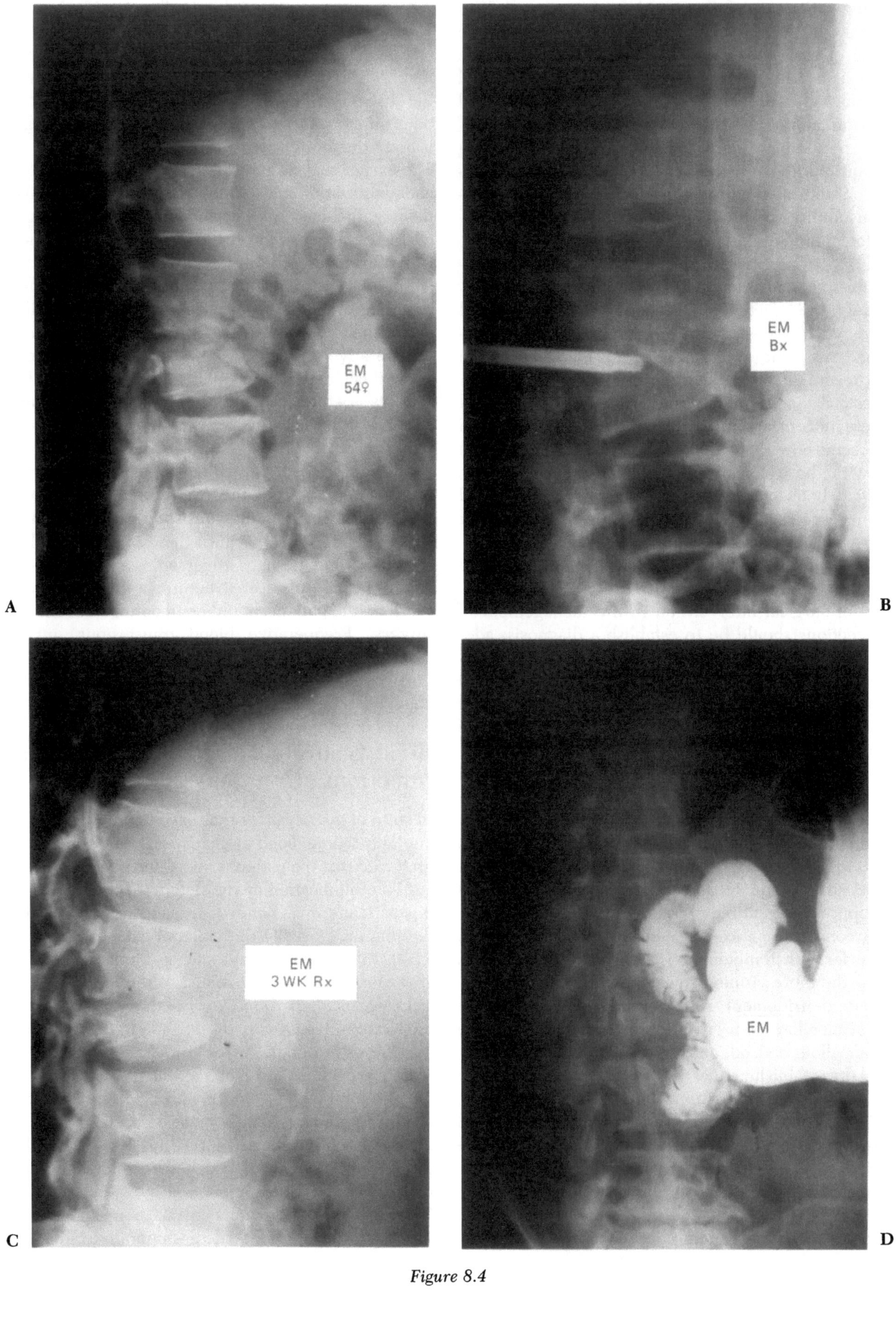

Figure 8.4

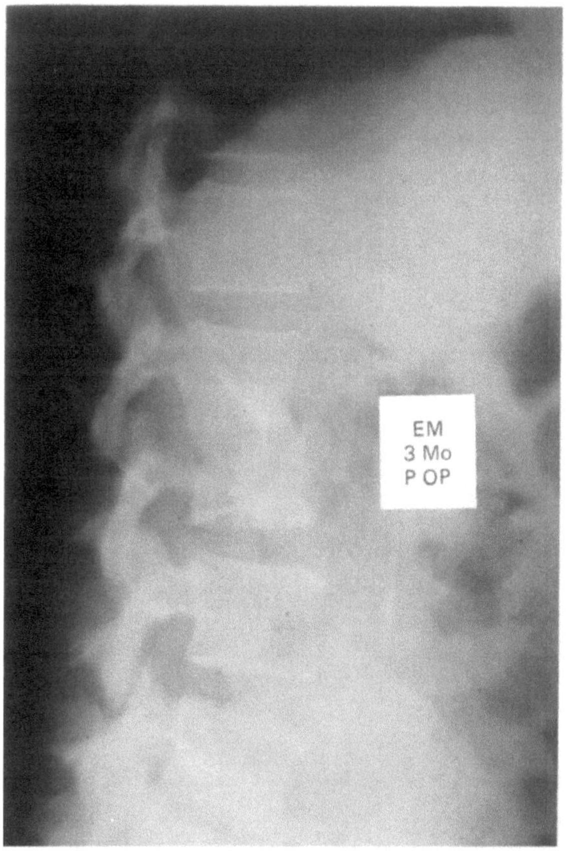

E

Figure 8.4. **A.** Vertebral infection following septicemia in 54-year-old diabetic woman. **B.** Craig needle biopsy revealed *E. coli* infection. **C.** Three weeks of gentomycin failed to control infection. **D.** Upper GI series demonstrated abscess displacing intestine anterior to area of destruction in spine. **E.** After debridement and fusion with iliac crest bone graft, infection cleared.

of the patient, should accomplish the architectural stability that is necessary.

We have not found it necessary to supplement the bone grafting with plates, screws, wires, or methylmethacrylate, and in fact it probably would be contraindicated to introduce a foreign body into an area of spinal infection. Vascularized rib grafts have been used in the thoracic area when it is possible to maintain a neurovascular bundle to the rib and rotate the rib to fill the defect of the spine.[13] I am not certain that this is absolutely necessary, as certainly a free autogenous graft seems to work well in most cases also. It appears that there is very little indication for a free vascularized bone graft to the spine with spinal infections, because the increased morbidity from such a procedure outweighs the advantage of having a vascularized piece of bone bridging the defect.

Specific Arthrodeses for Spinal Infections

Upper Cervical Spine

Infections of the upper cervical spine are relatively common, are difficult to treat, and are exceedingly dangerous. Tuberculosis and nontuberculous infections involving the occiput, C1 and C2 frequently present as severe upper cervical pain and limitation of motion. Palpation of the posterior pharynx with a gloved hand may reveal a retropharyngeal abscess. The diagnosis is usually established radiologically, and often subluxation of C1 on C2 is caused by destruction of the transverse alar ligaments by the infectious process. Treatment should be aimed at reducing the dislocation, debriding the abscess, and establishing arthrodesis of the upper cervical spine.

Fang[14] in 1962 described a method of draining upper cervical spine abscesses and creating an arthrodesis between C1 and C2 through an incision in the back of the pharynx. This requires a tracheostomy and halo immobilization. Morbidity and mortality for such a procedure can be quite high. An alternative method of treatment is to immobilize the spine in a halo, treat the infection with appropriate antibiotics and/or drainage, and accomplish arthrodesis through a posterior cervical fusion including the occiput if necessary. Most authors favor early decompression of upper cervical abscesses, because of the rapid onset of possible serious neurological sequelae and the frequency of subluxation of C1 on C2 from destruction of stabilizing ligaments.[15]

Although the cervical spine from C3 distally is readily approached through the same standard anterior approaches, as one approaches the upper cervical spine, it becomes progressively more difficult to expose the front of the vertebrae.[16,17] The parotid gland, cranial nerves VII, IX, X, XI, and XII, and branches of the external carotid artery interfere with the approach. Also the fixation of the internal jugular vein and internal carotid artery to the base of the skull makes it difficult to mobilize these structures without damage. The preferred method for approaching the C1 and C2 levels anteriorly is through the back of the pharynx. The preferred approach to the front of C2, C3, and C4 is the procedure described by DeAndrade and Macnab.[18]

Posterior Pharyngeal Approach to the Upper Cervical Spine

The C1 and C2 levels are readily approached through the mouth, and the C2, C3, and C4 levels can be approached through a transthyrohyoid posterior pharyngeal approach as described by Fang.[14,19] To approach the upper cervical spine through the oropharynx, a tracheostomy is performed after the head is stabilized with skull traction

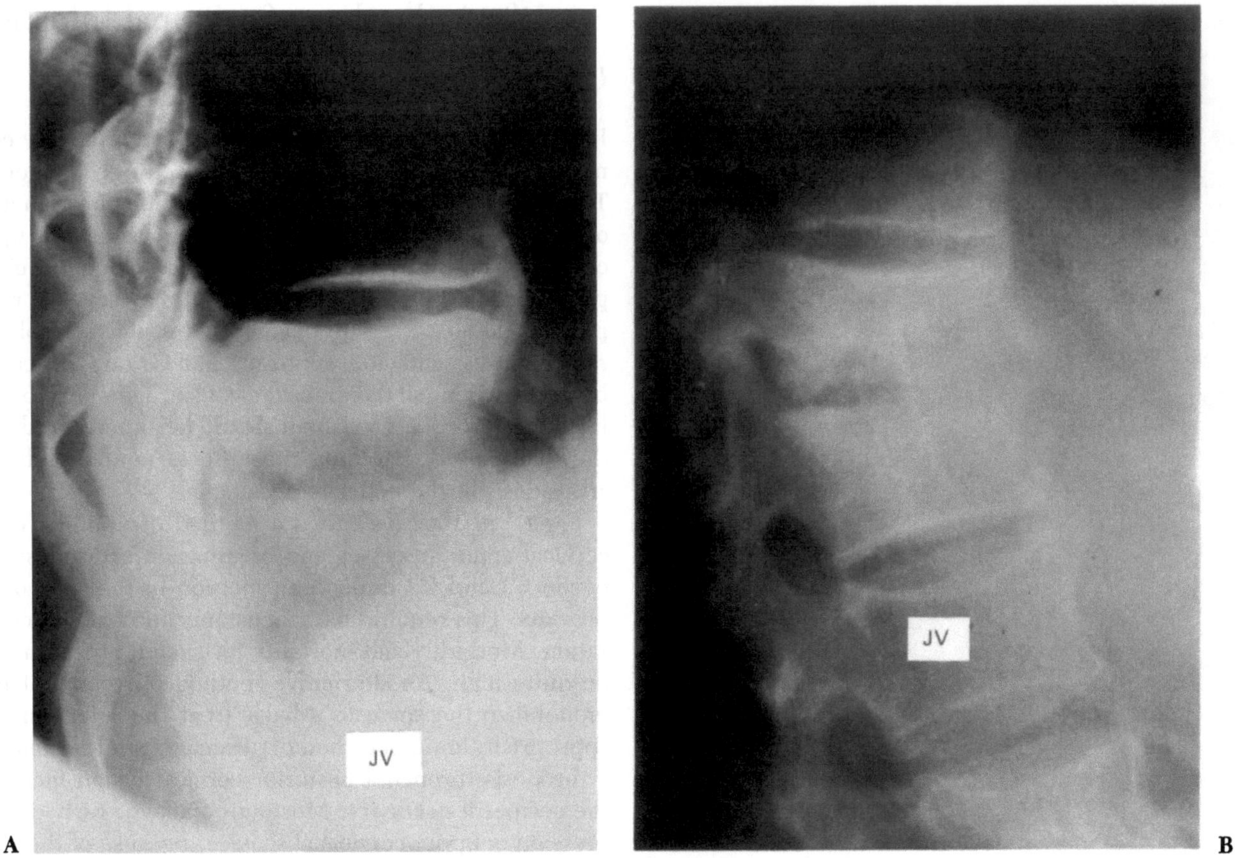

Figure 8.5. **A.** Progressive destruction of T11–T12 disk space and adjacent vertebral bodies by pseudomonas infection in 56-year-old diabetic woman. Infection remained active in spite of adequate doses of intravenous gentomycin for 15 days. **B.** Prompt control of infection and arthrodesis resulted from anterior spinal debridement and fusion with iliac crest bone graft.

or a halo. If there is preoperative subluxation of C1 on C2, correct this by positioning the head before or during the operative procedure. The back of the pharynx is exposed by using the palate retractor and sewing the uvula to the soft palate.

A 1.5-in. incision in the midline posteriorly directly over the abscess or over the anterior arch of C1 gives access to the front of the spine. There is very little bleeding in this area unless the patient is a child with a large amount of lymphoid tissue. Injecting this area with a dilute solution of epinephrine has been helpful. Elevation of the soft tissues laterally exposes the articular facets between C1 and C2. After evacuation of the abscess, removal of the cartilage on the articular surfaces can be completed and bone grafts can be placed across the facet joints to effect an arthrodesis. Careful closure of the wound in three layers should be accomplished to prevent leakage of the posterior pharyngeal wall. A feeding tube should be avoided in the postoperative period as it may erode through the operative site; also, the tracheostomy should be left in place until the wound is well healed.

A transpharyngeal approach to the more distal part of the upper cervical spine can be carried out through a transverse incision across the neck in the upper cervical crease extending from one carotid sheath to the other. The platysmas, sternohyoid muscles, and thyrohyoid muscles are divided in line with the incision. The thyrohyoid membrane is separated from the hyoid bone, and the separation continues laterally, taking care to avoid injuring the internal laryngeal nerve and the superior laryngeal arteries that pierce the thyrohyoid membrane laterally. The mucous membrane overlying the pharynx anteriorly is carefully divided, taking care not to injure the epiglottis. The posterior pharyngeal wall is opened and closed in the manner previously described. These two approaches to the upper cervical spine are occasionally necessary, but it should be pointed out that a large number of complications are associated with these procedures.

Anterior Approaches to the Cervical Spine

The cervical spine can be approached in the interval just anterior to the sternocleidomastoid muscle. If the area to be approached is in the upper half of the cervical spine,

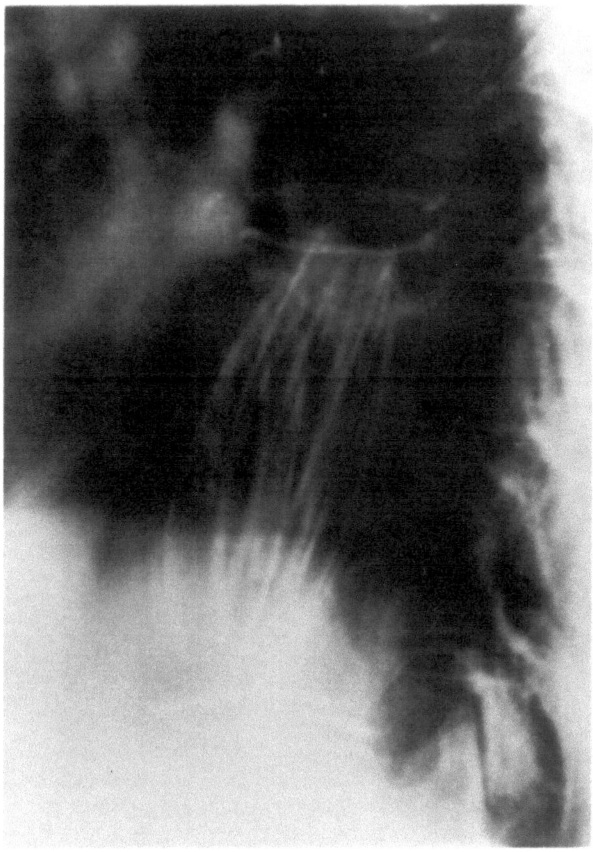

Figure 8.6. Multiple rib grafts used to arthrodese three thoracic vertebrae infected with tuberculosis.

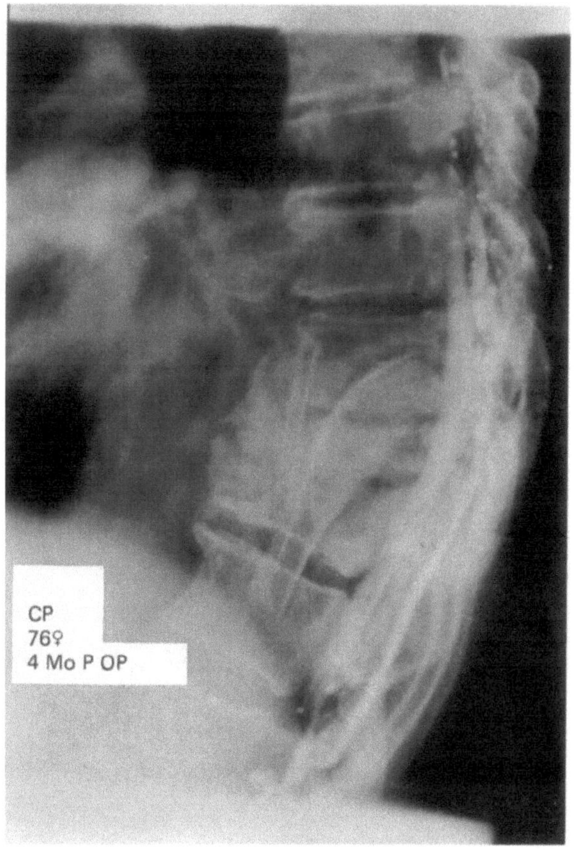

Figure 8.7. Iliac crest and rib graft used to arthrodese lower thoracic spine of 76-year-old woman with staphylococcal osteomyelitis of spine, following cholecystitis and septicemia. Debridement, arthrodesis, and intravenous methicillin controlled the infection.

an incision parallel to the anterior border of the sternomastoid will be satisfactory. A transverse incision in line with the creases of the neck or the mid- and lower cervical spine gives a much more cosmetically attractive appearance and allows easy access to the front of the spine. The platysma is divided in line with the incision.

In the upper cervical spine, take care to identify and ligate the superior thyroid artery and vein, which then gives you mobilization of the carotid sheath posteriorly and access to the midline of the upper cervical spine by retracting the esophagus, pharynx, and trachea toward the opposite side. When approaching the cervical spine anteriorly for an infectious process, it is quite often beneficial to pass a nasogastric tube down the esophagus thus if tissue planes are distorted, the esophagus may be palpated by feeling the plastic tube and damage to the esophagus can be avoided. An extension of this incision superiorly to expose C1 and C2 involves identification of the hypoglossal nerve and superior laryngeal nerves, which must be protected during this exposure. The superior thyroid artery and vein and facial artery can be ligated if necessary. In the mid- and lower cervical spine, the anterior approach is similar to that for discectomy and arthrodesis; the only difference is that occasionally tissue planes are difficult to identify. A nasogastric tube in the esophagus facilitates this identification.

Before opening any abscess, be certain you are not dealing with a mycotic aneurysm. If there is any question, a small aspiration needle should be placed into the presumed abscess to make sure it is not an aneurysm. After the pus has been evacuated and sequestered bone and disc fragments have been removed, appropriate notches are cut into good cancellous bone above and below the destroyed area of spine and corticocancellous grafts are keyed into place (Figs. 8.8A and 8.8B). A drain is usually placed in the wound for a day or so, and the patient's airway should be carefully observed postoperatively because postoperative swelling could compromise the patient's breathing.

This anterior cervical approach can be used to expose as far down as the T3 level by incising the sternal attachment of the sternocleidomastoid muscle and remaining

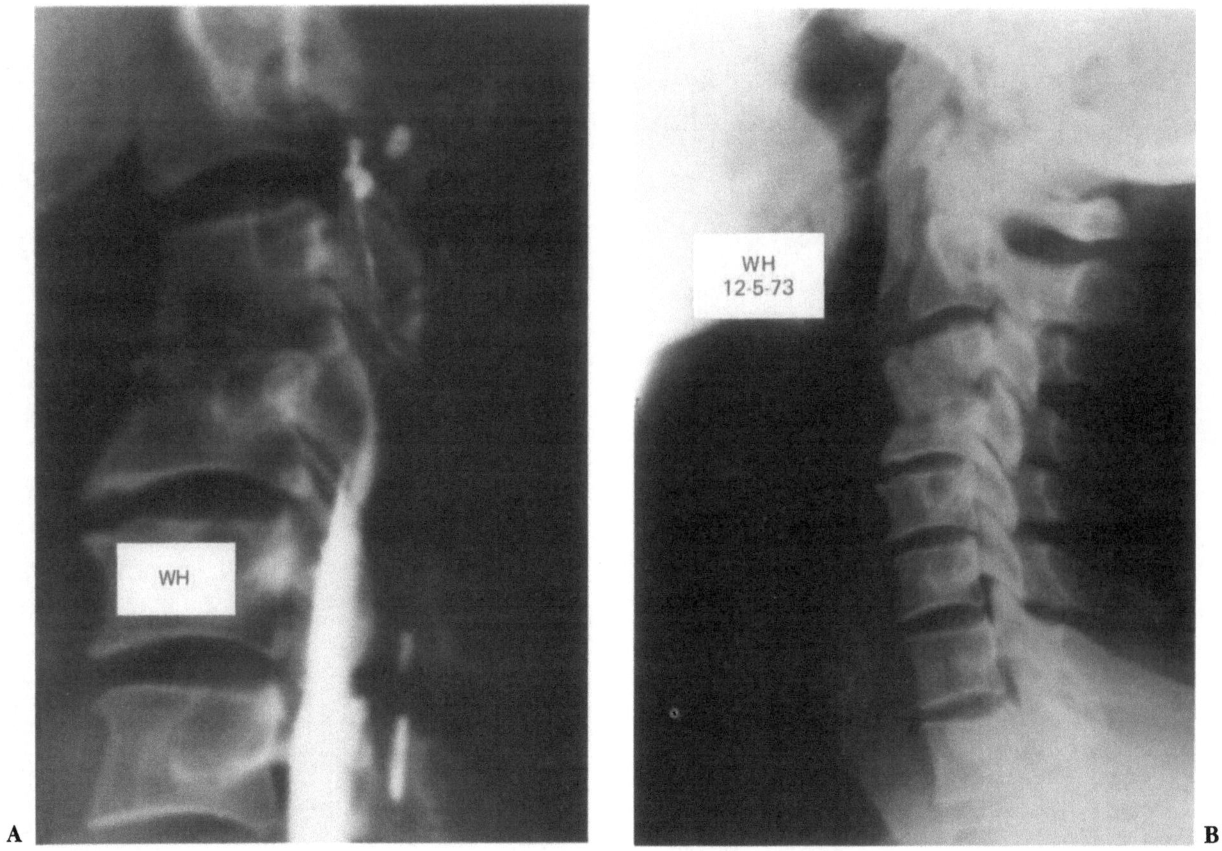

Figure 8.8. **A.** Preoperative myelogram of 26-year-old heroin addict with quadriplegia secondary to pseudomonas infection involving C3 and C4. **B.** After decompression and fusion, infection and quadriplegia promptly resolved even though upper edge of graft dislodged anteriorly. Arthrodesis was allowed to occur in this position.

close to the midline with the dissection.[16] In the erect position, the body of T4 is straight posteriorly from the sternal notch. Upper thoracic and cervicothoracic abscesses frequently can be drained through this anterior cervical approach without having to undertake a thoracotomy. If it appears that the destructive lesion is too great to manage through an anterior cervical approach, then a combined anterior cervical approach and high thoracotomy can safely expose the area and maintain control of the great vessels. The recurrent laryngeal nerve is more easily damaged on the right side, so the preferred approach is through the left side of the neck. At the lower portion of the cervical spine and upper portion of the thoracic spine, however, care must be taken not to injure the thoracic duct. If it is inadvertently cut, it should be tied off carefully.

Thoracotomy Approaches to Infections of the Thoracic Spine

It is much easier to visualize, decompress, and graft an anterior spinal destructive process with an intrapleural thoracotomy approach than it is to try to create an extrapleural approach or a costotransversectomy. Frequently, the extrapleural approach or costotransversectomy approach to the front of the spine results in an inadequate debridement and poor positioning of grafts for arthrodesis. The preferred approach is from the left side so that the aorta can be palpated and protected during the operation.[20] Occasionally it is necessary to go in the right side when an abscess points to the right or when an abscess extends into lung tissue on the right side.[21] The third-rib approach to the chest is used for upper thoracic lesions from T2 to T4. In the lower thoracic areas, the rib that crosses the middle or upper portion of the area of destruction in the midaxillary line is the rib to be resected for the thoracotomy. This places the surgeon just above the lesion. The ribs are more easily retracted distally than proximally. If extension of the thoracotomy is necessary, one must fracture a rib or resect another rib to gain adequate exposure.

In most cases when a thoracotomy is performed for an infectious process, the rib is resected from its bed and used for graft material. In the lower thoracic area it may be necessary to use an iliac crest graft to have enough strength and enough bone to fill the defect created by the debridement. Careful attention to placement of the grafts will prevent their dislodging and becoming free in the pleural cavity. If possible the parietal pleura is sewn back over the abscess cavity and grafts. Bed rest and immobilization are necessary to allow incorporation of the grafts or they will dislodge.

Unless there is definite neurological involvement or definite extension of the abscess into the epidural space, no attempts should be made to remove the posterior longitudinal ligament and thus risk injury to the dura. An area of pachymeningitis over the spinal cord, however, should be carefully removed with a blunt dissector because late contraction of the pachymeningitis can cause late neural compromise. Spillage of abscess material into the pleural cavity has not proven to be a source of infection with thoracotomy for spinal infections. Care is taken not to excessively soil the thoracic cavity, but when adequately evacuating the abscess and placing the patient on appropriate antibiotics, empyema has not been a problem. A chest tube is used for several days until the drainage is minimal and then is removed.

Thoracolumbar Spinal Infections

Thoracolumbar spinal infections are approached through the standard thoracolumbar incisions through the eleventh or twelfth ribs, detaching the diaphragm at its periphery and entering the retroperitoneal space.[17,20] Care should be taken to identify the ureter. When a retroperitoneal approach is contemplated, a preoperative IVP is quite helpful when infectious disease is present. The ureter usually mobilizes anteriorly with the peritoneum. Again, care must be taken to not enter into a mycotic aneurysm. Thus, the abscess cavity is palpated and occasionally aspirated to make certain that it is not full of blood. As with all anterior spinal procedures, ligation of the segmental vessels and mobilization of the great vessels before beginning the bony work renders the procedures less hazardous. The diaphragm is reattached in the usual manner, and the chest cavity is drained for several days with a chest tube. Usually an iliac crest graft is necessary to bridge the defects in the lower thoracic and lumbar spine.

Anterior Lumbar Debridement and Arthrodesis for Spinal Infection

If the spinal infection does not extend above the T12 vertebrae, it is possible to stay out of the pleural cavity by performing a standard anterolateral approach to the spine through the retroperitoneal space. Ligation of the segmental vessels across the involved vertebral bodies will allow for mobilization of the aorta, and if the segmental vessels are ligated halfway between the aorta and their division at the neural foramen, then the chance of interruption of their retrograde flow through the intercostals will be minimized. Preoperative evaluation of the spinal cord blood supply by arteriography has not proven useful, and although the chance of vascular interruption of the blood supply to the spinal cord does exist, it appears that with spinal infection the occurrence of paraplegia caused by vascular interruption is extremely rare. At the L4 level and distally, one must be very careful to identify and ligate the iliolumbar vein. Frequently this vein will exist as two or three separate veins, and all must be ligated before mobilization of the common iliac artery and vein.

In the lumbosacral area, the need for an anterior debridement and arthrodesis is extremely rare. The standard transperitoneal approach to this area would be contraindicated in an infectious process, and in most cases disease in this area is treated by conservative measures.

Posterior Spinal Arthrodesis for Infectious Disease of the Spine

Many of the goals of operative intervention cannot be met by posterior approach to the spine. Adequate debridement of infections, which in most cases involve the anterior and middle columns of the spine, cannot be fully accomplished through a posterior approach or a costotransversectomy approach. Posterior arthrodeses, however, are used in the treatment of spinal infections to stabilize the spine, to correct and prevent spinal deformity, and, on rare occasions, to biopsy and debride the rare posterior spinal infectious process.

The standard spinal arthrodesis can be used for infectious disease. In most cases it is preferred that the disease be brought under control with appropriate medical management and/or anterior spinal surgery. At a later date, a posterior arthrodesis may be performed. This often entails the use of hardware in addition to bone grafting to accomplish the correction of spinal deformity and stabilization of the spine. In young children who have had extensive destruction anteriorly from an infectious process, a posterior arthrodesis carried out over several more segments than are involved anteriorly will in some cases cause a tethering of the spinal column growth posteriorly and thus correct or prevent development of a severe kyphotic deformity. In the very young child with extensive disease mandating surgery anteriorly, at the same time that the anterior procedure is carried out, a posterior arthrodesis just using bone grafting and decortication is frequently carried out at the same operative session. If this appears to be too much surgery for the child, then certainly staging procedures are the safer course of management.

Late Spinal Correction and Arthrodesis Following Spinal Infections

Patients occasionally will have persistent pain after treatment for spinal infection from instability or mechanical derangement caused by the infection. A posterior arthrodesis by the standard methods has proven to be a very useful procedure in those cases.

Unacceptable deformity or late-onset paraplegia caused by chronic pressure on the spinal canal contents can lead to the necessity for anterior spinal debridement, correction of the deformity, and arthrodesis. These procedures are usually staged, and require rigid immobilization such as halo-pelvic traction or plaster treatment in recumbency during the recovery period, because spinal debridement, osteotomy, and correction will often produce a very unstable spine.[22,23] Whenever an area of old spinal infection is surgically approached, adequate antibiotic coverage should be carried out. In particular, old tuberculous infections should have antituberculous antibiotic coverage for 6 to 12 months following any surgical manipulation, even when the disease has been quiescent for a number of years.

Correction of spinal deformities can be done gradually with halopelvic or halofemoral traction, but must not be carried out until an anterior debridement has been done. Maintenance of correction always requires an anterior arthrodesis, because a posterior spinal arthrodesis will not maintain correction of a kyphotic deformity.

References

1. Sayre LA. Spinal Diseases and Spinal Curvature: their treatment and the use of the plaster of paris bandage. London: Smith, Elder, 1877.
2. Hibbs RA. A further consideration of an operation for Pott's disease of the spine with report of cases from the service of the New York Orthopaedic Hospital. Ann Surg 1912;55:682–688.
3. Albee FH. A report of bone transplantation and osteoplasty in the treatment of Pott's disease of the spine. NY Med J 1912;95:469–475.
4. McHenry MC. Vertebral osteomyelitis presenting as spinal compression fracture: six patients with underlying osteoporosis. Arch Intern Med 1988;148:417–423.
5. Ross PM, Fleming JL. Vertebral body osteomyelitis. Clin Orthop 1976;118:190–198.
6. Eismont FJ, Green BA, Brown MD, Ghandur-Mnaymneh L. Coexistent infection and tumor of the spine. A report of three cases. J Bone Joint Surg 1987;69A:452–458.
7. Jensen JE, Jensen TG, Smith TK, Johnston DA, Dudrick SJ. Nutrition in orthopaedic surgery. J Bone Joint Surg 1982;54A:1263–1272.
8. Smith TK. Prevention of complications in orthopaedic surgery secondary to nutritional depletion. Clin Orthop 1987;222:91–97.
9. Digby JM, Kersely JB. Pyogenic nontuberculous spinal inection. J Bone Joint Surg 1979;61B:47–55.
10. Frederickson B, Yuan H, Olans R. Management and outcome of pyogenic vertebral osteomyelitis. Clin Orthop 1978;131:160–167.
11. Eismont FJ, Bohlman HH, Soni PL, Goldberg VM, Freehafer AA. Pyogenic and fungal vertebral osteomyelitis with paralysis. J Bone Joint Surg 1983;65A:19–29.
12. Adendorff JJ, Boeke EJ, Lazarus C. Pott's paraplegia. South African Med J 1987;71:427–428.
13. Louw JA. Anterior vascular rib pedicle graft and posterior instrumentation in tuberculous spondylitis. A case report. South African Med J 1987;71:784–785.
14. Fang HSY, Ong GB. Direct anterior approach to the upper cervical spine. J Bone Joint Surg 1962;44A:1588–1604.
15. Ziegler JE, Bohlman HH, Robinson RA, Riley LH, Dodge LD. Pyogenic osteomyelitis of the occiput, the atlas, and the axis. A report of five cases. J Bone Joint Surg 1987;69A:1069–1073.
16. Kaplan EB. Surgical Approaches to the Neck, Cervical Spine and Upper Extremity. Philadelphia: Saunders, 1966.
17. Watkins RG. Surgical approaches to the spine. In: Chapman MW, ed. Operative Orthopaedics. Philadelphia: Lippincott, 1988:1861–1866.
18 DeAndrade JR, Macnab I: Anterior occipito-cervical fusion using an extra-pharyngeal exposure. J Bone Joint Surg. 51A:1621, 1969.
19. Fang D, Leong JC, Fang HSY. Tuberculosis of the upper cervical spine. J Bone Joint Surg 1983;65B:47–50.
20. Smith TK, Stallone RJ, Yee JM. The thoracic surgeon and anterior spinal surgery. J Thorac Cardiovasc Surg 1979;77:925–928.
21. Yau ACMC, Hodgson AR. Penetration of the lung by the paravertebral abscess in tuberculosis of the spine. J Bone Joint Surg 1968;50A:243–254.
22. O'Brien JP, Yau ACMC, Smith TK, Hodgson AR. Halopelvic traction: a preliminary report on a method of external skeletal fixation for correcting deformities and maintaining flexion of the spine. J Bone Joint Surg 1971;53B:217–229.
23. Yau ACMC, Hsu LCS, O'Brien JP, Hodgson AR. Tuberculous kyphosis: correction with spinal osteotomy, halopelvic distraction and anterior and posterior fusion. J Bone Joint Surg 1974;56A:1419–1434.

9

Fusion Techniques for Degenerative Disease

A. Alexander M. Jones, Richard H. Rothman, and Richard A. Balderston

Introduction

The era of spinal fusion surgery began with the first reports of Hibbs and Albee in 1911.[1,2] Since that time many types of fusion have been described, but the specific indications for performing fusion in the setting of degenerative disease have remained less well defined. Despite some more recent articles that have attempted to clarify the role of fusion in the treatment of degenerative spinal disease,[3–11] there still exist areas of confusion regarding this controversial subject. The goal of this chapter is to provide a selection of recommended techniques of spinal fusion that may be used to stabilize the spine following degenerative disease. In addition, an attempt is made to describe what the authors believe are the indications for which spinal fusion should be considered.

Degenerative spinal disease represents a continuum, beginning with the derangement of the disc and alteration of the motion segment biomechanics and leading to subsequent abnormal stresses and degenerative changes in the facet and intervertebral joints. As a consequence of degeneration, instability and subluxation, intervertebral disc space narrowing and osteophyte formation can occur, and may cause neural compression. Degenerative changes in the vertebral column can be part of "normal" osteoarthritic aging. It may occur locally, secondary to post traumatic arthritis, or be a more diffuse and uniform process as part of a systemic disease such as rheumatoid arthritis. The final common pathway of these various degenerative processes is an alteration of the biomechanics of the spine and its subsequent adaptive changes, which in turn may lead to spinal instability and/or neurocompression.

Indications

Historically, surgical decompression of symptomatic and documented neurocompressions producing radicular or myelopathic complaints has yielded good results.[12–19] The results of decompression either with or without the addition of a fusion for the treatment of predominantly axial back or neck pain have been more disappointing.* The poor results following spinal fusion that have been reported in the literature[7,20,23–27] are probably multifactorial but result in large part from the difficulty of the clinician in precisely localizing that element or elements of the spine complex responsible for the production of pain in a particular patient.[9] The poor correlation between radiographic findings and axial spine pain is well known,[11,28–32] but radiographs document only "static" findings. Spinal fusion provides nothing more than a permanent immobilization of a spinal motion segment. If the origins of a patient's radicular or (less likely) axial complaints can be traced to abnormal spinal segment motion, then the addition of a fusion to the surgical intervention seems logically indicated. Therefore, abnormal spinal motion kinetics or more simply, spinal instability from whatever cause including degenerative change, is a problem that can be treated well by fusion.

Degenerative Instability

Instability can be subdivided into three categories to facilitate analysis: dynamic, "fixed," and anatomic.

Dynamic instability is readily documented by objective means. In the cervical spine work by Fielding[32–34] and also by White et al.,[35] these objective radiographic markers of clinical instability have been defined as greater than 3.5 mm of anteroposterior translation on flexion-extension views or greater than 11° of angular deformity as measured between the endplates of adjacent vertebral bodies. In the lumbar spine these types of objective criteria are less well defined.** Recent work by Friberg[37] has shown a

* 9,15,18,20–24.
** 11,28,29,30,36

correlation between instability and symptomatology in patients with spondylolisthesis. This instability was measured by comparing axial load and traction films of the lumbar spine of military recruits. The authors found a positive correlation between greater instability and greater complaints of low back pain. Also, work by Dupuis[38] evaluating frontal and lateral dynamic radiographs provides guidelines for documentation of lumbar instability: translation at one spinal motion segment that exceeds 3 mm at L3–L4 or L4–L5 or 5 mm at L5–S1, or 10° or more at angulation between vertebral bodies of a motion segment defines instability. McAfee and Bohlman[39] have suggested the use of the magnetic resonance imaging (MRI) as useful in documenting evidence of myelopathic compression, particularly in degenerative conditions of the cervical spine when one compares flexion and extension images.

The categories of fixed and anatomic represent situations of potential instability. "Fixed" instability is illustrated by an immobile subluxation or malalignment. Normally, because of this "self-fused" arrangement stability is already present, and a formal attempt at fusion is not necessary. If, however, further progression of the deformity can be either documented or readily predicted, then a fusion may need to be considered. Such is the situation with anatomic instability. In this situation, instability can be predicted because of iatrogenic removal of structural elements. This is typically seen following the treatment of spinal stenosis by surgical decompression including removal of the medial articular facets.[3,4,24] The authors consider resection of both facet joints at one level to meet the definition of anatomic instability. The spine can be anticipated to demonstrate either gross dynamic instability or progressive malalignment and deformity with time, and a fusion procedure is indicated.

After documentation of instability it is also recommended to supplement these studies with computerized tomography,[31,32,39,40] myelography,[31,39,41] and perhaps magnetic resonance imaging[40,42,43] to confirm nerve root or cord compression and to more precisely define the location of that compression. When instability has been documented in the symptomatic patient with degenerative disease, fusion can be contemplated with greater confidence of success.

Surgical Approaches and Fusion Types

When the decision to treat by fusion has been made, the surgeon is then faced with the choice of the anatomic approach and surgical technique of fusion to be employed. In addition, the anatomic extent of the proposed fusion must be decided.

The decision of an anterior versus posterior approach in the cervical spine as well as the lumbar spine should be dictated by the clinical problem to be treated. In general, when both decompression and subsequent fusion are anticipated, the surgical approach should be from the direction of the predominant neural compression.* This route is chosen to enhance exposure and facilitate removal of the compressing structures. Balanced against this advice to "go where the money is" is the caveat that most anterior approaches to the spine involve a more extensive dissection. If there is a reasonable choice between an anterior or posterior approach to the spine, the posterior choice is to be recommended because of its relative simplicity. Certain clinical situations tend to lend themselves to a particular approach, and in the following sections the authors have outlined their preferences.

When deciding the anatomic extent of the proposed fusion, we recommend that no more segments of the spine should be fused than necessary. This has been a particular problem in the lumbosacral spine with respect to the large mechanical loads with which this region must contend.

Cervical Spine: Indications and Recommendations

In the setting of degenerative disease, the primary indication for an anterior approach to the cervical spine seems to be for the excision of an anteriorly placed cervical disc herniation or treatment of an anteriorly placed cervical spondylotic bar and subsequent intervertebral fusion using a Smith–Robinson type of bone graft.** There exists enthusiasm among some neurosurgeons for the Cloward dowel type of intervertebral fusion. However, the Smith–Robinson graft or "keystone" construct is thought to provide superior immediate postoperative stability and is, therefore, preferred[50] (Fig. 9.1).

In the neurosurgical literature are reports[14,51] documenting excellent results using simple posterior foraminotomies for decompression of lateral nerve root compressions by both hard and soft disc herniations (Fig. 9.2). Therefore, anterior disc excision for lateral herniations with or without intervertebral fusion is not absolutely mandated.

In the unlikely event of such extensive degenerative change that a vertebral body corpectomy would be required, we advocate the tricortical T-shaped iliac graft method as outlined by Bohlman, again utilizing an anterior approach.[48,52]

In the rheumatoid patient, atlantoaxial subluxation (AAS) and atlantoaxial impaction (AAI) may require posterior stabilization.[53,54] In the situation of AAI in conjunction with upper cervical instability, an occiput-to-C2 fusion

* 13,15,16,17,21,44–47.

** 12,13,17,19,47,49.

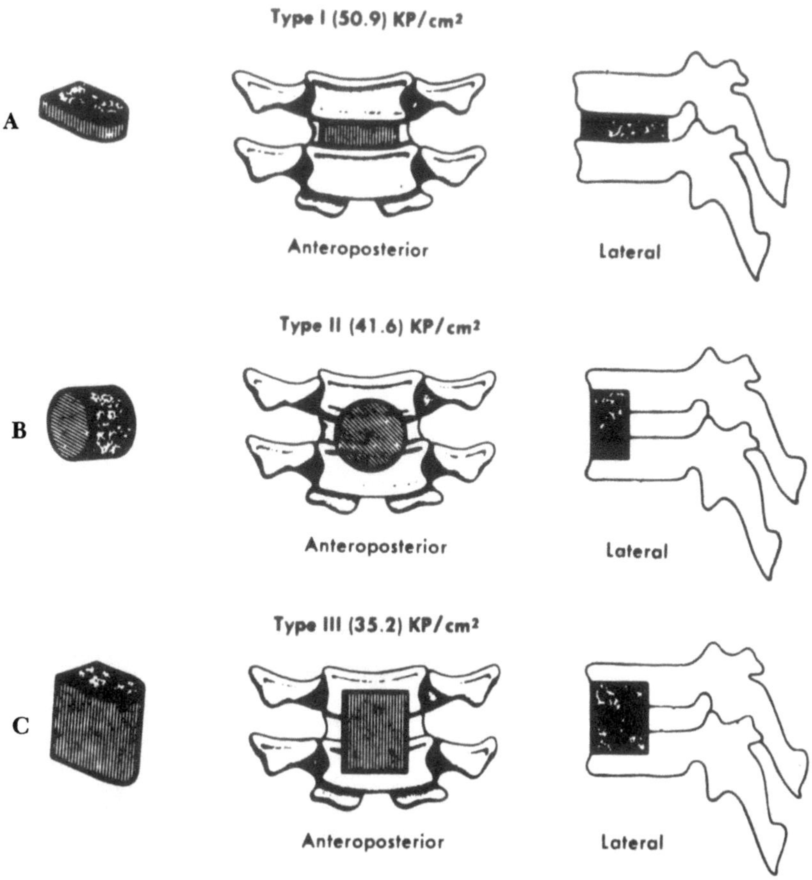

Figure 9.1. Stability of several types of anterior cervical fusions to axial load. **A.** Smith–Robinson fusion. **B.** Cloward fusion. **C.** Bailey–Badgley fusion. (Reproduced with permission from White AA, III, et al. Clin Orthop 1973;91:22.)

utilizing corticocancellous bone grafts secured with sublaminar wires, or alternatively a Luque rectangle contoured to match the occipitocervical junction to augment the fusion, is recommended. With the C1–C2 subluxations commonly found in the rheumatoid patient, the recommended technique would be a posterior fusion of the Brooks type.[25]

For the treatment of degenerative cervical spondylolisthesis, various posterior fusion techniques are suggested. Recent work by Zigler[55] suggests that a simple intertransverse wiring technique with bone grafting without decortication of the posterior lamina is all that is required. Bohlman has described a posterior triple-wire technique with autogenous iliac corticocancellous grafts wired into place, a technique that provides tremendous immediate postoperative stability.[48] Callahan[56] has described facet wiring techniques with lateral autogenous bone grafting that is of particular use following laminectomy of the cervical spine.

Anterior cervical instrumentation has been advocated in selected settings, particularly trauma,[57,58] and for reconstruction following resection of neoplasms.[59] Its use has been associated with significant complications, and its role in the treatment of degenerative cervical disorders is poorly defined at this time.

The use of polymethylmethacrylate cement as a stabilization technique without bone grafting cannot be advocated, as documented by the works of Whitehill[60] and McAfee,[61] and the use of banked bone also is not recommended for the use of augmentation of a posterior cervical fusion, as supported by the work of Stabler et al.[62]

Lumbar Spine: Indications and Recommendations

In the degenerated lumbar spine, anterior approaches are perhaps indicated for the treatment of higher grades of spondylolisthesis,[15,21,26] while a posterior approach and fusion will provide effective treatment for both the lower and higher grades.[8,63,64]

In the area of lumbar instrumentation, the technique that has aroused the greatest interest of late is the use of transpedicular fixation, particularly when attempting fusion of the lumbosacral junction. Transpedicular fixation allows the surgeon to gain control of the posterior, middle, and anterior columns[65,66] simultaneously and thereby gain greater purchase for added fixation of the lumbar vertebra. For low-grade spondylolisthesis without exacerbating factors of obesity and excess activity, our recommendation is for an intertransverse fusion alone using autograft, or

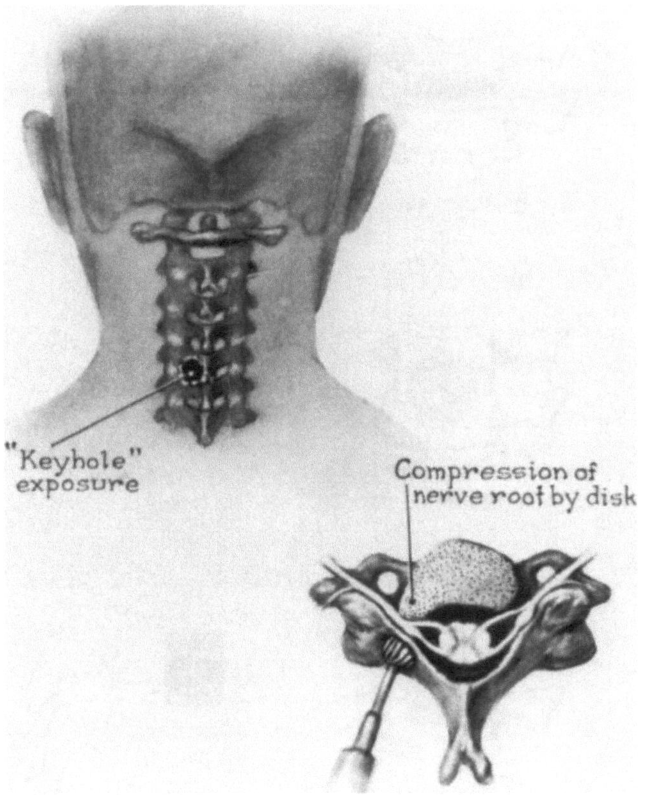

Figure 9.2. Posterior laminotomy-foraminotomy exposure of the cervical nerve root. (Reproduced with permission from Robinson RA, Southwick WO. Surgical approaches to the cervical spine. In: American Academy of Orthopaedic Surgeons: Instructional Courses Lectures, Vol. XVII. St. Louis: Mosby, 1960. Drawing modified after "keyhole" exposure of Scoville WB. Discussion. J Neurosurg 1958;15:614.)

allograft if autograft is not considered sufficient. Posterior fusions that were used in the past for the treatment of spondylolisthesis have been shown in various biomechanical studies to be associated with decreased mechanical efficiency[64] and, in addition, have at long-term follow-up been associated with the problem of overgrowth spinal stenosis, a particularly difficult problem to treat.[67]

Summary

Therefore, in overview, the recommended indication for fusion in the setting of degenerative disease is that of instability. This instability should be documented by objective radiographic means. The recommended approaches for cervical fusion are predominantly posterior, with the exception of anterior cervical fusion for central herniations of the disc and removal of more focal cervical spondylotic bars. In the degenerated lumbar spine, anterior approaches are perhaps indicated for treatment of extremely high grades of spondylolisthesis thought to be refractory to posterior fusion attempts.[26] The recommended posterior techniques in the cervical spine predominantly are those of bone grafting and wiring without need of additional instrumentation. In the lumbar spine, the recommended techniques constitute primarily the intertransverse fusion; if additional fixation is required, use of a transpedicular internal fixation system is currently advocated.[68]

As an adjunct to all spinal surgical procedures we recommend the use of head lights for improved illumination. In addition, for cases requiring neural decompression and manipulation of the spinal cord, nerve roots, or cauda equina, we strongly recommend the use of a loupe magnification (usually 2–3.5× power magnification) to enhance visualization and decrease the risk of inadvertent dural or neural laceration.

Surgical Techniques: Cervical Spine

Technique of Anterior Cervical Fusion (Robinson Technique)[17,49,70]

The patient is positioned supine with the head supported on the Mayfield "U-shaped" head holder, with axial traction applied either through Gardner–Wells two-point skull tongs or alternatively with a head halter cervical traction sling. The neck should be rotated slightly to the right to facilitate surgical exposure (Fig. 9.3). Approximately 4 kg of traction is applied initially, and the weight is increased at half-hour intervals until a total of approximately 15 kg is applied. This traction is applied to help distract the intervertebral disc space and facilitate later placement of the intervertebral bone graft.

General anesthesia is recommended for this procedure and is usually administered either through naso- or endotracheal intubation. The left side of the neck is chosen for the surgical approach because of the variability in the course of the recurrent laryngeal nerve on the right side. The skin incision is made following Langer's lines or alternatively in a line paralleling the anterior border of the sternocleidomastoid muscle (Figs. 9.4A and 9.4B).

Infiltration of the subcutaneous tissue and skin with epinephrine in saline solution (1:500,000) may be used to help control local hemorrhage. The use of the incision paralleling the anterior border of the sternocleidomastoid muscle is useful if a multiple-level exposure of the cervical spine is required. For single-level exposure, particularly of the mid- and lower cervical spine, the more transverse incision using Langer's lines is preferred (Fig. 9.5). If the local infiltration with epinephrine is not used, it is

Figure 9.3. Correct position for anterior cervical fusion using left-sided approach to cervical spine and left iliac crest graft. Note that folded sheet is placed beneath scapula and also beneath left iliac crest. Hair is covered with sterile towel or cap. (Reproduced with permission from Rothman RH, Simeone FA. The Spine. Philadelphia: Saunders, 1982;1:480, Fig. 7.37.)

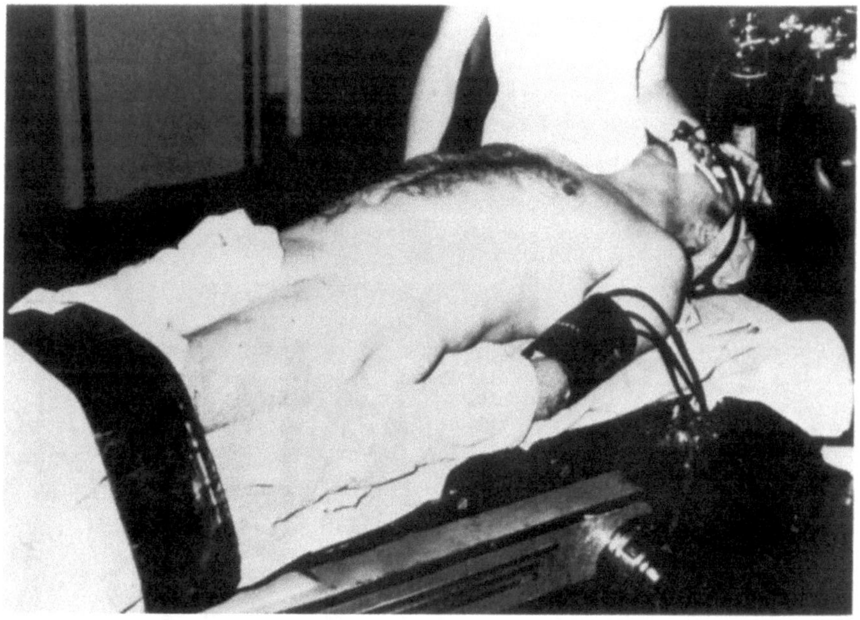

A

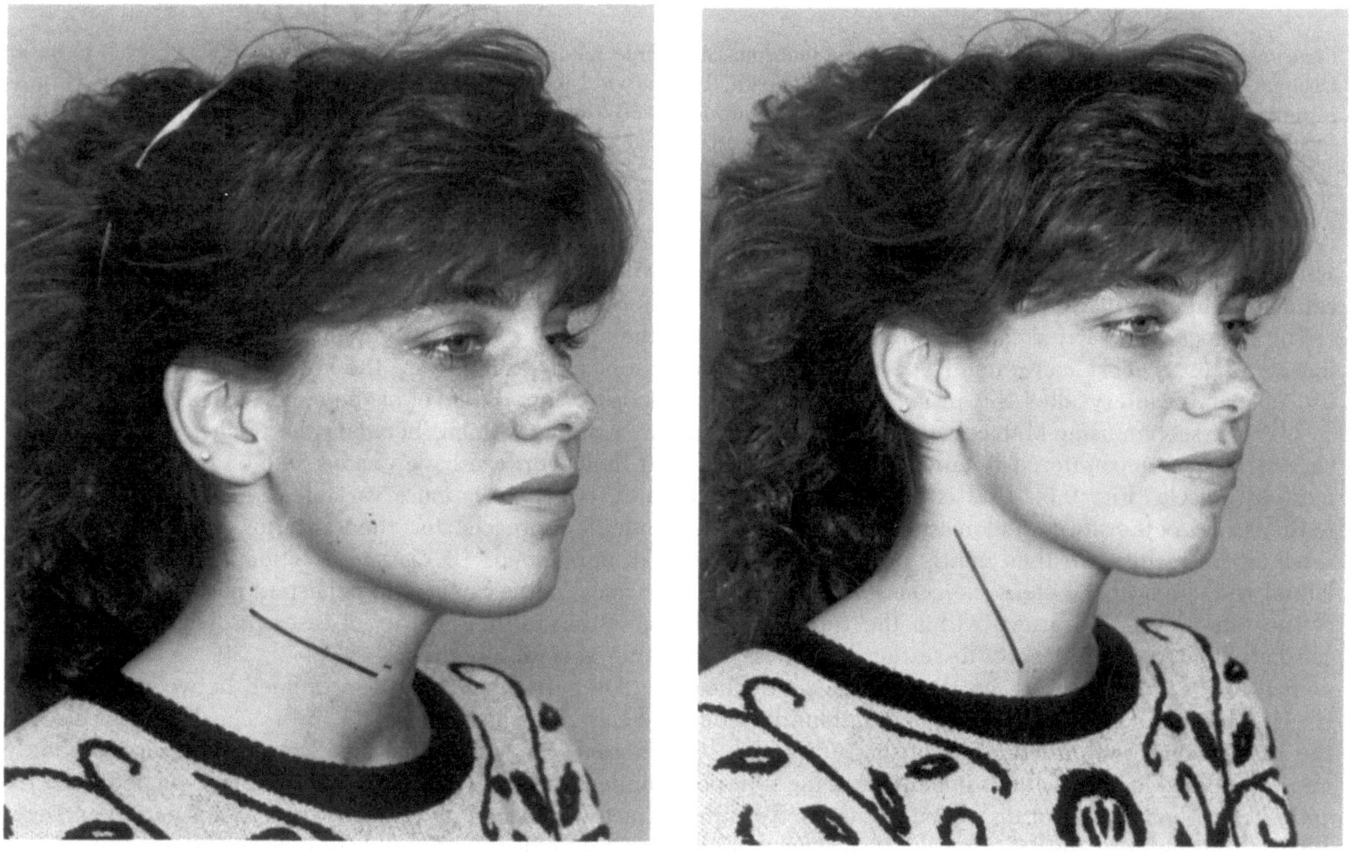

B

Figure 9.4. **A.** Horizontal incision for anterior cervical fusion. This is usually cosmetically acceptable, but is not an extensile approach. **B.** Oblique incision for anterior cervical fusion. This produces less satisfactory cosmetic appearance, but is a more extensile approach.

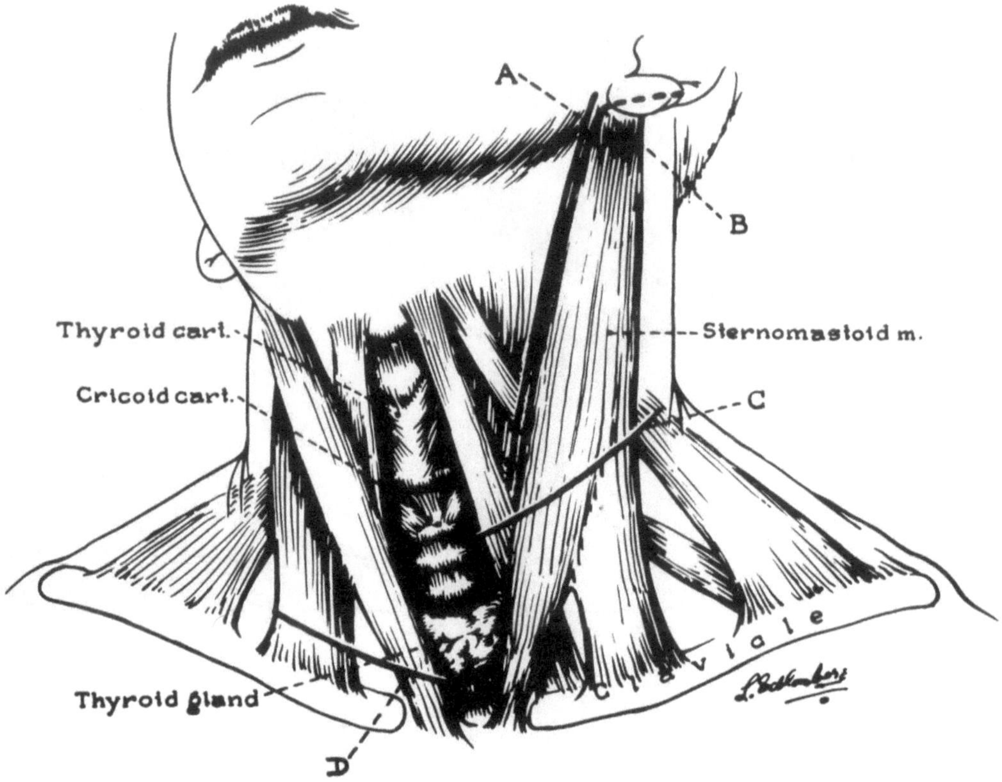

Figure 9.5. Anterior approaches to cervical spine; incisions. **A.** Occiput and upper cervical spine medial to carotid sheath. **B.** Anterior approach to first and second vertebrae lateral to carotid sheath. **C.** Anterior approach to middle and lower cervical vertebrae medial to carotid sheath. **D.** Anterior approach to lower cervical and upper thoracic vertebrae. (Reproduced with permission from Rothman RH, Simeone FA. The Spine. Philadelphia: Saunders, 1982;1:97, Fig. 4.29.)

recommended that multiple subcutaneous curved hemostats be placed for hemostasis and self-retaining Weitlaner retractors then be placed to aid exposure.

The dissection is carried sharply through the platysma muscle. This is most conveniently performed with the use of electrocautery after the plane has been defined by blunt dissection using Metzenbaum scissors. The deep cervical fascia is encountered as it invests the sternocleidomastoid muscle (Fig. 9.6). This is divided just anterior to the border of the sternocleidomastoid muscle. The self-retaining retractors are then gently positioned to allow lateral retraction of the sternocleidomastoid. The pulses of the internal carotid artery within the carotid sheath can be palpated. The plane of dissection is then carried medial to the carotid sheath on through the pretracheal fascia. This dissection is best performed bluntly along the tissue planes with a minimum of sharp dissection to minimize blood loss. It is at this juncture that the superior and inferior boundaries of dissection are defined by the superior and inferior thyroid arteries. If, however, additional exposure is necessary superiorly, the superior thyroid artery may be ligated.

The recurrent laryngeal nerve descends in the neck within the carotid sheath after branching off the vagus nerve. On the left side it emerges and loops underneath the arch of the aorta to ascend between the trachea and esophagus to innervate the vocal chords. On the right it loops below the level of the subclavian artery to ascend, in a similar fashion, between the trachea and esophagus. It, however, can have various take-off points on the right and its course is more variable; and therefore, the left-sided approach to the anterior cervical spine is recommended.[49] Excessive traction on the recurrent laryngeal nerve can lead to persistent postoperative hoarseness that in the majority of cases resolves spontaneously after several months.

After the plane has been defined between the carotid sheath and the trachea, the pretracheal fascia is sharply incised. Further medial dissection is then carried bluntly underneath the esophagus. A hand-held angled knee retractor is placed underneath the esophagus to gently retract it medially. The anterior surface of the spinal column can then be visualized. The prevertebral fascia overlies the anterior cervical column and through it the longus

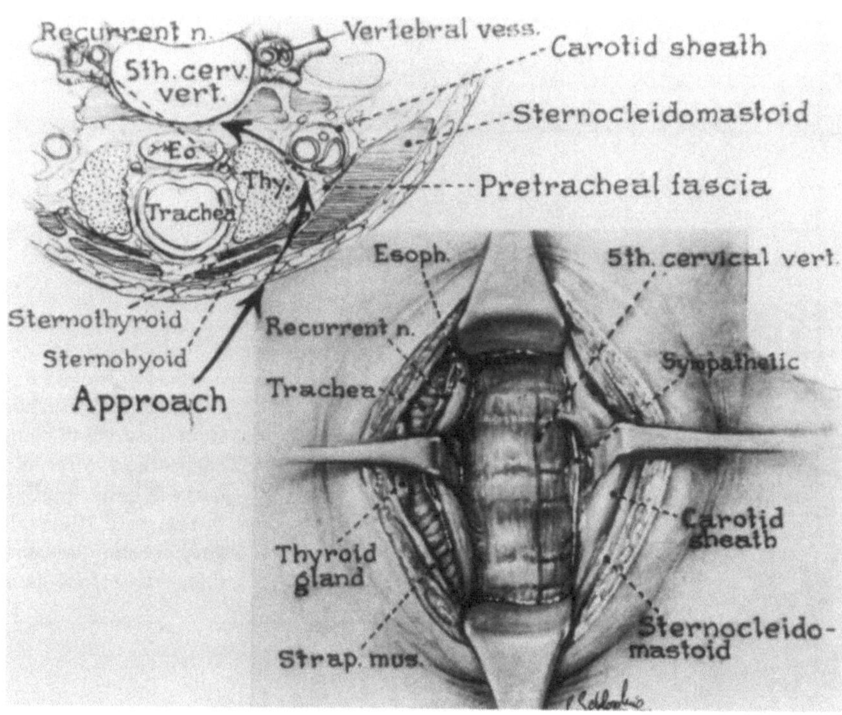

Figure 9.6. Anterior approach to mid- and lower cervical vertebrae, deep dissection. (Reproduced with permission from Southwick WO and Robinson RA. Surgical approaches to the vertebral bodies in the cervical and lumbar regions. J Bone Joint Surg 1957;39A:634, Fig. 4.42.)

colli and/or lateral splenius capitus muscles can be seen flanking the vertebral bodies. The longitudinal masses of the sympathetic chain can be seen on the anterior surface of the longus colli.

Because of the generous vascular supply to the prevertebral fascia, it is recommended to electrocauterize a longitudinal tract in the midline of the vertebral bodies between the intervertebral discs. Subsequently the prevertebral fascia can be elevated both medially and laterally using a periosteal elevator. The edges of a Cloward self-retaining retractor are then placed underneath the edges of the prevertebral fascia to provide exposure. Care is taken to place the tips of the retractor subperiosteally to avoid direct traction on the esophagus, recurrent laryngeal nerve, or sympathetic chain. The superficial temporal arterial pulse should be palpated at intervals by the anesthesiologist. Loss of this pulse may indicate excessive pressure on the internal carotid, and the self-retaining retractor would need to be repositioned.

The particular vertebral disc is identified by an intraoperative cross-table cervical spine radiograph. An 18-gauge spinal needle can be used as a marker for the intraoperative radiograph, but it should have two successive 90° bends placed to prevent accidental penetration of the posterior longitudinal ligament and possible dural laceration (Fig. 9.7). In addition, the marker should be placed in as cephalad an interspace as possible (i.e., C3–C4 or C4–C5) to prevent any difficulty confirming vertebral levels, which may be obscured by the superimposed images of the shoulders on the lateral radiograph.

The intervertebral annulus is sharply incised, and the disc material is removed in piecemeal fashion using a combination of straight and angled pituitary-type rongeurs and small straight and curved curettes. The attempt is made not to violate the continuity of the posterior longitudinal ligament and risk possible spinal cord injury. In similar fashion, no particular effort is made to remove posterior lip osteophytes. We agree with Robinson that the natural history is for spontaneous resorption of the osteophytes after solid fusion is achieved.[17] There are, however, differing opinions.[69]

After the disc has been removed, measurements of the intervertebral space are made using a malleable silver probe, and the requisite bone graft dimensions are determined. The bone graft is harvested from one of the anterior iliac crests. It is a tricortical "horseshoe" graft using the inner and outer tables of the iliac crest as well as the iliac ridge (Fig. 9.8) and is approximately 7–9 mm thick. Before placing the graft the superior and inferior endplates of the adjacent vertebral bodies are decorticated with a diamond-tipped burr, and care is taken to create a small groove transversely on the superior endplate to create a notch to help lock the graft into place. The graft is gently tamped into place with a narrow bone tamp. Care is taken to recess the anterior surface of the graft some 1–2 mm posterior to the anterior cortex of the superior vertebral body. Additional care is taken to avoid splitting of the cortex of the graft, which may promote resorption of the graft and collapse of the intervertebral space. The last proviso regarding the graft is the obvious need to avoid

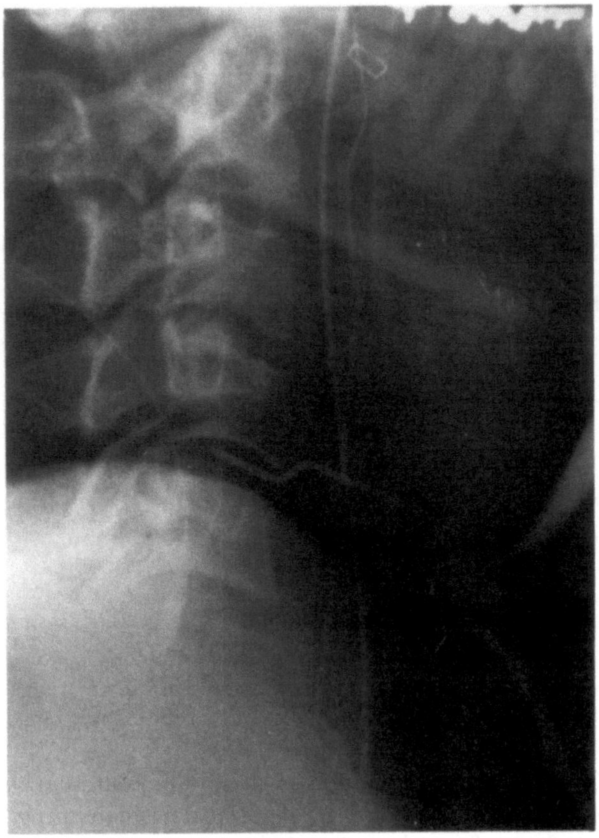

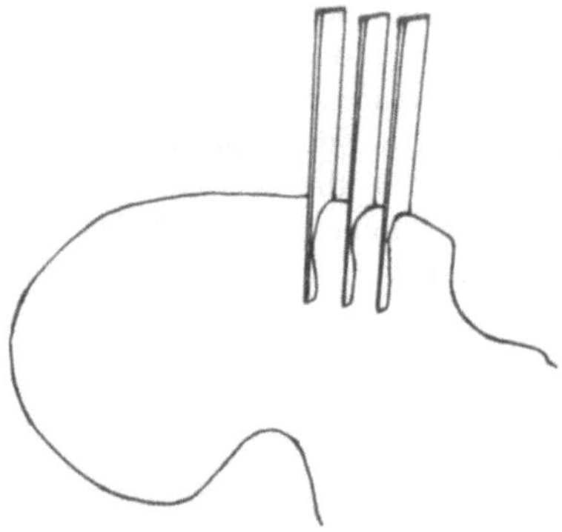

Figure 9.8. Horseshoe-shaped corticocancellous bone graft is obtained from iliac crest using oscillating osteotomes positioned parallel to each other. Alternatively, an oscillating power saw may be used to harvest bone graft. Use of saw may create fewer "microfractures" in the graft. (Reproduced with permission from Lumbar Spine Surgery: Techniques and Complications, White AA, Rothman RH, Ray CD, eds. St. Louis: Mosby, 1987: 437, Fig. 39.2.)

◁
Figure 9.7. Note 18-gauge spinal needle with two successive 90° bends used as intraoperative marker in the C3–C4 interspace. See text for additional discussion.

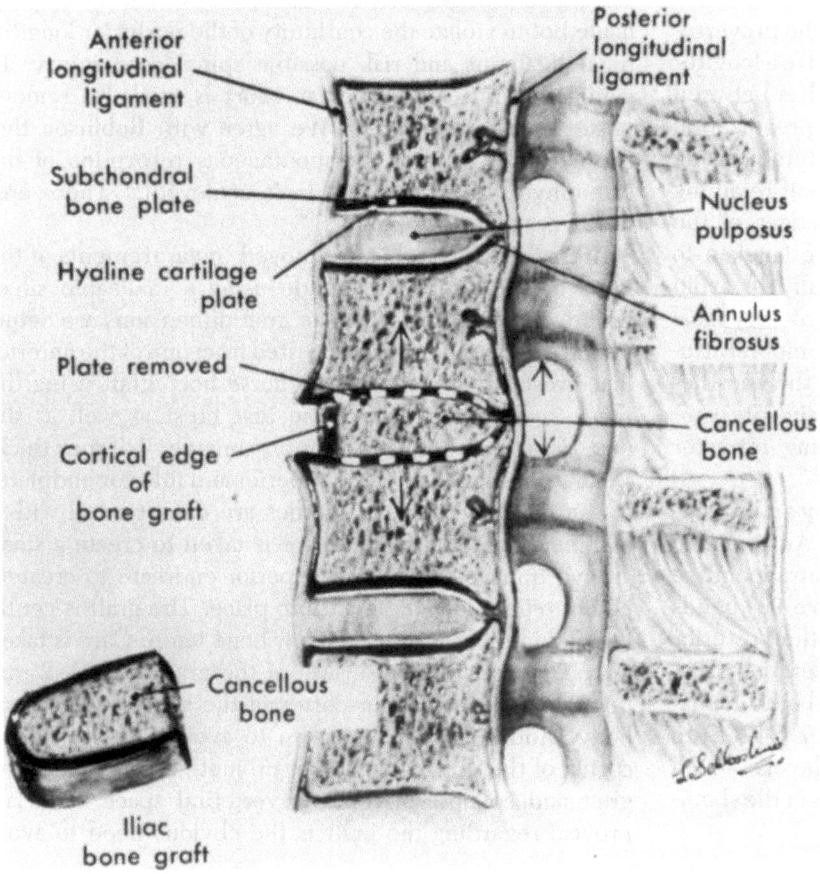

Figure 9.9. Technique of Robinson et al. for anterior fusion of cervical spine (see text). [Reproduced with permission (modified) from Robinson RA, et al. J Bone Joint Surg 1962;44A:1569, Fig. 70.3.]

iatrogenic cord compression by either too large a graft (as measured in the A-P dimension) or displacement of the graft posteriorly by overly vigorous tamping. At this point most of the cervical traction is discontinued (approximately 12 kg) and the graft is assessed for stability (Fig. 9.9).

The wound is then well irrigated and the subcutaneous tissue and dermis are closed in layers. Because of the stability of this construct with the intact middle and posterior columns, postoperative immobilization with a hard collar for 6–8 weeks is thought sufficient.

It should be noted that for all anterior cervical spine fusions, intraoperative neurological monitoring with the use of somatosensory evoked-response potentials for the assessment of the dorsal columns and the intraoperative wake-up test for assessment of anterior motor columns is advocated.[55,71]

Posterior Cervical Approach and Atlantoaxial Fusion Technique (Brooks Technique)[25,72]

The patient is placed in the prone position after induction of anesthesia, which may be either general or local according to the surgeon's preference; the use of local anesthetic technique allows for easy direct monitoring of the patient's neurological status.[55] The head is supported by the Mayfield three-pin head holder or alternatively by the simple U-shaped Mayfield head rest (Figs. 9.10–9.12). With use of the U-shaped head rest, care must be taken to avoid undue pressure on the patient's eyes. The dorsal skin of the neck can be infiltrated with an epinephrine and saline solution (1:500,000) for hemostasis. Following skin incision the plane of dissection is carried down directly in the midline, using the relatively avascular plane of the ligamentum nuchae. Self-retaining retractors are placed for additional exposure. Intraoperative radiographs may

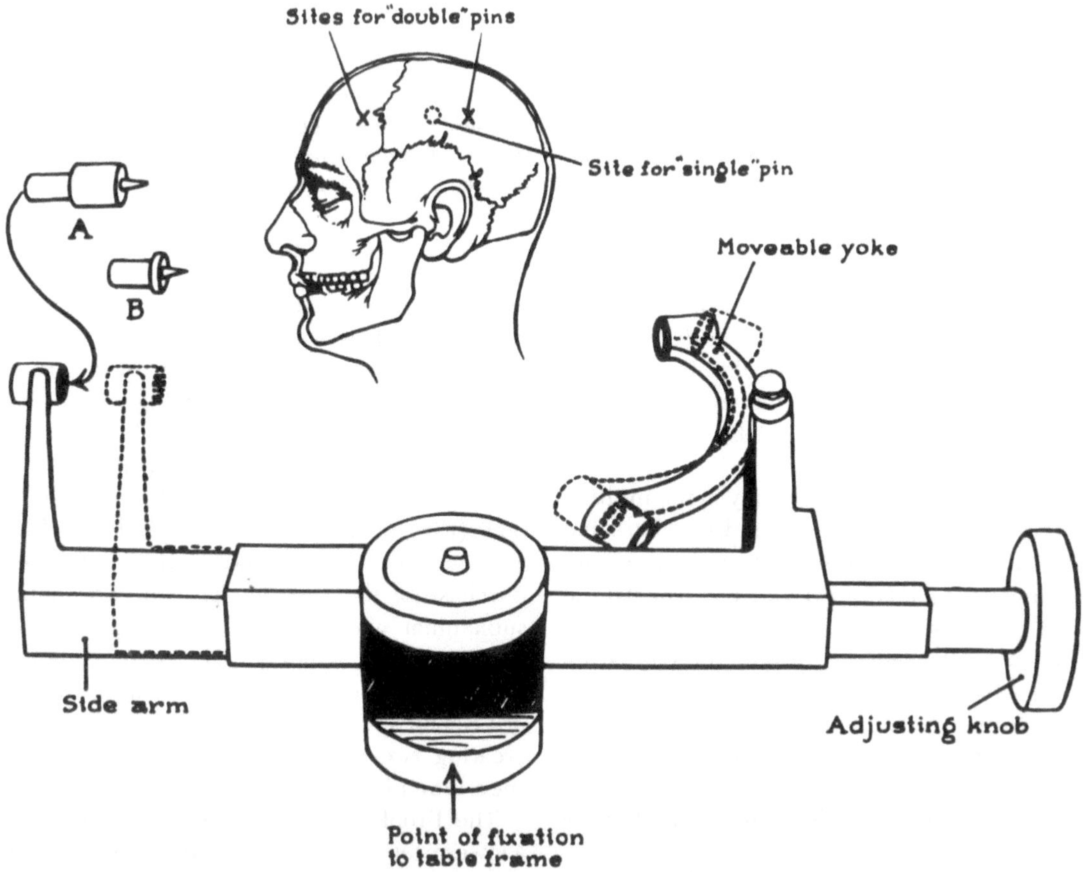

Figure 9.10. Three-point headrest is U-shaped frame that is adjustable in width. Two pins are fixed to hinged yoke on one side of frame; third pin is fixed to opposite side. These are placed just above ear of the patient at widest point of the skull. Pediatric pins (A) are available with longer shank, and should be used for children or adults with narrow head. These decrease distance between pins and provide satisfactory fixation even when skull is narrow. (Reproduced with permission from Rothman RH, Simeone FA. The Spine, Philadelphia: Saunders, 1982:102, Fig. 4.34.)

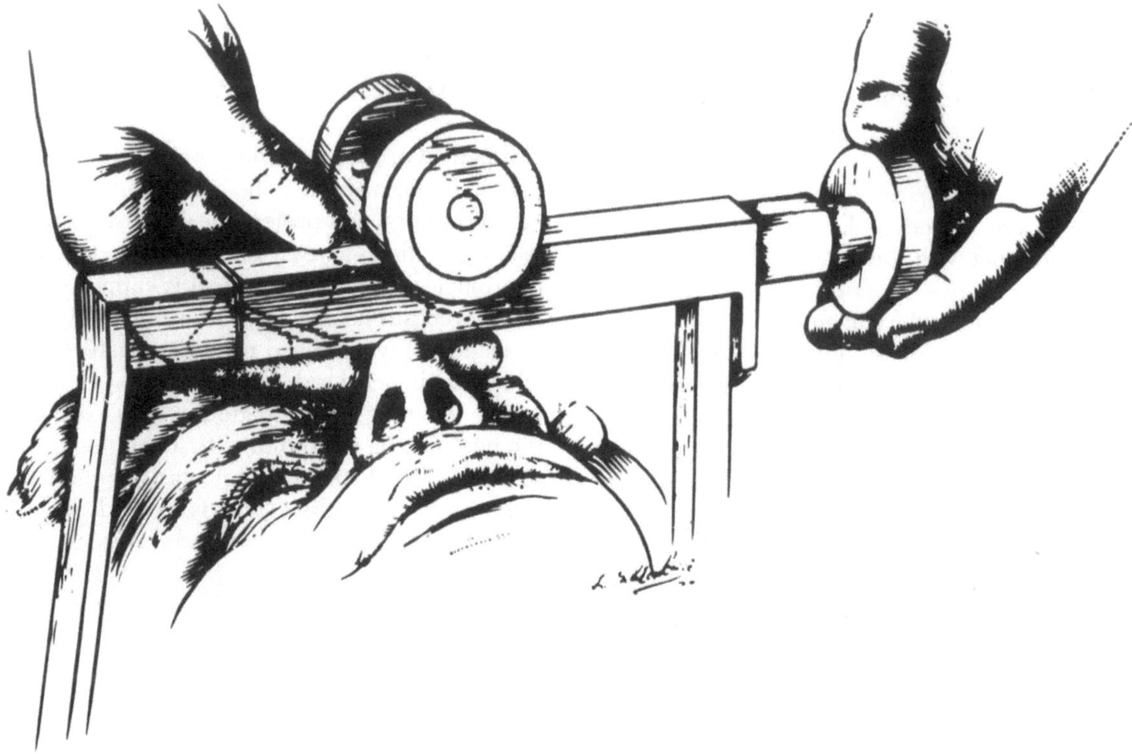

Figure 9.11. To place pin headrest on patient, surgeon holds center of frame in one hand with fingers resting on patient's forehead to ensure frame does not press against patient's skin. Pins are placed just above ear at widest portion of skull; frame is closed firmly using turning knob until pins are well seated in outer table of skull. Frame should be moved to check that all pins are well fixed to bone and do not move within soft tissues. (Reproduced with permission from Rothman RH, Simeone, FA. The Spine, Philadelphia: Saunders, 1982:103, Fig. 4.35.)

be obtained to help ascertain vertebral levels; however, this is usually not necessary, and levels may be determined by palpation of bony landmarks. In particular, the absence of the spinous process of C1 and the large, easily palpated bifid spinous process of C2 provide readily confirmable landmarks.

The dissection is carried further ventrally in the midline down to the level of the lamina of C1 and C2. Utilizing subperiosteal dissection technique, exposure is carried laterally exposing the lamina of C1 and C2. The lateral limits of dissection are determined by the vertebral artery as it travels superiorly through the foramen transversarum and then at the level of the atlas courses medially and then anteriorly to plunge through the posterior atlanto-occipital membrane to contribute blood supply to the spinal cord (Figs. 9.13 and 9.14). The vertebral arteries are present usually some 2 cm laterally from the midline of C1.

Using gentle subperiosteal dissection techniques, a plane of dissection is then developed underneath the lamina of C1 and C2, and two doubled 20-gauge wires are passed underneath the lamina of C1 and C2 (Fig. 9.13). Care is taken not to exert any anterior pressure on the cervical spinal cord, which may cause neurological damage. This is accomplished by maintaining constant pressure between the doubled loop of wire and the bony undersurface of the lamina during wire passage.

The bone grafts are harvested from the posterior iliac crest and are shaped into wedge-shaped blocks with an intact posterior cortex and an anterior wedge of cancellous bone (Figs. 9.15–9.18). Notches are created at the superior and inferior edges of the cortical endplate to improve purchase of the wire loops. The two doubled 20-gauge sublaminar wires are passed into the midline and then gently moved laterally. The two wedge-shaped bone blocks are then positioned dorsally between the lamina of C1 and C2. The looped end of the wire is snipped, creating two wires for each bone graft. The wires are then individually tightened to secure the grafts.

The Brooks atlantoaxial fusion is documented to have a lower pseudarthrosis rate[25] than the Gallie-type fusion.[73] However, the Gallie fusion entails the passage of a single, double wire underneath the lamina of C1 and requires no wire passage under the lamina of C2. Because of this decreased risk of neurological injury, the Gallie fusion may be preferred.

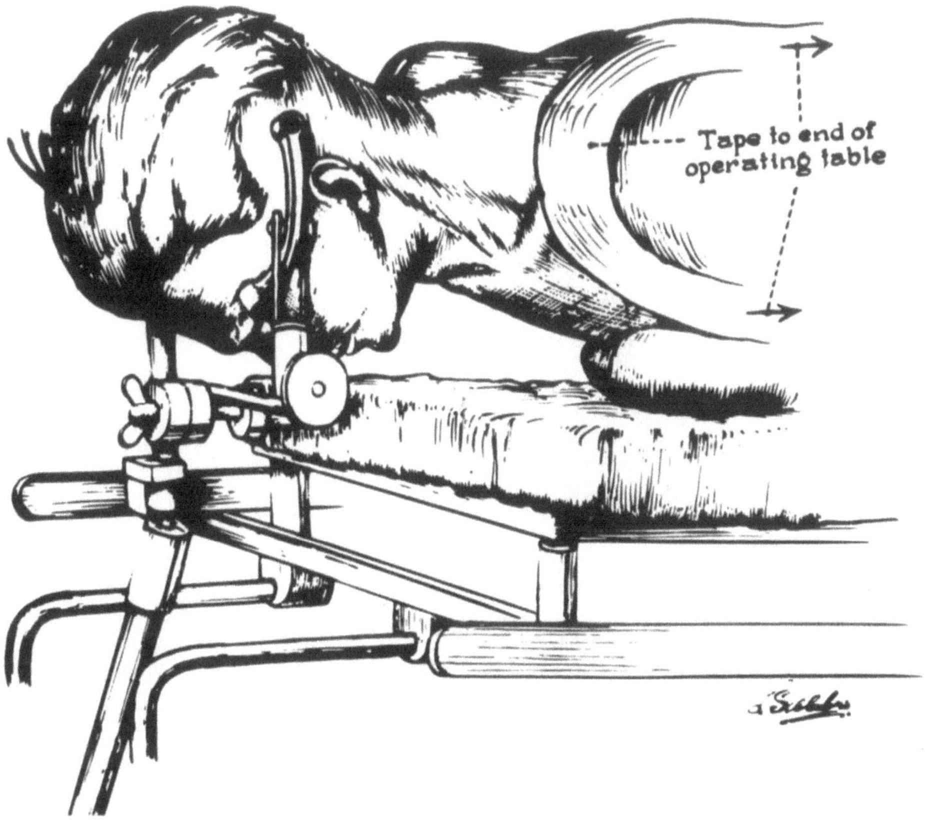

Figure 9.12. Patient is turned onto operating table with surgeon controlling head and neck by holding pin headrest. Surgeon places head and neck in desired position, and assistant secures frame to operating table. Countertraction is then applied to neck by taping shoulders to distal end of operating table. Lateral roentgenogram is made to verify that vertebrae are properly aligned. (Reproduced with permission from Griswold DM et al. Atlantoaxial fusion for instability. J Bone Joint Surg 1978;60A:285–292, Fig. 1.)

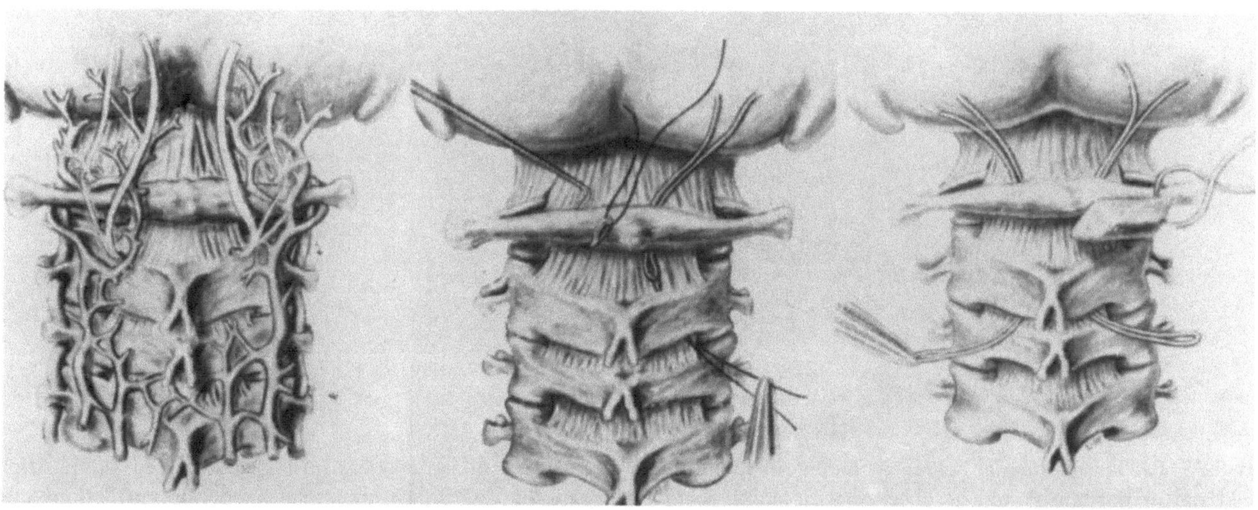

A B C

Figure 9.13. Brooks and Jenkins technique of atlantoaxial fusion. **A.** Position of vertebral arteries and occipital nerves. With midline approach, they are fairly well protected by neck muscles. **B.** Insertion of wires under atlas and axis. **C.** Wires are in place, and one graft is being inserted. (Reproduced with permission from Brooks AL, Jenkins EB. J Bone Joint Surg 1978;60A:279, Fig. 1–3.)

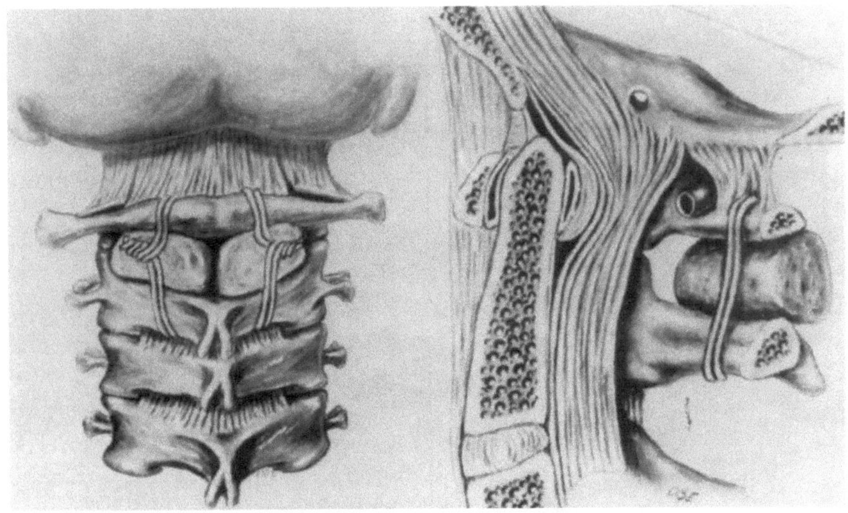

A B

Figure 9.14. Brooks and Jenkins technique of atlantoaxial fusion, **A** and **B.** Grafts are secured by wires. Note relationship of sublaminar wires to vertebral arteries. (Reproduced with permission from Brooks AL, Jenkins EB. J Bone Surg 1978;60A:279, Figs. 4 & 5.)

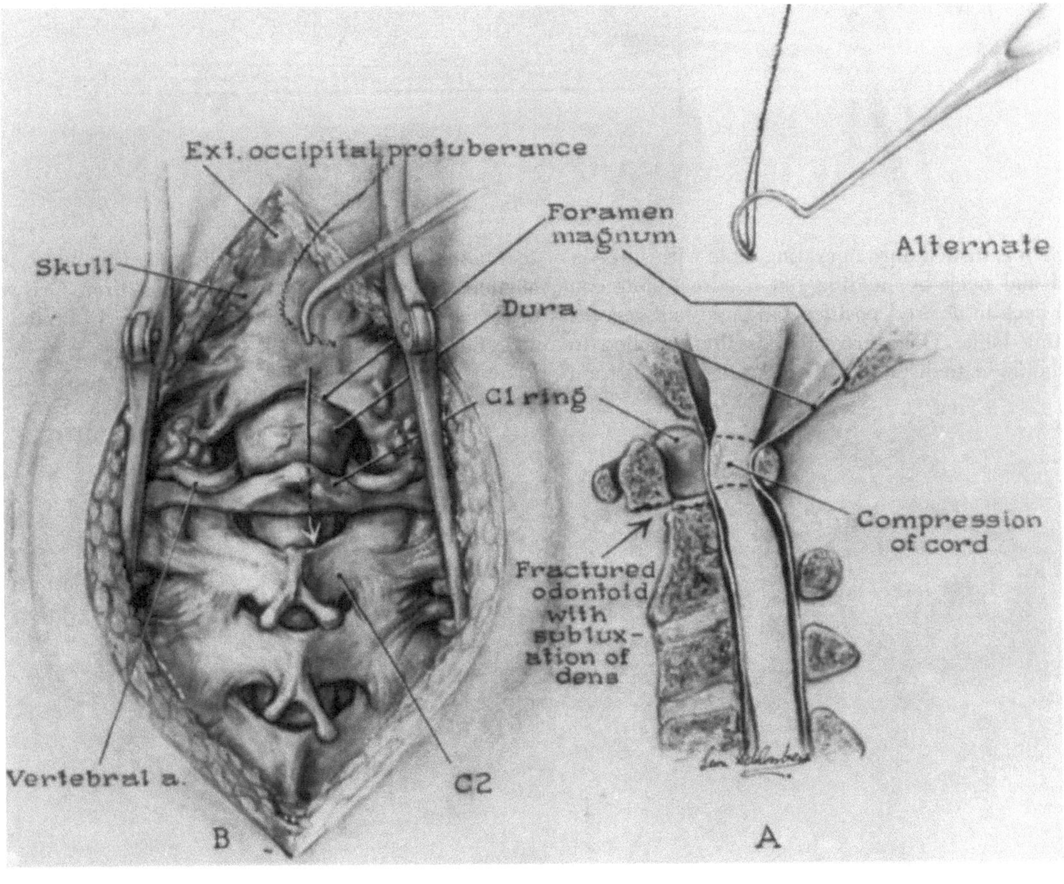

Figure 9.15. Brooks atlantoaxial fusion. **A.** Odontoid should be reduced and its position should be checked with lateral roentgenogram made in operating room before preparing or draping patient. This must be done before dissecting around posterior elements or passing wires to prevent injury to spinal cord or medulla. **B.** Posterior ring of atlas and lamina of axis are cleared of soft tissue by gentle subperiosteal dissection. Base of occiput is not dissected free, as shown, to avoid inadvertent fusion to skull. Twisted 24-gauge stainless steel wires are passed beneath ring of atlas and lamina of axis using right-angled clamp. Alternative method is to pass aneurysm needle around lamina of axis from above. A heavy silk suture is threaded into eye of aneurysm needle, needle is withdrawn upward, and suture is retrieved. Silk suture is passed in similar manner beneath posterior ring of atlas. Wires then may be attached to silk suture and passed atraumatically beneath both posterior rings. (Reproduced with permission from Griswold DM et al. Atlantoaxial fusion for instability. J Bone Joint Surg 1978;60A:285–292, Fig. 2A & B.)

Figure 9.16. **A,B,C.** Two 24-gauge twisted wires are passed beneath the posterior atlantoaxial rings, two on each side of midline to hold grafts in place. (Reproduced with permission from Griswold DM et al. Atlantoaxial fusion for instability. J Bone Joint Surg 1978;60A:285–292, Fig. 2C, D, & E.)

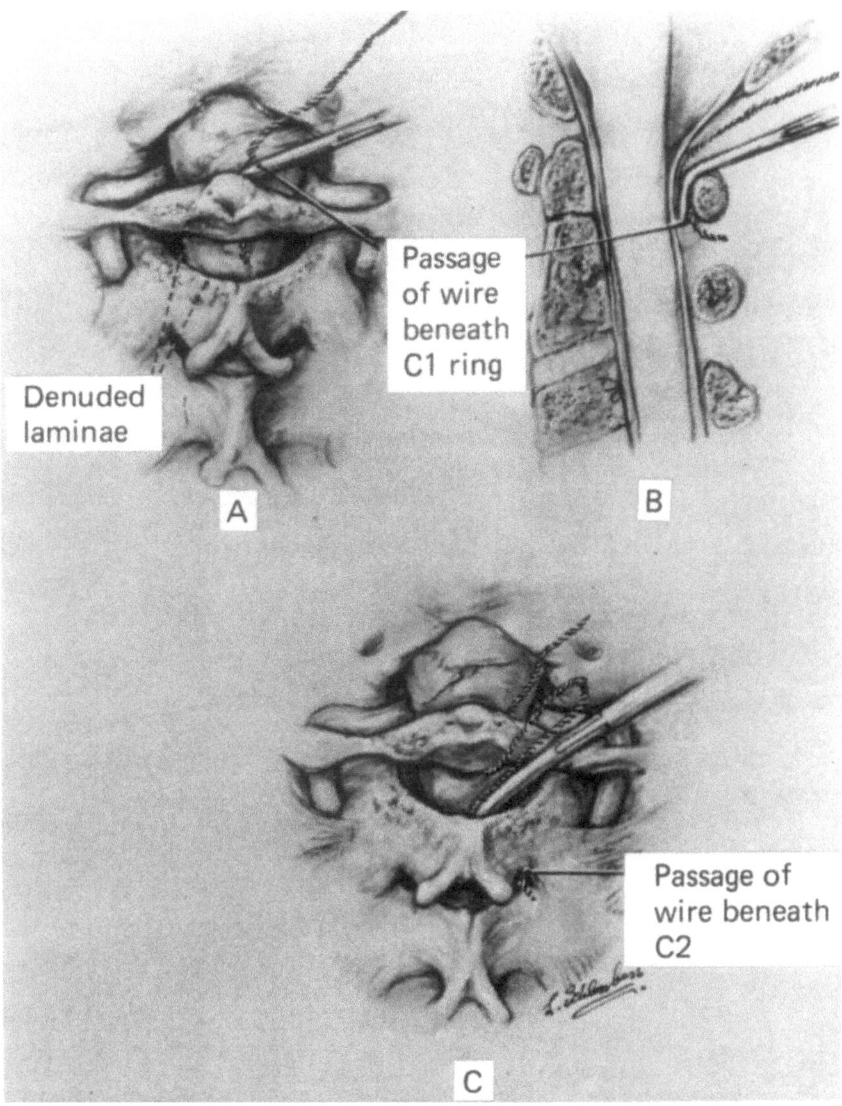

Gallie Technique for Posterior Atlantoaxial Fusion[33,73]

The technique for the Gallie fusion is identical to the Brooks technique in terms of patient position and surgical exposure. The major difference is in the fashioning of the corticocancellous graft and the technique of fixation.

An approximately 1 × 3 × 1 cm corticocancellous graft is harvested from the patient's iliac crest and then fashioned into an H shape with notching superiorly and inferiorly of the posterior cortical plate (Fig. 9.19). A small notch is also prepared in the superior surface of the C2 spinous process to help lock the graft in position. A doubled 20-gauge wire is passed in an inferior to superior direction underneath the lamina of C1. The free ends of the wire are then passed through the loop of the 20-gauge wire. The H-shaped graft is placed between the undersurface of the lamina of C1 and the superior surface of the lamina of C2. The graft is fitted into the notch created on the superior surface of the spinous process of C2. The loose ends of the wire are brought around and tightened underneath the spinous process of C2 to secure the graft.

The decision to drain or not drain these fusions is left to the discretion of the surgeon. Drainage of surgical procedures utilizing metallic internal fixation is recommended. We routinely drain the necks of our patients in whom metal has been used to help secure the grafts. Closure is in layers, and skin closure is accomplished by a running subcuticular absorbable suture. Postoperative immobilization of the Brooks fusion is probably adequate, as mentioned, with a Philadelphia-type collar. The Gallie fusion construct is less intrinsically rigid, and particularly when attempting fusion in patients with osteopenia, we recommend postoperative immobilization in a halo orthosis for some 8–12 weeks. The halo is removed after radiographic evidence of fusion is seen. Detailed description of halo techniques and applications are available elsewhere.[74]

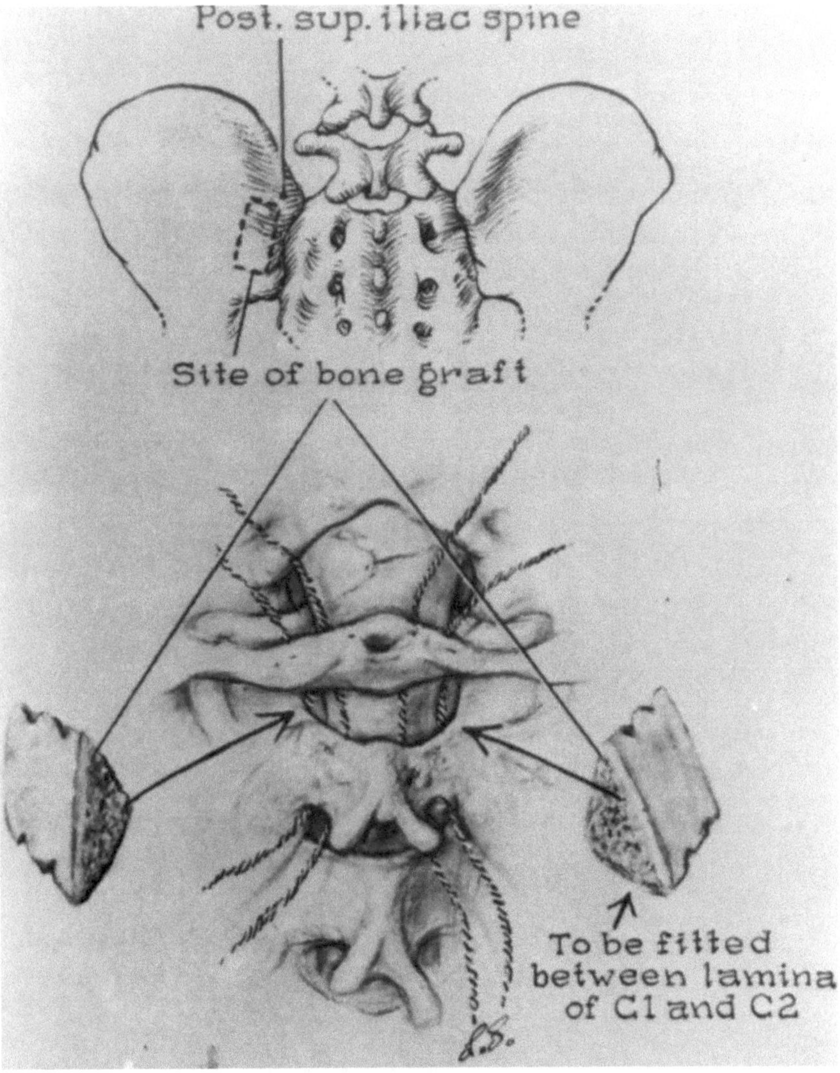

Figure 9.17. Rectangle of bone graft 2 × 4 cm is taken from posterior ilium superficial to sacroiliac joint and includes only outer cortex. Rectangle is centered over longitudinal ridge, normally present over posterior ilium. Graft is divided into two prism-shaped pieces, 1.5 × 2.0 cm long and 1 cm deep. Deep surface should be carved to create triangle, apex of which will fit snugly between posterior vertebral rings. Grafts are notched at upper and lower ends to hold wires and to keep them from slipping. (Reproduced with permission from Griswold DM et al. Atlantoaxial fusion for instability, J Bone Joint Surg 1978;60A:285–292, Fig. 2F.)

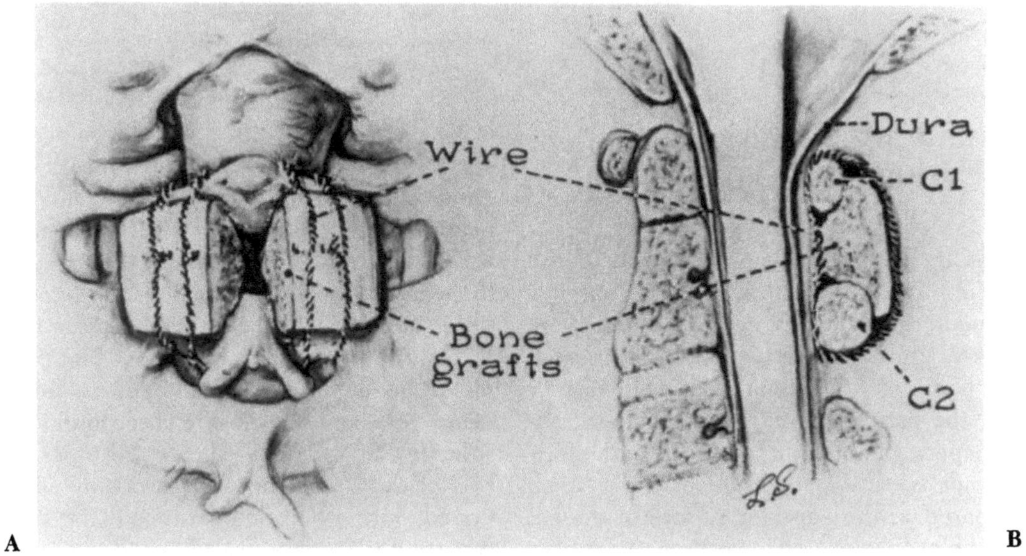

Figure 9.18. **A, B.** Two wires on either side are separated as far as possible without injuring vertebral vessels. Wires are then tightened and twisted to wedge grafts in place between vertebral rings. This creates secure bone block, which effectively limits motion in all planes. (Reproduced with permission from Griswold DM et al. Atlantoaxial fusion for instability. J Bone Joint Surg 60A:285–292, Fig. 2G & H.)

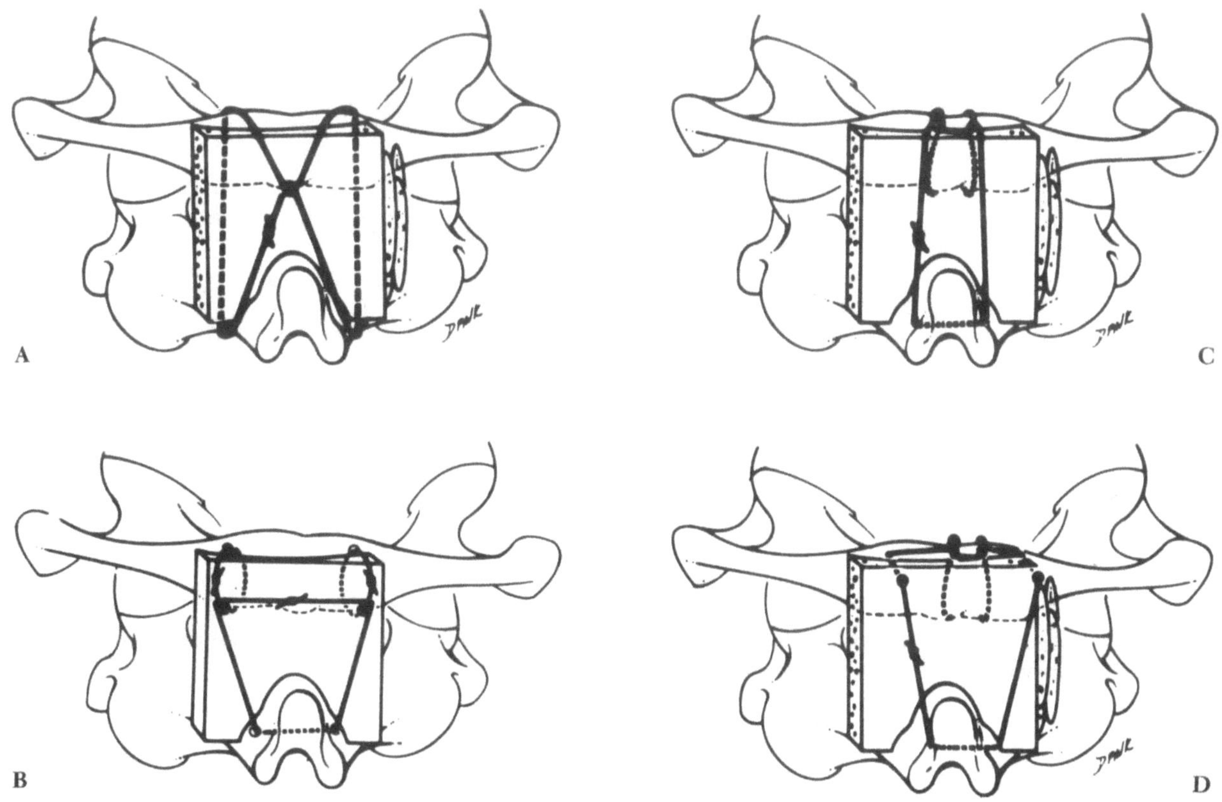

Figure 9.19. Drawings demonstrate various methods of using wire to hold graft in place. **A.** Wire passes under lamina of atlas and axis and is tied over graft. **B.** Wire passes through holes drilled in lamina of atlas and through spine of axis; holes are drilled through graft. This is method we use most frequently. **C.** Wire passes under lamina of atlas and through spine of axis and is tied over graft. **D.** Wire passes under lamina of atlas and through spine of axis: holes are drilled through graft. (Reproduced with permission from Fielding JW, Hawkins RJ, Ratzan SA. J Bone Joint Surg 1976;58A:400, Fig. 3A–D.)

Posterior Cervical Interspinous Fusion

The technique of interspinous process fusion as originally described by Rogers[75,76] is quite simple and as modified by Zigler[55] is an even more simple technique. The patient is positioned prone as described for atlantoaxial fusion. These posterior cervical fusions may be performed under local anesthesia, allowing for direct assessment of the patient's neurological status.

Dissection is made through the midline, utilizing the avascular plane of the ligamentum nuchae. The spinous processes of the affected cervical levels are exposed in a subperiosteal fashion, and a simple wire loop of 18-gauge wire is then passed through and around the superior spinous process using a hole created by a towel clip at the juncture of the spinous process with the lamina (Fig. 9.20). Care is taken not to penetrate the spinal canal and risk possible dural laceration. The wire is then looped around the inferior spinous process and tightened. Corticocancellous grafts fashioned into "matchsticks" are laid directly on the posterior cortices and spanning the gap between the adjacent lamina (Fig. 9.20). Zigler reports uniformly good incorporation of the grafts without decortication of the posterior lamina.[55] The wound is drained and closed in layers. Postoperative immobilization and a hard collar for 8–12 weeks are advised.

Multilevel Posterior Cervical Stabilization

If stabilization of a degenerated cervical spine is indicated, such as after wide decompressive laminectomy for the treatment of diffuse spondylosis, the posterior grafting and wire stabilization technique of Callahan et al[56] is suggested. A posterior cervical approach as previously outlined is used. A careful debridement of the capsules overlying the facet joints is carried out. A small flat elevator is placed into the facet, and a power burr is used to create a drill hole through the inferior facet. A small flat elevator is positioned within the facet joint to intervene between the tip of the burr and the superior facet and protect the subsequent anterior structures of the vertebral artery and nerve roots (Fig 9.21). A 20-gauge wire is passed, as is shown in Fig. 9.22, between adjacent ipsilateral facets and tied down. If bone grafting is thought to be necessary, two long, approximately 2 × 5 cm, corticocancellous grafts

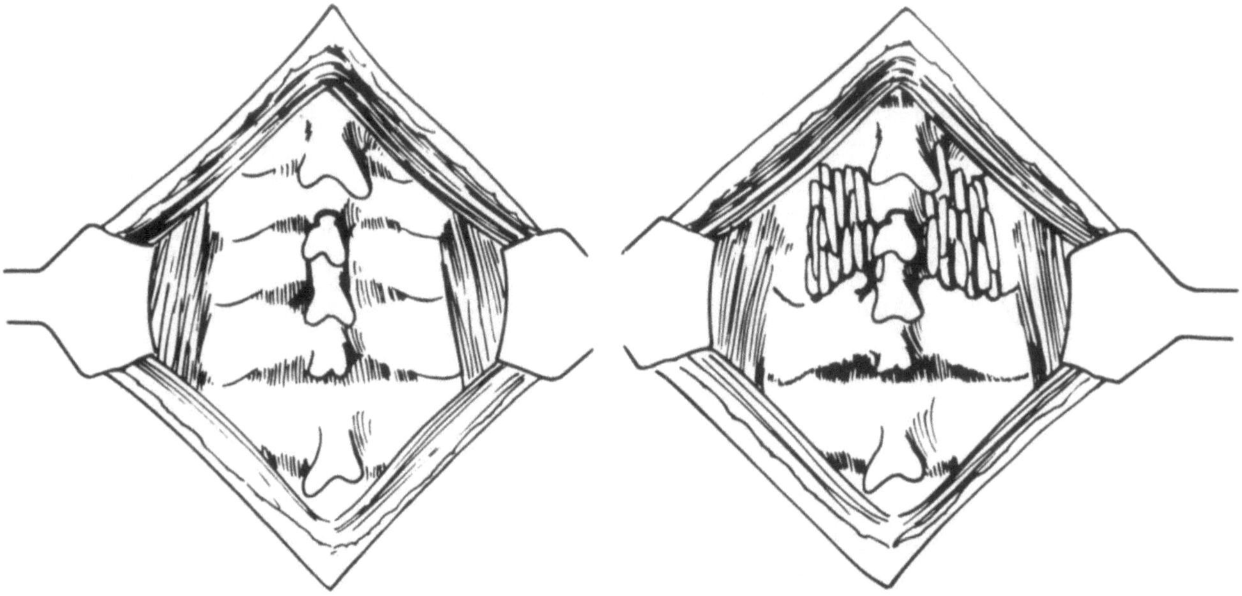

Figure 9.20. Correct placement of matchstick is illustrated cancellous grafts bridging adjacent laminae. (Reproduced with permission from Rothman RH, Simeone FA. The Spine. Philadelphia: Saunders, 1982:426, Figs. 7–31 & 7–32.)

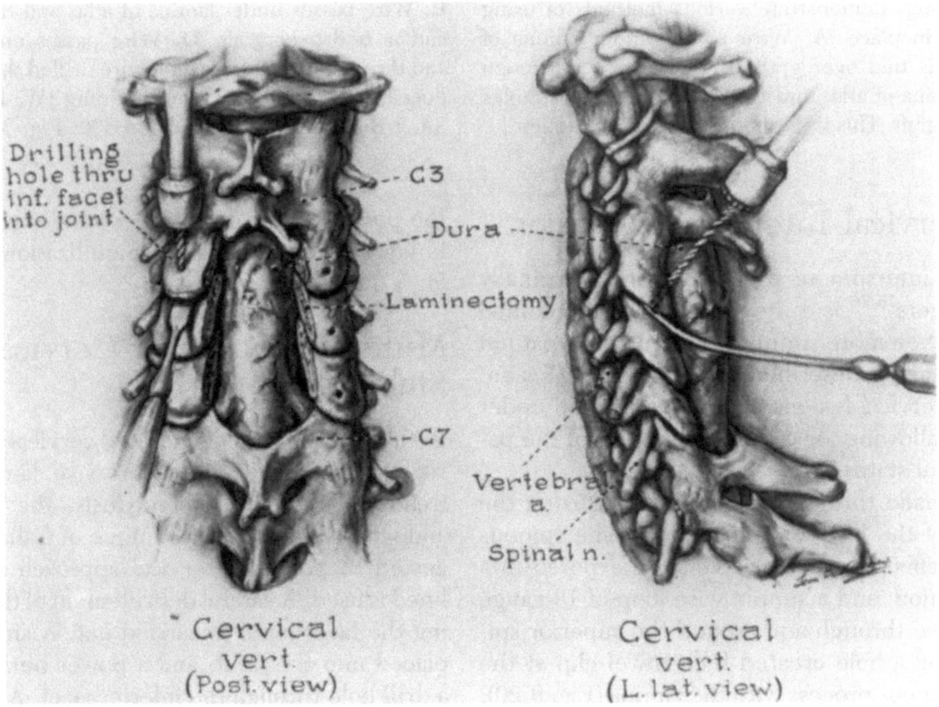

A B

Figure 9.21. **A** and **B.** Facet fusion: Soft tissues and capsular ligaments are cleared from facets and posterior pillars, and facet joints are pried open using small curved elevator. Drill holes are made in posterior pillars, using 3-mm drill, at right angle to plane of facet joints. **B.** These holes are made eccentrically toward midline so that grafts ultimately may rest on large area of posterior pillar. During drilling, flat elevator is left between facets to protect facet below and vertebral artery and nerve roots to front. (Reproduced with permission from Callahan RA, Johnson RM, Margolis RN, et al. Cervical facet fusion for control of instability following laminectomy. J Bone Joint Surg 1977;59A:991–1002, Fig. 1A & B.)

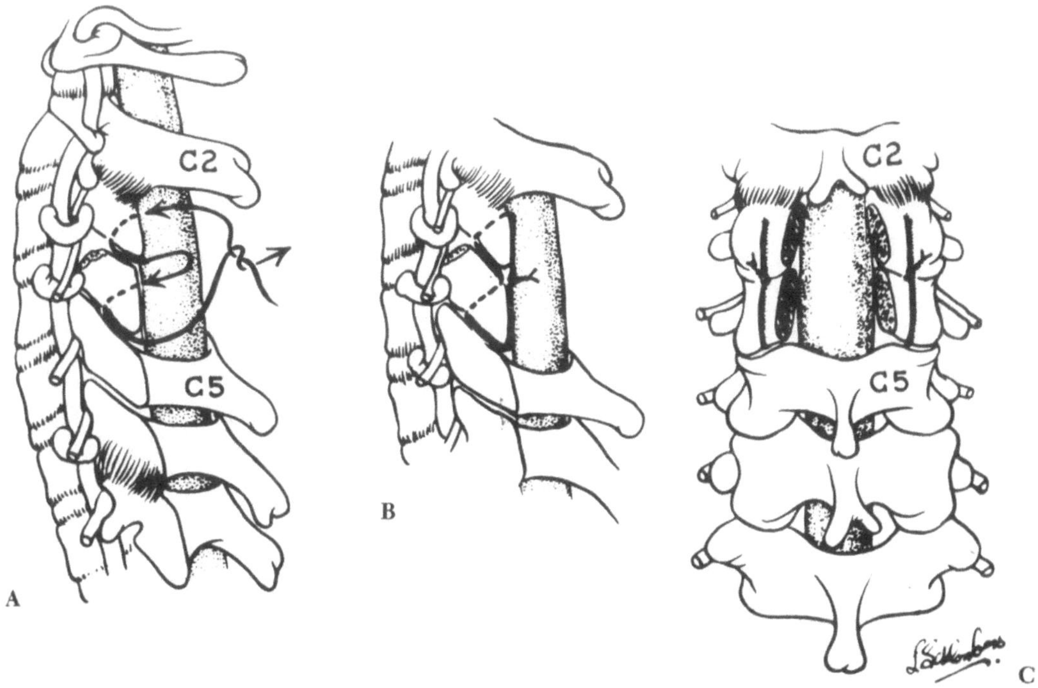

Figure 9.22. Drill holes are made in posterior pillars of involved facets using 3-mm drill directed at right angles to plane of facet joint. Curved elevator is placed within facet joint to protect lower facet and vertebral artery and nerve roots to front. Holes are made in facets at level of instability and facet below. Single strand of 18-gauge wire is passed through hole in upper facet pillar (**A**) and retrieved within joint using fine-angled clamp. Wire is advanced by pushing wire into hole within facet pillar with one hand while pulling wire from facet joint with clamp. When sufficient wire has been retrieved, free end is introduced into hole within next lower facet pillar, and wire is retrieved from that joint. Wire is pulled snugly; facet joints are reduced in fully apposed position. (**B** and **C**) Wire is then tightened and twisted. Lateral roentgenogram is obtained in operating room to ensure that satisfactory stabilization is provided and there is not too much extension or posterior overriding of facets. Excessive overriding will compromise spinal canal and neural foramina. Wire that leaves facet joint and is then passed posteriorly to next lower facet pillar provides horizontal buttress (**B**) that effectively prevents anterior translation of one vertebra forward on next. (Reproduced with permission from Rothman RH, Simeone FA. The Spine. Philadelphia: Saunders, 1982;1:141, Fig. 4.53.)

can be harvested from the outer table of the iliac crest. Wires are passed at each level around the graft and through each individual facet. Each bone graft is then wired down to the facets on both sides as illustrated (Fig. 9.23).

A complication of multilevel laminectomies can be a progressive "swan neck" deformity[77] characterized by a proximal occipitocervical hyperlordosis and more distal cervical or cervicothoracic increasing kyphosis. For treatment of this structural deformity we suggest pre- and intraoperative cervical traction to provide some reduction of the curves followed by posterolateral facet wiring and fusion, using corticocancellous grafts as described.[56]

Technique for Stabilization of Cervical Spondylolisthesis

An additional technique for stabilization of the cervical spine in situations of degenerative spondylolisthesis is the so-called triple-wire technique described by Bohlman[48] and similar to the technique described by Rogers[75,76] (Fig. 9.24). Again, approach to the cervical spine is subperiosteal dissection after a posterior midline incision. Holes are created through the bases of the spinous processes just at their juncture with the lamina of the two or three adjacent vertebral levels to be fused. Wires are passed first in an interspinous fashion to provide immediate stability, and secondary wires are also passed through the previously created fenestrations to secure longitudinal, unicortical, iliac crest bone grafts. One suggested advantage of this particular type of fusion is the postoperative stability that is conferred by the construct. Postoperative immobilization with the Philadelphia hard collar is recommended.

The technique of occipitocervical fusion using a Luque-type rectangle with fixation to the occiput by a wire fixation through the outer table of the calvarium and fixation to the cervical spine with the passage of sublaminar wires is an experimental one, and is best left in the hands of

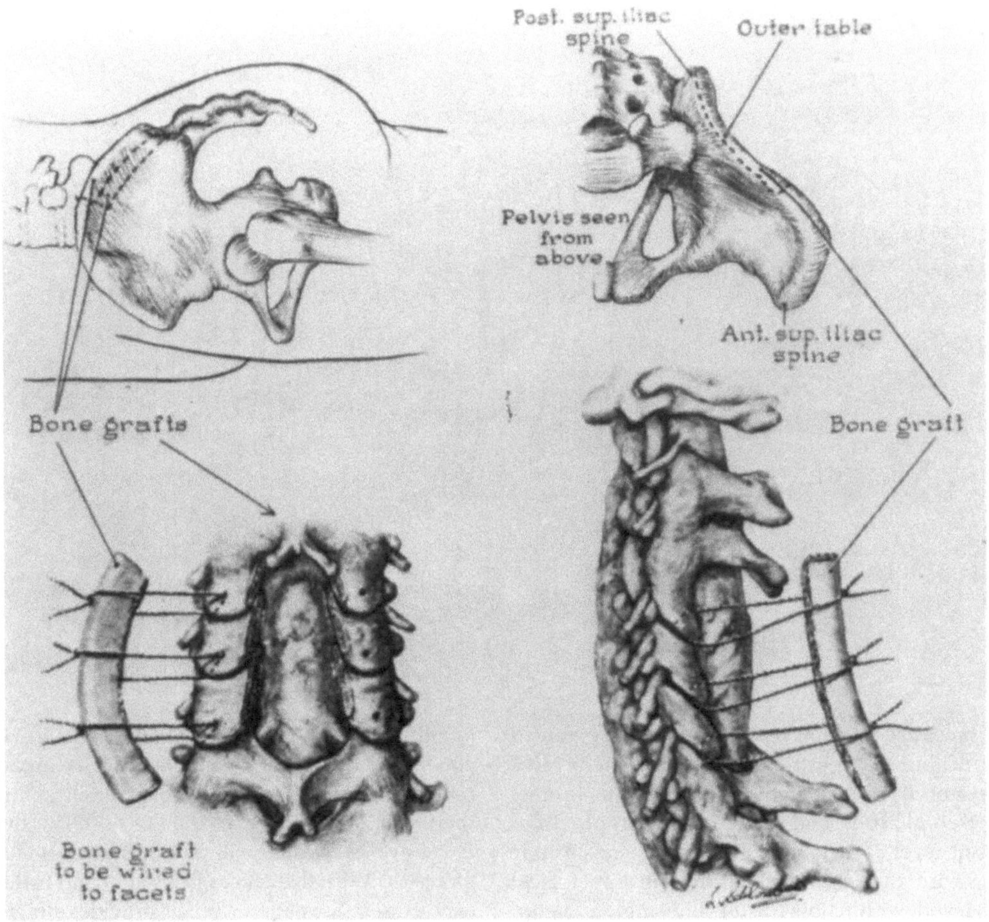

Figure 9.23. Bone graft curved in two planes is taken from posterior iliac crest. Posterior ilium is normally curved in two planes. One of these curves (**A** and **C**) keeps graft from impinging on exposed dura and spinal cord; other (**B** and **D**) conforms with normal cervical lordosis. Two biconcave grafts are taken from outer table of ilium. These are notched laterally at upper and lower poles to keep wires from slipping. **C** and **D.** Twisted 24-gauge stainless steel wire is then inserted into each hole, and tip of wires is grasped within joint space using fine, curved clamp. Wires are placed at each level of intended fusion bilaterally. Grafts are then placed along posterior facet pillars, and wires are tightened and twisted around grafts. This is usually started at midpoint of fusion so that graft will rest snugly against apex of lordotic curve. Wire that extends through hole in facet pillar is passed medially about graft (**C**); wire that emerges from facet joint is passed laterally. This prevents graft from drifting medially toward exposed spinal canal. (Reproduced with permission from Callahan RA, Johnson RM, Margolis RN, et al. Cervical facet fusion for control of instability following laminectomy. J Bone Joint Surg 1977;59A:991–1002, Fig. 1C–F.)

experienced spinal surgeons familiar with its particular indications and techniques.

Lumbar Spinal Fusion Techniques

Anterior Retroperitoneal Approach to the Thoracolumbar Junction and Lumbar Spine

The anterior retroperitoneal operative approach, as described, was originally developed to provide enhanced exposure of the kidney.[15,21,49,78] It evolved from a costotransversectomy procedure when it became apparent that it gave better exposure with less tissue damage. This exposure provides an extraperitoneal approach to the anterior thoracolumbar junction and upper lumbar spine, and as such is useful for anterior bone grafting or possibly anterior instrumentation from T11 to L4, although its major use is an exposure of the upper lumbar spine (L1–L2). The lateral two-thirds of the twelfth rib is resected subperiosteally, avoiding the pleural cavity and division of the anterior abdominal musculature. The major dissection takes advantage of the potential space behind the kidney between the renal fascia (or Gerota's fascia) and the quadratus lumborum and psoas muscles. Retraction in this interval

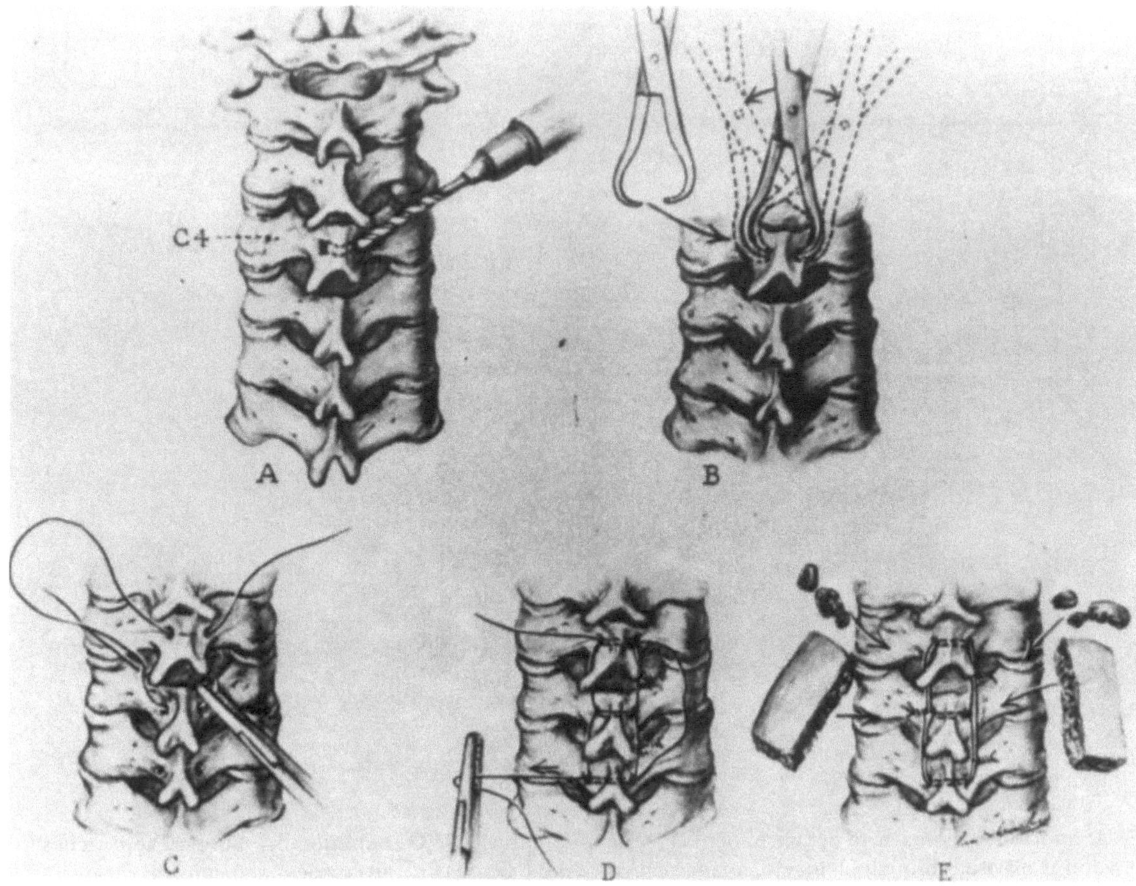

Figure 9.24. Method of interspinous process wiring and fusion. **A.** Drill makes initial hole at base of spinous process. **B.** Towel clip used to enlarge hole should be "locked" in a superior-inferior direction to prevent additional contusion of neural elements. **C.** Wires passed between adjacent spinous process. **D.** Secondary wires passed to "lock" whole construct together. **E.** Corticocancellous grafts positioned. Alternatively, holes can be created in grafts and secondary wire used to secure grafts on either side of spinous process, adding to strength of the fusion. (Reproduced with permission from Rothman RH, Simeone FA. The Spine. Philadelphia: Saunders, 1982;1:135, Fig. 4.51.)

provides exposure of most of the lumbar vertebral bodies and sufficient working space for extensive excision, grafting, and possibly instrumentation.

For exposure of the lower lumbar spine and lumbosacral junction, a retroperitoneal approach with the skin incision placed inferior and parallel to the twelfth rib is used. The subsequent dissection is essentially the same as described, except that the rib and its periosteal bed are not disturbed.

One of the major complications of the retroperitoneal approach through the periosteal envelope of the twelfth rib is damage to the parietal pleura and inadvertent violation of the thoracic cavity. The twelfth rib is variable in length, ranging from 1.5 to some 14 cm, most often between 11 and 14 cm. The pleura attaches to the undersurface of the posterior 6 cm of the rib and then extends anteriorly over the T11–T12 interspace for some 10 to 11 cm from the midline. If a shorter twelfth rib is encountered, it should be considered to be covered with pleura for its entire length. Suggestions to help prevent perforation of the pleura include studying maximum inspiration chest roentgenograms to locate the lowest extent of the pleura and making the longitudinal incision in the periosteum and inner aspects of the last rib sufficiently far out to be below the pleural reflection.

Technique

The patient is placed in the right lateral decubitus position with the left side up and the twelfth rib positioned over the break in the operating room table, which allows the table to be flexed and extended to provide an increased working space between the thorax and the left iliac crest (Fig. 9.25).

The skin is sharply incised along the twelfth rib from the costotransverse junction to within 1 cm of the tip of

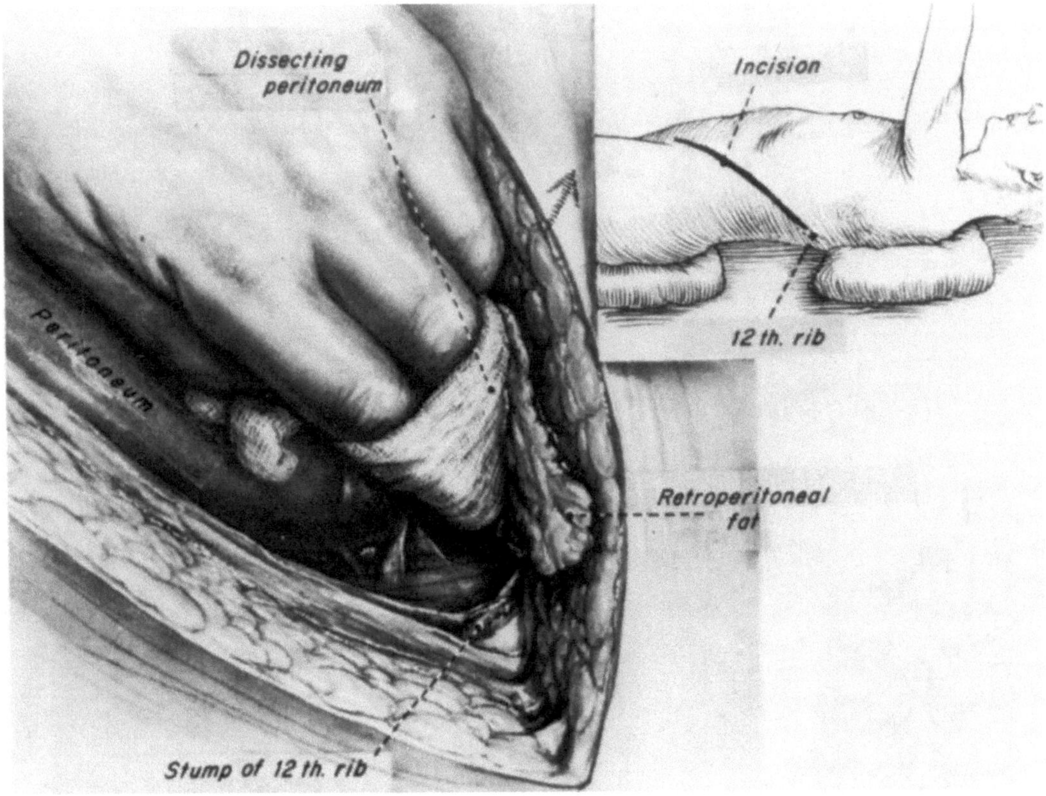

Figure 9.25. Anterolateral approach to bodies of lumbar vertebrae. Peritoneum is exposed through oblique flank incision beginning over twelfth rib. (Reproduced with permission from Southwick WO, Robinson RA. Surgical approaches to the vertebral bodies in the cervical and lumbar regions. J Bone Joint Surg 1957;39A:638, Fig. 5–A.)

the twelfth rib. The dissection is then carried through the subcutaneous tissue, and the intervening muscle layers (latissimus dorsi and serratus) superficial to the rib. Care should be taken to keep the skin incision and subsequent deeper dissection directly in line with the curve of the rib. The dissection is carried down through the periosteum. Care should be taken to avoid sliding off the rib inferiorly and damaging the subcostal neurovascular bundle. The rib is dissected subperiosteally and is disarticulated from its costotransverse attachment with a Cobb

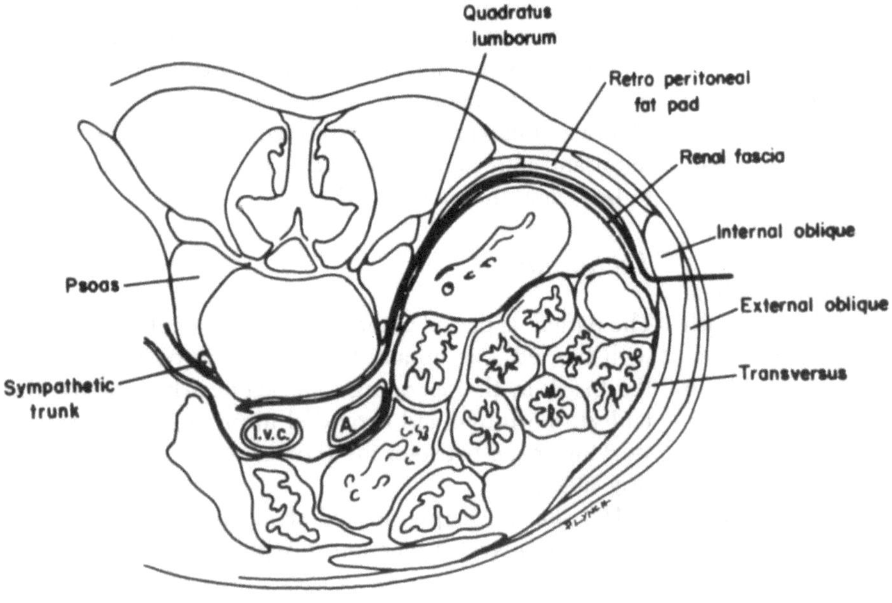

Figure 9.26. Transverse section through midlumbar vertebrae illustrates plane of dissection to vertebral bodies between renal fascia anteriorly and retrorenal fat pad, quadratus lumborum, and psoas muscles posteriorly. (Reproduced with permission from Rothman RH, Simeone FA. The Spine. Philadelphia: Saunders, 1982;1:173, Fig. 4.85.)

periosteal elevator. The rib is then sectioned at the costotransverse junction. Using a bone clamp, the rib is elevated and dissected free of the rib bed moving from dorsal to ventral. It is important to remember that the diaphragm is attached to the superior edge of the twelfth rib. The tissue at the tip is then gently split while elevating the rib and dissected free, again taking care to avoid violating the parietal pleura or diaphragm.

In the periosteal bed from which the rib has been dissected, note the transverse abdominal musculature inferiorly and the diaphragmatic insertion superiorly, and gently retract the diaphragmatic insertion cephalad and the abdominal musculature caudad. A thin layer of the retroperitoneal space fat should then be identified. This is opened carefully using Metzenbaum scissors in a gentle cutting and spreading fashion until the peritoneum is encountered. Bluntly dissect the peritoneum from the undersurface of the abdominal wall.

The incision is extended through the external oblique and internal oblique muscular layers using electrocautery. At this point, the transverse abdominal musculature is identified. This muscle layer is gently spread to expose the transversalis fascia. The peritoneum is retracted anteriorly and the retroperitoneal space revealed (Fig. 9.26). The transversalis fascia is then bluntly dissected from the left psoas muscle, the posterior renal fascia, perinephric fat, and left kidney, and the peritoneal contents are safely retracted anteriorly with a large abdominal pad and Dever retractor. This maneuver exposes the left crus of the diaphragm and the origin of the left psoas muscle, and facilitates ligation of the segmental vertebral vessels. With the kidney retracted forward, identify the ureter on the undersurface of the peritoneum. The ureter need not be dissected out and is retracted away from the operative field with the peritoneum. A Finochietto rib retractor is placed between the eleventh rib and the iliac crest (Fig. 9.27).

By palpating the spine, the soft prominent intervertebral discs are located. The overlying retroperitoneal soft tissue is bluntly spread, and excess bleeding is avoided by staying on the surface of the disc and not on the vertebral body where the intercostal vessels are located. The aorta can be mobilized anteriorly and protected with a malleable retractor. Then using meticulous subperiosteal dissection, the crus of the diaphragm superiorly and the psoas muscle inferiorly can be elevated off, exposing the first lumbar vertebral body. If the vertebral body must be removed, it is advisable to remove the T12–L1 and L1–L2 intervertebral discs first to clearly establish the limits of dissection, and then remove the vertebral body

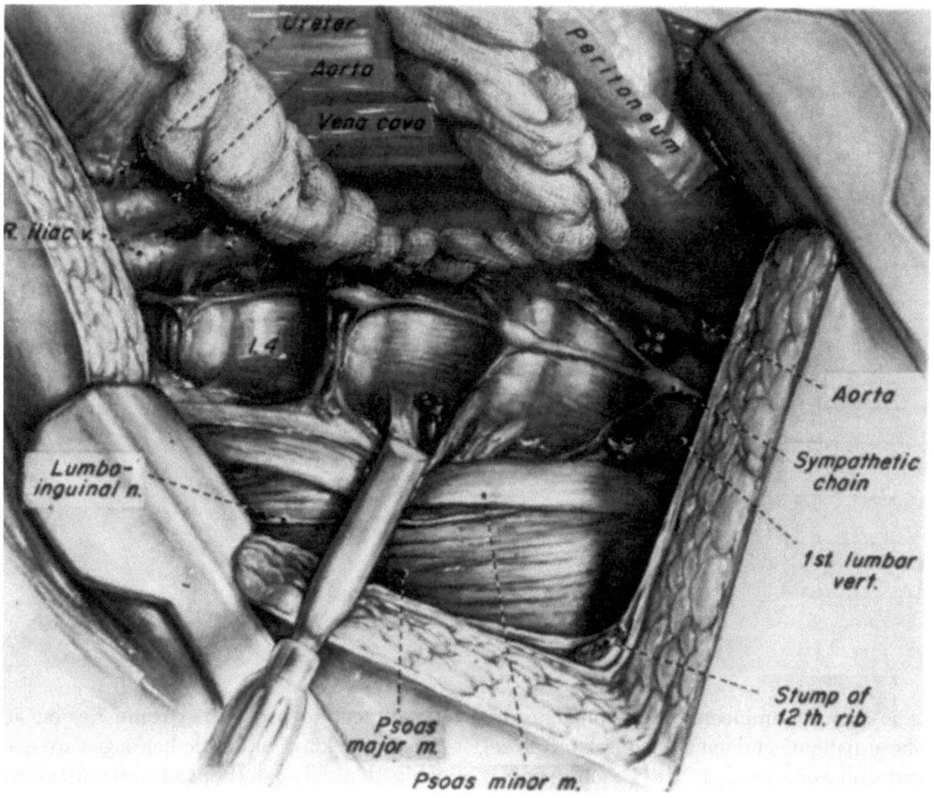

Figure 9.27. Chest retractor opens wound longitudinally. Peritoneal contents are retracted medially, exposing vertebral bodies. (Reproduced with permission from Southwick WO, Robinson RA. Surgical approaches to the vertebral bodies in the cervical and lumbar regions. J Bone Joint Surg 1957;39A:639, Fig. 5–B.)

in piecemeal fashion. Grafting techniques including the tricortical iliac crest graft for vertebral body replacement or tricortical iliac crest grafts for replacement of intervertebral discs, which have been described earlier, can be used. In addition, anterior console type grafting techniques may be used but are not thought to be as inherently stable. As with all intervertebral grafting techniques, careful removal of all the intervertebral disc and decortication of the sclerotic endplates of the vertebral body will enhance graft incorporation.

The wound incision is closed by reapproximating the rib bed and then subsequently closing each abdominal muscle layer in turn.

Posterior Lumbar Spine Fusion Techniques

Lumbar Intertransverse Posterolateral Fusion[24,70]

The patient is brought to the operating room and can usually undergo operation with only a spinal anesthetic, avoiding the complications of general anesthesia. We advocate the kneeling position using an Andrews-type frame for patient positioning to decrease intraoperative blood

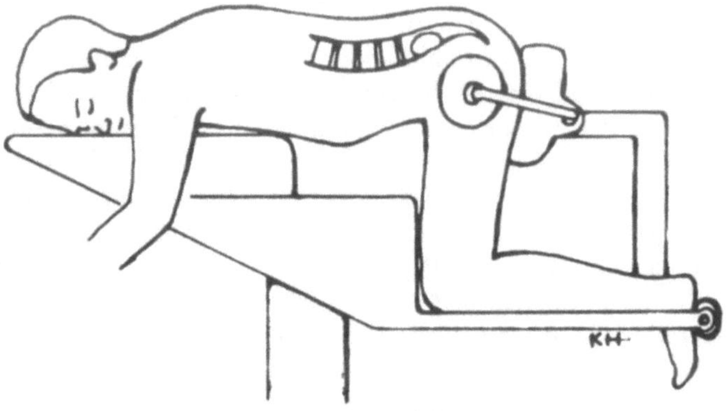

Figure 9.28. Note: Abdomen is freely dependent to allow for venous pooling and decompression of epidural veins, and to facilitate exposure and minimize operative blood loss. (Reproduced with permission from White AA, Rothman RH, eds. Lumbar Spine Surgery: Techniques and Complications. St. Louis: Mosby, 1987:302, Fig. 30.6.)

loss (Figs. 9.28 and 9.29). This decreased blood loss is effected by the dependency of the abdominal cavity and panniculus, allowing for venous decompression particularly of the epidural veins by venous pooling in the abdominal cavity. After the patient has been placed in the kneeling position and prepared and draped in a sterile fashion,

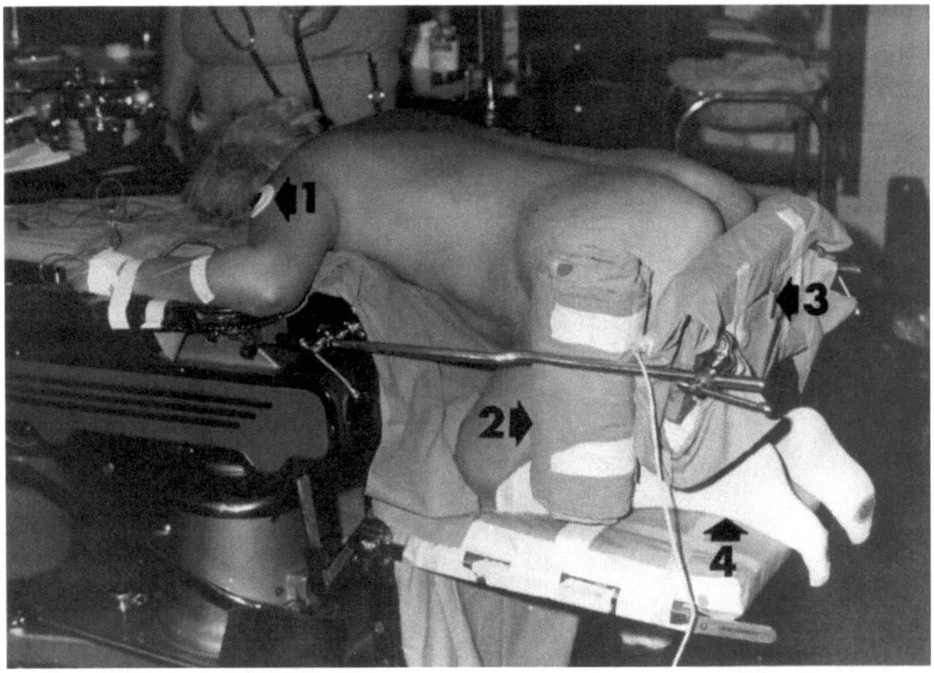

Figure 9.29. Kneeling position for laminectomy and spinal fusion. Note how, even in obese patient, abdomen is completely free, preventing any pressure on vena cava. 1. EKG monitoring is used because of difficulty of listening to heart sounds in this position. 2. Lateral padding is used to stabilize patient and prevent pressure on side bars. 3. Patient is stabilized caudally by use of seat to prevent extreme flexion at knees and hips. 4. Elastic stockings or elastic bandages are used to prevent pooling of blood in calf area. (Reproduced with permission from Rothman RH, Simeone FA, eds. The Spine. Philadelphia: Saunders, 1982;1:615, Fig. 9–116.)

the skin overlying the midline lumbar region may be infiltrated with a solution of epinephrine in saline (1:500,000) to aid local hemostasis.

The incision is carried sharply through the skin and subcutaneous tissues down to the level of the lumbar dorsal fascia. If the surgeon has elected to omit use of epinephrine solution, he may alternatively place subcutaneous hemostats and self-retaining retractors for hemostasis and to further facilitate exposure. The spinous processes can be palpated through the lumbar dorsal fascia, and incision is made through the fascia to connect the spinous processes. Either sharp scalpel dissection or electrocautery can then be used to transect the Sharpey's fibers of the lumbar dorsal fascia as they attach to the spinous processes. Using large subperiosteal elevators (either the Cobb or Kermison type), the erector spinae musculature is then dissected down and off the spinous processes and lamina using a subperiosteal technique. The musculature is retracted laterally to the facet complexes. In degenerative spondylolisthesis in which there is no defect of the pars interarticularis, a facetal and intertransverse fusion can be carried out alone without need for instrumentation.

The facets are exposed using a subperiosteal elevator to gently retract the musculature and soft tissue further laterally beyond the facet joints. Electrocautery can be used to strip the joint capsule off the facet, exposing the joint line. The facet surfaces are denuded of their articular cartilage using the narrow double-action rongeurs. Dissection is carried laterally to define transverse processes of the vertebral bodies adjacent to the spondylolisthetic slip. Corticocancellous graft, primarily cancellous graft, is harvested from the posterior iliac crest. This can be accomplished through the existing incision by elevation of the subcutaneous tissue off the lumbar dorsal fascia and through a separate incision through the lumbar dorsal fascia or through an entirely separate incision through the skin subcutaneous tissue and lumbar dorsal fascia overlying the iliac crest. Alternatively the skin incision can be angled toward the particular crest to facilitate exposure (Fig. 9.30).

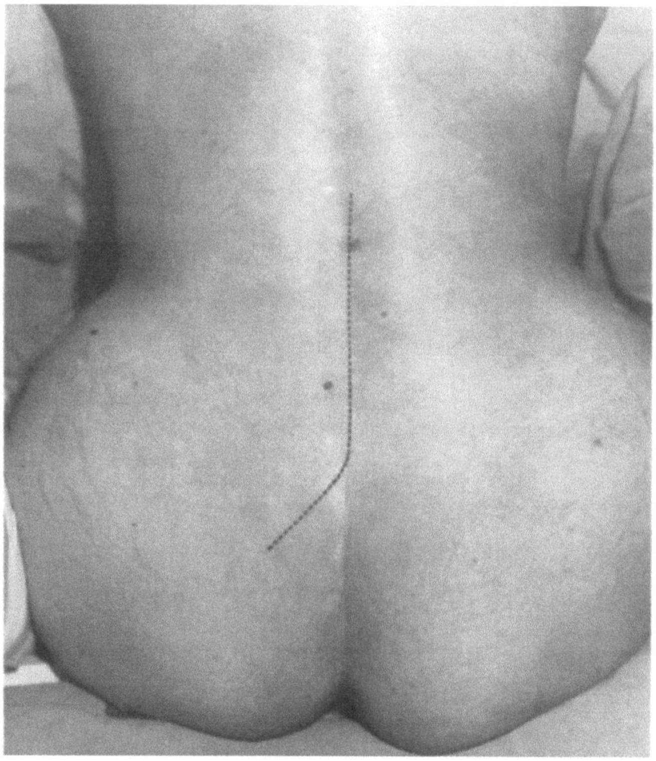

Figure 9.30. Hockey stick incision used for two-level spinal fusion from L4 to the sacrum. Incision extends from third lumbar spinous process to sacrum and then deviates laterally to iliac crest to facilitate exposure for obtaining bone graft. (Reproduced with permission from Rothman RH, Simeone FA. The Spine. Philadelphia: Saunders, 1982;1:615, Fig. 9.117.)

Corticocancellous graft is carefully tamped within the denuded facet surfaces of each facet joint. The dorsal surfaces of the transverse processes are decorticated using the Leksell double-action rongeur, care being taken not to fracture the transverse processes, and corticocancellous "matchsticks" are placed in the lateral gutters which have been created lateral to the facet complexes (Fig. 9.31). Care is taken to span the gap between the adjacent transverse processes with corticocancellous bone graft. When closing, the self-retaining retractors are removed and the erector spinae musculature is allowed to fall toward the midline, helping to hold the graft masses in position. Care is taken not to decorticate or to place bone graft posterior to any of the laminae or spinous processes that remain after neural decompression, in an attempt to prevent posterior fusion and possible later overgrowth spinal stenosis[67] (Fig. 9.32).

If the isthmic spondylolisthesis involves a discontinuity bilaterally of the pars interarticularis, a slightly different approach to fusion is carried out. A similar surgical approach is made after the erector spinae musculature has been retracted laterally. If there is evidence of neurological compression at the level of the spondylolisthesis, a Gill-type procedure is carried out, removing the detached posterior element consisting of the lamina and spinous process of the affected vertebral body (Fig. 9.33). The Gill procedure is performed by gently developing a plane between the ligamentum flavum and superior and inferior edges of the lamina of the detached posterior element. A large curette is used, with care being taken to keep its bowl directed toward the dura at all times as the curette is swept in a side-to-side fashion using its sharp edges to detach the soft tissue from the undersurface of the lamina. A long-bladed Frazer nerve probe can be used intermittently to assess the adequacy of the dissection and the detachment of the ligamentum flavum and epi-

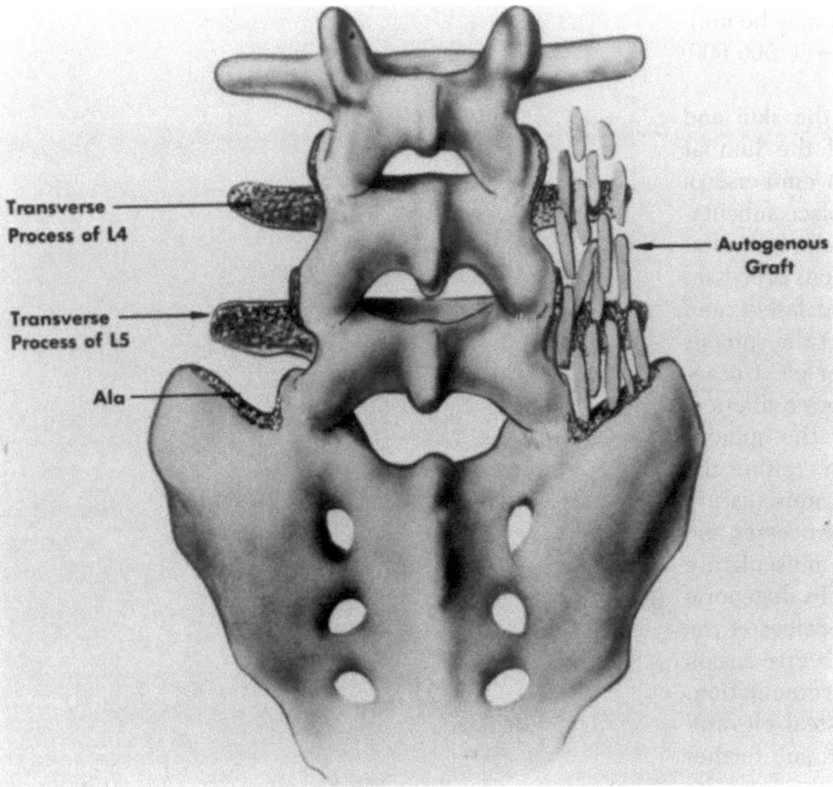

Figure 9.31. Area of bed or raw cancellous bone for lateral spine fusion from L4 to sacrum. Bed is shown on left and graft material is in place on right. In actuality, much larger volume of graft material is used. Bed includes transverse processes, ala of sacrum, lateral portion of pedicle, and lateral portion of superior articular facets. (Reproduced with permission from Rothman RH, Simeone FA. The Spine. Philadelphia: Saunders, 1982;1:617, Fig. 9.119.)

dural fat from the undersurface of the lamina. The tip of the spinous process is then firmly grasped with a Coker clamp, and the capsule of the facet complex and hypertrophic scar, which surrounds the pars interarticularis defect on one side, is incised. Care is taken to identify and

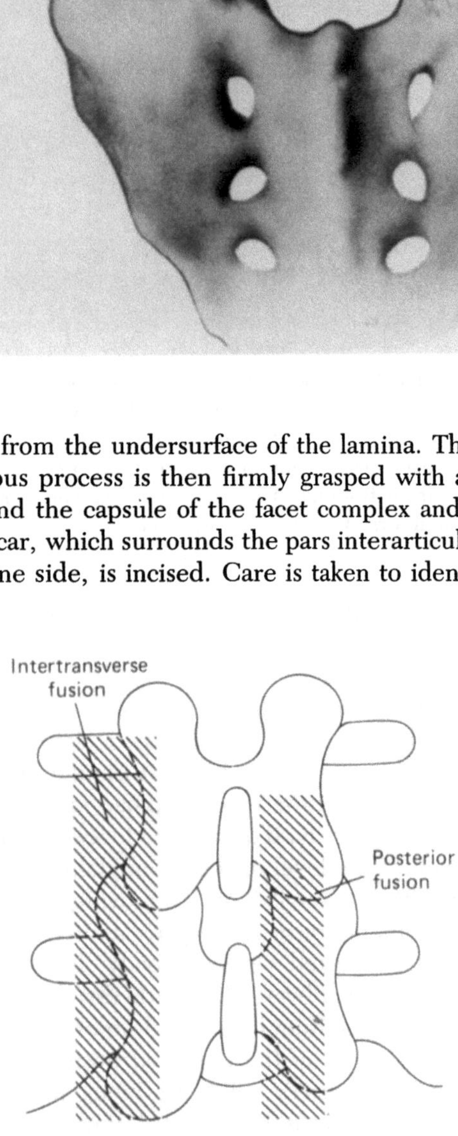

Figure 9.32. Comparison of beds prepared for intertransverse and posterior fusions. Posterior fusion is currently not recommended because of secondary overgrowth spinal stenosis. (Reproduced with permission from Macnab I, Dall D. J Bone Joint Surg 1971;53B:628, Fig. 2.)

protect the adjacent nerve root. The spinous process is then gently levered to the opposite side and in this fashion the posterior elements of the affected level can be detached in continuity. Alternatively, the posterior elements of the olisthetic vertebral body can be removed in piecemeal fashion using a Schlessinger-type Kerrison rongeur. This perhaps is the safer technique, avoiding possible nerve root damage that may be caused by levering of the intact posterior neural arch.

After the posterior arch has been removed, the nerve roots are explored in standard fashion and carefully dissected free from any enveloping or compressing fibrous scar. The transverse processes are exposed and decorticated, as previously described, and corticocancellous graft placed in the posterolateral gutters. The incision is closed in layers. The fusion and bone graft donor sites are drained separately. Postoperative immobilization in a molded thoracolumbar sacral orthosis (TLSO) is recommended for 8–12 weeks.

Transpedicular Fixation with Posterolateral Fusion

If additional stabilization is thought to be required by the initial degree of spondylolisthetic slip or concern for increased rate of pseudarthrosis, additional stability can be provided by the use of transpedicular fixation. As au-

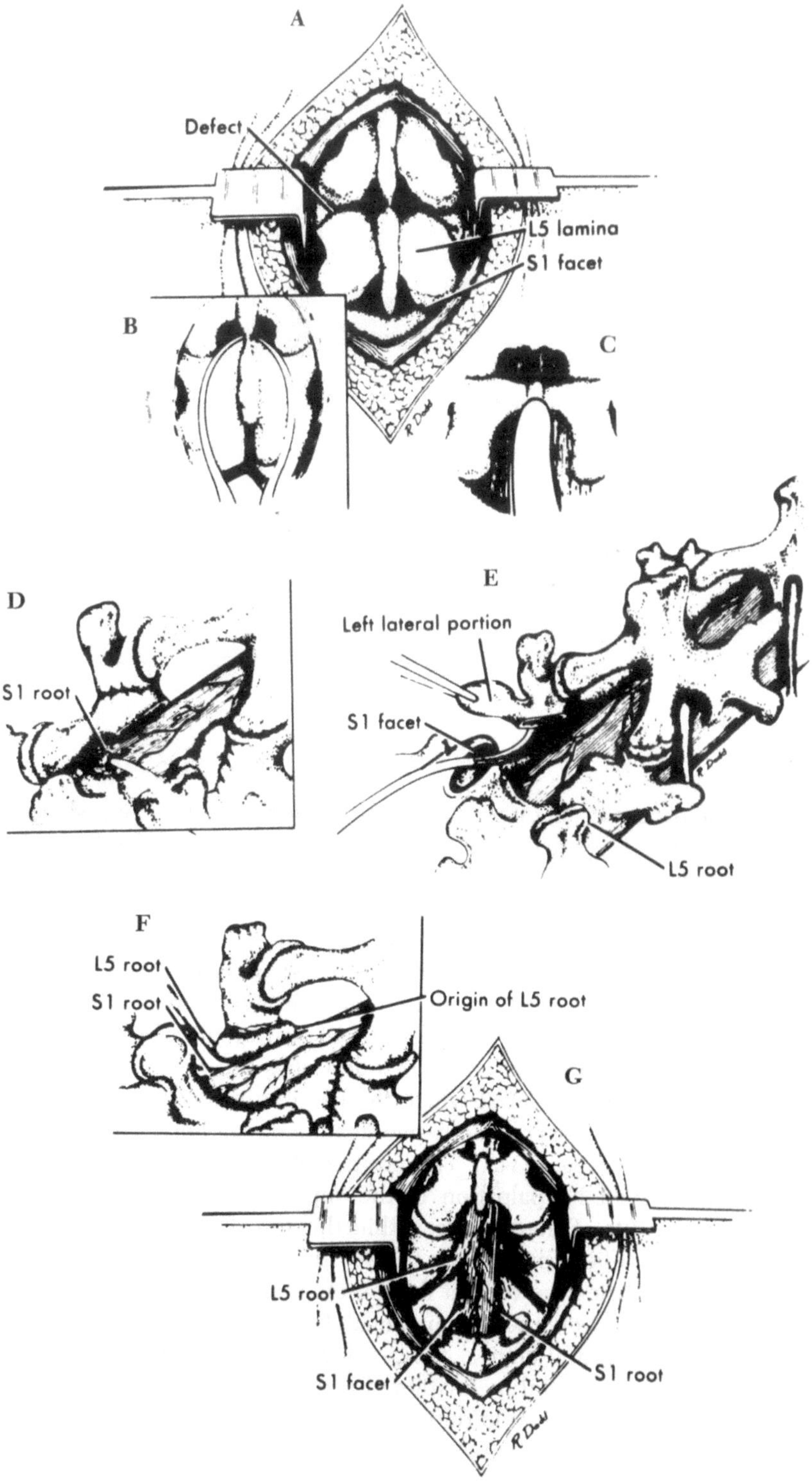

Figure 9.33. Operation of Gill, Manning, and White for spondylolisthesis. **A, B,** and **C.** Exposure of posterior elements. **D, E,** and **F.** Removal of "loose" lamina and spinous process of L5. Note impingement of L5 nerve root by hypertrophic callus and pseudarthrosis of L5 pars interarticularis. (Reproduced with permission from Gill G, Manning JG, White HL. J Bone Joint Surg 1955;37A:493, Fig. 1–3.)

thors have emphasized, transpedicular fixation is not a new concept, having been originally described in the American literature in 1949 by Michele and Krueger.[79]

The technique of transpedicular fixation is an exacting one and should be practiced in the laboratory before in vivo usage. The pedicle is located in the following fashion. After the appropriate posterior elements and facets have been identified, the pedicle is located by the intersection of two landmark lines. The first landmark line is defined horizontally by the midpoints of the widths of the

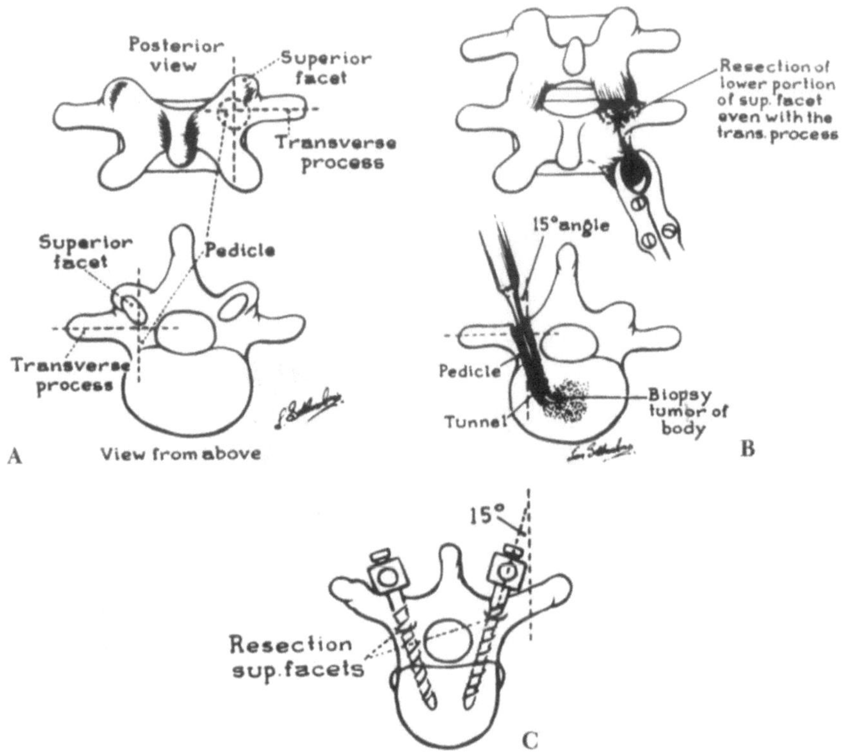

Figure 9.34. Transpedicular fixation. **A.** At every level of thoracolumbar spine, transverse processes are in same transverse plane as pedicles. **B.** Most investigators recommend probing rather than drilling through pedicle to ensure intraosseous placement. Fluoroscopic visualization is helpful for orientation in obtaining biopsies of vertebral body. **C.** Use of 15° angle with sagittal plane, starting from superior articular processes, can aid in placement of fixation devices. (Reproduced with permission from McAfee PC. Orthopaedic Knowledge Update 2: Home Study Syllabus. Park Ridge, Illinois: American Academy of Orthopaedic Surgeons, 1987:306, Fig. 5.)

transverse processes on either side of the particular vertebral body. The intersection of this transverse line with a longitudinal line that is defined by a line which runs from one facet joint line to an adjacent facet line on the same side of the patient identifies the location of the pedicle. To clarify, the superior and inferior articular processes that constitute each facet form a joint line that is roughly longitudinal. Connecting the midpoints of two of these joint lines of adjacent facet complexes describes the perpendicular line. The point at which the longitudinal and transverse lines intersect directly overlies the dorsal border of the pedicle (Fig. 9.34A). This position of the pedicle can be confirmed by palpation of the superior medial and inferior walls of the pedicle within the spinal canal with a blunt Penfield probe (Fig. 9.34B). In the lumbar region, the pedicles are oval in cross section and in the superior inferior dimension, approximately one-half the height of the vertebral bodies. Progressing caudally, one notes an increased sacral inclination of the lumbar spine secondary to the lumbar lordotic curve (Fig. 9.35). In addition, the pedicles are inclined approximately 15° to the sagittal plane converging towards the anterior vertebral body (see Fig. 9.34C).

The lower portion of the superior facet, even with the transverse processes, is resected with a rongeur or diamond-tipped burr; then by gentle probing within the pedicle using a small curette or pedicle probe, a channel is created that extends through the pedicle into the vertebral body. The position of these channels within the pedicles is checked by intraoperative lateral radiographs. By placing sharp-tipped Steinman pins within the pedicle channels on the patient's one side and drill bits on the other, the location and direction of each pedicle "channel" can be confirmed (Figs. 9.36 and 9.37). The pin placements can then be adjusted accordingly.

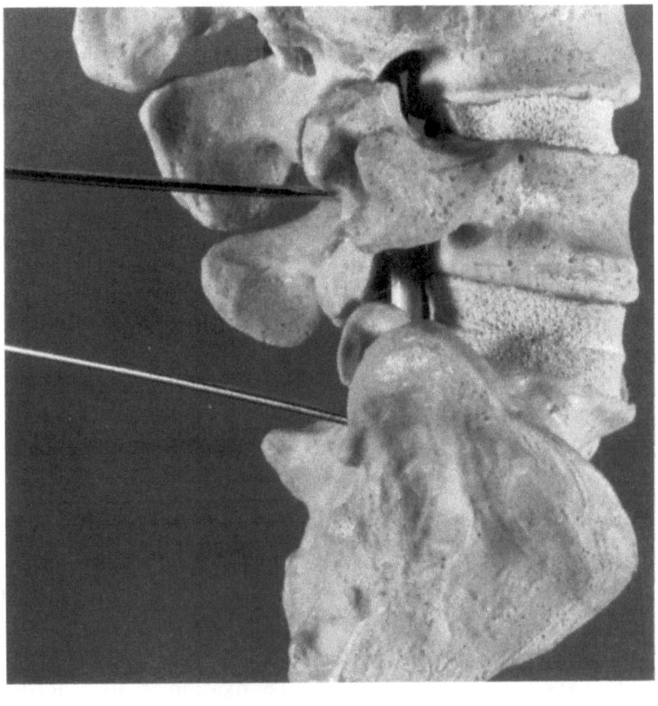

Figure 9.35. Steinman pins placed in pedicles of L5 and S1. Note increased lumbar lordosis caudally.

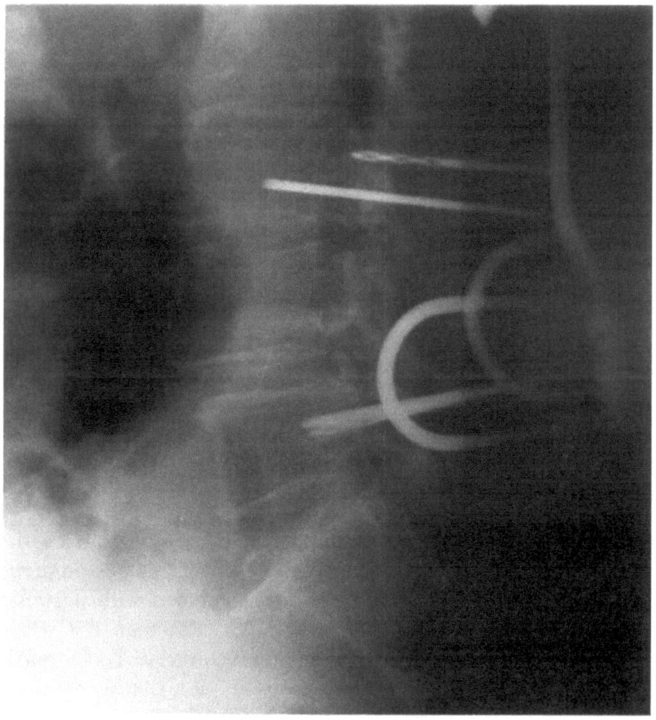

Figure 9.36. Pointed Steinman pins ipsilaterally and 3/32-in.-long drill tips contralaterally are placed in pedicles before tapping and placing screws to reconfirm placement within pedicle. In this example, superior drill bit in L3 is placed too far superior in pedicle and should be repositioned.

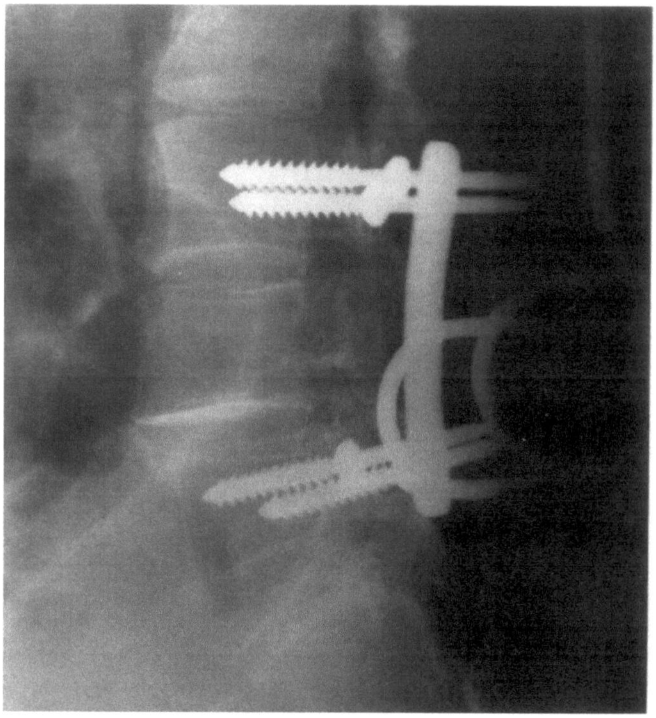

Figure 9.37. Patient with L4–L5 degenerative spondylolisthesis following wide decompression. Patient was stabilized with VSP plates L3–L5. Previous improper position of drill bit in L3 pedicle (Figure 9.36) was corrected. Radiograph shows good positioning of transpedicular screws. Note lordotic nerve bent into plate.

The course of the spinal nerve root is medial and inferior to each pedicle. If an error in pin placement within the substance of the pedicle is to be made, it should be made superiorly and laterally to avoid nerve damage. Once proper pin placement has been confirmed, the pedicles are tapped. After tapping, the walls of the transpedicular channel should be palpated in all four quadrants to reconfirm cortical wall integrity and prevent subsequent extraosseous screw placement (Figs. 9.38–9.40). Either 6- or 7-mm transpedicular screws can be used. If 6-mm screws are used and the threads are accidentally stripped while tapping the larger 7-mm screws could still gain adequate purchase and may be used. It should be noted that the use of 5-mm transpedicular screws is not advocated secondary to reports of premature bending and fracture with physiological loads.[80]

In the sacrum the process of pin location, tapping, and placement of the pedicle screw is similar. The major exception is that the tapping is carried out all the way to and through the ventral cortex of the sacrum, with the pedicle screw gaining purchase on the ventral cortex. In the ventral bodies, the purchase through this anterior cortex of the vertebral body is not recommended for fear of damage to the overlying anterior vascular structures including the aorta and vena cava.

Before placing the pedicle screws, the transverse processes have been exposed and decorticated. Corticocancellous bone graft strips are now placed laterally over and between the transverse processes and the plates or rods connected to the protruding pedicle screw ends. Minimal contouring may be necessary to help preserve lumbar lordosis; however, no particular attempt is made to reduce any olisthesis with the transpedicular screw system (Fig. 9.37). It should be noted, however, that some reduction of the olisthesis may be affected by patient positioning. Both the fusion area and the graft area should be closed and drained separately. In addition, we recommend the placement of small free-fat grafts, approximately 1 × 1 × 0.5 cm adipose tissue, usually harvested just superficial to the lumbar dorsal fascia, be placed over the nerve roots to help prevent postoperative nerve fibrosis and scarring.[81]

After the intertransverse fusion, with or without the addition of the transpedicular fixation system, there is little need for postoperative immobilization. We currently allow patients up and out of bed, weight-bearing as tolerated, on approximately the third postoperative day, while wearing a molded polyethylene lumbosacral corset. With the use of instrumentation we do recommend postoperative drainage, and with all our fusions we use both pre-

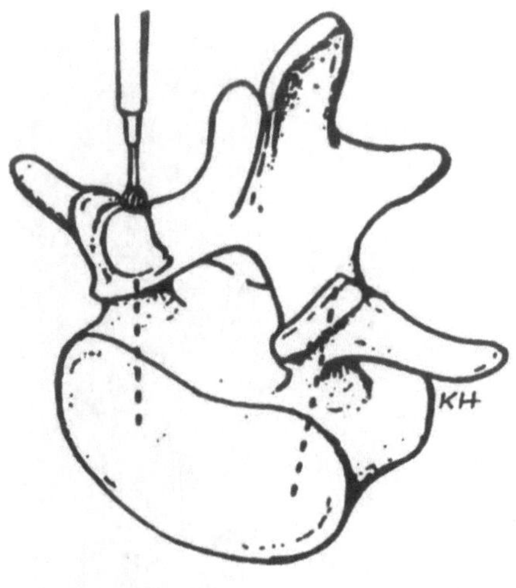

Figure 9.38. Power burr is used to decorticate dorsal entry point into pedicle. (Reproduced with permission from White AA, Rothman RH, Ray CD, eds. Lumbar Spine Surgery: Techniques and Complications. St Louis: Mosby, 1987:327, Fig. 33.8.)

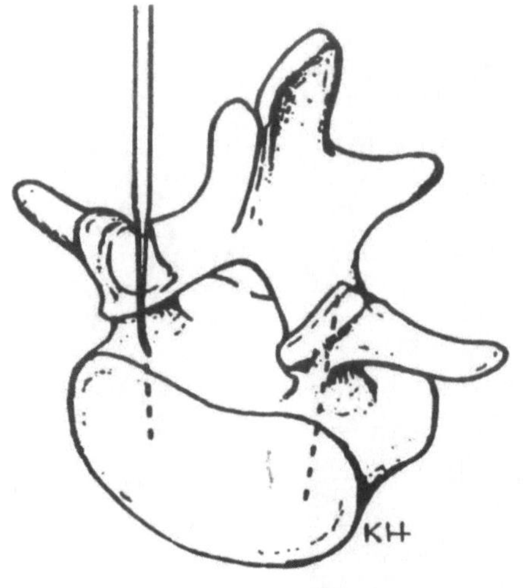

Figure 9.39. Pedicle probe is advancing through pedicle into vertebral body. (Reproduced with permission from White AA, Rothman RH, Ray CD, eds. Lumbar Spine Surgery: Techniques and Complications. St. Louis: Mosby, 1987:329, Fig. 33.10.)

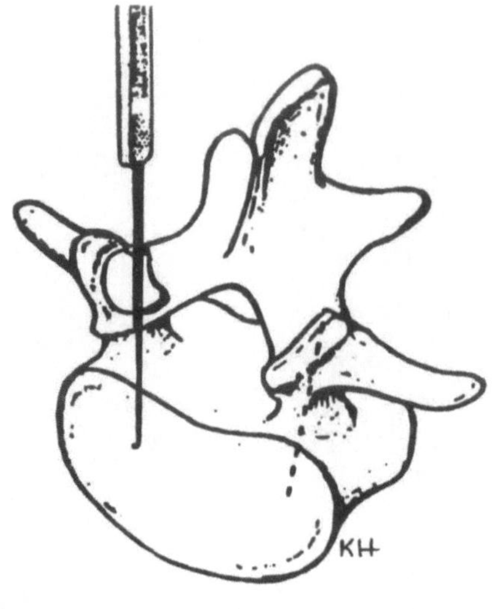

Figure 9.40. Hole in pedicle is probed with depth gauge to be sure it is surrounded by bone 360°. (Reproduced with permission from White AA, Rothman RH, Ray CD. Lumbar Spine Surgery: Techniques and Complications. St. Louis: Mosby, 1987:329, Fig. 33.12.)

and postoperative antibiotics, discontinuing antibiotics approximately 48 hours postoperatively. Various fixation systems are currently available to augment the intertransverse fusion, particularly for use in the treatment of spondylolisthesis. These include, among others, the "Fixateur Interne,"[82] and the Edwards, the VSP,[68] the Vermont,[83] and the Roy-Camille system,[84] all of which utilize the principle of the transpedicular fixation. As all these systems are relatively new with limited follow-up available, we are unable to recommend one system as being superior to another.

Conclusion

This chapter has attempted to provide an overview of the topic of spine fusion in the setting of degenerative disease. In this controversial area of spinal surgery, many widely differing opinions exist. Many of the questions causing controversy in this evolving field do not now have definitive answers. Recognizing this limitation, we have tried to represent the consensus opinion of the spine surgeons at one institution. As with all fusions, attention to intraoperative detail, careful placement of graft, and the use of sufficient quantities of bone graft (both allograft and autograft) are necessary. In addition, postoperative attention to good nutrition and the avoidance of factors known to be associated with increased rates of pseudarthrosis, such as anemia[47] and smoking,[85] as well as judicious preoperative patient selection should enable the surgeon to enjoy predictably good results when using spine fusion for the treatment of instability of the spine secondary to degenerative disease.[86] The various wiring constructs and instrumentation systems should be viewed merely as adjuncts to help promote successful bony fusion, which has been shown to be a cornerstone of successful treatment.

References

1. Albee FH. Transplantation of a portion of the tibia for Pott's disease. JAMA 1911;57:885–886.
2. Hibbs RA. An operation for progressive spinal deformities. NY State J Med 1911;93:1013–1016
3. Boumphrey FS. Fusion in the Lumbar Spine in Lumbar Disc Disease. New York: Raven Press: 1982:177–192.
4. Ehni G. The role of spine fusion: question 9. Spine 1981;6:308–310.
5. Frymoyer JW. The role of spine fusion, question 3. Spine 1981;6:284–290.
6. Frymoyer JW, Selby DK. Segmental instability: rationale for treatment. Spine 1985;10:280–286.
7. Lehmann TR, Spratt KF, Tozzi JE, Weinstein JN, Reinarz SJ, El-Khoury GY, Colby H. Long-term follow-up of lower lumbar fusion patients. Spine 1987;12:97–104.
8. Lombardi JS, Wiltse LL, Reynolds J, Widell EH, Spineur C. The treatment of degenerative spondylolisthesis. Spine 1985;10:821–827.
9. Mooney V. Where is the pain coming from? Spine 1987;12:754–759.
10. Nachemson A. Towards a better understanding of low back

pain. A review of the mechanics of the lumbar disc. Rheumatol Rehabil 1975;14:129–143.
11. Stokes IAF, Frymoyer JW. Segmental motion and instability. Spine 1987;12:688–691.
12. Bohlman HH. Cervical spondylosis with moderate to severe myelopathy. A report of seventeen cases treated by Robinson anterior cervical discectomy and fusion. Spine 1977;2:151–162.
13. Gore DR, Sepic SB. Anterior cervical fusion for degenerated or protruded discs. A review of one hundred forty-six patients. Spine 1984;9:667–671.
14. Henderson CM, Hennessy RG, Shuey HM, Shackelford EG. Posterior-lateral foraminotomy as an exclusive operative technique for cervical radiculopathy: a review of 846 consecutively operated cases. Neurosurgery 1983;13:504–512.
15. Hodgson MB, Wong SK. A description of a technique and evaluation of results in anterior spinal fusion for deranged intervertebral disc and spondylolisthesis. Clin Orthop 1968;56:133–162.
16. Lunsford LD, Bissonette DJ, Jannetta PJ, Sheptak PE, Zorub DS. Anterior surgery for cervical disc disease. Part I: Treatment of lateral cervical disc herniation in 253 cases. J Neurosurg 1980;53:1–11.
17. Robinson RA, Walker AE, Ferlic DC, Wiecking DK. The results of anterior interbody fusion of the cervical spine. J Bone Joint Surg 1962;44A:1569–1587.
18. Spangfort EV. The lumbar disc herniation. A computer-aided analysis of 2,504 operations. Acta Orthop Scand (Suppl) 1972;142:1–95.
19. White AA, Southwick WO, DePonte RJ, Gainer JW, Hardy R. Relief of pain by anterior cervical fusion for spondylosis. J Bone Joint Surg 1973;55A:525.
20. Crock HV. Observations on the management of failed spinal operations. J Bone Joint Surg 1976;58B:193–199.
21. Flynn JC, Hogue MA. Anterior fusion of the lumbar spine. End-result study with long-term follow-up. J Bone Joint Surg 1979;61A:1143–1150.
22. Hirsch C. Efficiency of surgery in low back disorders. J Bone Joint Surg 1965;47A:991.
23. Stauffer RN, Coventry MB. Anterior interbody lumbar spine fusion, analysis of Mayo Clinic Series. J Bone Joint Surg 1972;54A:756–768.
24. Stauffer RN, Coventry MB. Posterolateral fusion of the lumbar and lumbosacral spine. J Bone Joint Surg 1972;54A:1195–1204.
25. Brooks AL, Jenkins EB. Atlantoaxial arthrodesis by the wedge compression method. J Bone Joint Surg 1978;60A:279–284.
26. Jones AAM, McAfee PC, Robinson RA, Zinreich SJ, Wang H. Failed arthrodesis of the spine for severe spondylolisthesis. Salvage by interbody arthrodesis. J Bone Joint Surg 1988;70A:25–30.
27. White AH, von Rogov P, Zucherman J, Heiden D. Lumbar laminectomy for herniated disc: a prospective controlled comparison with internal fixation fusion. Spine 1987;12:305–307.
28. Frymoyer JW, Newberg A, Wilder PG, Clements J, MacPherson B. Spine radiographs in patients with low-back pain. J Bone Joint Surg 1984;66A:1048–1055.
29. Kellgren JH, Lawrence JS. Osteo-arthrosis and disc degeneration in an urban population. Ann Rheum Dis 1958;17:388–397.
30. Park WM. The place of radiology in the investigation of low back pain. Clin Rheum Dis 1980;6:93–132.
31. Bell GR, Rothman RH, Booth RE, Cuckler JM, Garfin S, Herkowitz H, Simeone FA, Dolinskas C, Hans SS. A study of computer-assisted tomography. II. Comparison of Metrizamide myelography and computed tomography in the diagnosis of herniated lumbar disc and spinal stenosis. Spine 1984;9:552–556.
32. Weisel SW, Tsourmes M, Feffer HL, Citrin CM, Patronas N. A Study of computer assisted tomography. The incidence of positive CAT scans in an asymptomatic group of patients. Spine 1984;9:549–551.
33. Fielding JW, Cochran GVB, Lawsing JF, Hohl M. Tears of the transverse ligament of the atlas. J Bone Joint Surg 1974;56A:1683.
34. Fielding JW, Hawkins RJ, Ratzau SA. Spine fusion for atlanto-axial instability. J Bone Joint Surg 1976;58A:400.
35. White AA, Johnson RM, Panjabi MM, Southwick WO. Biochemical analysis of clinical stability in the cervical spine. Clin Orthop 1975;109:85.
36. Macnab I. The traction spur: an indication of segmental instability. J Bone Joint Surg 1971;53A:663–670.
37. Friberg O. Lumbar instability: a dynamic approach by traction-compression radiography. Spine 1987;12:119–129.
38. Dupuis PR, Yong-Hing K, Cassidy JD, Kirkaldy-Willis WH. Radiologic diagnosis of degenerative lumbar spinal instability. Spine 1985;10:262–276.
39. McAfee PC, Bohlman HH, Han JS, Salvagno RT. Comparison of nuclear magnetic resonance imaging and computed tomography in the diagnosis of upper cervical spinal cord compression. Spine 1986;11:295–304.
40. Modic MT, Masaryk T, Boumphrey F, Goormastic M, Bell G. Lumbar herniated disc disease and canal stenosis: prospective evaluation by surface coil MR, CT, and myelography. Am J Neuroradiol 1986;7:709–717.
41. Fon GT, Sage MR. Computed tomography in cervical disc disease when myelography is unsatisfactory. Clin Radiol 1984;35:47–50.
42. Masaryk T, Modic MT, Geisinger MA, et al. Cervical myelopathy: a comparison of magnetic resonance and conventional myelography. J Comput Assist Tomogr 1986;10:184–194.
43. Modic MT, Masaryk TJ, Mulopulos GP, Bundschuh C, Han JS, Bohlman HH. Cervical radiculopathy: prospective evaluation with surface coil MR imaging, CT with metrizamide, and metrizamide myelography. Radiology 1986;161:753–759. Vol. 3, Dec 1986.
44. Lunsford LD, Bissonette DJ, Zorub DS. Anterior surgery for cervical disc disease. Part 2: Treatment of cervical spondylotic myelopathy in 32 cases. J Neurosurg 1980;33:12–19.
45. McAfee PC, Bohlman HH, Yuan HA. Anterior decompression of traumatic thoracolumbar fractures with incomplete neurologic deficit using a retroperitoneal approach. J Bone Joint Surg 1985;67A:89–104.
46. Robertson JR, Whitesides TE, Jr. Surgical reconstruction

of late post-traumatic thoracolumbar kyphosis. Spine 1985;10:307–312.
47. Rothman R, Klemek JS and Toton JJ. The effect of iron deficiency anemia on fracture healing. Clin Orthop 1971;77:276–283.
48. Bohlman H. Cervical spine and cord: trauma. Operative techniques in orthopaedic knowledge update 2: home study syllabus. Park Ridge, Illinois: American Academy of Orthopaedic Surgeons, 1987:275–276.
49. Southwick WO, Robinson RA. Surgical approaches to the vertebral bodies in the cervical and lumbar regions. J Bone Joint Surg 1957;39A:631–643.
50. Johnson RM, Owen JR, Panjabi MM, Bucholz RW, Southwick WO. Immediate strength of certain cervical fusion techniques. Orthop Trans 1980;4:42.
51. Scoville WB. Discussion. J Neurosurg 1958;15:614.
52. Bohlman HH and Eismont FJ. Surgical techniques of anterior decompression and fusion for spinal cord injuries. Clin Orthop 1981;54:57–67.
53. Lipson SJ. Cervical myelopathy and posterior atlanto-axial subluxation in patients with rheumatoid arthritis. J Bone Joint Surg 1983;67A:575–583.
54. Lipson SJ. Rheumatoid arthritis of the cervical spine. Clin Orthop 1984;182:143–149.
55. Zigler J, Rockowitz N, Capen D, Nelson R, Waters R. Posterior cervical fusion with local anesthesia. The awake patient as the ultimate spinal cord monitor. Spine 1987;12:206–208.
56. Callahan RA, Johnson RM, Margolis RN, Keggi KJ, Albright JA, Southwick WO. Cervical facet fusion for control of instability following laminectomy. J Bone Joint Surg 1977;59A:991–1002.
57. Bohler J, Ganderhak T. Anterior plate stabilization for fracture-dislocation of lower cervical spine. J Trauma 1980;20:3.
58. Olivera JC. Anterior plate fixation of the lower cervical spine. Spine 1987;12:324–329.
59. Carroll CC, McAfee PC. Anterior cervical plating: An initial experience. Orthop Trans 1987;11(1):8–9.
60. Whitehill R, Stowers SF, Fechner RE, Ruch WW, Drucker S, Gibson LR, McKernan DJ, Widmeyer JH. Posterior cervical fusions using cerclage wires, methylmethacrylate cement and autogenous bone graft: an experimental study of a canine model. Spine 1987;1:12–22.
61. McAfee PC, Bohlman HH, Ducker T, Eismont FJ. Failure of stabilization of the spine with methylmethacrylate. A retrospective analysis of twenty-four cases. J Bone Joint Surg 1986;68A:1145–1157.
62. Stabler CL, Eismont FJ, Brown MD, Green BA, Malinin TI. Failure of posterior cervical fusion using cadaveric bone graft in children. J Bone Joint Surg 1985;67A:370–375.
63. Harris IE, Weinstein SL. Long-term follow-up of patients with grade III and IV spondylolisthesis. J Bone Joint Surg 1987;69A:960–969.
64. Yang SW, Langrana NA, Lee CK. Biomechanics of lumbosacral spinal fusion in combined comparison-torsion loads. Spine 1986;11:937–941.
65. Denis F. Spinal instability as defined by the three-column spine concept in acute spinal trauma. Clin Orthop 1984;189:65–76.
66. Zindrick MR, Wiltse LL, Widell EH, Thomas JC, Holland WR, Field BT, Spencer CW. A biomechanical study of intrapeduncular screw fixation in the lumbosacral spine. Clin Orthop 1986;203:99–112.
67. Brodsky AE. Post-laminectomy and post-fusion stenosis of the lumbar spine. Clin Orthop 1976;115:130–139.
68. Steffee AD, Biscup RS, Sitkowski DJ. Segmental spine plates with pedicle screw fixation: a new interval fixation device for disorders of the lumbar and thoracolumbar spine. Clin Orthop 1986;203:45–54.
69. Simeone FA. Personal communication, 1987.
70. Robinson RA, Southwick WO. Surgical approaches to the cervical spine. In: American Academy of Orthopaedic Surgeons: Instructional Course Lecture, Vol. XVII. St. Louis: Mosby, 1960.
71. Lueders H, Gurd A, Hahn J, Andrish J, Weiker G and Klem G. A new technique for intraoperative monitoring of spinal cord function: multichannel recording of spinal cord and subcortical evoked potentials. Spine 1982;7:110–115.
72. Griswold PW, Albright JA, Schiffman E, Johnson RM, Southwick WO. Atlantoaxial fusion for instability. J Bone Joint Surg 1978;60A:285–292.
73. Gallie WE. Fractures and dislocations of the cervical spine. Am J Surg 1939;46:495.
74. Perry J. Surgical approaches to the spine. In: Pierce DH, Nickel VH, eds. Total Care of Spinal Cord Injuries. Boston: Little Brown, 1977.
75. Rogers WA. Treatment of fracture-dislocation of the cervical spine. J Bone Joint Surg 1942;24A:254–258.
76. Rogers WA. Fractures and dislocations of the cervical spine and end-result study. J Bone Joint Surg 1957;39A:2.
77. Mikawa Y, Shikata J, Yammuro T. Spinal deformity and instability after multilevel cervical laminectomy. Spine 1987;1:6–11.
78. Capener N. The evolution of lateral rachotomy. J Bone Joint Surg 1954;36B(2):173–179.
79. Michele AA, Krueger FJ. Surgical approach to the vertebral body. J Bone Joint Surg 1949;31A:873–878.
80. McAfee PC. What's new in spinal instrumentation. American Academy of Orthopaedic Surgeons, San Francisco, California, 1987.
81. Langenskold A and Kiviluoto O, et al. Prevention of epidural scar formation after operation on the lumbar spine by means of a free fat transplant. Clin Orthop 1976;115:92–95.
82. Dick W. The "Fixateur Interne" as a versatile implant for spine surgery. Spine 1987;12:882–900.
83. Krag MH, Beynnon BD, Pope MH, Frymoyer JW, Hough LD, Weaver DL. An internal fixator for posterior application to short segments of the thoracic, lumbar or lumbosacral spine: design and testing. Clin Orthop 1986;203:75–98.
84. Roy-Camille R, Saillant G, Mazel C. Interval fixation of the lumbar spine with pedicle screw plating. Clin Orthop 1986;203:7–17.
85. Brown CW, Orme TJ, Richardson HD. The rate of pseudarthrosis (surgical nonunion) in patients who are nonsmokers: a comparison study. Spine 1986;11:942–943.
86. DePalma A, Rothman R. The nature of pseudarthrosis. Clin Orthop 1968;59:113–118.

10

Fusion Techniques for Tumors

Franklin H. Sim, Frank J. Frassica, and Rudolph A. Klassen

The most common malignant tumors of the spinal column are multiple myeloma and metastatic lesions. Primary bone tumors, such as osteosarcoma, chondrosarcoma, and chordoma, do occur. Approximately 15% of bone tumors occur in the spinal column. The relative frequencies and locations of the 11 common malignant bone tumors that may occur in the spinal column are shown in Table 10.1. Understanding the epidemiology, pathophysiology, and prognosis of the various spinal column tumors is important in developing the optimal treatment plan. The development of modern oncological principles, techniques of spinal column reconstruction, and surgical team approach has resulted in increasing survival of these patients.

Identification and Clinical Evaluation

Identification of the presence of a tumor of the spinal column requires a high index of suspicion. The most frequent early symptom is pain, an almost universal complaint. Unusual pain patterns, however, should be recognized. In children and adolescents, spine pain is uncommon. Pain at rest, night pain, radicular distribution of pain, and neurological deficits need complete evaluation to determine their source. Because of the anatomical structure of the spine and spinal cord, the only effective treatment is to excise the tumor when it is small.

In children, malignant lesions are more likely to be primary, such as a neuroblastoma, Ewing's sarcoma, or histiocytosis X, whereas the more common benign tumors are osteoid osteoma, osteoblastoma, and aneurysmal bone cysts. Middle-aged patients are more likely to have lesions such as chordoma, myeloma, lymphoma, giant-cell tumor, or malignant giant cell tumor, chondrosarcoma, and osteosarcoma. The elderly patient will usually have metastatic lesions or myeloma. Infection may often mimic any of these tumors. Some tumors are commonly associated with systemic signs, such as fever, night sweats, and loss of weight. Neurological symptoms may occur rather abruptly and may require emergency decompression of the spinal cord. Initial evaluation should consist of a thorough history and physical examination and the appropriate plain roentgenograms of the affected region. A differential diagnosis is then established, and additional studies can be undertaken. These studies include an isotope scan of the spinal column to help define the lesion. Some lesions, such as myeloma and histiocytosis, may be nonreactive, as are some early symptomatic lesions such as osteoid osteoma and osteoblastoma. Magnetic resonance imaging (MRI) and computed tomography (CT) with or without myelography, other visualization techniques of the digestive and urogenital systems, and angiography may be helpful in further defining the site and size of the lesion, as well as in determining its primary source.

Malignant lesions of the spinal column are found most frequently in the vertebral body and pedicle, and less frequently in the posterior elements; the reverse is true with benign lesions.[2] When a lesion of the spinal column has been identified, a diagnosis must be accurately established in order to classify the lesion. Frequently either a needle biopsy specimen can be taken under radiographic or CT visualization, or the vertebral body can be approached by a transpedicular route.

The Lichtenstein classification modified by Dahlin, in which lesions are classified into histological subtypes from tissue origin, is uniformly accepted (Table 10.2). With primary tumors of the spinal column, 5-year survival rates are low if the lesion is curetted; however, if complete excision is achieved, a 75% survival rate can be expected. For patients undergoing incomplete resection, the survival rate is less that 20%. Simple biopsy of these lesions results in a longer survival rate than does curettage.

After diagnosis, a plan is formulated on the basis of the histological findings and the size of the lesion. Most

Table 10.1. Malignant spinal lesions in Mayo Clinic series.[a]

Tumor	Total	Spinal Column		Location			
		No.	%	Cervical	Thoracic	Lumbar	Sacrum
Myeloma	556	205	37	19	121	41	24
Lymphoma	469	67	14	4	24	18	21
Chondrosarcoma	634	55	9	9	18	12	16
Osteosarcoma	1274	37	3	7	10	8	12
Paget's sarcoma	50	2	4	0	1	1	0
Postradiation sarcoma	103	20	19	3	2	5	10
Ewing's sarcoma	402	31	8	1	1	10	19
Malignant fibrous histiocytoma	52	5	10	2	0	0	3
Fibrosarcoma	207	19	9	1	3	3	12
Chordoma	262	165	63	15	7	10	133
Hemangioendothelioma	60	10	17	0	4	6	0
Total	4069	616	15	61	191	114	250

[a] Data are from Dahlin DC, Unni K. Bone Tumors: general aspects and data on 8,542 cases. 4th Ed. Springfield, Illinois: Thomas, 1986:552.

metastatic bone or myeloma lesions are radiosensitive. Radiation and chemotherapy also may be used as adjunctive treatment to surgery. The patient with mechanical pain may be supported with braces through the healing period. Surgical intervention is indicated in patients with spine tumors when evaluation reveals:[3] (1) the possibility that the lesion can be totally excised and a cure can be achieved; (2) progressive neurological deficits; (3) destruction of the spinal column by the tumor or intractable pain from mechanical instability of the spinal column; and (4) progressive deformity secondary to previous attempts at decompression of the spinal cord.

Although the indications for surgery outlined in the preceding paragraph may be met, there are circumstances when surgery may not be the best treatment.[4] Elderly debilitated patients with metastatic bone disease, multiple myeloma, or primary bone tumors are not good candidates for a major surgical procedure. Patients with tumors that are associated with a very poor prognosis (survival less than 3 months) are also poor surgical candidates. High-dose therapeutic radiation is a relative contraindication. The surgical procedure can be performed after high doses (50 Gy), although the patient must understand that the incidence of significant wound complications is high. A

Table 10.2. Classification of 8542 primary tumors of bone in Mayo Clinic patients.[a]

Histologic Type	Total Cases	Benign	Cases	Malignant	Cases
Hematopoietic	3401 (39.8%)	—	—	Myeloma	2932
				Malignant lymphoma	469
Chondrogenic	1822 (21.3%)	Osteochondroma	727	Primary chondrosarcoma	545
		Chondroma	245	Secondary chondrosarcoma	89
		Chondroblastoma	79	Dedifferentiated chondrosarcoma	79
		Chondromyxoid fibroma	39	Mesenchymal chondrosarcoma	19
Osteogenic	1638 (19.2%)	Osteoid osteoma	245	Osteosarcoma	1274
		Osteoblastoma	63	Parosteal osteosarcoma	56
Unknown origin	878 (10.3%)	Giant cell tumor	425	Ewing's tumor	402
				Malignant giant cell tumor	28
				Adamantinoma	23
Histiocytic origin	62 (0.7%)	Fibrous histiocytoma	10	Malignant fibrous histiocytoma	52
Fibrogenic	315 (3.7%)	Metaphyseal fibrous defect (fibroma)	99	Desmoplastic fibroma	9
				Fibrosarcoma	207
Notochordal	262 (3.1%)	—	—	Chordoma	262
Vascular	147 (1.7%)	Hemangioma	80	Hemangioendothelioma	60
				Hemangiopericytoma	7
Lipogenic	7 (0.1%)	Lipoma	6	Liposarcoma	1
Neurogenic	10 (0.1%)	Neurilemoma	10		
Total	8542 (100.0%)		2028		6514

[a] Data are from Dahlin DC, Unni K. Bone Tumors: general aspects and data on 8,542 cases. 4th Ed. Springfield, Illinois: Thomas, 1986:552.

history of multiple previous surgical procedures is also a relative contraindication. Resection of the lesion is possible, but the patient and family must understand that the procedure can be hazardous because of scarring and distortion of the anatomy. An unresectable lesion is also a relative contraindication to surgery. Surgical adjuvants such as chemotherapy and radiation therapy may palliate and occasionally cure the patient after incomplete tumor removal. Adjunctive therapy such as radiation or chemotherapy is delayed until the graft material is well on the way to incorporation.

Technique for Posterior Fusion

In general, after extensive resections, it is necessary to fuse the spine with posterior or anterior instrumentation and graft material along the entire length of the fixation devices. For thoracic and thoracolumbar lesions, Harrington rods or the Cotrel–Dubousset (C-D) systems are most often used. When necessary, sublaminar wires are added to improve the fixation. In the lumbar spine, some of the newer fixation devices with pedicle screws, such as Steffee plates and the Cotrel–Dubousset system, have been used. The cortices of the posterior elements are decorticated, and the graft material is placed around both sides of the instrumentation devices.

For massive resections in the lumbosacral region, the fixation technique is customized to the remaining bony anatomy. Contoured Harrington rods with fixation to the ilium is a useful technique (see Case 9).

The patient must be thoroughly apprised of the magnitude of reconstructive surgery of the spinal column. Surgery usually consists of both anterior and posterior approaches. If the size of the tumor permits, en bloc excision is the ideal treatment. Frequently, the tumor has expanded so much that its excision is difficult because the tumor has invaded the spinal canal and migrated along its course.[5] The extensive venous distribution of the spinal column permits easy spread of the tumor.[6] Because massive bleeding may occur, adequate supplies of blood replacement must be available. The patient also should be informed that the problem is serious, that the intervention may cause the lesion to spread, and that cure may not be possible.

Primary Malignant Bone Tumors

Primary malignant bone tumors of the spinal column are rare. In patients with such bone tumors, the goal of operative treatment is to resect the lesion en bloc with a wide surgical margin. Stener[7] and Stener and Johnson[8] have described total spondylectomy and fusion in the treatment of selected patients with chondrosarcoma and giant-cell tumors. Because of anatomical restraints, the tumor often cannot be resected without entering it, thus precluding a wide margin. The malignant lesions that are most amenable to resection are low-grade chondrosarcomas and chordomas. Preoperatively, it is important to determine the surgical stage so as to define the anatomy of the tumor and to exclude metastatic disease. If the tumor is high grade, consideration is given to preoperative chemotherapy to reduce the tumor burden, to lessen the chance of spread intraoperatively, and to test the tumor's response to chemotherapy.

For small lesions that are located posteriorly, a limited resection, followed by a posterior fusion covering the involved levels, often can be performed. For unilateral lesions the fusion often can be achieved without instrumentation.

Unfortunately, most lesions are extensive, requiring major resection and reconstruction. Frequently, the largest lesions have primarily anterior involvement. The surgical procedure is staged into anterior and posterior portions separated by 1 to 3 weeks, depending on the patient's medical condition. If an anterior resection is performed, it is almost always necessary to fuse the spinal column posteriorly because the anterior and middle columns are destroyed.

Cervical Spinal Column Tumors

The most common lesion of the cervical spinal column are multiple myeloma and metastatic disease. Both primarily involve the anterior and middle columns of the spinal column. Destruction of the vertebrae may require halo traction and bracing for immobilization of the skull. Roentgenograms should always be taken before application of a halo so that smaller lesions of the skull can be avoided. After immobilization, appropriate treatment may be undertaken.

Patients with extensive destructive lesions not amenable to surgical reconstruction have been maintained as long as 2 years in halo vests. In many instances, reconstruction of the spinal column with bone struts, such as rib, fibula, or iliac crest, can be achieved both anteriorly or posteriorly. Wiring with the addition of methylmethacrylate[9] and the use of a special occiput plate also have been devised for this purpose.[10] The anterior approach to the spinal column may include a transoral approach for high C1 and C2 lesions, but this entails a great risk of infection.[11,12] When the prognosis is favorable, fixation with a halo vest until the graft is incorporated is very successful.

If a single vertebral body is involved, the standard anterolateral approach is used, and the entire vertebral body and adjacent discs can be excised and stabilized with a graft or methylmethacrylate and sometimes metal struts (Fig. 10.1). Multiple levels of involvement require the anterior placement of struts of ribs or fibula. Grafts also may be fixed with a small plate. If bone healing can be achieved and the prognosis is good, the use of methylmethacrylate should be avoided wherever possible.

Thoracic and Lumbar Spinal Column Tumors

McAfee et al.[13] reported failure of stabilization in 24 patients who had metastatic disease. The structural failure began most frequently at the bone–cement interface. Other authors have described both metallic and ceramic vertebral body prostheses that are inserted and combined with methylmethacrylate. Although several authors[9,15] have reported the use of methylmethacrylate constructs posteriorly, we tend not to use the acrylic cement posteriorly for several reasons. First, the cement is weakest in tension, making its use posteriorly biomechanically unsound. Second, the highest infections rates have been when cement is used as a posterior construct. Of serious concern were the six (25%) infections in the series reported by McAfee et al.[13] In all six patients, cement was used as a posterior construct. McAfee et al. concluded that (1) methylmethacrylate should be used for spinal fixation only as a salvage procedure; (2) only patients with a life expectancy of less than 1 year should be considered for stabilization with methylmethacrylate; and (3) the methylmethacrylate should be supplemented with bone graft when possible. This has also been our experience.

Bone graft should be added to the area in which the cement is applied. Because thoracic and lumbar regions of the spinal column are similar, treatment goals are the same for both regions: excision, decompression, and reconstruction of the deformity. All levels of the spinal column are readily approached retroperitoneally or through an extended thoracotomy. The site of the lesion, whether

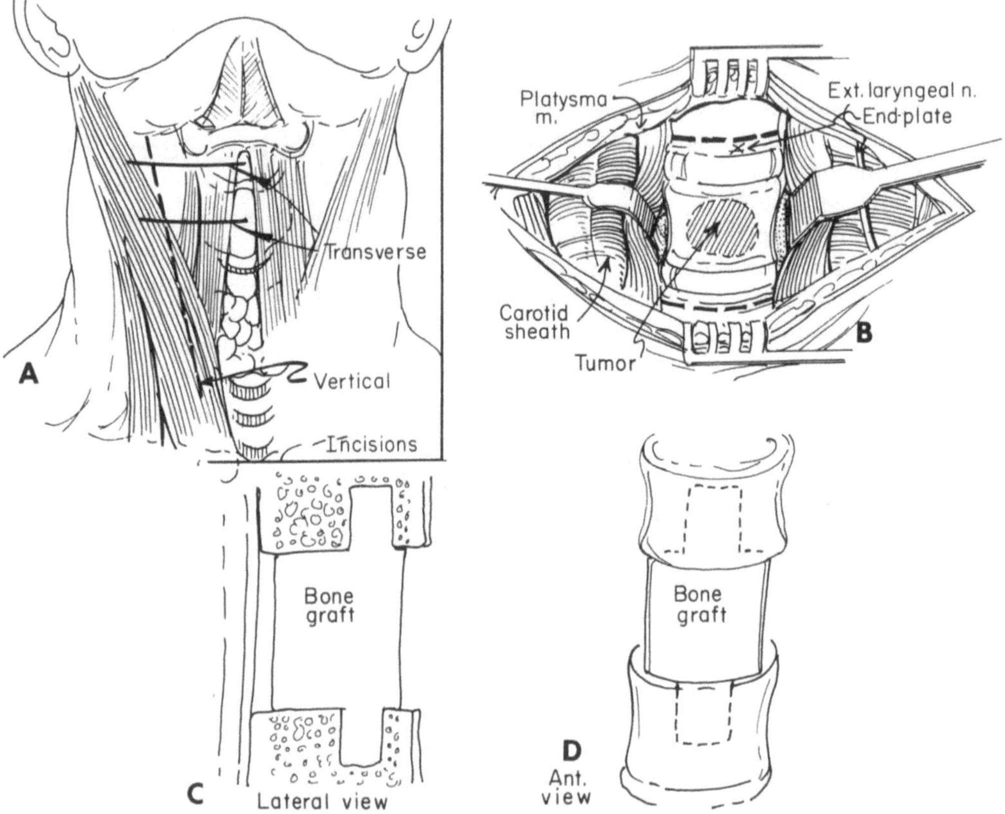

Figure 10.1. **A.** Transverse incisions are used most commonly for single-level involvement. For more extensive lesions that span more than one vertebral body, vertical incision is used. **B.** In general, approach anteriorly is medial to carotid sheath. Involved vertebral bodies are exposed and the tumor is removed. Intervertebral discs, above and below lesion, are removed. Superior and inferior vertebral endplates are cut to accept bone graft. **C.** Interval is opened using laminar spreader, and bone graft is locked into place. **D.** Anterior view shows bone graft locked into place.

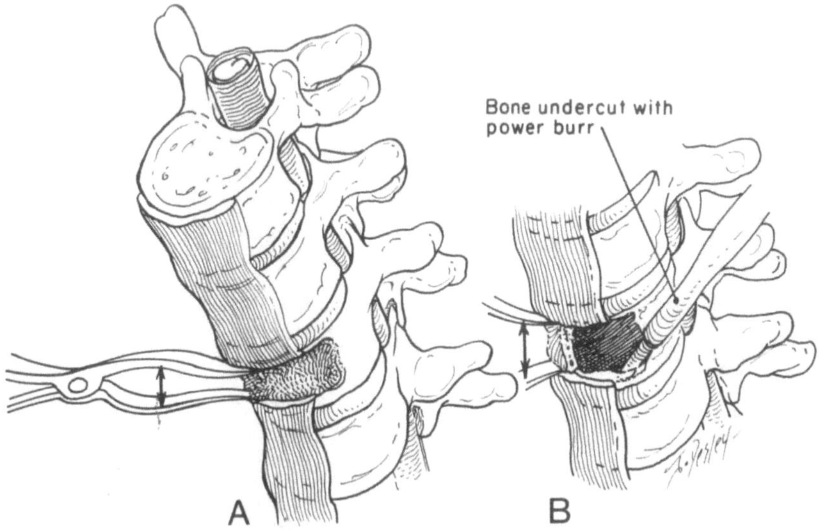

Figure 10.2. **A** and **B**. Involved vertebral body is exposed. Anterior longitudinal ligament is sectioned. Deformity is corrected using laminar spreader. Vertebral body is undercut in preparation for receiving bone graft and methylmethacrylate. **C**. For single-level involvement, vertebral body is often replaced with methylmethacrylate. **D**. When more than one level is involved, Harrington or Knodt rods are used to achieve rigid fixation. After rigid fixation is achieved, methylmethacrylate construct is fashioned. Methylmethacrylate increases contact surfaces.

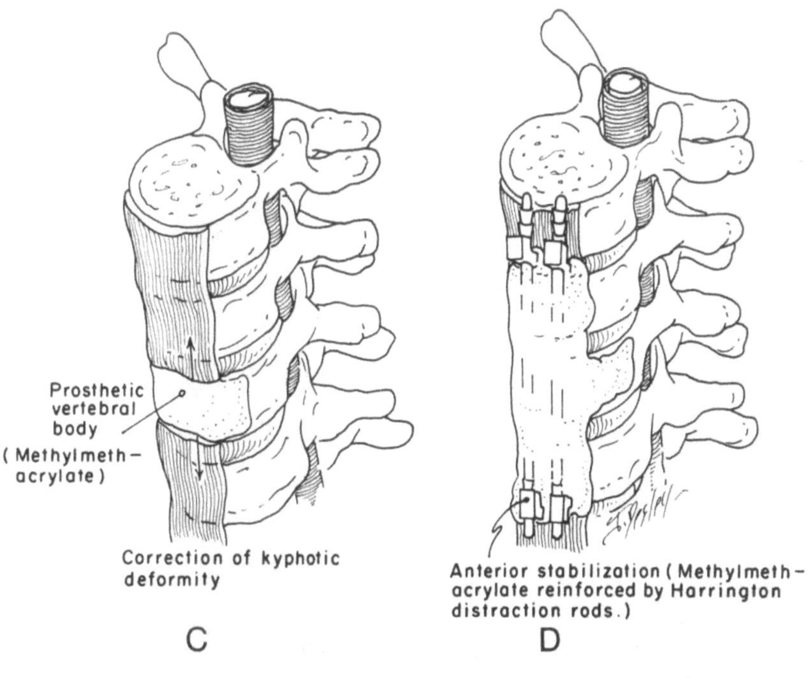

it is eccentrically placed or not, determines the surgical approach. If possible, en bloc excision of the lesion should be done, and sufficient margins of excision frequently can be determined by frozen-section study of the adjacent tissue. We prefer to use autogenous bone struts of fibular or iliac crest to reconstruct the spinal column. However, ceramic, metal, and methylmethacrylate have been utilized to fill the defect, and fixation devices such as plates, Harrington rods, hooks, and Zielke instrumentation also have been used anteriorly to help stabilize the spinal column. The deformity[16] is corrected using a laminar spreader (Figs. 10.2A and 10.2B). For a lesion at a single level, the vertebral body is reconstructed using methylmethacrylate (Fig. 10.2C). Involvement at multiple levels requires either a rib or fibular strut graft or methylmethacrylate construct. Harrington or Knodt rods (Fig. 10.2D) are used to achieve rigid fixation before applying methylmethacrylate to increase the contact areas.

Depending on the extent of the surgery undertaken, the posterior elements also may be removed at the same sitting or at a second operation. Fixation devices such as the Luque system with sublaminar wires, C-D system with multiple hooks or pedicle screws, or Steffee plates with pedicle screws can be applied posteriorly. Pedicle screws and plates are best applied in the thoracolumbar and lumbar regions.

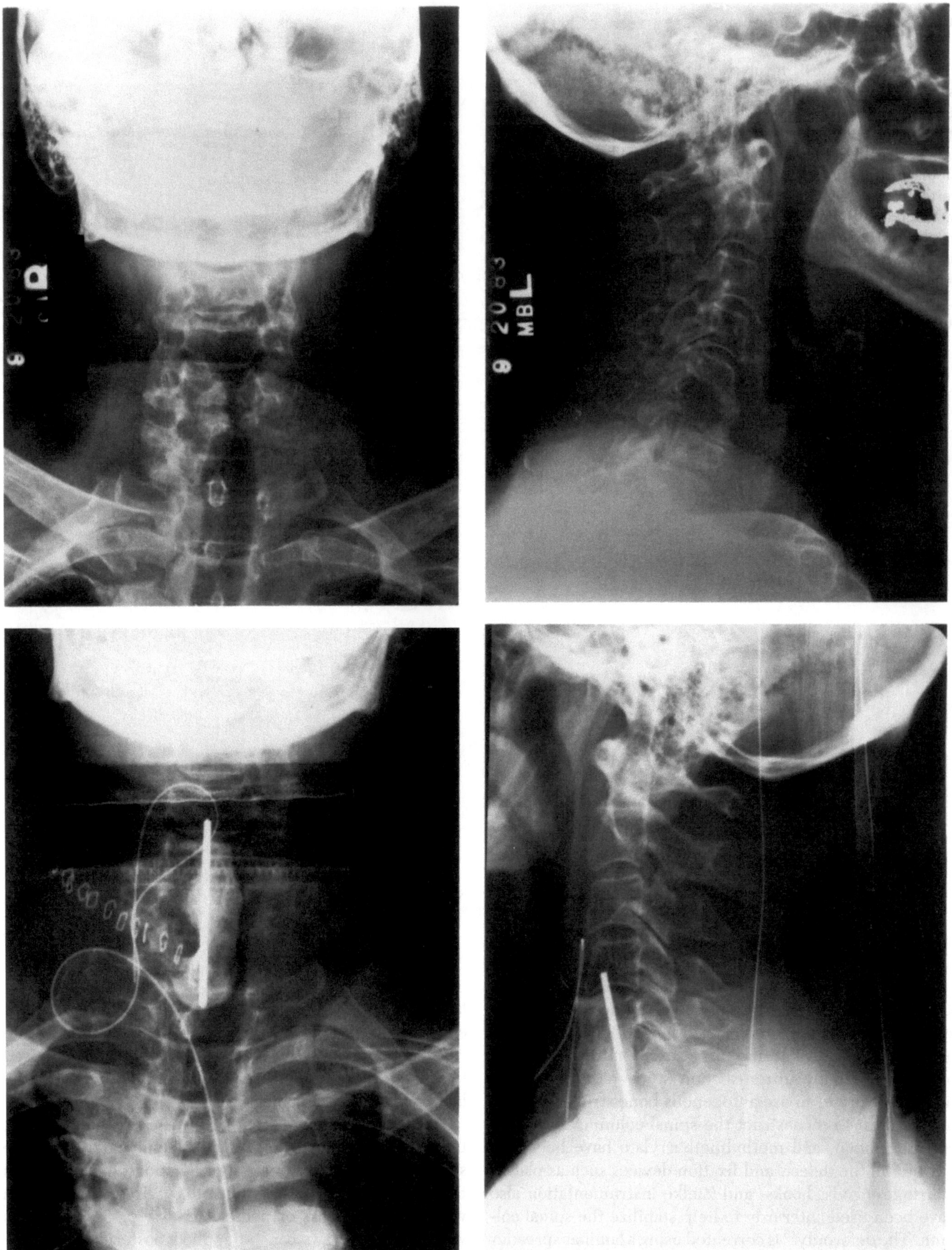

A B C D

During the reconstructive portion of the surgical procedure, a suitable graft material must be selected. Although prosthetic systems are being developed, we generally use autogenous bone grafts supplemented when necessary by allograft bone. The diaphysis of the fibula is the strongest strut and the one that we use most frequently. The rib is readily harvested and may serve as a useful strut graft. When locally feasible, a vascularized rib graft can be utilized for rapid healing, but when used alone, it does not offer much structural support, necessitating that other graft material also be used. For small defects, a graft can be fashioned from the iliac crest. Femoral head allografts can also be used to reconstruct the small defects. In general, we do not use large allografts because they require years to revascularize and the revascularization can be unpredictable.

For extensive posterior fusions, we often combine morselized autogenous graft with morselized allograft bone. In our experience, allograft bone used alone in the adult patient is associated with high failure rates. In general, we try not to exceed a ratio of two parts of allograft bone to one part of autogenous graft. It is important to coat the graft material with blood, as this has been shown in animal studies to improve incorporation (the blood adds a layer of fibronectin to the graft material).

Cases Illustrating Operative Technique in Metastatic Disease and Myeloma

Case 1: A 62-year-old man with renal disease was initially seen because of complaints of shoulder pain and paresthesia in the left thumb and index finger. Neurological examination was consistent with a left C6 and C7 radiculopathy. Anteroposterior and lateral radiographs demonstrated lytic destruction of C5, C6, and C7 (Figs 10.3A and 10.3B). There was also moderate compression of the vertebral body of C7 on the left. A CT scan showed destruction of the left lateral vertebral bodies of the fifth, sixth, and seventh cervical bodies. Both the plain radiographs and the CT scan were consistent with metastatic disease or hematological malignancy such as multiple myeloma or lymphoma.

Open biopsy through a standard anterior approach revealed grade 4 adenocarcinoma. The body of C7 was resected completely to decompress the neural elements. The bony destruction at C4, C5, and C6 was primarily on the left. A threaded Steinmann pin was fashioned to span the gap and was inserted into anchoring holes made with a motorized burr. Avitene was then placed over the dura to control the bleeding and to serve as a buffer between the methylmethacrylate and the spinal cord. The curetted area was then filled with methylmethacrylate (Figs 10.3C and 10.3D). As the cement hardened, the wound was copiously irrigated with normal saline. The wound was closed in a routine fashion. Postoperative irradiation (3,000 rad in 10 fractions) was used to halt tumor progression at the bone–cement interface.

Case 2: A 46-year-old man presented with a 12-month history of progressive weakness in both lower extremities. One month before presentation, he noticed increasing difficulty with gait and numbness in both lower extremities. Plain radiographs showed destruction of the body of T3 and T4 and the inferior aspect of T2. Tomography confirmed the destruction of T3 and T4 (Figs. 10.4A and 10.4B) and a myelogram showed a complete block at T4. Preoperative staging studies were consistent with multiple myeloma. Because of the severity of the patient's neurological compromise, it was decided to decompress the spinal cord and to fuse the spinal column if necessary.

The patient was placed in the left lateral decubitus position, and a thoracotomy was performed through the bed of the nonresected fourth rib. Open biopsy of T3 and T4 was consistent with multiple myeloma. The spinal canal was decompressed. Overall, enough of the anterior and middle columns were preserved so that fusion was not necessary. Postoperatively, the patient was treated with irradiation (total dose, 4000 rad).

Although the initial response to irradiation was good, 6 months later the patient's pain and neural compromise recurred. A two-stage anterior and posterior procedure was planned. The patient was positioned in the right lateral decubitus position. A left posterolateral thoracotomy was performed, and the posterior aspect of the left third rib was resected. The pleural cavity was entered, and the first four vertebral bodies were identified. The parietal pleura overlying the area from T2 to T5 was incised. The recurrent tumor in the area from T2 to T5 was removed with curettes and rongeurs. Slots were then made in the second and fifth vertebral bodies for the placement of a rib strut graft. The rib stumps were then wired over the rib strut graft.

Fresh gowns and instruments were used, and the left iliac crest was exposed and a graft harvested. The iliac crest graft was also slotted into the second and fifth vertebral bodies. The chest was then closed in a routine fashion.

Figure 10.3. **A** and **B.** Anteroposterior and lateral radiographs of cervical region of 72-year-old man demonstrate destruction of anterior and posterior aspects of C5 and C6 vertebral bodies. **C** and **D.** Anteroposterior and lateral radiographs demonstrate methylmethacrylate construct. Steinmann pin is locked to vertebra of C4 superiorly and to vertebra of C7 inferiorly. Right side of vertebral bodies was preserved. Methylmethacrylate was used to fill in defect.

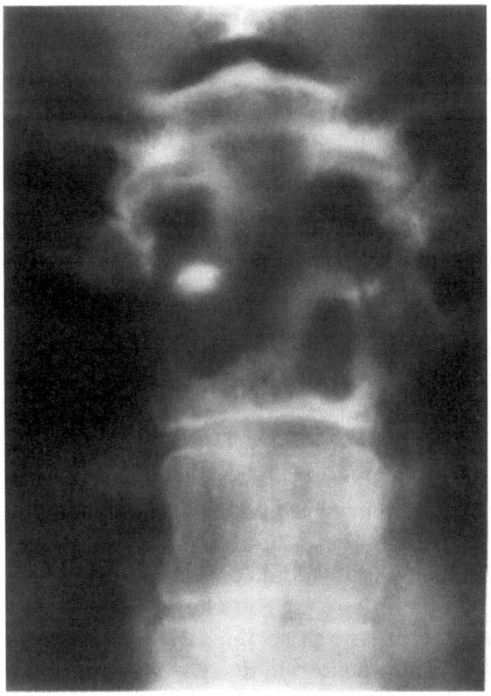

A

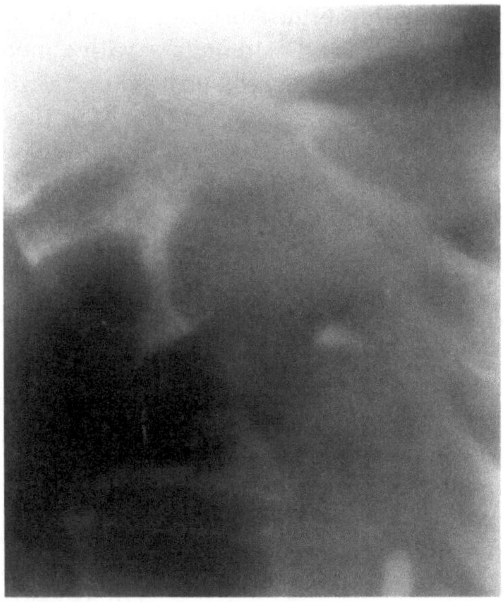

B

Figure 10.4. **A** and **B.** Anteroposterior and lateral tomograms show extensive destruction of vertebrae of T3 and T4. T4 vertebra has collapsed with resultant deformity. **C.** Postoperative radiograph demonstrates posterior fixation with compression hooks placed over lamina of T1 into facets of T5 and T6 using Wisconsin hooks.

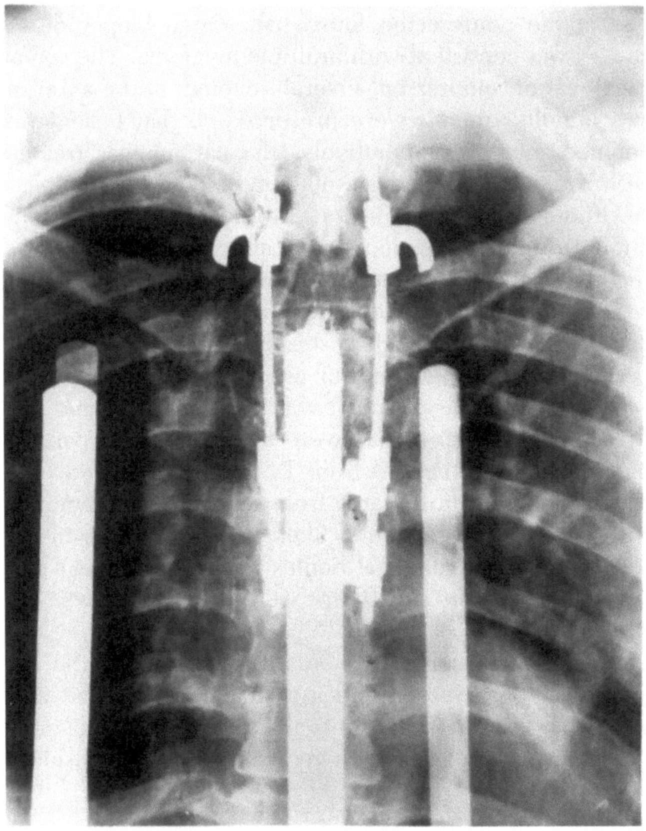

C

One week later, the posterior portion of the procedure was performed. The posterior elements from C7 to T7 were exposed. Compression hooks were placed on the lamina of T1 and the transverse processes of T3 and into the facets of T5 and T6 using the Wisconsin hooks (Fig. 10.4C). Compression rods were then inserted, and maximal compression was achieved.

Separate instruments and gowns were used, and the right iliac crest was exposed and a bone graft taken. The graft was placed over the transverse processes and along the gutter between the spinous processes from T1 to T6. The incisions were then closed in a routine fashion.

Case 3: A 70-year-old man presented with a 7-month history of increasing low back pain. Seven years before, he had undergone a thyroidectomy because of follicular cell carcinoma. Plain radiographs showed lytic destruction of T11. A needle biopsy was consistent with grade 3, metastatic follicular cell carcinoma of the thyroid. A radioactive tracer study showed that the patient's metastatic bone disease was not amenable to radioactive iodine treatment. Therapeutic irradiation (3000 rad) was administered in 10 fractions. Two years later, he presented with weakness in both lower extremities and difficulty in walking. Radiographic and CT studies showed progression of the metastatic disease at T11 (Figs. 10.5A–10.5C). A two-stage procedure was planned to decompress the spinal cord and fuse the spine.

The patient was placed in the lateral decubitus position,

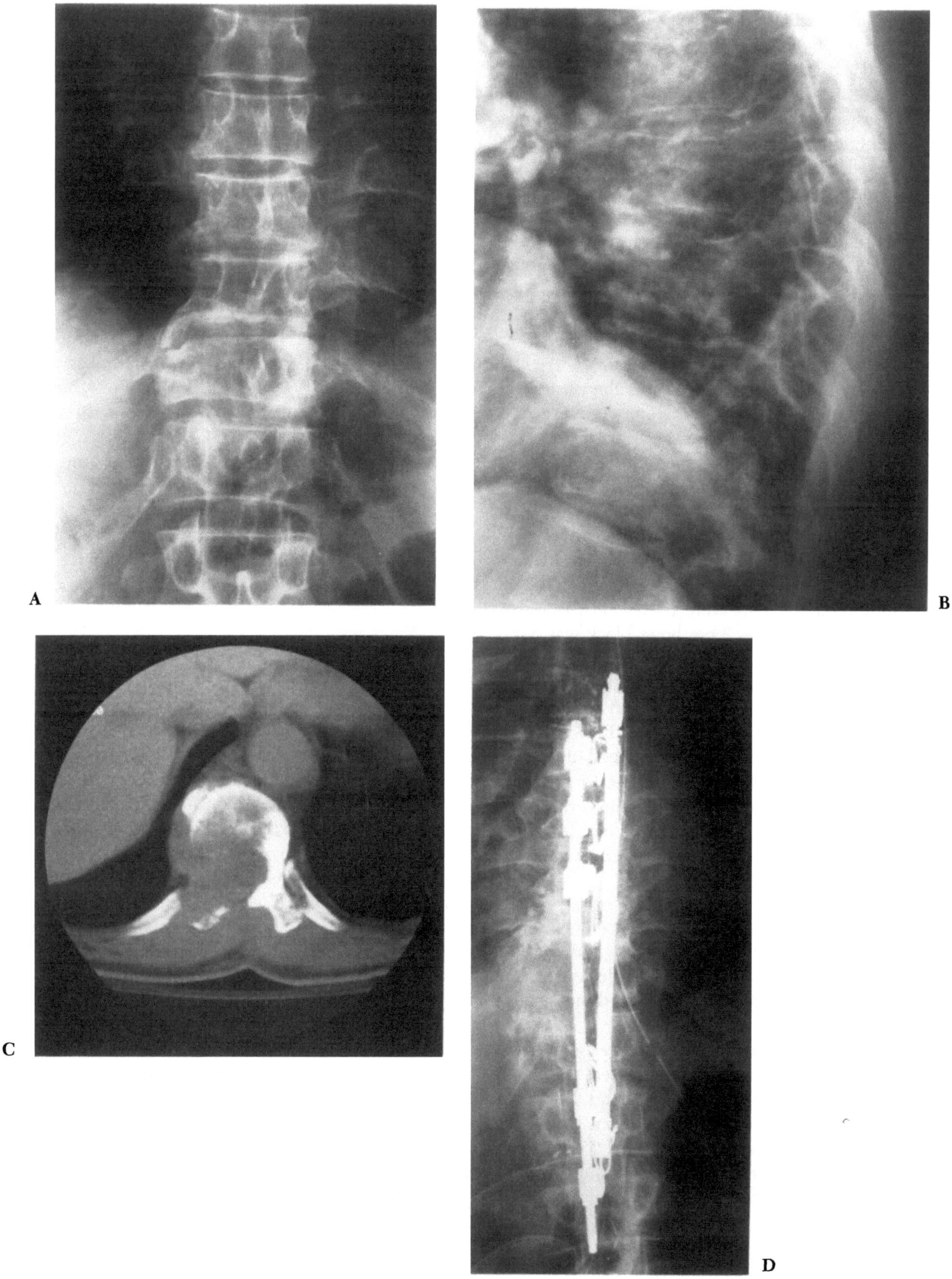

Figure 10.5. **A** and **B.** Anteroposterior and lateral radiographs demonstrate destruction of vertebra of T11 with complete absence of pedicle on right and also moderate collapse of vertebra. **C.** CT scan demonstrates destruction of anterior and middle columns and also destruction of posterior elements in pedicle on right. **D.** Postoperative radiograph demonstrates compression hooks placed under lamina of T7, T8, T9, L1, and L2, and compression rod. Distraction hooks were placed at T6 and T2 and distraction rod were inserted. Sublaminar wires were tied over rod.

and a longitudinal incision was made along the course of the right tenth rib. The eighth rib was prepared to serve as a vascularized rib graft. The parietal pleura overlying the thoracic vertebra was incised.

The tumor was seen destroying the eleventh vertebral body and invading the soft tissues on the right. The tumor cavity was opened and a vertebrectomy performed. The inferior and superior intervertebral discs were also removed. The tumor was very vascular and bled profusely. The right T11 pedicle was removed. Because of profuse bleeding, it was decided to fashion a graft from an allograft femoral head to fill the dead space and tamponade the bleeding points rather than to insert the vascularized rib graft. The graft was fashioned and slotted into place. The wounds were then closed in a routine fashion.

Two weeks after the anterior procedure, the posterior fusion was performed. The posterior elements were exposed from T8 to L2. A laminectomy was performed at T11 and all remaining tumor was removed.

The transverse processes were then exposed. Compression hooks were placed under the laminae of T7, T8, T9, L1, and L2. Sublaminar wires were placed at the same levels. A compression rod was contoured to fit the spinal column and inserted.

New instruments and gowns were used, and the right iliac crest was exposed. A 2 × 2 cm bone block was harvested and shaped to fit into the anterior interbody space on the left. Distraction hooks were placed at T6 and L2 on the left, and a distraction rod was inserted. The sublaminar wires were then tied over the rod (see Fig. 10.5D). Bone struts were also fashioned, and were placed to bypass the area from which the vertebral body had been removed. Additional bone graft was laid over the transverse processes. The autogenous bone graft was supplemented with bone bank bone. The incisions were closed in a routine fashion.

Case 4: A 40-year-old woman was initially seen with a 10-month history of pain in her right buttock. Plain radiographs and CT scan showed a destructive lesion at L2 (Figs. 10.6A–10.6C). A needle biopsy revealed metastatic adenocarcinoma.

An anterolateral retroperitoneal exposure was performed. The inferior vena cava was identified and protected. The spinous processes of L1, L2, and L3 were identified. The soft tissues were stripped from the bony processes. The tumor was centered on the L2 vertebra. As much of the tumor was removed as possible, leaving a rim of bone along the left side of the vertebral body. The L1, L2, and L2, L3 disc spaces were then removed. The right L2 pedicle was removed, protecting the nerve root of L2.

Attention was then directed to the right calf to harvest the fibular graft. A new set of gowns and instruments were used to preclude spreading the tumor to the donor site. A 10-cm length of fibula was harvested.

The bodies of L1 and L3 were cut to accept the fibular graft, and the graft was impacted into place. Autogenous graft was packed into the contact surfaces between the fibula and the vertebral bodies. A piece of subcutaneous fat was placed between the dura and the bone grafts. The retroperitoneal exposure was closed in routine fashion.

Two weeks after the anterior procedure, the posterior procedure was performed. The posterior elements of L1 to L4 were exposed. Screws were passed into the pedicles of L2, L3, and L4 on the left. The remainder of the posterior element of L2 was removed. A small amount of remaining tumor was removed. A plate was placed on screws at the L2, L3, and L4 levels. Four hooks were placed over the lamina of L3 and were directed over the laminae of L1 and L4. A C-D rod was inserted and maximally tightened. A wire was placed around the plate at L1 (Figs. 10.6D and 10.6E).

The left iliac crest was exposed. Again new gowns and instruments were used. The graft was harvested and placed over the posterior element bilaterally from L1 to L4. A subcutaneous fat graft was placed over the exposed dura at L2.

Cases Illustrating Operative Techniques in Primary Bone Tumors

Case 5: An 18-year-old man presented with a 4-month history of left lower back pain and paresthesia over the left lower extremity. Physical examination was consistent with mild radiculopathy of L4. Plain radiographs revealed a 3-cm mineralized mass arising from the transverse process of L5 (Fig. 10.7A). A CT scan confirmed that the lesion arose from the transverse process of L5 and impinged on the nerve of L5 (Fig. 10.7B). Open biopsy showed a low-grade (grade 1) chondrosarcoma. The operative plan was to remove the tumor en bloc while protecting the nerve root of L4 and L5. A fusion from L4 to the sacrum was planned.

A curved incision was made over the lateral border of the sacrospinalis muscles. The lumbosacral fascia was split along the lines of the incision, and the paraspinal muscles were reflected off their bony attachments. The mass was easily seen at the L5 level.

The tumor appeared to arise from the left superior facet of L5 and the transverse process of L5. A hemilaminectomy at L5, with transection of the facet joint, was performed. The inferior articular facet at L5 was also excised. The ligamentum flavum was excised, and the nerve root of L5 was identified and protected. The L5 pedicle was then

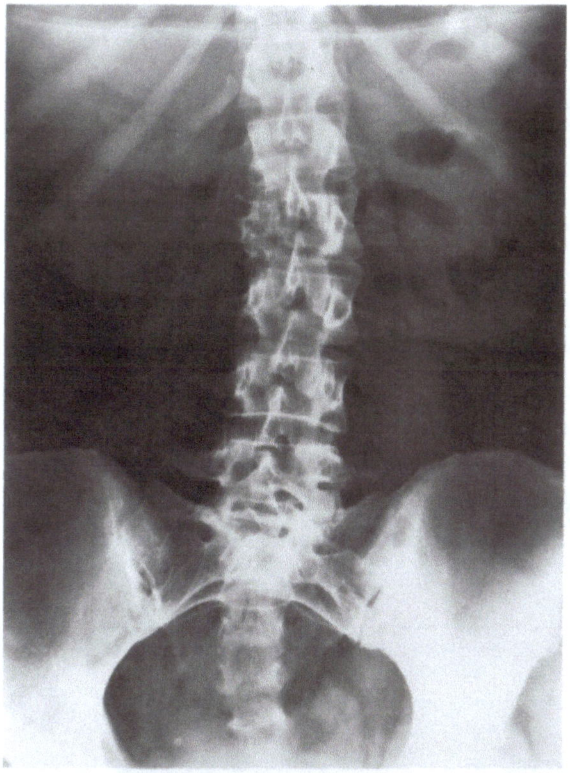

A

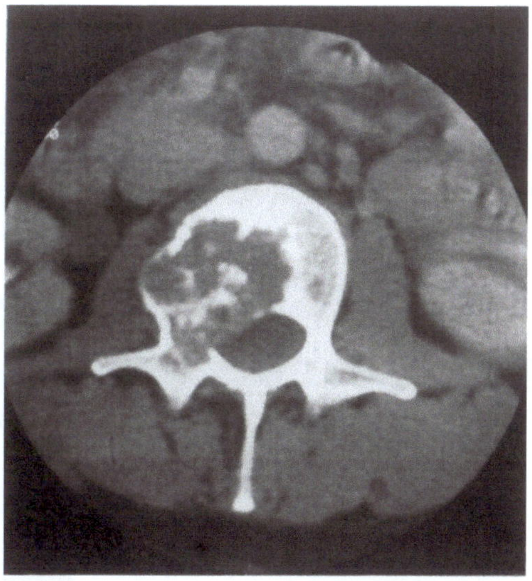

B

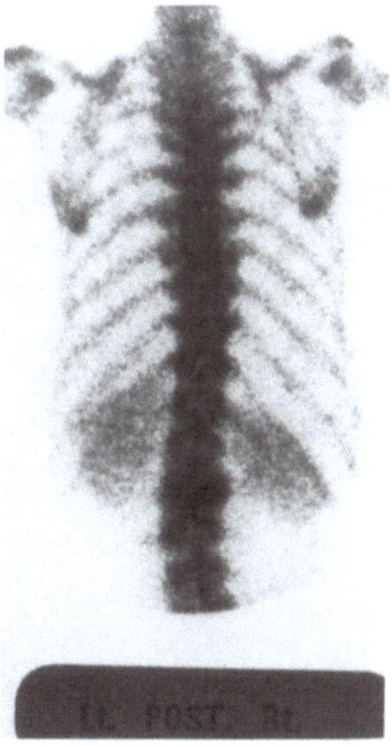

C

Figure 10.6. **A.** Anteroposterior radiograph demonstrates destruction of vertebra of L2 along with collapse. **B.** CT scan demonstrates lytic destruction of vertebral body with compression of spinal cord. **C.** Technetium bone scan shows increased uptake at single level, **D** and **E.** Postoperative anteroposterior and lateral radiographs demonstrate screws placed at L2, L3, and L4. Plate was used as fixation. Hooks were placed in lamina of L1, L3, and L4; C-D rod was inserted and maximally tightened. Wire was placed around the plate at L1.

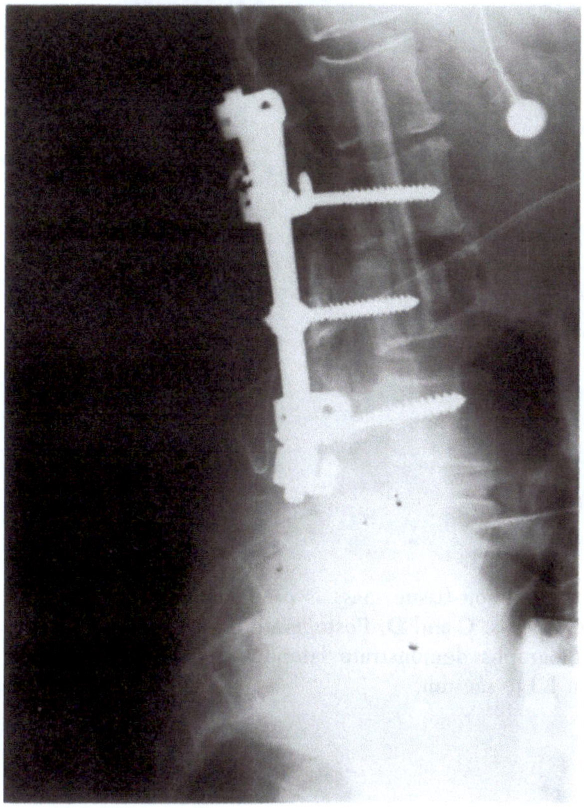

D

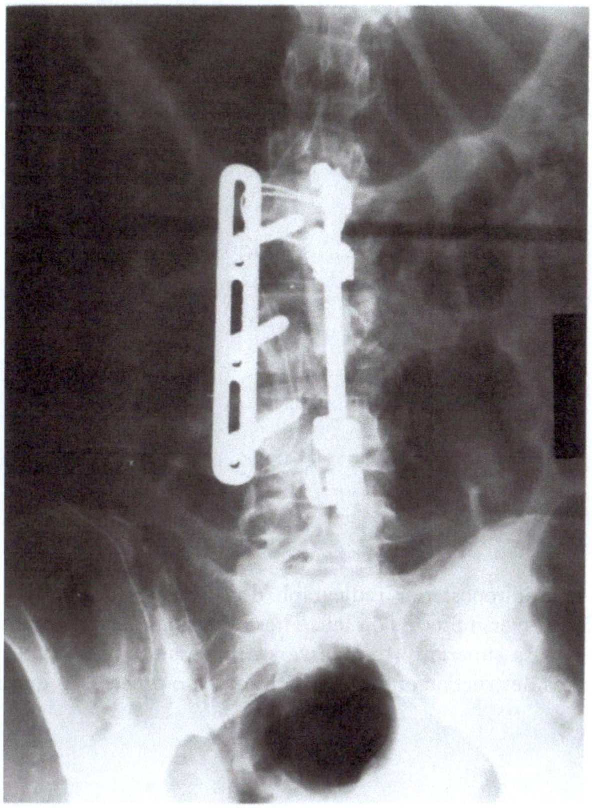

E

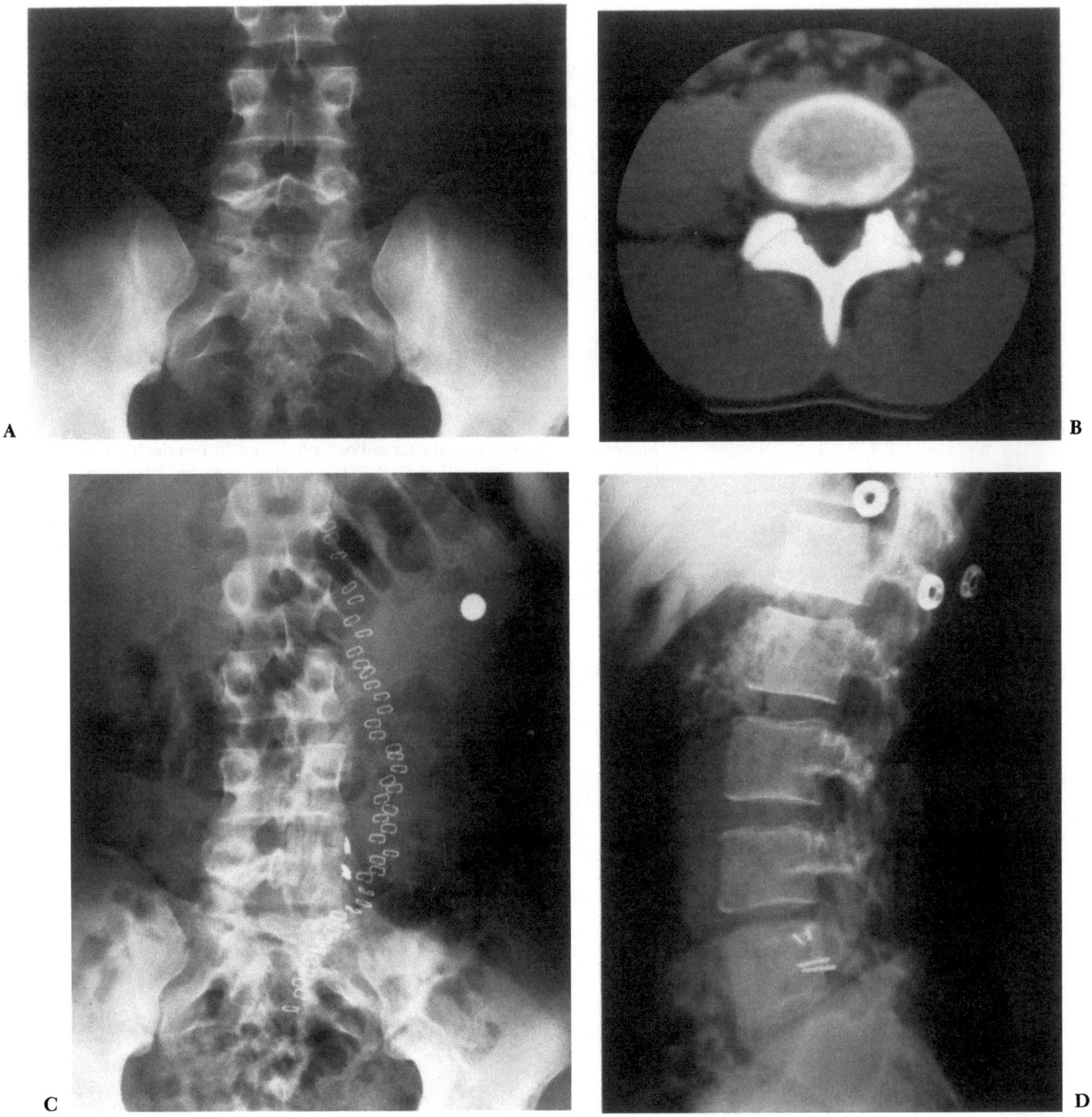

Figure 10.7. **A.** Anteroposterior radiograph demonstrates destruction of L5 transverse process on left. There is also mineralized soft-tissue mass superiorly to transverse process. **B.** CT scan demonstrates destruction of the left L5 transverse process. The mineralized soft-tissue mass is predominantly anterior to transverse process. **C** and **D.** Postoperative anteroposterior and lateral radiographs demonstrate lateral fusion with bicortical grafts from L3 to sacrum.

transected with an osteotome. The tumor was then elevated away from the L4 nerve root and removed after the L5 transverse process was osteotomized.

The left iliac crest was exposed. A new set of instruments and gowns was used for the harvest of the bone graft to avoid contaminating the donor site. Bicortical grafts were harvested. The facet joint between L3 and L4 was curetted and packed with cancellous graft. A motorized burr was used to remove all the soft-tissue attachments from L4, L5, and the sacrum. The bicortical grafts were then placed along the spinous processes and from the transverse process of L3 to the sacrum (Figs. 10.7C and 10.7D).

On the seventh postoperative day, a well-padded body cast with a left leg extension was placed and was to be worn for 3 months. Radiographs at 3 months showed a satisfactory fusion, and the patient was placed in a corset for 3 more months.

Case 6: A 62-year-old woman presented with a 10-month history of progressive neck pain. At presentation, she had severe paresthesia in both hands. A myelogram revealed complete block at the second cervical interspace. Open biopsy revealed a chordoma. Decompressive laminectomies were performed at C1, C2, and C3 (Figs. 10.8A and 10.8B). Despite oral steroids and irradiation (total dose, 6000 rad), she presented to the Mayo Clinic 6 months later with increasing pain and weakness of both arms and hands. Her neurological examination revealed spastic quadriplegia. MRI showed the extensive nature of the lesion (Fig. 10.8C).

The patient was placed in the prone position, and the posterior elements were exposed from the occiput to C7. The scar tissue from the previous laminectomies was removed, and the posterolateral dural sac was identified. The dural sac was opened because recurrent chordoma had infiltrated the dura. A large portion of the tumor was removed. A large dural defect resulted from the tumor excision. The dural defect was reconstructed with a fascia lata graft. Subcutaneous fat grafts were placed on both sides of the dura.

Wires were then placed beneath the laminae of C5 and C6. Four burr holes were placed in the occiput on either side of the midline so that 18-gauge wires could be passed.

An incision was then made over the tip of the right scapula exposing the posterior portion of the fourth and fifth ribs. A 15-cm segment of each was excised in a subperiosteal fashion. The two rib struts were then fashioned to fit against the occiput and the posterior elements of C5 and C6. The struts were placed centrally to cover the defect over the cord. The rib struts were then wired into place (Fig. 10.8D). The grafts were augmented with autogenous iliac crest grafts. The reconstruction was protected with a halo vest.

Case 7: A 52-year-old man presented with a history of back pain and weakness in both legs. Plain radiographs demonstrated a destructive process with collapse of L1 (Figs. 10.9A and 10.9B). The CT scan showed sclerosis and destructive changes in the vertebral body, with a soft-tissue mass to the right of the L1 vertebral body. The largest dimension of the mass was 5 × 3 cm. An open biopsy revealed a chordoma.

A two-stage anterior and posterior procedure was planned. The patient was placed in the left lateral thoracotomy position, and the entire right side of the chest, the abdomen, and the flank were prepared. An incision was made based on the twelfth rib. The twelfth rib was removed and saved for later bone grafting. An obvious mass growing into the lateral attachments of the diaphragm was apparent on the right lateral aspect of the L2 vertebral body. A portion of the posterolateral diaphragm and the overlying viscera and partial pleura were resected along with the tumor. The psoas muscle fibers were divided at their origin to permit identification of L2 and L3. The inferior vena cava and right ureters were identified and protected.

The anterior border of the spinal column was further cleared of soft tissues. Osteotomes were used, and a tumor-free margin was identified above and below the mass. The transverse processes of T12 and L1 and the pedicle of L1 were transected with osteotomes. The vertebral body and the soft-tissue extension of the tumor were removed.

The intervertebral discs of T12, L1, and L1, L2 were completely removed. A 14-cm length of fibular graft was harvested. The inferior aspect of T12 was undermined with a motorized burr, and a slot was cut in the vertebral bodies at L2 and L3. The fibular graft was then augmented with the twelfth rib graft. The grafts were further held in place with a Dwyer staple, cortical screw, and suture. The wounds were then closed in a routine fashion.

Two weeks after the anterior procedure, the posterior procedure was performed. The posterior elements were exposed from T10 to L4. The posterior elements of L1 were removed completely. The spinal column was then fused posteriorly. Distraction hooks were placed under the lamina of T11 superiorly, and a Leatherman hook was placed under the lamina of L4 inferiorly on the left. Wires were placed under the laminae of L2 and L3 inferiorly and under the lamina of T12 superiorly. Wires were also placed around the spinous processes of L3, L4, and T11, T12. A distraction rod was inserted, and the spinal column was distracted under radiologic control to be sure that the anterior strut was not disengaged. Compression hooks were placed under the laminae of T11 and T12 superiorly and under the laminae of L3 and L4 inferiorly (Fig. 10.9C). Maximal compression was achieved.

The left iliac crest was exposed. New instruments and

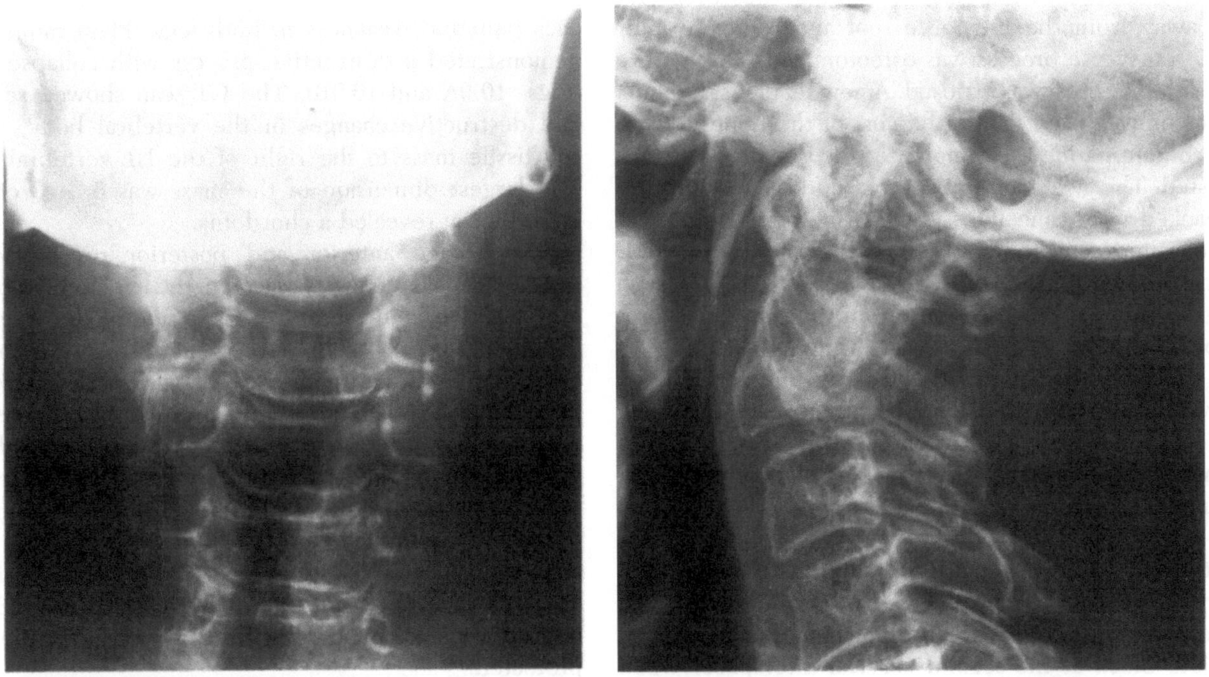

A B

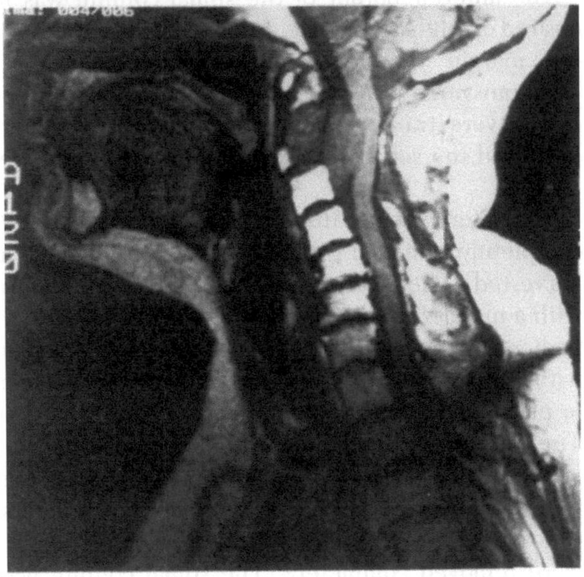

C

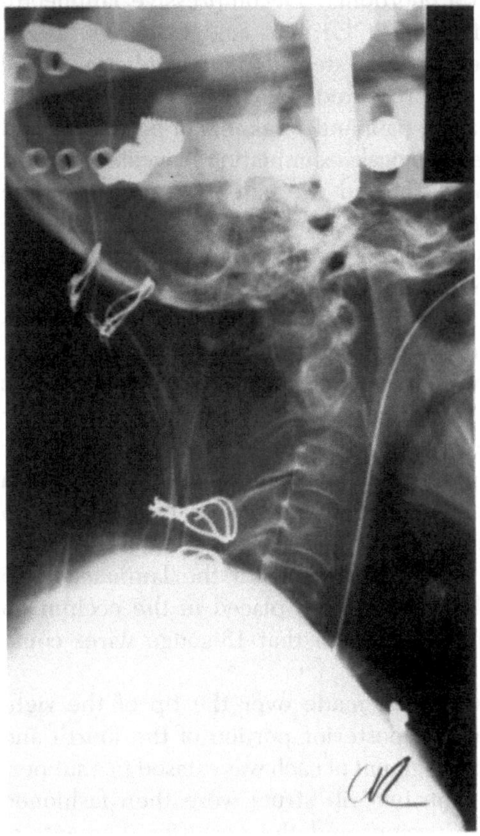

D

Figure 10.8. **A** and **B.** Anteroposterior and lateral radiographs demonstrate laminectomies performed at C1, C2, and C3. **C.** Lateral MRI demonstrates extensive destruction of C2. There is also large soft-tissue mass extending posteriorly and compressing spinal cord, primarily at C2. **D.** Postoperative radiograph demonstrates resection of posterior elements and fusion of cervical spine from occiput to C4 and C5 using conduit rib strut grafts. Halo immobilization was used to protect reconstruction.

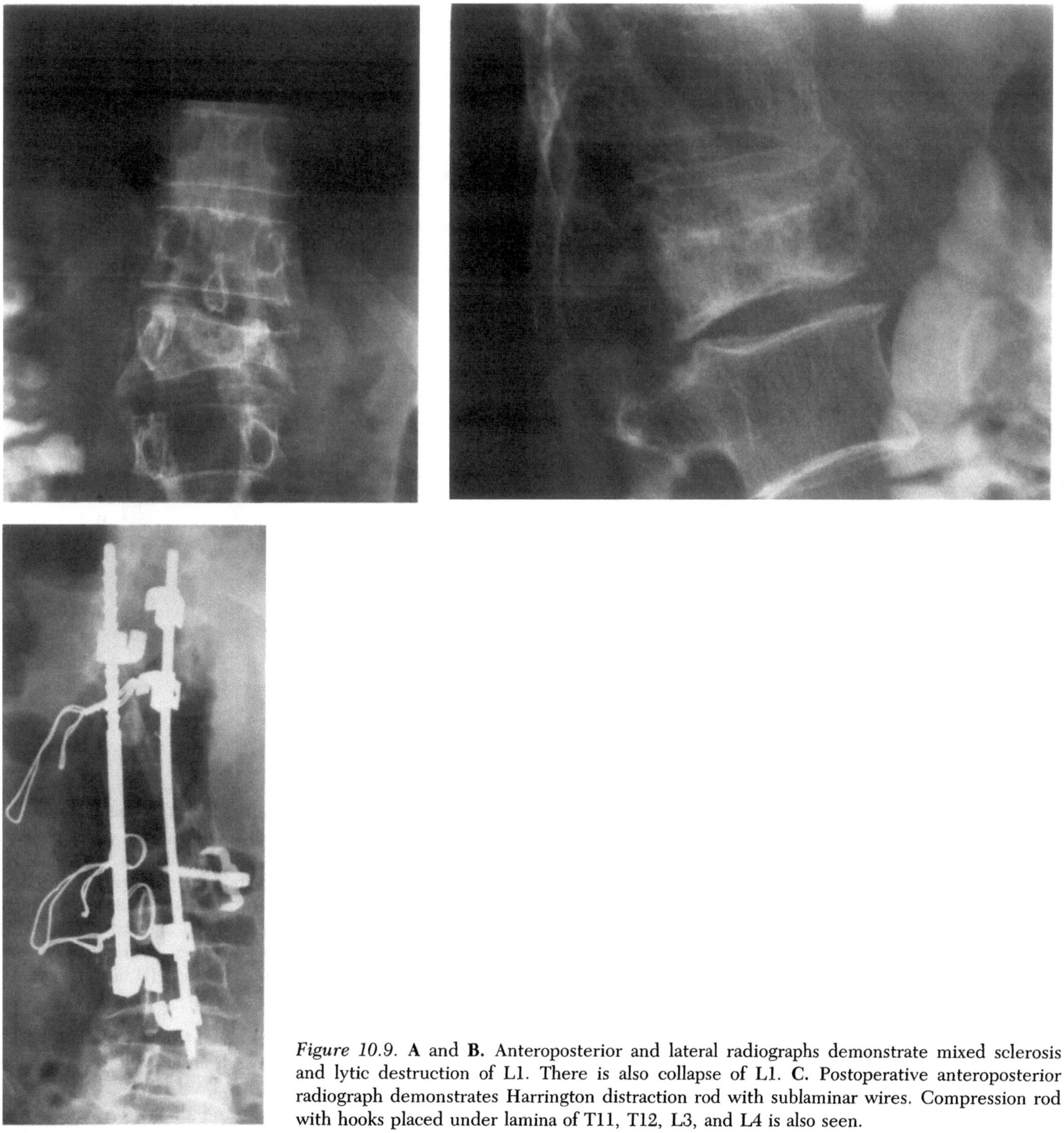

A B C

Figure 10.9. **A** and **B.** Anteroposterior and lateral radiographs demonstrate mixed sclerosis and lytic destruction of L1. There is also collapse of L1. **C.** Postoperative anteroposterior radiograph demonstrates Harrington distraction rod with sublaminar wires. Compression rod with hooks placed under lamina of T11, T12, L3, and L4 is also seen.

gowns were used. The bone graft was slotted under the transverse processes from T11 to L4 bilaterally. The wound was then closed in a routine fashion.

Case 8: A 62-year-old woman presented with a 12-month history of low back pain. Plain radiographs revealed a mixed lytic/sclerotic lesion in the spinous processes and lamina of L3 (Figs. 10.10A and 10.10B). A CT scan showed encroachment into the posterolateral aspect of the spinal canal in addition to the bony destruction (Fig. 10.10C). A myelogram confirmed the compression of the dural sac.

Open biopsy showed a grade 3, fibroblastic osteosarcoma. A two-stage anterior and posterior approach was planned to remove the tumor. The anterior procedure was performed first. The patient was placed in the right

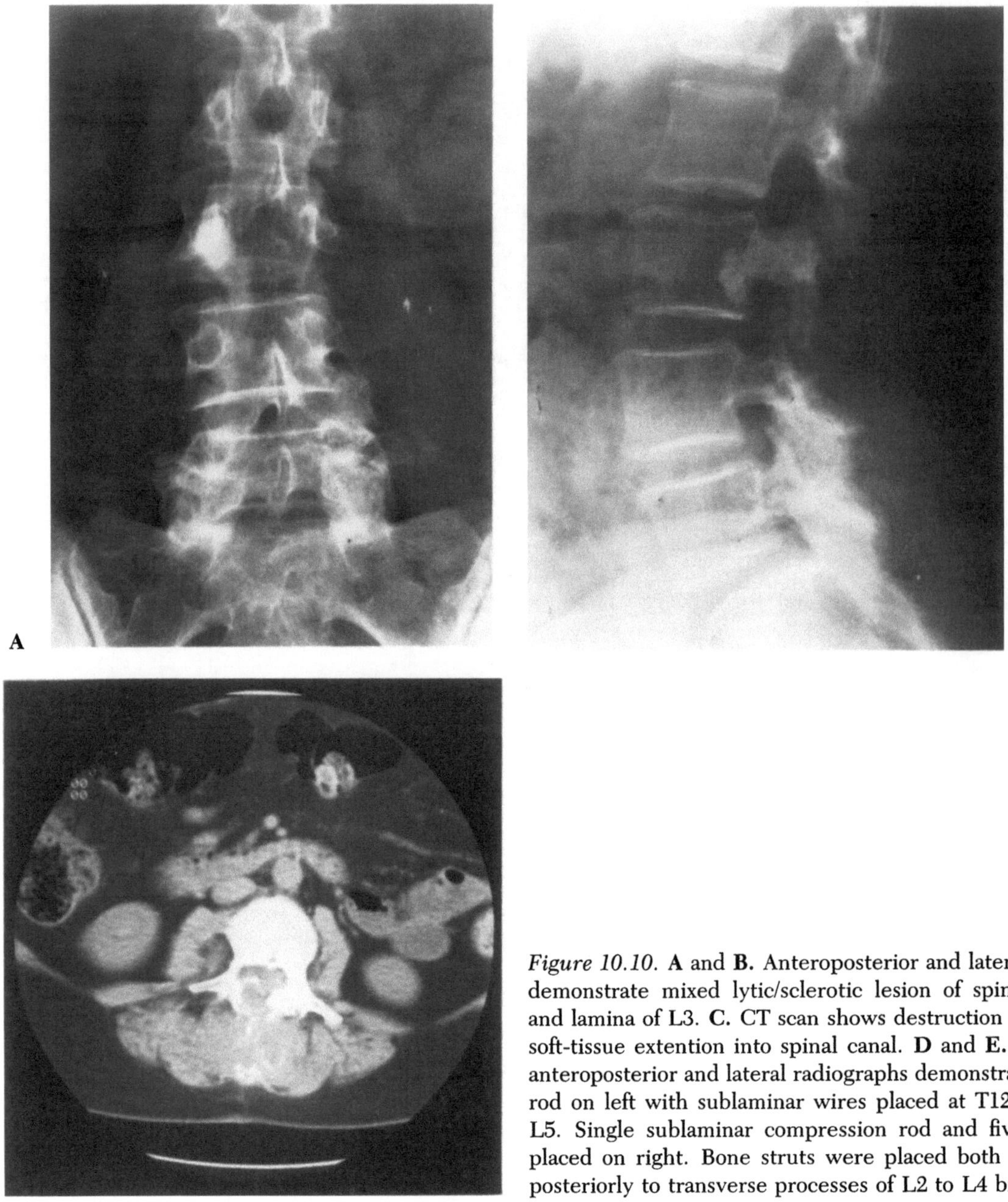

Figure 10.10. **A** and **B.** Anteroposterior and lateral radiographs demonstrate mixed lytic/sclerotic lesion of spinous processes and lamina of L3. **C.** CT scan shows destruction of lamina with soft-tissue extention into spinal canal. **D** and **E.** Postoperative anteroposterior and lateral radiographs demonstrate Harrington rod on left with sublaminar wires placed at T12, L1, L4, and L5. Single sublaminar compression rod and five hooks were placed on right. Bone struts were placed both anteriorly and posteriorly to transverse processes of L2 to L4 bilaterally.

lateral decubitus position. A diagonal flank incision was outlined midway between the pubis and the umbilicus and was extended superiorly and laterally to the twelfth rib. The retroperitoneal space was developed. The aorta was mobilized, and segmental arteries were divided as necessary. Adequate exposure was gained from L1 to L5.

The fascia overlying the L3 vertebral body was incised, and the intervertebral discs above and below L3 were sectioned. The L3 vertebral body was removed. Tumor was encountered at the level of both pedicles. The nerve roots were identified and traced to their respective foramina.

New gowns and instruments were used, and an 18-cm segment of fibula was removed from the left leg. The left iliac crest was then exposed, and several bone staves (5 × 1 cm) were harvested.

The body of L2 superiorly and the bodies of L4 and L5 inferiorly were slotted to accept the fibular graft. The fibula was then slotted into place, and the autogenous iliac graft was placed around the contact areas. Additional graft was placed into the defect created by removal of the L3 vertebral body, and was held in place with three heavy sutures. The wound was then closed in layers.

Eight days after the anterior procedure, the posterior procedure was performed. The area of the previous posterior biopsy incision was excised. The initial exposure was

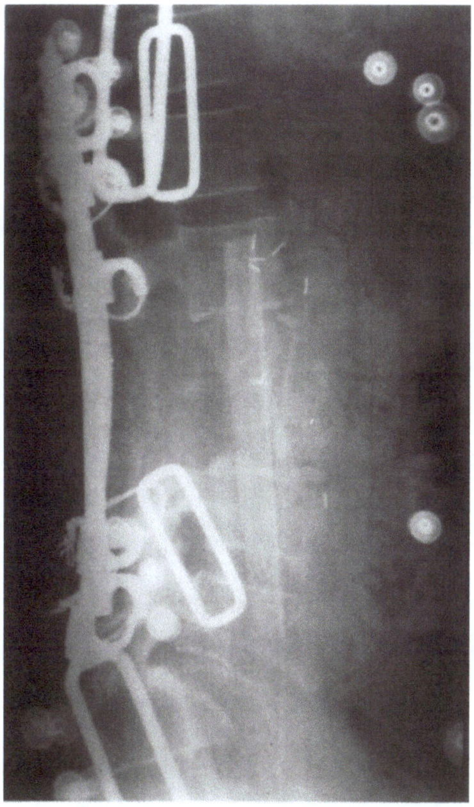

D

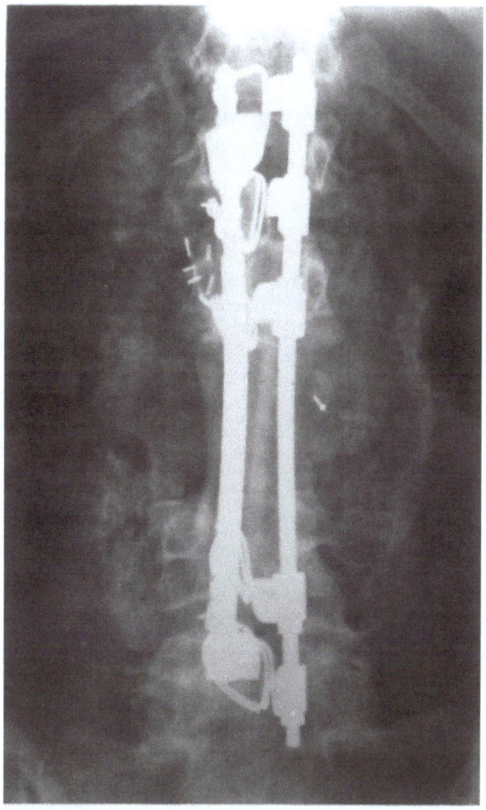

E

from only L1 to L4 to avoid contaminating the entire spinal column with tumor. The tumor was peeled easily from the dura and carefully removed. Both pedicles were removed at L3, as were the inferior and superior facets and the tranverse processes. Both inferior facets at L2 were also removed.

New instruments, drapes, and gowns were used, and the left iliac crest was exposed. Four bone struts (1.5 × 6.0 cm) were harvested along with additional cancellous grafts. The posterior elements from T12 to S2 were exposed. Wires were passed under the laminae of T12, L1, L2, L4, and L5 on the left. A Harrington distraction rod was fashioned to conform to the normal lumbar lordosis, inserted, and minimal distraction applied. The wires were then tightened over the rod. Laminotomies were performed at T12, L1, L2, and L5 on the right. A heavy compression rod with five hooks was inserted and maximal compression achieved. Radiographs were taken to verify the position of the anterior graft and the alignment of the spinal column. Bone struts were placed anteriorly and posteriorly to the transverse processes of L2 to L4 bilaterally (Figs. 10.10D and 10.10E). The facet joints were resected and packed with bone graft. A subcutaneous fat graft was placed over the dura. The wound was then closed in a routine fashion.

Case 9: A 39-year-old man presented with a history of multiple posterior surgical procedures to control a neurofibrosarcoma of the sacrum. A large local recurrent lesion was found.

The plain radiographs showed destruction of the upper portion of the sacrum and the posterior half of L5 (Fig. 10.11A). A CT scan showed destruction of L5 and the sacrum, along with a large, anterior, presacral soft-tissue mass (Fig. 10.11B).

The goal of the surgical procedures was to remove the tumor en bloc. This would entail removing the entire sacrum, L4, and L5. Reconstruction would require fusion of L3 to the ilium.

Entrance to the abdominal cavity was achieved through a lower midline incision. The lateral attachments of the sigmoid colon were taken down, and the rectum was freed down to the sacral promontory. A large tumor adherent to the sacrum and rectum was palpated below the sacral promontory. The midrectum was resected in anticipation of a sigmoid colostomy. The right and left internal iliac arteries and veins were mobilized, transected, and ligated.

The femoral nerve was isolated and tagged. The psoas muscles were mobilized off the spinal column, and a silastic sheet was placed posterior to them to allow identification of the anterior structures in anticipation of the posterior osteotomy. The sigmoid colostomy was then completed. The anterior wound was closed in a routine fashion.

The patient was placed in the prone position, prepared,

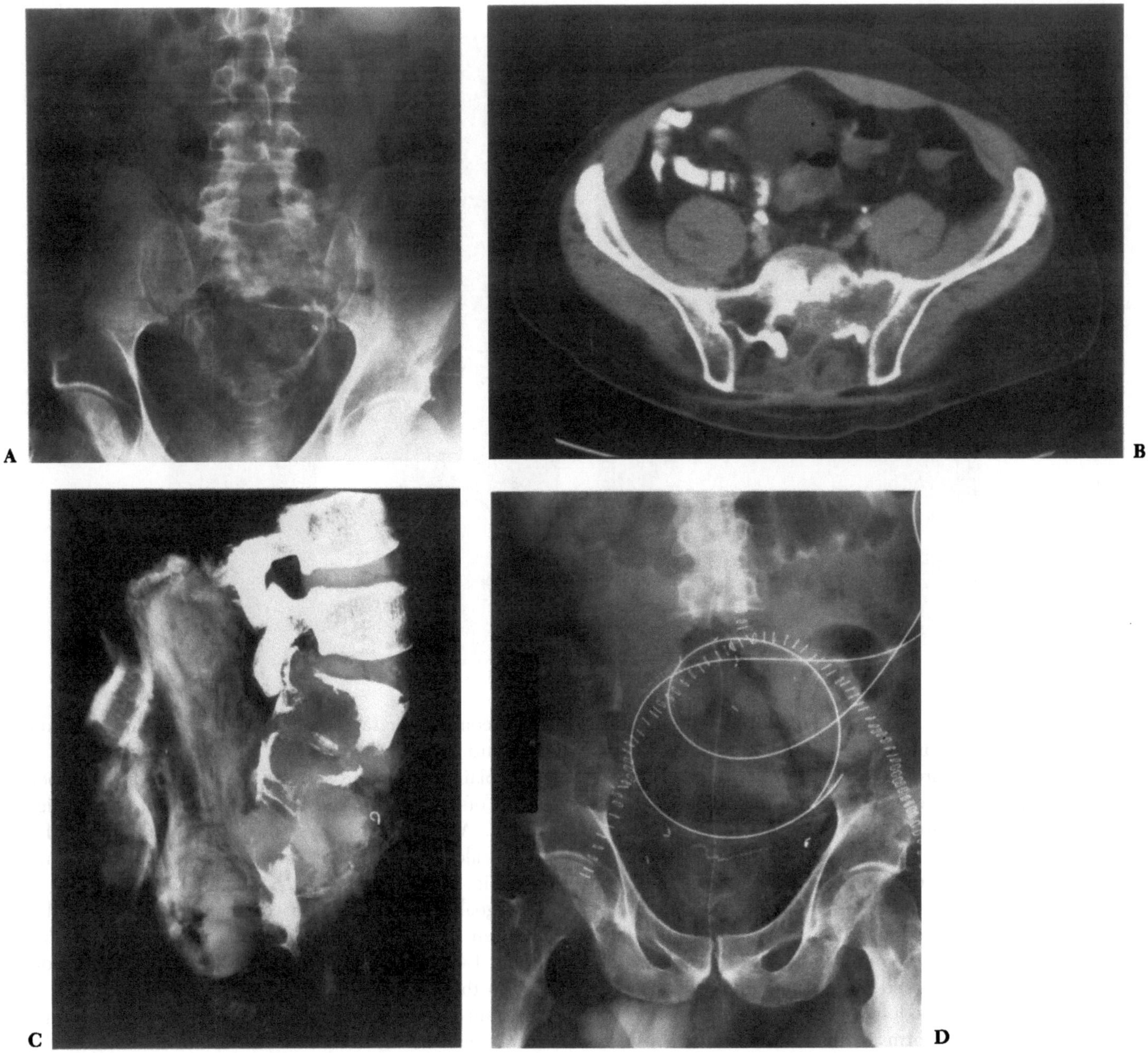

Figure 10.11. **A.** Plain film demonstrates extensive destruction of sacrum and L5. **B.** CT scan shows destruction of left sacrum. Further cuts of same scan demonstrate large anterior presacral mass. **C.** Lateral radiograph demonstrates resected specimen. Almost entire sacrum is destroyed, along with much of posterior half of L5 vertebral body. **D.** Postoperative radiographs demonstrates extent of resection. **E** and **F.** Postoperative anteroposterior and lateral radiographs demonstrate reconstruction using contoured Harrington rods and split fibular strut grafts.

and draped. The patient had a previous incision that curved across his sacrum. The area of the previous incision was excised. The incision was supplemented by a vertical limb extending to L2. Wide, distally based skin flaps were fashioned. The gluteus maximus was divided laterally to the sciatic notch. The sciatic nerve was isolated, ligated, and divided lateral to the notch. The posterior surface of the ilium was exposed lateral to the sciatic notch. The paraspinal muscles were divided just inferior to S1, and the muscle attachments to the pelvis were divided.

The lamina of L4 was removed. The nerve roots of L4 were identified bilaterally. Extensive foraminotomies were necessary to fully visualize and protect the nerve roots of L4 as they entered the femoral nerves. After

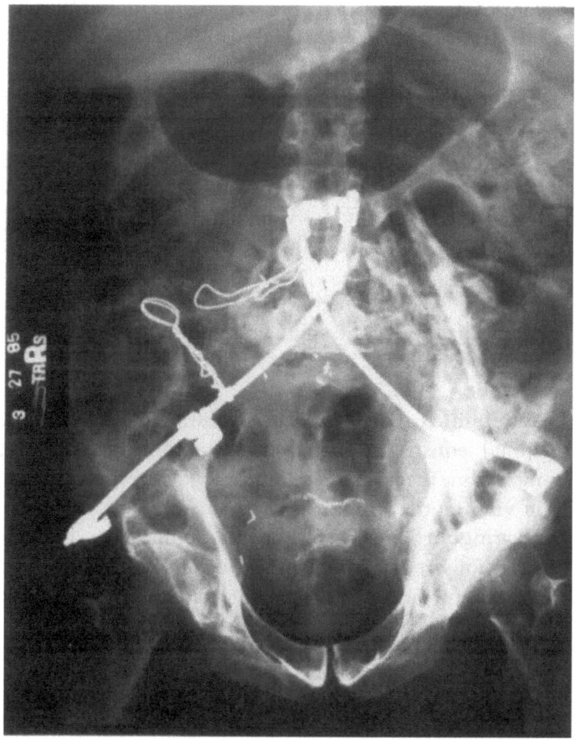

E

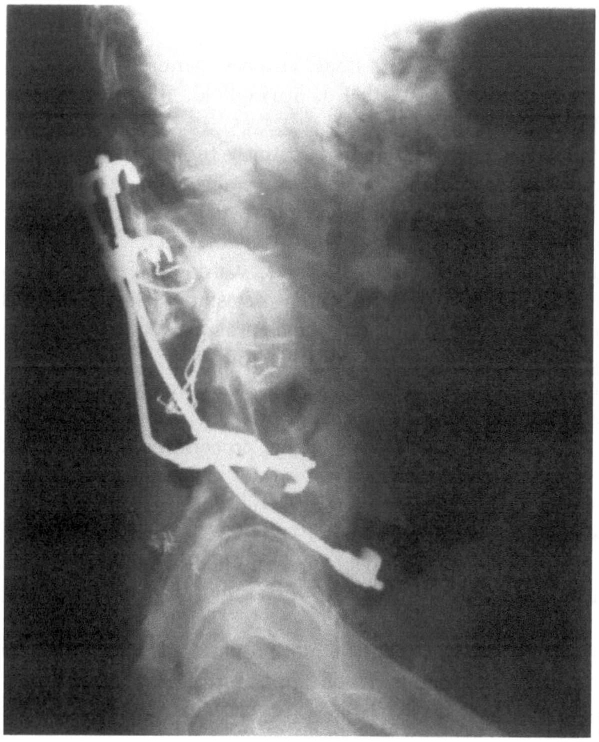

F

the foraminotomies, ligatures were placed around the dural sac below the exit of the nerve roots of L4. The ligatures were secured, and the dura was sectioned below them at the level of the L4 intervertebral disc. The intervertebral disc and the anterior longitudinal ligament were divided.

The femoral and obturator nerves had been preserved. The sacrum was then mobilized anteriorly and laterally along with the rectum and anus. The tumor was completely removed. The extent of the resection is demonstrated by a lateral radiograph of the specimen (Fig. 10.11C) and the postoperative radiograph (Fig. 10.11D). The wound was then closed in a routine fashion.

Two weeks after the anterior procedure, the posterior fusion was performed. A 15-cm segment of fibula was harvested from the left leg. The anterior defect (in the area where L4, L5, and the sacrum had been removed) was reconstructed using a panel of Vicryl mesh.

Two large, threaded Harrington rods were fashioned to clamp around the iliac wings bilaterally, crossed in the midline, and clamped to the L2 and L3 vertebrae bilaterally. The rods were simultaneously tightened. The diastasis between the iliac wings was thus reduced, and the spine was approximated to the iliac wings. The upper ends of the iliac wings were then split over an area of 5 × 3 cm, and this segment was swung medially and anteriorly over the transverse processes of L2 and L3. On the left side, it was necessary to wire the bone segments in place to maintain position. The fibula was split, and two struts were fashioned. The struts were placed from the iliac wing to the transverse process of L3 bilaterally. The remainder of the fibula was cut into small corticocancellous pieces and packed into the various contact areas between the strut grafts and the ilium and transverse processes. The grafts were augmented with bank bone. The wound was closed in a routine fashion after the skin flaps were reduced (Figs. 10.11E and 10.11F).

Summary

Although primary bone tumors of the spinal column are rare, metastatic disease and multiple myeloma are very common in the spinal column. Most patients with metastatic disease or multiple myeloma can be managed nonoperatively, while patients with primary bone tumors often require resection and fusion. In patients with a favorable prognosis, resection followed by bone grafting and rigid fixation is the preferred treatment. In patients with a poor prognosis, methylmethacrylate/metal composites may be used.

Resection and reconstructions are formidable procedures that require a team approach. Spinal cord monitoring is employed to decrease the incidence of neurological complications. Adjuvant treatment with chemotherapy or irradiation is utilized as appropriate. Preoperatively, the patient is counseled as to the goals of treatment and the difficulty of the surgical procedure.

References

1. Dahlin DC, Unni KK. Bone Tumors: general aspects and data on 8,542 cases. 4th Ed. Springfield, Illinois: Thomas, 1986:552.
2. Weinstein JN, McLain RF. Primary tumors of the spine. Spine 1987;12(9):843.
3. Harrington KD. Current concepts review: metastatic disease of the spine. J Bone Joint Surg 1986;68A:1110.
4. Barcena A, Lobato RD, Rivas JJ, Cordobes F, De Castro S, Cabrena A, Lamas E. Spinal metastatic disease: analysis of factors determining functional prognosis and the choice of treatment. Neurosurgery 1984;15:820.
5. Siegel T, Tiqva P, Siegal T (Tali). Vertebral body resection for epidural compression by malignant tumors: results of forty-seven consecutive operative procedures. J Bone Joint Surgery 1985;67A:375.
6. Batson OV: The role of the vertebral veins in metastatic processes. Ann Intern Med 1942;16:38.
7. Stener B: Total spondylectomy in chondrosarcoma arising from the seventh thoracic vertebra. J Bone Joint Surg 1971;53B:288.
8. Stener B, Johnsen OE: Complete removal of three vertebrae for giant-cell tumour. J Bone Joint Surg 1971;53B:278.
9. Clark CR, Keggi KJ, Panjabi MM. Methylmethacrylate stabilization of the cervical spine. J Bone Joint Surg 1984;66A:40.
10. Fidler MW. Pathologic fractures of the cervical spine: palliative surgical treatment. J Bone Joint Surg 1985;67B:352.
11. Fang HSY, Ong GB. Direct anterior approach to the upper cervical spine. J Bone Joint Surg 1962;44A:1588.
12. Crockard HA: The transoral approach to the base of the brain and upper cervical cord. Ann R Coll Surg Engl 1985;67:321.
13. McAfee PC, Bohlman HH, Ducker T, Eismont FJ: Failure of stabilization of the spine with methylmethacrylate: a retrospective analysis of twenty-four cases. J Bone Joint Surg 1986;68A:1145.
15. Whitehill R, Barry JC. The evolution of stability in cervical spinal constructs using either autogenous bone graft or methylmethacrylate cement: a follow-up report on a canine in vivo model. Spine 1985;10:32.
16. Harrington KD. The use of methylmethacrylate for vertebral-body replacement and anterior stabilization of pathological fracture-dislocations of the spine due to metastatic malignant disease. J Bone Joint Surg 1981;63A:36.

11

Fusion Techniques for Traumatic Injuries

Paul R. Meyer, Jr. and Howard B. Cotler

Introduction

Agreement over the most appropriate method of managing spinal column and spinal cord injuries is legitimately controversial, and opinion is strongly divided between nonoperative and operative approaches. Much of the disagreement centers on the definition of stability.[1–19a,b,c,d] Nonoperative management was popularized and in vogue when early patient retrieval was not a factor, patients arrived at spinal centers weeks after injury, postural reduction was the only alternative, and rehabilitation the primary and single remaining option.* This approach, however, resulted in prolonged hospitalization, pain, lasting spinal deformity and disability.[25–33] With the coming of operative intervention, the length of hospitalization was shortened, spinal deformities were prevented or corrected, decompression of neural tissue compromise provided for the preservation of neurological function, and early patient mobilization was possible.** It is now recognized that the analysis of the mechanism of injury, pathology, biomechanics, and pathophysiology of the spine and spinal cord provides the best opportunity for arriving at the most appropriate management scheme.

The need for the establishment of emergency medical services and trauma centers is now, in the nonpolitical environment, well recognized.[24,40–45] Acute spinal cord injury trauma units have developed within trauma centers.[46,47] Such well-designed units bring together a critical mass of patients that provides the managing staff an opportunity to maintain proficiency while developing disease management expertise, and, ultimately, the enhancement of disease-related research. Through a multidisciplinary approach to the problem of spinal trauma and spinal cord injury, the goals of managing services can be more rapidly and consistently attained. The patient becomes the beneficiary, demonstrated through an ever-decreasing injury-related morbidity[48,49] and mortality rate. This is exemplified by observing, over time (Fig. 11.1), the reduction in annual mortality from 13% in 1972 to 2.51% in 1988. Collectively, the mortality rate is 4.41% for the period 1972 through 1988 (Figs. 11.2 and 11.3).

Treatment goals include (1) the saving of life, (2) the prevention of neurological injury extension, (3) enhanced neurological recovery whenever possible, (4) restoration of spinal alignment and stability while maintaining spinal mobility wherever possible, and (5) maximizing the patient's functional, emotional, and gainful societal reinvolvement through aggressive rehabilitation.

Spinal Stability

The basic unit of spinal anatomy is the motion segment, also known as the functional spinal unit (FSU), which consists of two adjacent vertebrae, an intervening disc, the facet joints, and the connecting ligamentous structures. Spinal instability might be described as a condition in which a functional spinal unit (FSU) is unable to resist or withstand physiological forces. The result of excessive loading would be failure of the column and potential neurological injury. White and Panjabi[18] further defined clinical instability as an inability of the spine, under physiological loads, to maintain a relationship between adjacent vertebrae in such a way that there is neither damage nor subsequent irritation to either the spinal cord or its nerve roots, nor development of incapacitating pain or deformity secondary to structural deformation. Several systems for prognosticating clinical vertebral column instability have been developed* and modified (Tables 11.1–11.3). Also of bene-

* 1, 9–11, 14, 20–24.
** 17, 27, 29, 34–39.

* 4, 12, 18, 51, 52.

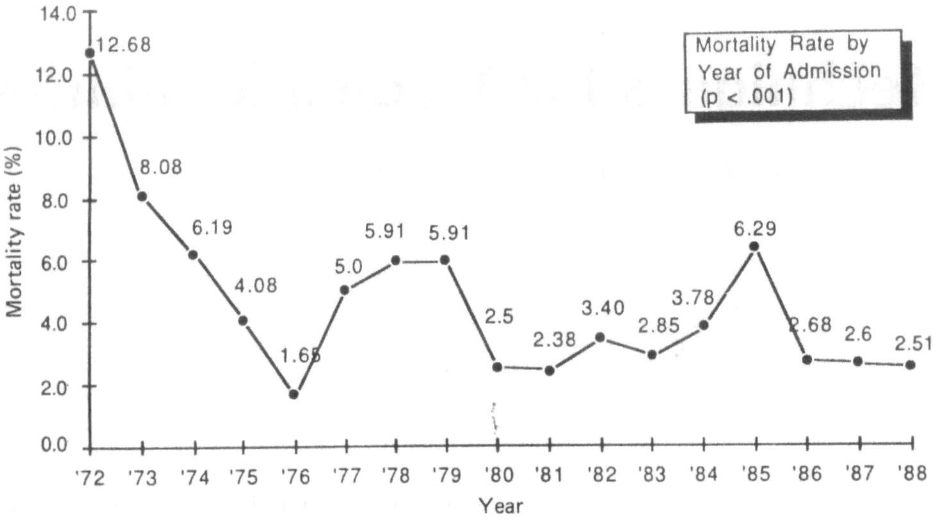

Figure 11.1. Mortality rate by year of admission, June 1972–October 1988, at Northwestern University Acute Spine Injury Center. In 1972, most patients admitted to acute spine injury service were not acute by definition; average time between injury and admission was weeks. In 1988, average time is 6.6 hours. Chart reveals gradual but consistent improvement in mortality rate, year by year, separated by unexplained (chance or reasoned) fluctuations.

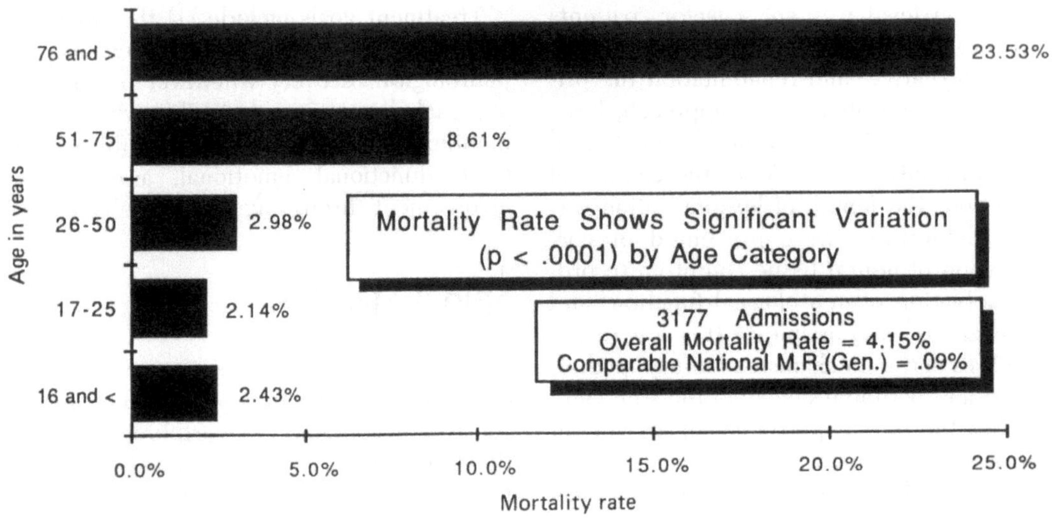

Figure 11.2. Mortality rate by age for 3177 admissions, Northwestern University Acute Spine Injury Center, June 1972–October 1988. Mortality rates vary with both severity of neurological injury (see Fig. 11.3) and age of patient at onset of spine injury. The "pediatric" population (247, 8%) is small but, as anticipated, its mortality rate is close to that seen for 17–25 age group (largest and most mobile population) and 26–50 age group (more often the employed-industrially related population). As age of patient increases above 51 years, pathology other than trauma (pulmonary, urinary, gastrointestinal) significantly influences patient morbidity and mortality. With mortality rate of 0.09% for general population above age of 15 and rate of 4.15% for spinal cord patients whose average age is 32.5, chances of dying as result of or after spinal cord injury are 28 times greater than national mortality incidence.

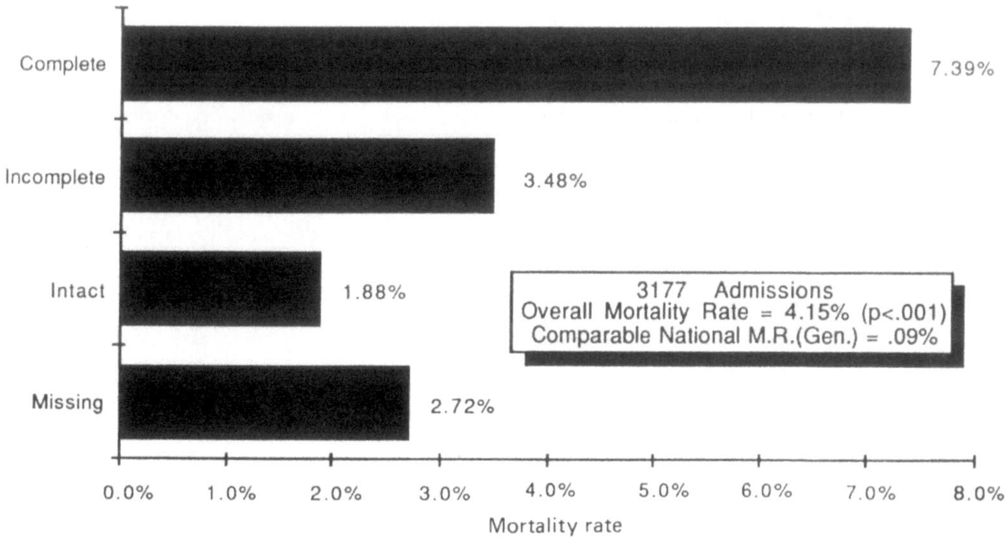

Figure 11.3. Mortality rate by extent of neurological injury at admission, Northwestern University Acute Spine Injury Center, June 1972–October 1988. Significance of the p value is validated by size of overall population and extremes found between those admitted COMPLETE and those INTACT. With mortality rate of 0.09% for general population above age of 15 years and rate of 4.15% for spinal cord patients whose average age is 32.5 years, chances of dying as result of or after spinal cord injury are 28 times greater than national mortality incidence.

Table 11.1 Clinical instability of the cervical spine.[a]

Element	Weighted Value
Anterior elements destroyed or unable to withstand axial loading	2
Posterior elements destroyed or unable to withstand flexion or axial loading	2
Relative sagittal plane translation (subluxation) >3.5 mm	2
Relative sagittal plane rotation >11°	2
Incomplete spinal cord injury	2
Nerve root injury	2
Abnormal disc narrowing	1
Total of 5 or more = ? instability	

[a] Modified from White AA, Southwick WO, Panjabi MM. Clinical instability in the lower cervical spine. A review of past and current concepts. Spine, 1:15, 1976.

Table 11.2. Clinical instability of the thoracic and thoracolumbar spine[a]

Element	Weighted Value
Anterior elements destroyed or unable to undergo axial loading	2
Posterior elements destroyed or unable to undergo axial loading	2
Unacceptable vertebral element loading	2
Compression fracture of vertebral body >25%–35%	2
Sagittal plane translation >2.5 mm	2
Disruption of costovertebral articulations	2
Spinal cord or cauda equina injury	2
Total of 5 or more = ? instability	

[a] Modified from White AA, Panjabi MM. Clinical Biomechanics of the Spine. Philadelphia: Lippincott, 1978.

Table 11.3. Suggestive evidence of lumbar spine instability[a]

Element	Weighted Value
Neural canal compromise with cauda equina (incomplete) injury	3
Abnormal displacement (translation of 25%) of sagittal or frontal plane diameter of subadjacent vertebral body	2
Anterior elements compression >25%–35% with inability to withstand axial loading	2
Burst fracture of vertebral body with inability to withstand axial loading	2
Posterior element fracture or diastasis	3
Total of 5 or more = ? instability	

[a] Modified from White AA, Panjabi MM. Clinical Biomechanics of the Spine. Philadelphia: Lippincott, 1978.

fit in diagnosing vertebral column instability is the radiological imaging of acute spinal injuries. These techniques allow the identification and analysis of deformities and pathological load conditions. When coupled with neurological involvement and assessment, these studies serve as good predictors of spinal instability.

Holdsworth[12,52] classified spinal instability on the basis of the fracture pattern observed on plain roentgenograms; simple wedge fractures, burst fractures, and extension injuries were classified as stable injuries, and dislocations, rotational fracture-dislocations, and shear fractures were classified as unstable. Kelly[53] and Whitesides[54] were of the opinion that burst fractures were unstable because of the increased frequency of associated neurological injury. Their "column" theory was a two-column model

Table 11.4. Column theory: spinal stability.

Two-Column Theory (Holdsworth)	Three-Column Theory (Denis)
Posterior bone–ligament complex Posterior laminar arch Supraspinous ligament Interspinous ligament Posterior capsule Ligamentum flavum	Posterior bone–ligament complex as in two column theory[a]
	Middle column[a] Posterior longitudinal ligament Posterior annulus fibrosis Posterior vertebral body wall
Anterior column Anterior vertebral body Anterior longitudinal ligament Anterior annulus fibrosis	Anterior column as in two-column theory[a]

[a] Disruption of any two indicates instability.

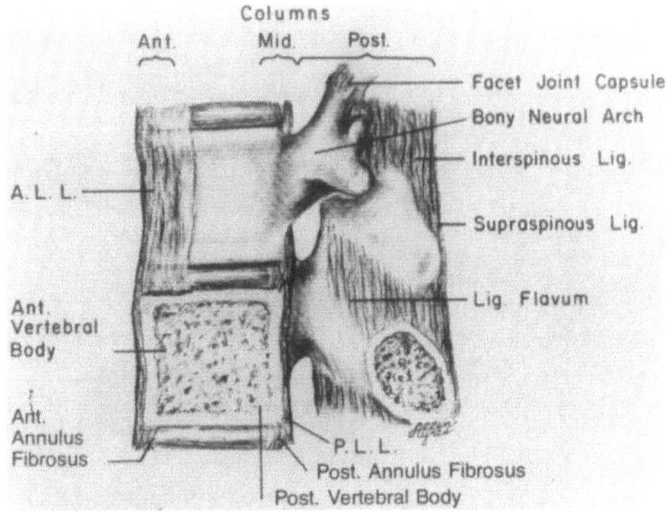

Figure 11.4. The three columns. Anterior column includes anterior longitudinal ligament (A.L.L.), anterior two-thirds of vertebral body, and disc; middle column includes posterior one-third of vertebral body, annulus fibrosis, and posterior longitudinal ligament; posterior column includes facet joint capsules, ligamentum flavum, neural arch, supraspinous ligament, interspinous ligament, and articular processes. (Reprinted with permission from McAfee PC, Yaun HA, Fredrickson BE, et al. The value of computed tomography in thoracolumbar fractures. An analysis of 100 consecutive cases and a new classification. J Bone Joint Surg 1983;65A(4):461–473.)

with an anterior weight-bearing (compression) column that was composed mainly of the vertebral bodies, and the posterior (tension-resisting) column of the neural arches.

Denis'[4,51] "three-column model" called attention to the formerly unheralded midvertebral element structures (Table 11.4). By studying computerized axial tomography (CAT) scans, McAfee[55] thought that he could substantiate the three-column principle. He was able to identify each of the following structures: (1) the anterior column, to include the anterior two-thirds of the vertebral body and disc; (2) the middle column, including the posterior one-third of the vertebral body, the annulus fibrosis, and the posterior longitudinal ligament; and (3) the posterior column, which included the remaining posterior structures (interlaminar and interspinous ligaments, facet joints, and capsules)[56] (Fig. 11.4). It is the middle column that most frequently fails with extreme axial loads. The posterior column fails with injury to the posterior ligamentous structures following excessive flexion (or tension loads), and the anterior vertebral body complex fails with compression loads. Rupture of the anterior longitudinal ligament and the anterior intervertebral disc may occur with excessive extension forces (Figs. 11.5A and 11.5B). Translational injuries are infrequent, but cause gross anatomical disruption (facet fractures and/or ligament tears). The injuries that often affect all three columns are vertebral translation (Figs. 11.6A–11.6D), subluxation, and/or frank dislocation injuries. Because the middle column rarely fails alone, the rule is: "When any two of the three vertebral columns fail, spinal column instability exists and surgical stabilization is indicated!"

Louis[57,58a] proposed an articular "orthogonal triangulation" theory based on anatomical data in which the functional spinal unit (FSU) is formed by a set of three joints located at the apex of each angle of a triangle and lying in perpendicular planes. The three joints include the (a) intervertebral disc and (b) the two zygapophyseal (facet) joints. In this theory, stability is the result of "coupling" of the osteoligamentous articular buttresses and the ligamentous brakes. For reconstruction of the columns, it becomes necessary that stability be gained through internal fixation and bone grafting until a stable montage is obtained.[58b]

An important aspect of vertebral column injury, and the presence or absence of "stability," is that there is no direct relationship between spine "stability" and the presence of "neurological injury." The rationale for this association, although infrequent, is that neurological injury may follow or be the consequence of injury, while the vertebral column fails to demonstrate any evidence of either bone or ligamentous injury.

Classification of Spinal Injuries

Multitudes of spine injury classification systems have been proposed.* Few have gained general recognition or accept-

* 4, 7, 12, 30, 52, 53, 55, 59–71a,b.

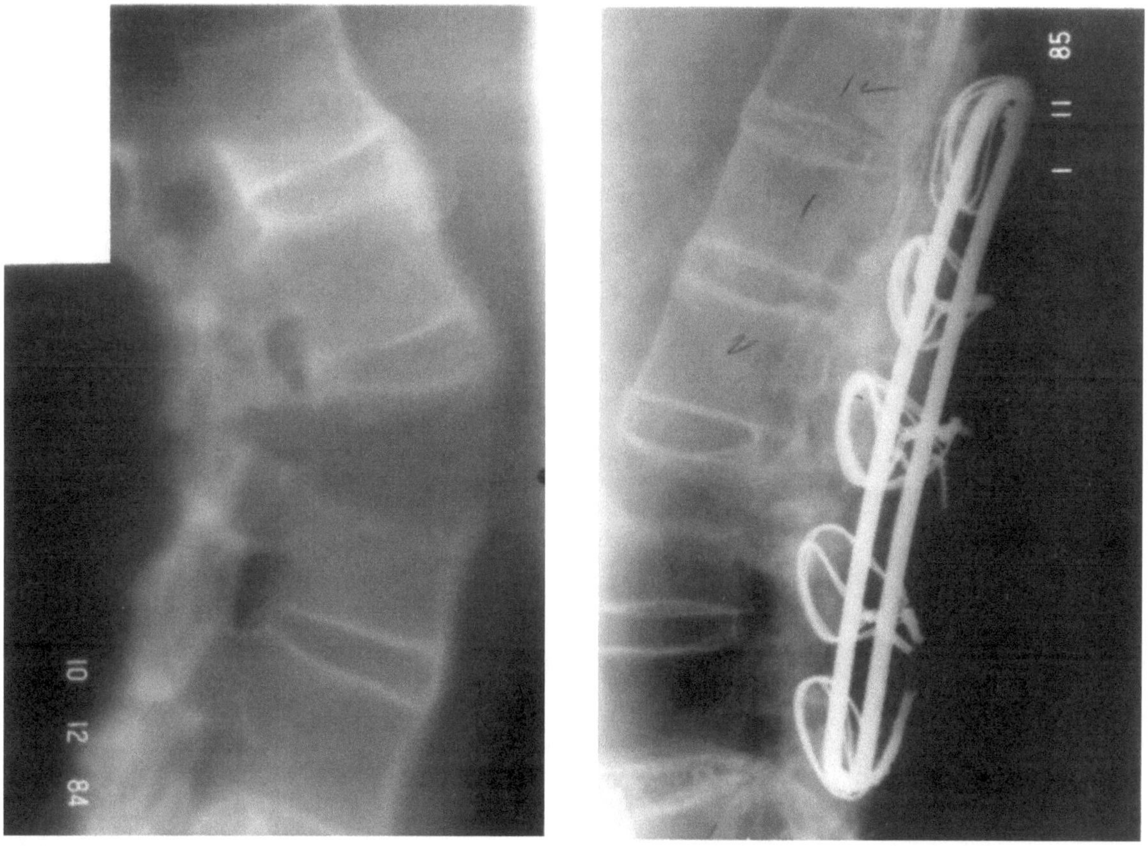

A B

Figure 11.5. **A.** Lateral radiograph of an extension injury in patient with ankylosing spondylitis. **B.** Same patient treated by Luque rod stabilization and posterolateral spine fusion.

ance because of their inability to simultaneously satisfy each of the disciplines working in the field. In general, the classification systems most appropriate for spinal trauma are those based on the biomechanical forces which, when applied to the spine, result in injury or tissue failure. These include the classification systems of Harris et al.,[65] Holdsworth,[52,12] Denis,[51,4] and Ferguson and Allen.[7] Each is based on the mechanism of injury: compressive flexion, distractive flexion, lateral flexion, translational, torsional flexion, vertical compression, and distractive extension.

The basic purpose of a uniform classification of vertebral column injuries, whether cervical or thoracolumbar, is to provide an international definition of the injury being managed, and to describe or assign an appropriate surgical/nonsurgical management scheme. Such a classification need not specifically assign a particular (or popular) surgical internal fixation apparatus.

Management of Spinal Trauma

The management of the patient with a spinal fracture often presents the clinician with a multitude of simultaneous problems requiring prioritization. Multiple trauma is frequently (43%) associated with the spinal injury may require resuscitation before treatment of the fracture (Figs. 11.7 and 11.8).

What is done in the first few hours after spinal column and/or cord injury—at the scene of the injury, during transportation to the hospital, and through management in the emergency room—is generally accepted as more important than all subsequent management efforts. Following emergency resuscitation (ABC) in the field, careful attention is directed toward the anticipation or recognition of a spine injury and its immobilization. The cervical spine is immobilized using a Philadelphia (or other hard cervical) collar, and the patient is "log rolled" onto a long spine board with the head, neck, and body secured to the board using sandbags, straps, and tape. The patient's history and mechanism of injury should be ascertained in the field to evaluate the cause of the pathology. Head injury, particularly with loss of consciousness, alcohol or drug intoxication, and associated fractures or injuries may impair the diagnosis of spinal column or even spinal cord injury. The presence of facial and scalp lacerations, abrasions, or contusions may suggest the presence of a cervical spine injury as well as its mechanism. Palpation of a posterior hematoma, a gibbus, a large gap between the spinous

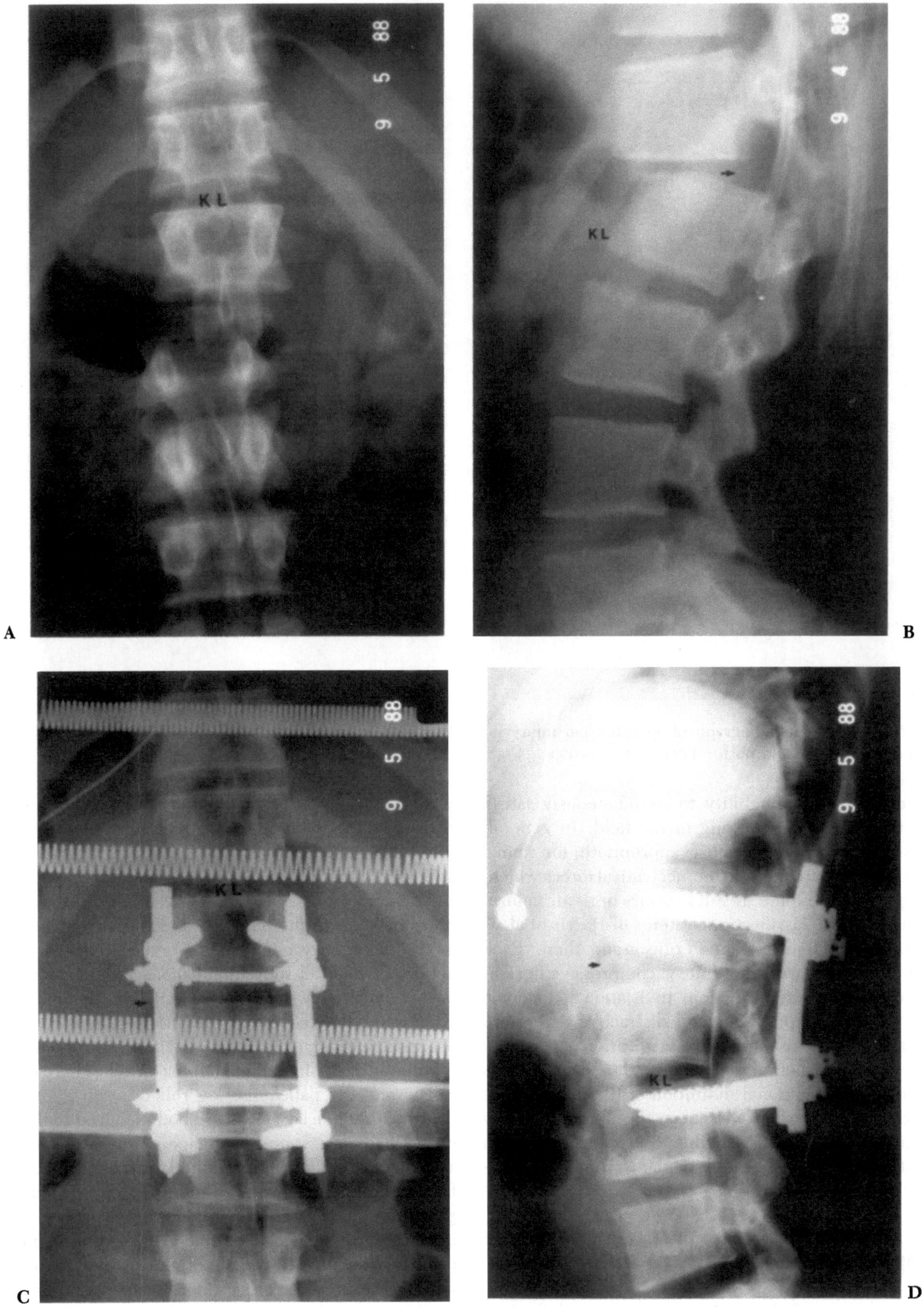

Figure 11.6. **A** and **B.** T12–L1 translational injury. **C** and **D.** Stabilization of T12–L1 translational injury using Cotrel–Dubousset instrumentation and fusion.

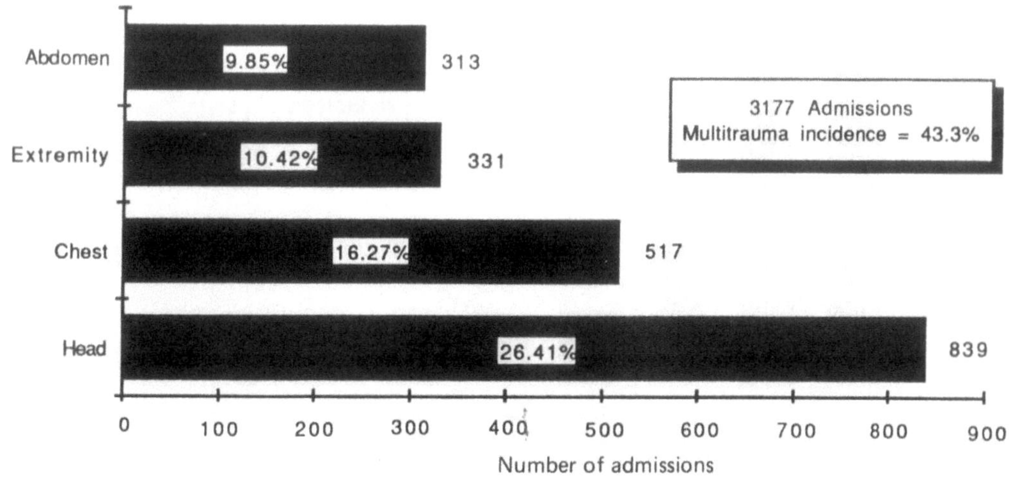

Figure 11.7. Incidence of secondary system injury at Northwestern University Acute Spine Injury Center, June 1972–October 1988. Of 3177 patients admitted to spine injury service between June 1972 and October 1988, 43.4% sustained multiple-system (other than spine or spinal cord) injury. Within that group, head injury (26% of 43%), followed by chest, extremity, and abdominal injuries, were most frequent.

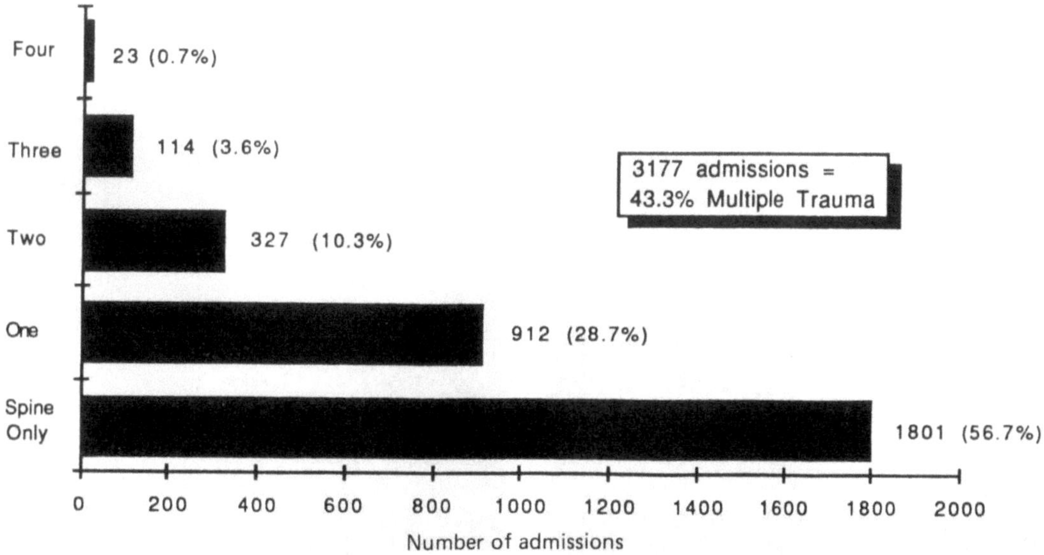

Figure 11.8. Incidence of systems injured by admissions at Northwestern University Acute Spine Injury Center, June 1972–October 1988. Of 3177 patients admitted with spine injuries, 43% were involved in multiple trauma. Largest representation were patients sustaining one system (spine) injury, followed in logical sequence by those sustaining multiple systems injuries (head, 37.1%; chest, 15.1%; extremity, 10%; abdomen, 7.5%).

processes, or malalignment of the spinous processes on physical examination may be a significant sign of vertebral column injury and instability. An accurate baseline neurological examination, including a rectal examination, must be performed as soon as possible after stabilization to determine the presence or absence of neurological involvement. If a neurological deficit is present, an attempt should be made to classify it as either a complete or incomplete neurological injury and, if incomplete, to determine whether the injury is an anterior cord, posterior cord, Brown–Sequard, central cord, or root-escape syndrome[72] (Fig. 11.9). The presence of a neurological lesion is usually indicative of a high-energy spinal column injury, and spinal instability must be suspected.

The definitive diagnosis of the type of spinal column trauma is made by radiological assessment. Biplane or anterior/posterior and lateral roentgenograms are required for accurate assessment of all areas suspected of injury.

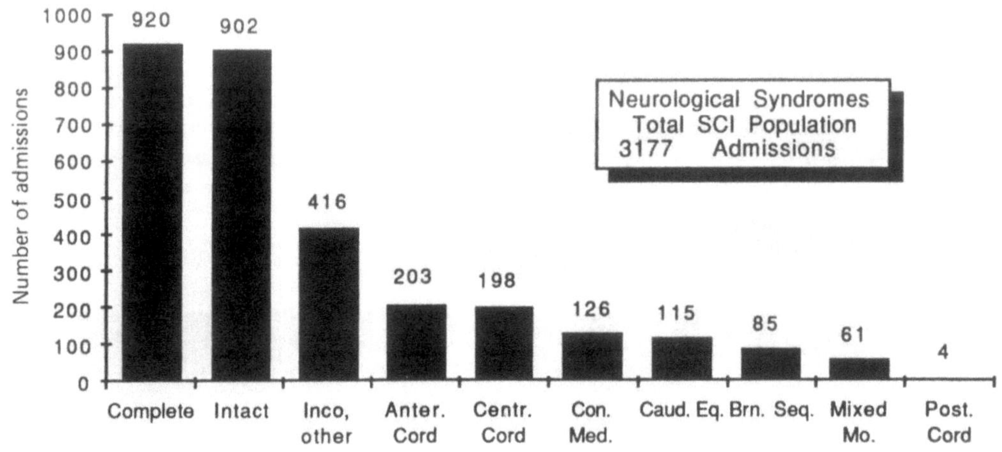

Figure 11.9. Neurological findings (injuries and syndromes) at Northwestern University Acute Spine Injury Center, June 1972–October 1988. Within general spinal cord injury population, there is significant evidence that number of intact and incomplete neurological (syndrome) patients "doubles" number admitted with complete or irreversible neurological injury. There is also very convincing evidence of improvement in number of intact and neurologically incomplete patients admitted to Acute SCI service since 1972. In that year, 76% revealed presence of complete neurological injury; in 1987, this figure had been reduced to 15%. Abbreviations: incomplete, other; anterior cord; central cord; conus medullaris; cauda equina; Brown Sequard; mixed motor; posterior cord.

A

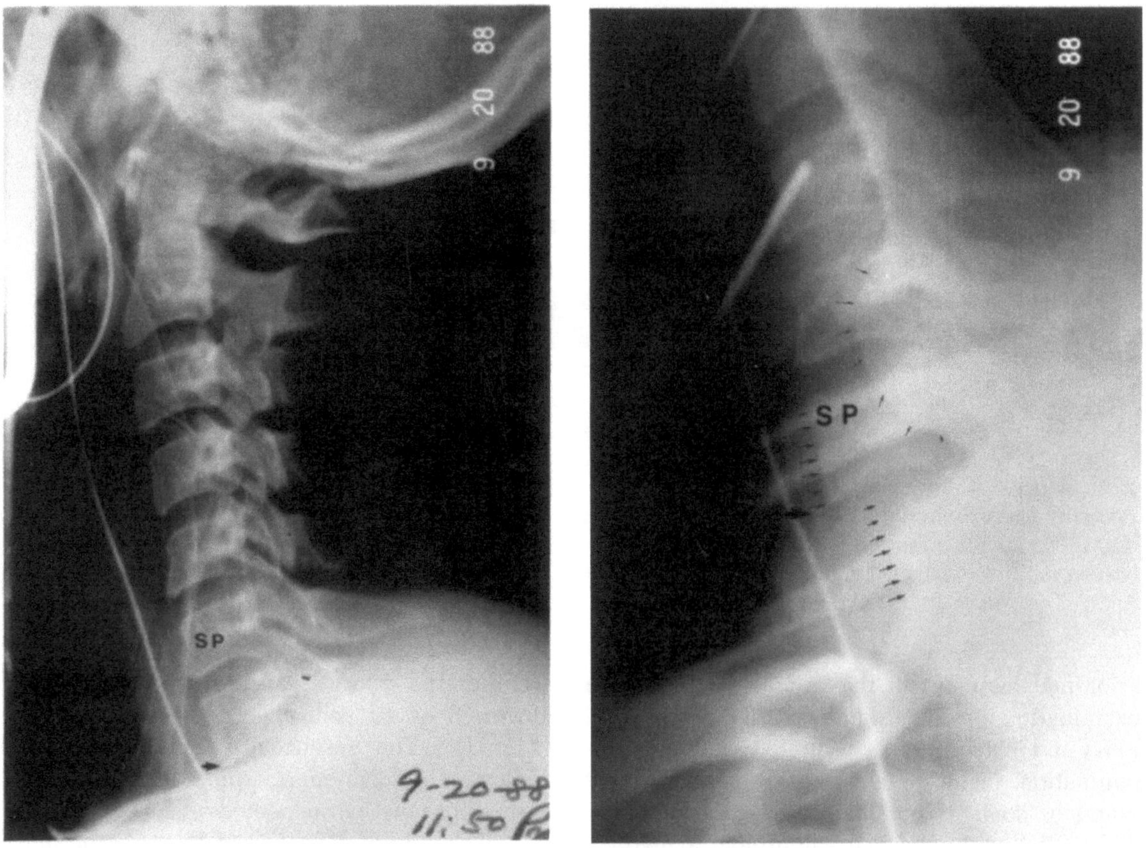

B

Figure 11.10. **A.** Lateral cervical roentgenogram. **B.** "Swimmer's" view shows C7–T1 dislocation (*arrows*). **C.** MRI displays C7–T1 dislocation and associated herniated discs. **D** and **E.** Treatment by reduction, anterior discectomy, interbody fusion, and stabilization with A-O plate (*arrow*).

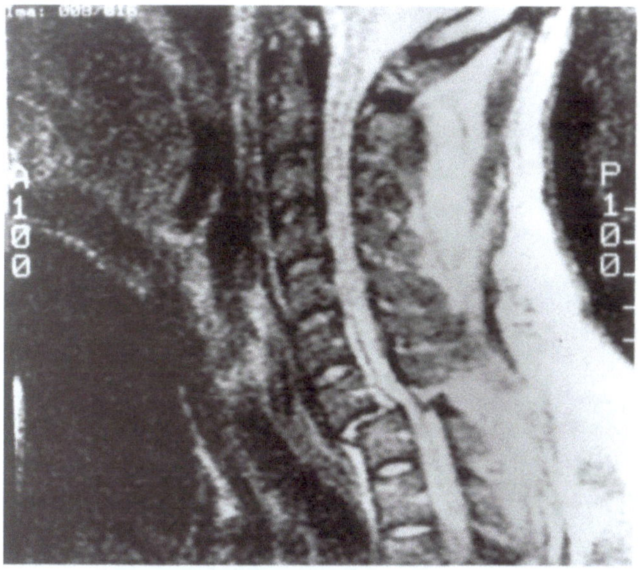

C

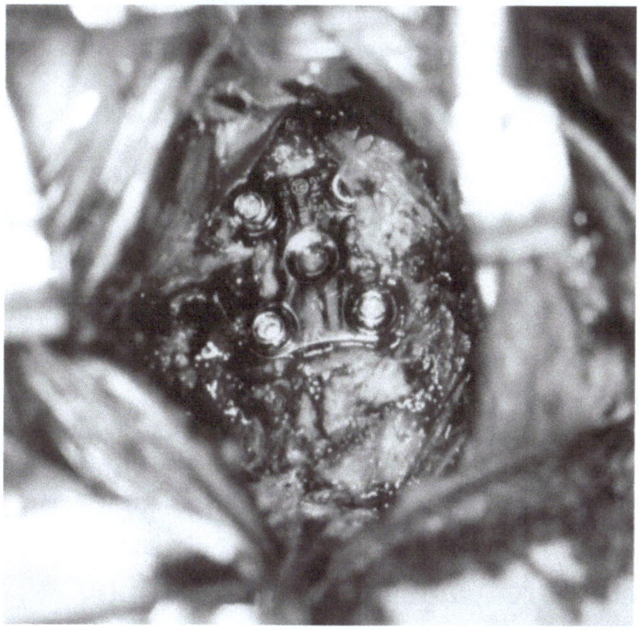

D

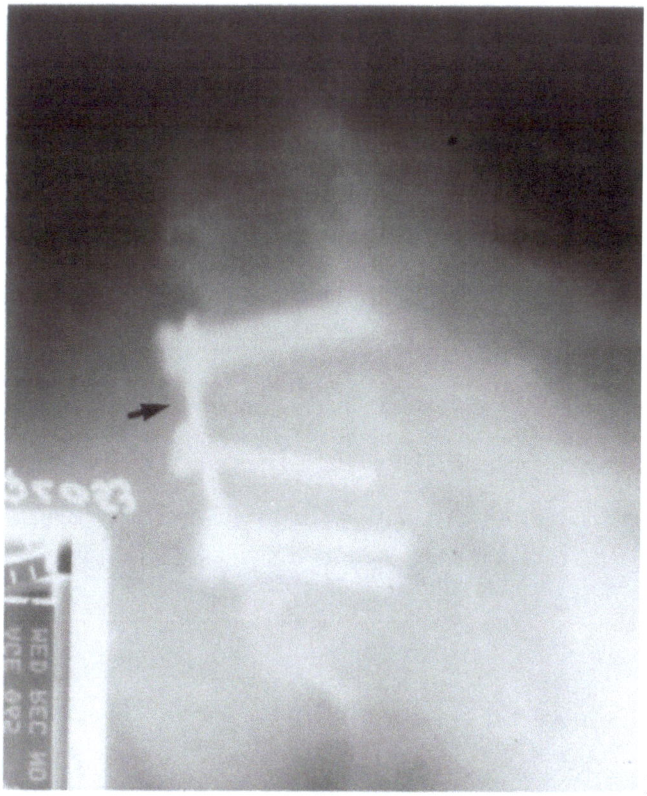

E

Figure 11.10

In the area of the cervical spine, the cross-table lateral view is the most helpful for visualization of all seven vertebrae. A lateral radiograph revealing less than seven cervical vertebrae is unacceptable (Fig. 11.10A). When one is unable to visualize all seven cervical vertebra, traction on the arms and continued immobilization of the head and neck (as with Gardner–Wells skull tongs) and/or a "swimmer's view" (Fig. 11.10B) is required. While other radiological views may be contributory, those studies found most helpful during initial assessment of a cervical spine injury include a standard anterior/posterior (AP) (Figs. 11.11A and 11.11B) and lateral roentgenogram, flexion-extension lateral tomograms (Figs. 11.12A and 11.12B), CAT scan (Fig. 11.13), and magnetic resonance imaging (MRI) (Figs. 11.10C–11.10E). The open-mouth view is an additional film always obtained with the standard AP and lateral roentgenograms of the cervical spine. Oblique views and "cone-down" views of specific areas of the spine help later, but are not included in the initial assessment phase. Flexion and extension lateral roentgenograms of the cervical spine are obtained during the initial assessment in those situations in which no obvious bony injury exists in a patient who is alert, usually intact or incomplete neurologically, and in which undue hazards of produced neurological injury do not exist. For injuries of the cervical spine at the C6, C7, T1, or T2 levels, admission lateral tomograms are extremely helpful. After the level of injury has been identified, CAT scan views of the injury site provide excellent horizontal definition of the fracture pattern, assessment of the size of the spinal canal, and evidence of bony encroachment of neural elements.

Metrizamide myelogram or metrizamide enhanced CAT scanning may be indicated in the following circumstances:

1. When there is evidence of neurological deterioration in the neurologically incomplete or intact spine-injured patient;
2. For the preoperative evaluation of the spinal canal in the incomplete patient who is undergoing a spine stabilization procedure;
3. When a vertebral column lesion does not correlate with the presence of a neurological deficit;

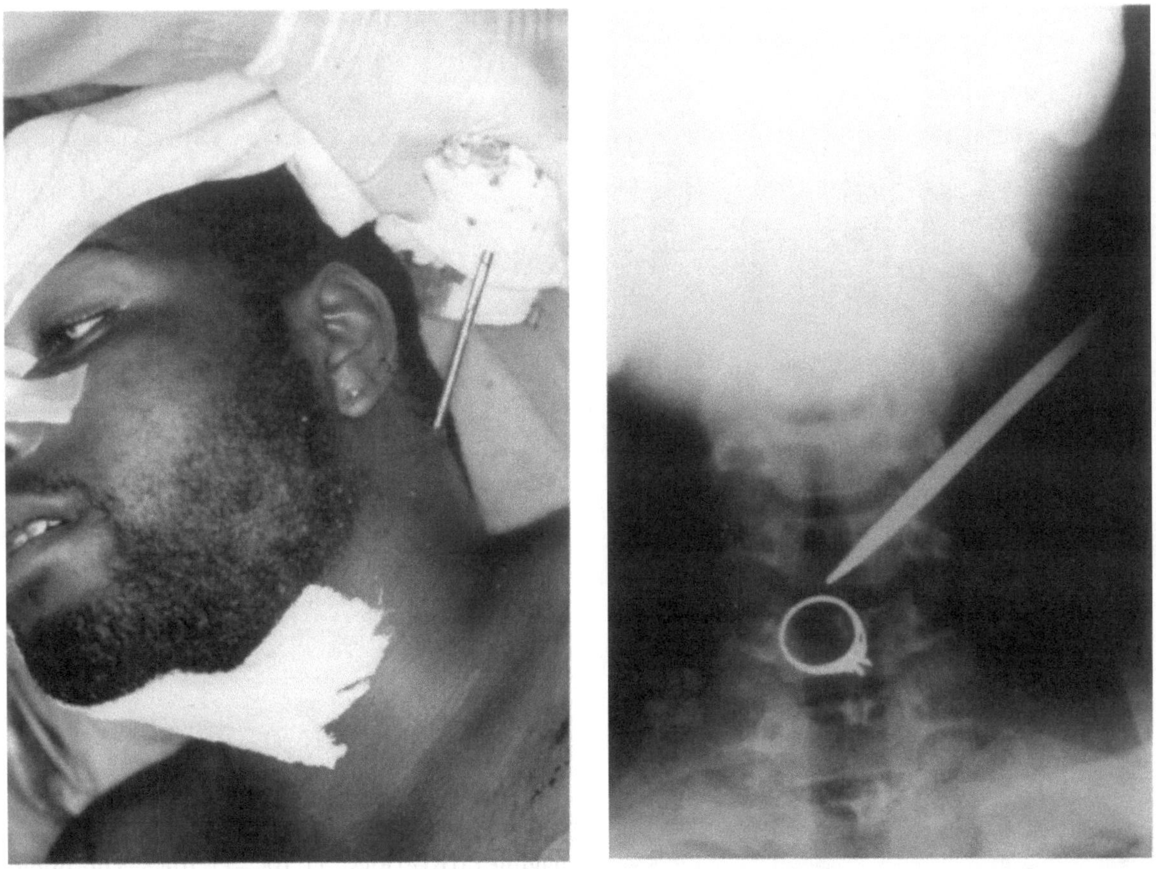

Figure 11.11. **A.** Ice-pick injury of neck. **B.** AP roentgenogram of ice-pick injury. CAT scan (not shown) demonstrated ice pick traversing spinal canal. Surgical exploration of neck, but not spinal canal, was required.

4. The somatosensory-evoked potential (SSEP) does not correlate with the neurologic deficit; and
5. The patient with a neurological injury shows evidence of recovery and plateaus early.

Some authors think that a myelogram is helpful in the patient suspected of having a dural tear; however, dural tears per se are not surgically explored except under unusual situations. For example, low-velocity gunshot wounds to the vertebral column producing a complete neurological injury can be anticipated as having sustained a dural injury, but the information derived by a myelogram will not support a decision for surgical intervention.

MRI is more frequently employed to evaluate acute spinal trauma. It provides a noninvasive opportunity to assess ligamentous, disc, spinal cord, and nerve root structures, and simultaneously may have some predictive value relative to the potential for neurological recovery.[73,74] MRI has not been found to be satisfactory for evaluation of fracture patterns of the spine. Likewise, the study has been found ineffective in those patients requiring spinal canal reassessment after the insertion of metal internal fixation devices. The procedure is difficult to obtain in those patients requiring the continuous use of life support systems and monitoring in the presence of a strong magnetic field.

Fracture Management: Philosophy

Most injuries to the vertebral column can be managed conservatively or nonoperatively. This is specifically true for fractures occurring at the level of C1 and C2 (Table 11.5). The rationale for conservative care in this area of the vertebral column is that the spinal canal is widest at this area (1.95–2.1 cm) and generally can be managed conservatively either at bed rest or immobilized in an appropriate orthosis (halo vest) for 6–12 weeks. Particularly for fractures of the odontoid, repeat follow-up radiographs are required to ensure against loss of position and evidence of instability. Should either occur, surgical stabilization may be required.

For injuries of the thoracic and lumbar spine (Table 11.5), the area of the spine most frequently managed con-

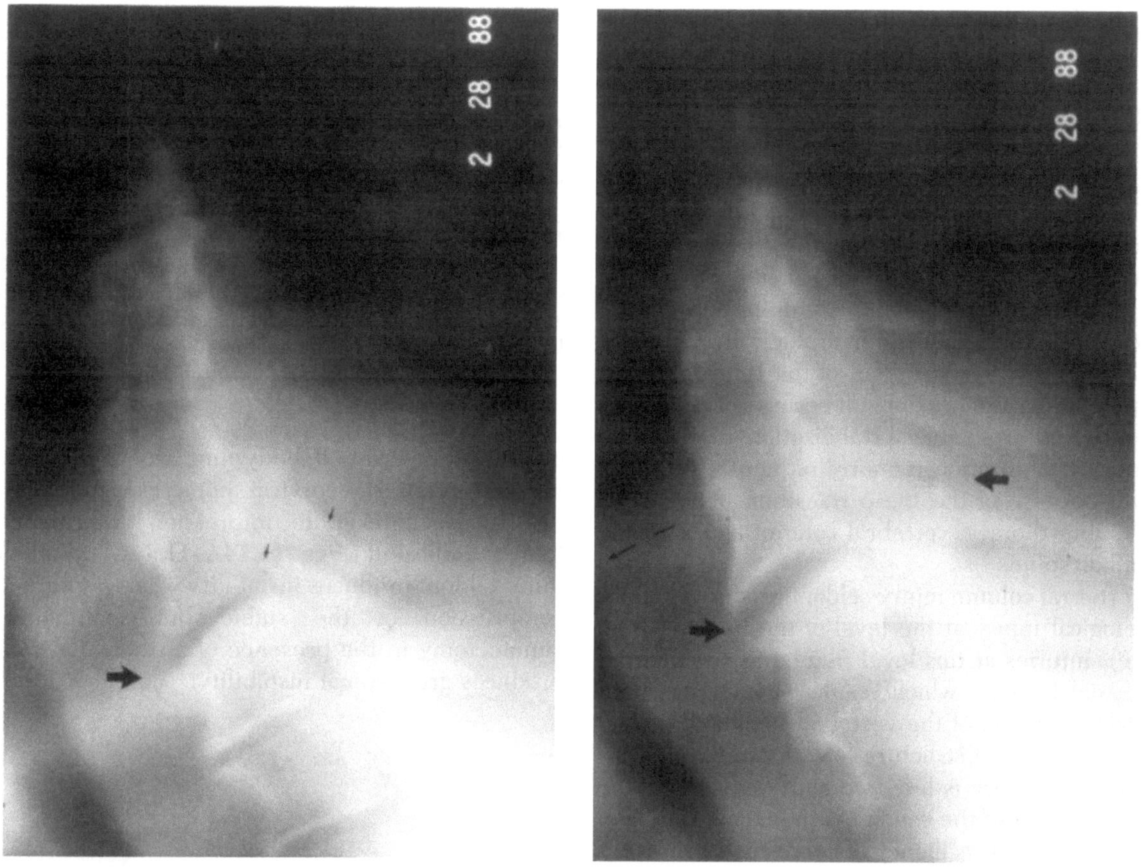

A B

Figure 11.12. Segmental instability (*arrows*) as seen on (**A**) lateral flexion and (**B**) extension tomograms.

Table 11.5 Management by level of spine injury[a]

	Surgery	Conservative	Total
Cervical	711 (43%)	951 (57%)	1662
Thoracic	143 (41%)	205 (59%)	348
Thoracolumbar	345 (67%)	170 (33%)	515
Lumbar/sacral	48 (51%)	46 (49%)	94
Total	1247 (48%)	1372 (52%)	2619

[a] The two levels of the vertebral column most amenable to conservative management are the cervical spine (C1–C3) and the thoracic spine (T1–T9). The rationale is the size of the spinal canal at the upper end of the cervical spine and the inherent stability associated with the "chest cage." The thoraco-lumbar junction (T10–L2) is the most unstable area of the vertebral column, thus most frequently in need of stabilization. In the lumbar spine (L3–L5), the fracture most often appearing is some form of compression or burst fracture. Internal fixation with fusion or conservative care can be used.

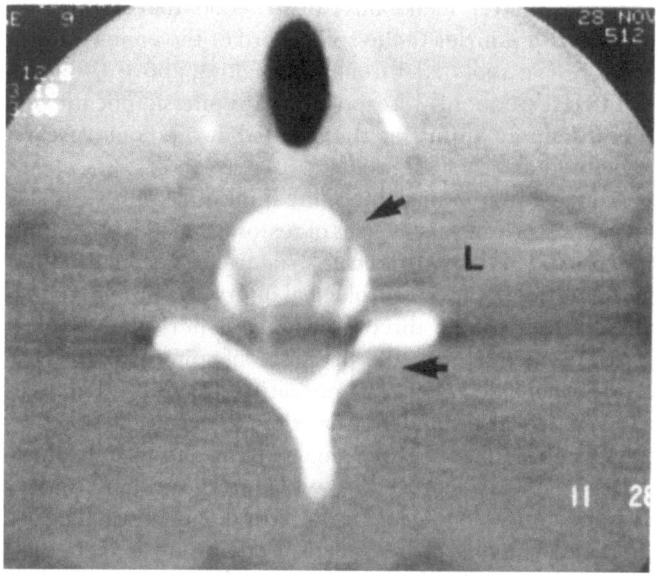

Figure 11.13. CAT scan of unstable cervical spine fracture (three-column injury).

servatively has been that between T1 and T9. The rationale for conservative care in this area in the thoracic spine is the inherent rigidity of the thoracic cage from the stability provided the vertebral column by the rib attachments bilaterally. A secondary reason for conservative care is that significant injury to the thoracic vertebral column often results in a complete neurological injury. While a surgical procedure may be required in the grossly unstable spine or one with existing neurological function in the presence of spine instability, spine stabilization per se will not be helpful in the already neurologically complete patient. Conservative management of the thoracolumbar junction spine injury is more difficult because of instability and frequently requires surgical stabilization (67%) (Table 11.5). Surgical stabilization is more frequently required at this level because of the sharp transition between an otherwise stable thoracic vertebral column and a highly mobile lumbar spine.

While vertebral column injury seldom produces significant neurological injury at the level of the lumbar spine (Table 11.6), injuries at this level frequently result from significant axial loading, which results in bursting, with significant compression of the vertebral body and reduction in the ability of that structure to withstand axial loading. Neurological injury is less frequently caused by the anatomical presence of the cauda equina below the level of L1 and the inherent resiliency of nerve roots to trauma resulting from their anatomical construction (axon sheath and axon). An additional rationale for the presence of residual neurological function with injury to the lumbar spine is that nerve roots (L1 through L4) start exiting the spinal cord at T10 and, therefore, frequently escape the gray matter (cell body) destruction that commonly occurs with injuries to the spinal cord or the conus medullaris. Nerve roots L1 through L3 exiting above the level of T12–L1 frequently escape injury despite significant vertebral column injury at the T12–L1 level. Such escape is defined as "root escape."

Management of unstable spine injuries requires consideration of the long-term goals of restoring vertebral column function. There is a delicate balance between mobility and stability. Where neurological injury is complete, spine stabilization has no direct relevance; where neurological injury is incomplete, the presence of spine instability is a major consideration. The operative procedure laminectomy, although a standard procedure in the past for decompression of injuries to the spinal column and its neurological contents, is a procedure with rare indications today. Laminectomy is indicated in patients demonstrating radiographic evidence of neurological compromise secondary to spinal stenosis of the neural canal (either cervical or lumbar) that results from spondylosis and produces enlargement of the posterior elements, hypertrophy of the ligamentum flavum, or osteophyte formation in the area of posterior vertebral body and articular facets. In the presence of anterior cervical spondylosis and acute cervical disc disease, anterior decompression rather than laminectomy is indicated (Figs. 11.14A–11.14E). While laminectomy seldom produces instability when performed for decompression of the stable but spondylitic spine, laminectomy in the presence of a traumatic spine injury produces gross spinal instability.*

Table 11.6. Neurological extent by level of injury[a]

	Complete	Incomplete	Intact	Total
Cervical	480	690	475	1645
Thoracic	213	88	44	345
Thoracolumbar	138	202	174	514
Lumbosacral	1	56	37	94
Total	832	1036	730	2598

[a] The area of the vertebral column most frequently associated with complete neurological injury after spine trauma is the thoracic (T1–T9) spine. The neurological injury rate in this area is greater than injury to the cervical spine. Because the spinal cord anatomically ends at the L1 vertebral body level, the least number of neurological injuries are found to occur in the area of the "cauda equina," L2–L5.

* 5, 12, 30, 75–77.

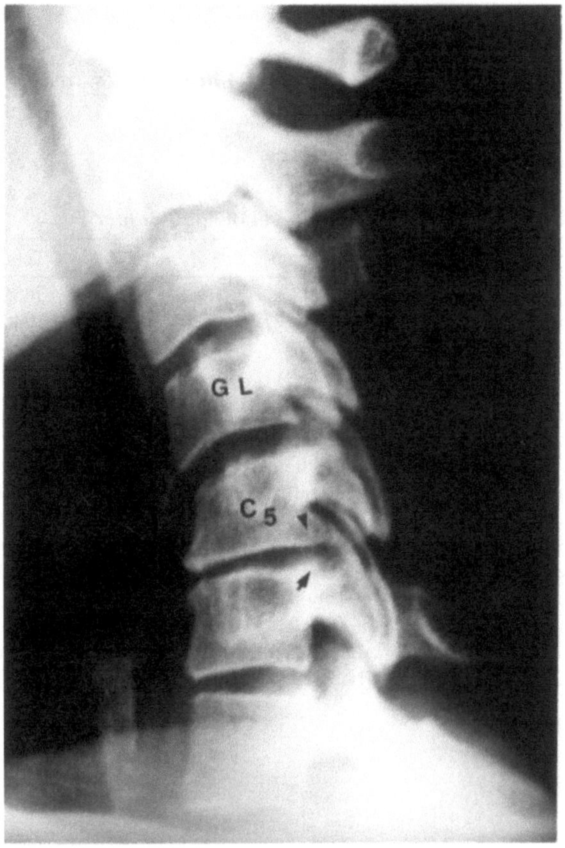

A

Figure 11.14

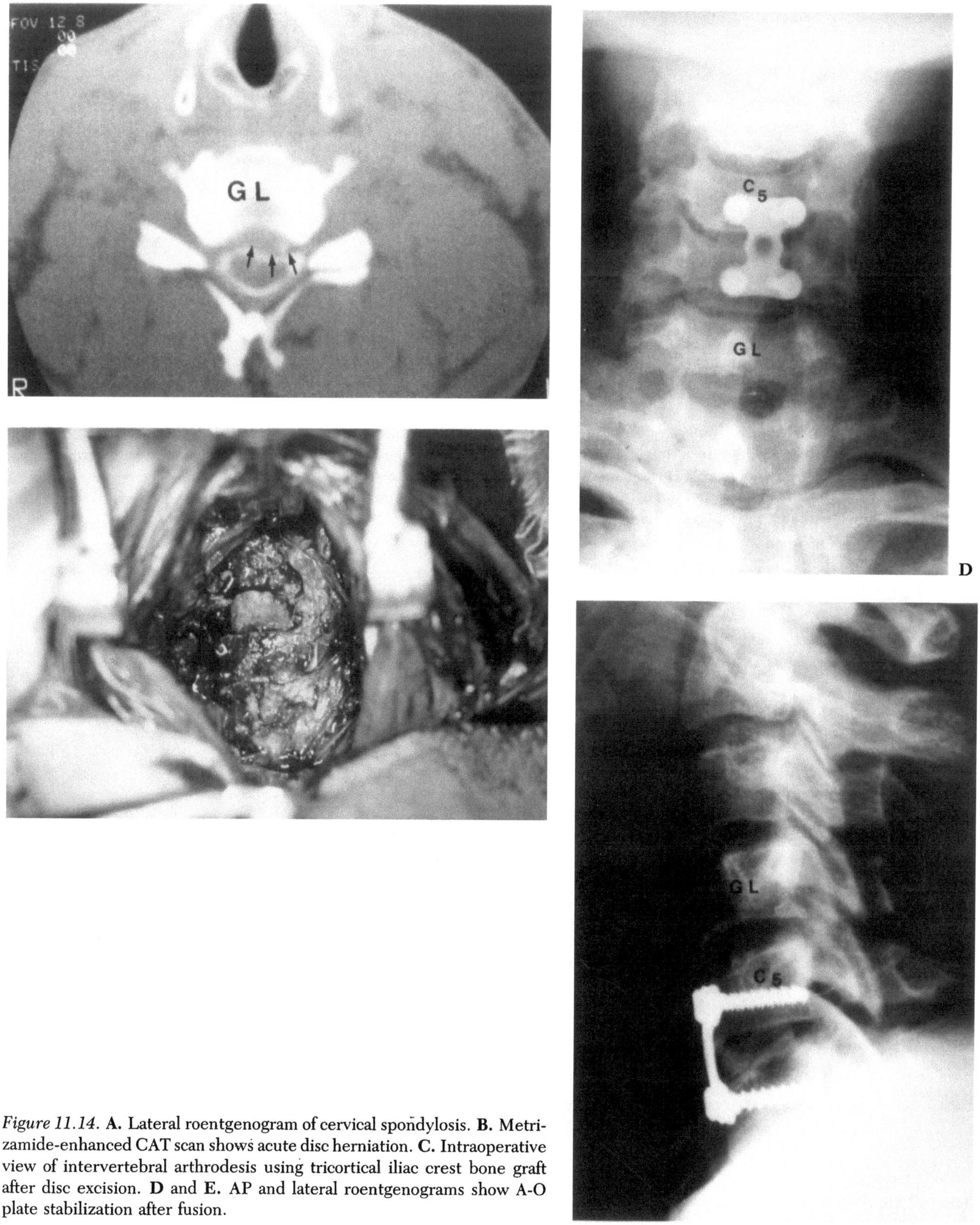

B

C

D

E

Figure 11.14. **A.** Lateral roentgenogram of cervical spondylosis. **B.** Metrizamide-enhanced CAT scan shows acute disc herniation. **C.** Intraoperative view of intervertebral arthrodesis using tricortical iliac crest bone graft after disc excision. **D** and **E.** AP and lateral roentgenograms show A-O plate stabilization after fusion.

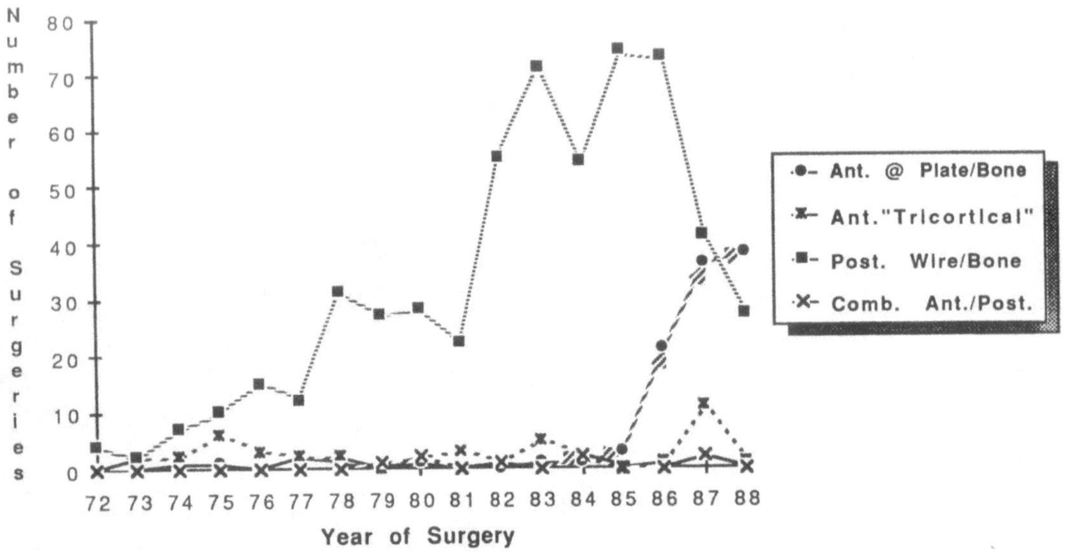

Figure 11.15. Trends in fusion and internal fixation techniques for cervical spine fractures, Northwestern University Acute Spine Injury Center, June 1972–October 1988. Customary fusion techniques used during early years included standard posterior wire bone graft fusion technique and anterior Robinson–Southwick tricortical interbody graft procedure. More recently, anterior cervical spine A-O plate and screws technique has become popularized. Latter procedure is accepted and effective method of obtaining immediate, rigid, multiple-level, cervical spine fixation.

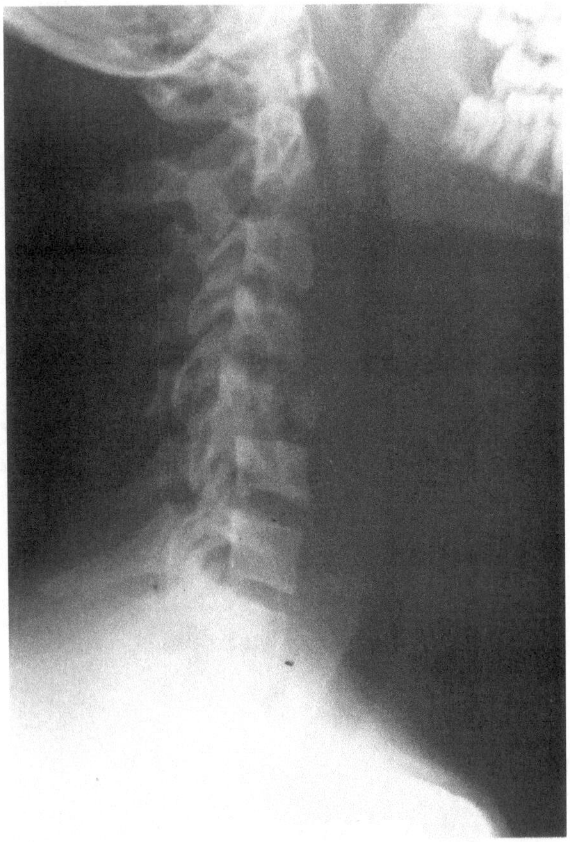
A

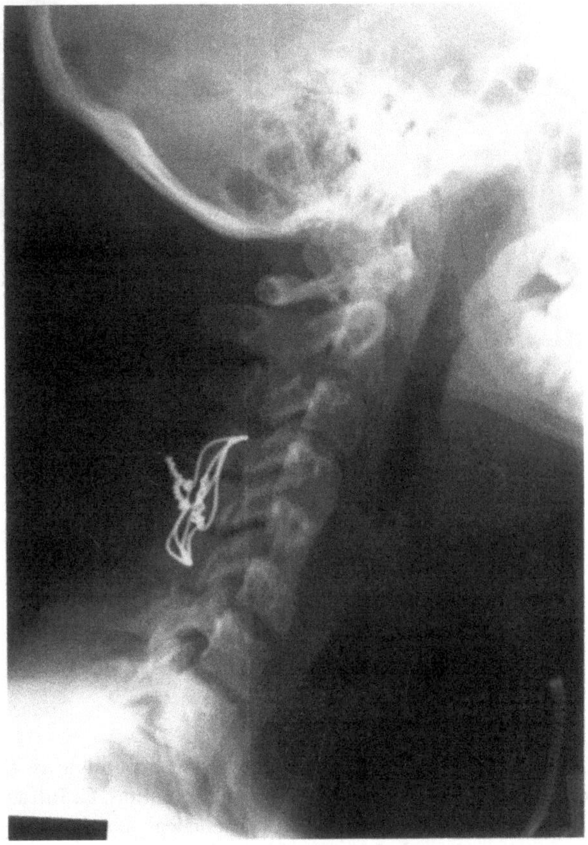
B

Figure 11.16. **A.** Lateral roentgenogram of compressive flexion injury of C5 in patient with incomplete quadriplegia. Note retrolisthesis of C5 body. **B.** Inadequate posterior stabilization required anterior C5 corpectomy and fusion for decompression and restoration of anterior column stability.

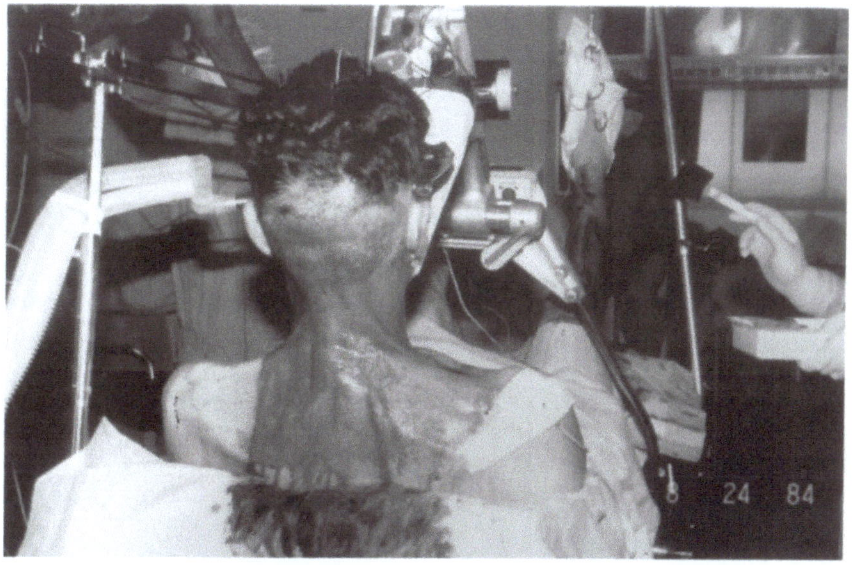

A

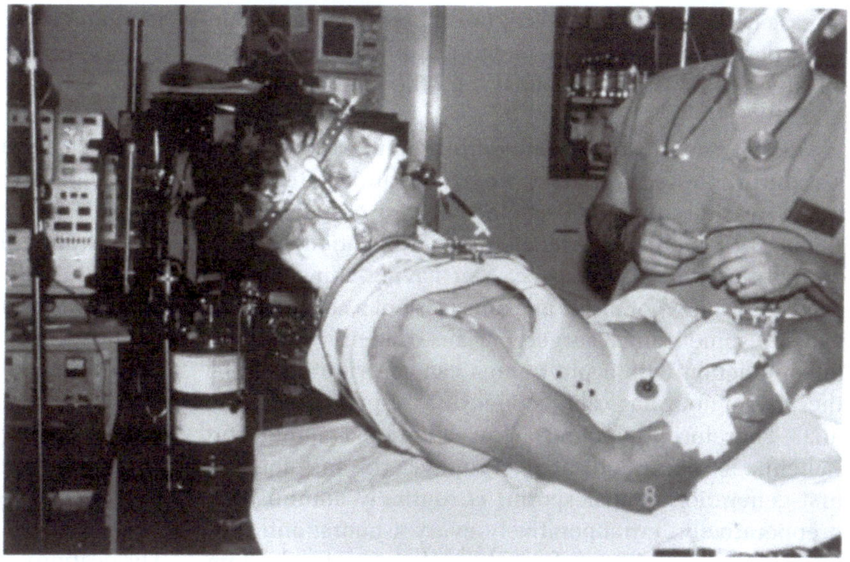

B

Figure 11.17. Patient with ankylosing spondylitis, C6–7 fracture dislocation, and no neurological deficit. **A.** Use of sitting position for posterior cervical surgery. **B.** Postoperative view of patient with deformity that mandated sitting position for surgery.

Surgical stabilization of the cervical spine was performed more frequently via the posterior approach and was reserved for those patients who had sustained flexion injuries resulting in posterior structure instability. This philosophy is changing (Fig. 11.15). While anterior decompression is the recommended approach for the neurologically incomplete patient with compromise of the neural canal anteriorly by posteriorly extruded disc or bony elements, the anterior approach can also be used for stabilization for injuries of the cervical spine resulting in gross instability from fracture of the posterior elements. This type of fracture is identified by the presence of retrolisthesis of the superior vertebra on the next inferior vertebra and is the sine qua non of a bilateral lamina injury (Fig. 11.16A). This particular cervical spine injury has been found to be insufficiently stabilized by a singular posterior procedure (Fig. 11.16B). If managed by posterior stabilization, this type of fracture requires the postoperative assistance of a halo vest for additional stabilization and support.

The patient is placed on the operating table for surgical stabilization of the spine in one of four positions. The prone position of the patient on a Stryker frame is the most utilitarian method of performing a posterior stabilization procedure on either the actue cervical or thoracolumbar spine The supine position for an anterior procedure on either the cervical or lumbar spine is best performed on a Stryker frame, although the standard operating table can be used. A lateral position is useful for those patients requiring decompression or fusion of either the thoracic or the thoracolumbar spine. Occasionally, the sitting position on the operating room table (Fig. 11.17A) is required for the cervical spine patient who has Marie Strumpel

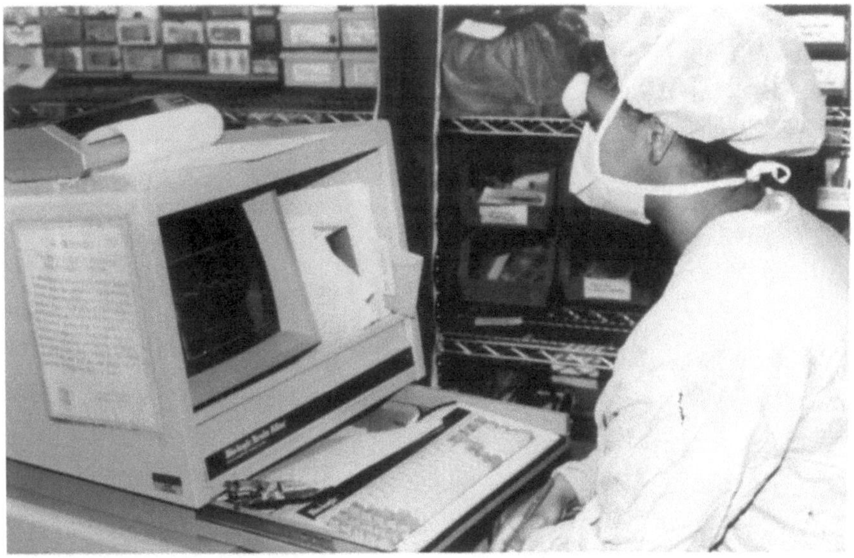

Figure 11.18. Somatosensory-evoked potentials (SSEPs) are used for all spine trauma surgeries in patients with partial or intact nervous systems.

disease (ankylosing spondylitis) or diffuse idiopathic skeletal hyperostosis caused by an acute kyphotic angular deformity of the spine secondary to the pathology (Fig. 11.17B).

The cell saver is commonly employed to capture blood lost during those procedures where the anticipated blood loss is greater than 1500 ml. SSEPs are employed as a spinal cord monitoring technique in all patients with a partially or intact nervous system having spine surgery (Fig. 11.18). Hypotensive anesthesia is not a consideration in acute spine trauma surgery because added hypotension in conjunction with acute trauma can contribute to a further loss of neurological function, due to spinal cord ischemia. Therefore, hypotension or additional spinal cord ischemia is contraindicated. Prophylactic antibiotics (a first-generation cephalosporin) is routinely administered preoperatively, intraoperatively every 4 hours, and postoperatively every 6 hours for 48 hours by parenteral administration.

Surgery on the spinal cord patient is performed emergently for one of three reasons: (1) the patient demonstrates the presence of some form of intact neurological function and evidence of progressive neurological deterioration; (2) the patient has injury to the vertebral column resulting in a fracture or dislocation that cannot be reduced closed and whose abnormal position is causing neurological tissue compromise; and (3) in open spinal injuries. While some authorities have suggested that gunshot wounds should be explored because of dural injury, the authors have found no indication for the exploration of a gunshot wound of the vertebral column by a low velocity missile unless there is perforation of the esophagus, trachea, or large bowel. More importantly, however, gunshot wounds of the neck require exploration because of potential injury to vascular structures, and gunshot wounds of the abdomen require exploration and irrigation because of the potential for bowel perforation and intraperitoneal fecal contamination.

Specific indications for elective spine surgery are frequently recommended for the injuries discussed in the remainder of this chapter.

Cervical Spine

Occipitoatlantal Dislocation

Dislocations of the occipitoatlantal level are frequently fatal. The resultant injury is usually an anterior displacement of the skull in relation to the atlas.[79] Death is the result of injury to the medulla oblongata or brain stem. Patients surviving such injuries are best managed by attempted reduction using carefully monitored skeletal traction (3 to 5 pounds). With attainment of a reduction, the patient's traction should be reduced to a minimum, and an in situ surgical stabilization from the occiput to C2 performed. Postoperative orthotic immobilization is best attained using a halo vest for 12 weeks.[18,80,81]

Surgical management of occipitoatlantal dislocations re-

Figure 11.19. Technique of occipitocervical fusion. **A.** Ridge is created on each side of external occipital protuberance using burr; hole is made in ridge. **B.** Wires are passed as illustrated. **C.** Corticocancellous graft is obtained from posterior iliac crest and horizontally divided; three holes are placed in each graft. **D.** Wires are passed through grafts. **E.** Wires are tightened to hold grafts in position. (Reprinted with permission from Wertheim SB, Bohlman HH. Occipitocervical fusion. J Bone Joint Surg 1987;69A(6):834–835.

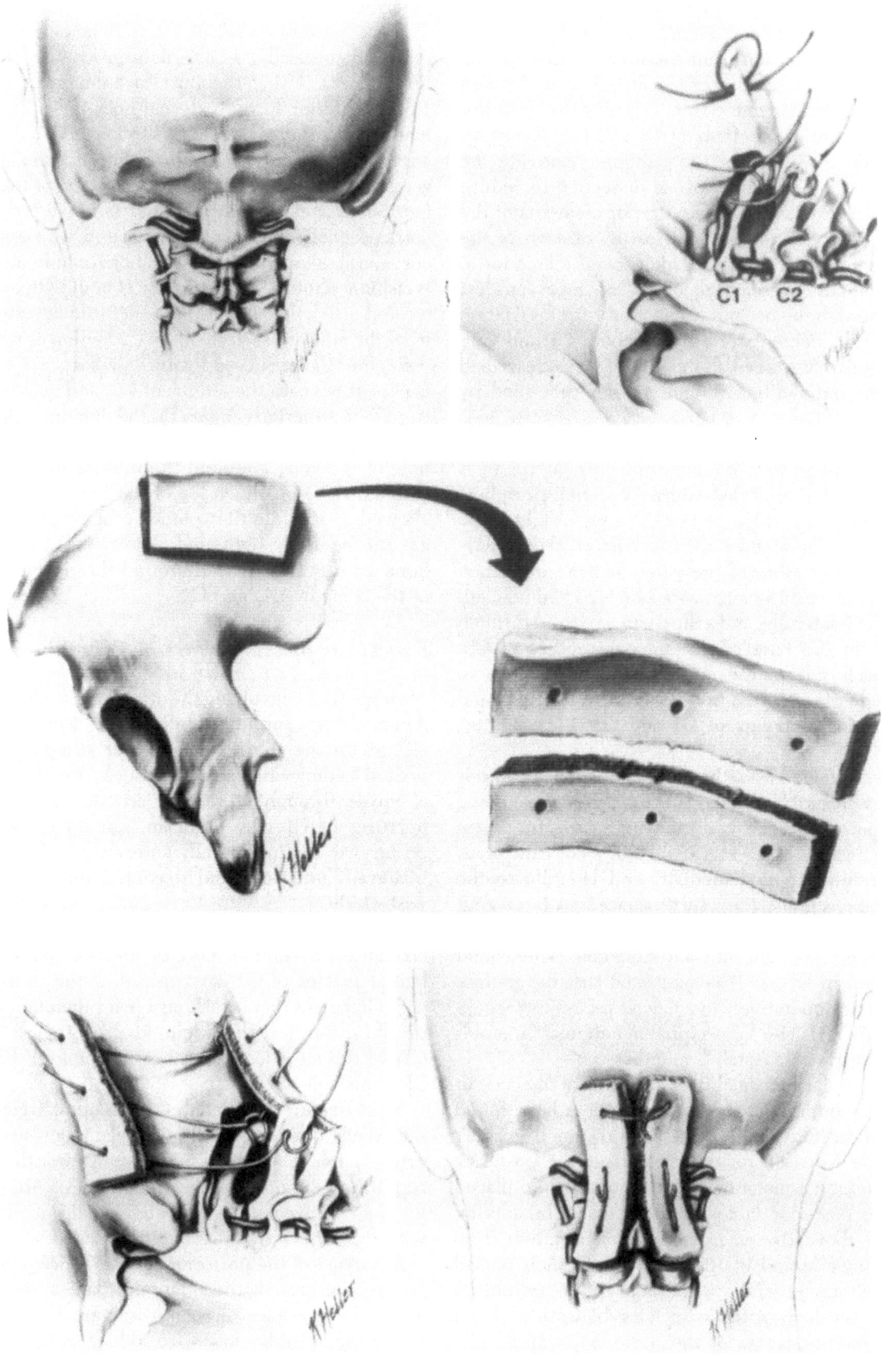

A B C D E

quires placing the patient in a prone position in traction on a wedge Stryker frame. Lateral radiographs of the cervical spine are obtained before starting the surgical fusion. A midline incision from the inion process of the occiput to the C3 spinous process is carried down through the skin to the subcutaneous tissue, exposing the posterior occiput and posterior elements of C1 and C2. Every attempt is made to remain in the midline, removing the paraspinal muscles by subperiosteal dissection to reduce bleeding. After exposure of the posterior elements of the occiput, C1 and C2, the external cortex of each of the structures is roughened using a high-speed diamond-tip burr. To facilitate the passage of an 18-gauge stainless steel wire through the occiput (to be used later for fixation to the posterior elements of either or both C1 and C2), two techniques have been found useful, one described by Weitheim and Bohlman[80] and another described by Meyer.[24]

Approximately 2 cm above the rim of the foramen magnum, using a high-speed diamond-tip burr, a trough is created on either side of the external occipital protuberance, thus making a ridge of bone. Using a right-angle high-speed burr or a towel clip, a hole is placed only through the outer table of the ridge of bone described previously. A second 18-gauge wire loop is passed beneath the arch of C1 bilaterally, and a third wire is passed through a drill hole in the base of the spinous process of C2. Thus, on each side of the midline of the spine, there are three wires to secure a bone graft to the occiput and to the posterior elements of C1 and C2 (Figs. 11.19A and 11.19B).

Bone graft obtained from the outer table of the posterior iliac wing is shaped and fixed in place after developing drill holes into the bone graft and tightening the wires bilaterally (Figs. 11.19C–11.19E). Additional cancellous bone is carefully applied medially and laterally to the corticocancellous grafts. This corticocancellous bone graft measures approximately 4 cm in length and is split longitudinally; each graft is 1 cm wide and 4 cm long. The wound is then closed in layers. It is suggested that the patient be managed postoperatively in a halo vest for 6 to 8 weeks and then a SOMI (sternal-occipital-mandibular immobilizer) for 4 to 6 weeks (total, 3 months).

If the congenital abnormality of flattening of the occiput and/or basilar impression exists, the authors have found it helpful to carefully use a high-speed diamond-tip burr with an angle Kerrison rongeur to enlarge the posterior rim of the foramen magnum. A drill hole is then placed through the posterior tables of the occiput, bilaterally, about 1 cm above the enlarged foramen magnum (Fig. 11.20). A single strand of 18-gauge wire is then passed beneath the foramen and out the hole in the occiput on either side, the loop of the wire lying beneath and just inside the inferior cortex of the posterior occiput. The remainder of the fixation procedure is as was previously described.

If the posterior ring of C1 is deficient, fractured, or removed surgically, an alternate procedure may be used (Fig. 11.21). Using the burr, a 4-cm transverse trough 1.5 cm inferior to the external occipital protuberance is made. A transverse burr hole is then made in the protuberance, through only the outer table of bone, and an 18-gauge wire is passed. The posterior part of the iliac crest is exposed and a tricortical graft is harvested; additional corticocancellous strips are harvested with a gouge. The corticocancellous bone is split horizontally and the graft is fashioned into a "hot pants" or H graft with one centrally located drill hole. Next, the ligamentum flavum is stripped from the anterior surface of the C2 lamina using a Penfield dissector. Using curved ligature passers, a #1 silk suture is passed beneath the lamina of C2, and an 18-gauge wire is pulled superiorly beneath the lamina using the silk suture. The looped wire is then passed through the central hole of the bone graft and the inferior wires are brought through the loop. Each leg of the hot pants or H graft is allowed to straddle the spinous process of C2. The wires are subsequently tightened. Additional corticocancellous bone graft is then placed around the posterior elements of the occiput, C1, and C2.

Fractures of C1 (Jefferson Fracture)

Most fractures, involving the atlas or C1 (Jefferson fracture) do not require surgical stabilization.[24] Fractures involving C1 usually are the result of either straight axial loading or axial loading with extension. Because of the transmission of forces through C1 to the articular processes of C2, fractures of C1 may occur in four areas: (a) bilaterally posteriorly, (b) ipsilaterally anteriorly and posteriorly, (c) bilaterally anteriorly, and (d) contralaterally anteriorly and posteriorly.

The only indication for fixation of the posterior ring of C1 and C2 is 7mm or more of lateral displacement of the lateral masses of C1, or rupture of the posterior transverse ligament that is responsible for maintaining the relationship between the odontoid process and the ring of C1. In this situation, the relationship of C1–C2 is considered unstable.[18]

Most fractures of C1 and C2 can be managed by Gardner–Wells traction for 4 to 6 weeks followed by a SOMI orthosis or a halo vest for 6 to 8 weeks. For those fractures requiring a surgical stabilization, a SOMI orthosis is worn for 8 to 10 weeks postoperatively, although this varies with the type of fracture being managed.

A fracture of the posterior ring of C1 frequently accompanies fractures of the odontoid. The authors have not found the presence of such a fracture to be a deterrent to the use of sublaminar wire so long as the fracture does

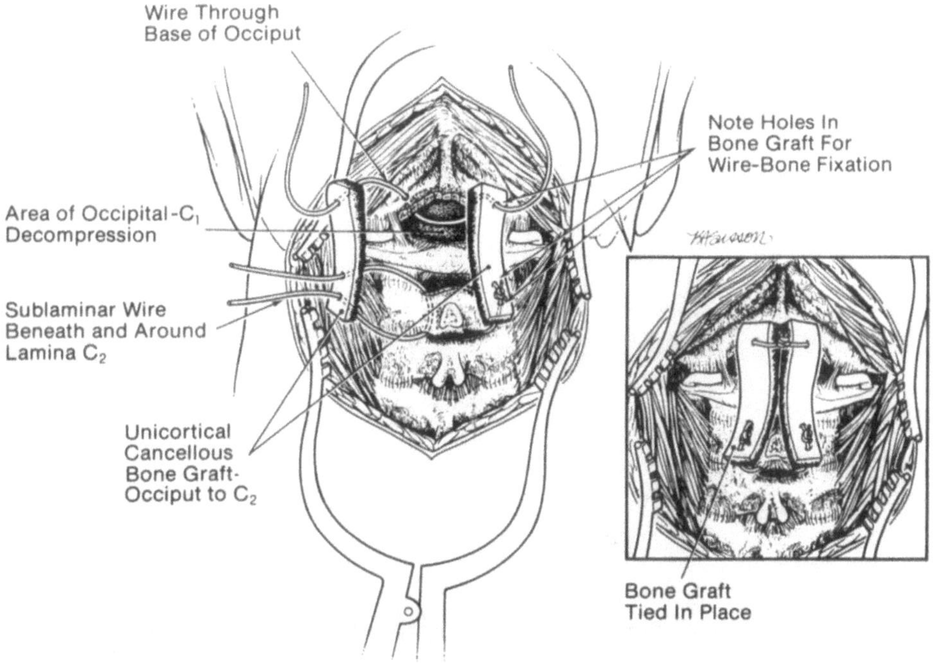

Figure 11.20. Technique of occipitocervical fusion after enlargement of foramen magnum. (Reprinted with permission from Meyer PR Jr, ed. Surgery of Spine Trauma. New York: Churchill Livingstone, 1989:489, Fig. 15–52.)

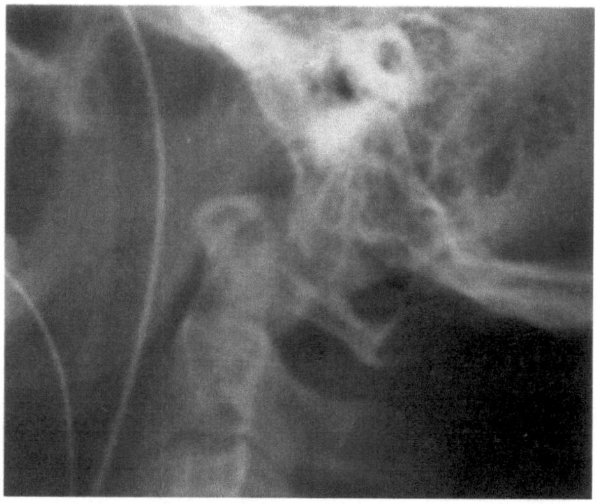

A

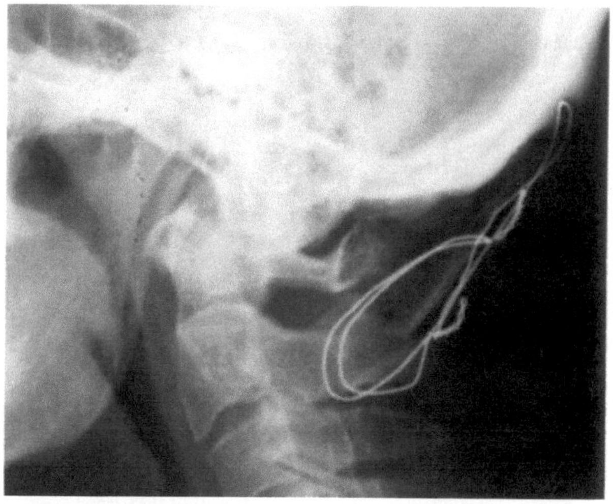

B

Figure 11.21. **A.** Posterior occipitoatlantal dislocation. **B.** Due to C1 fracture, alternate wiring technique was performed to stabilize occipitoatlantal articulation.

not occur through both sides of the posterior ring of C1. When 3 to 4 months of conservative management has failed to result in fracture union, either a C1–C2 fusion (Figs. 11.22A and 11.22B) or screw fixation of the odontoid fracture (Figs. 11.23A–11.23D) may be done. In those situations where the foramen magnum-proximal end of the odontoid process relationship poses a problem, an occiput to C2 fusion may be required.

Fractures of the Odontoid Process

Odontoid fractures are divided into three basic types.[82] Type I is a fracture through the upper third of the odontoid and probably represents an avulsion fracture of the odontoid produced by the apical and alar ligament attachments. The fracture is rare and in fact may not be a fracture at all. The defect may represent a developmental abnormality

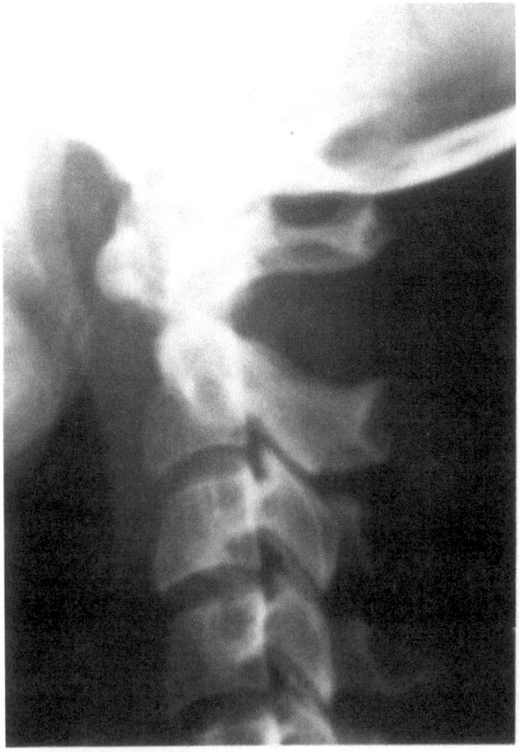

A

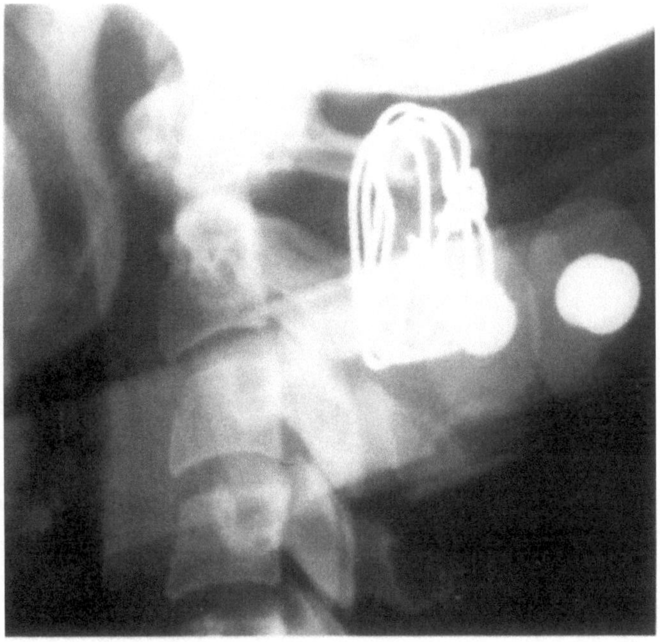

B

Figure 11.22. **A.** Nondisplaced fracture of C1 associated with rupture of transverse ligament. **B.** Posterior cervical fusion using Brooks technique was performed after continued instability was demonstrated.

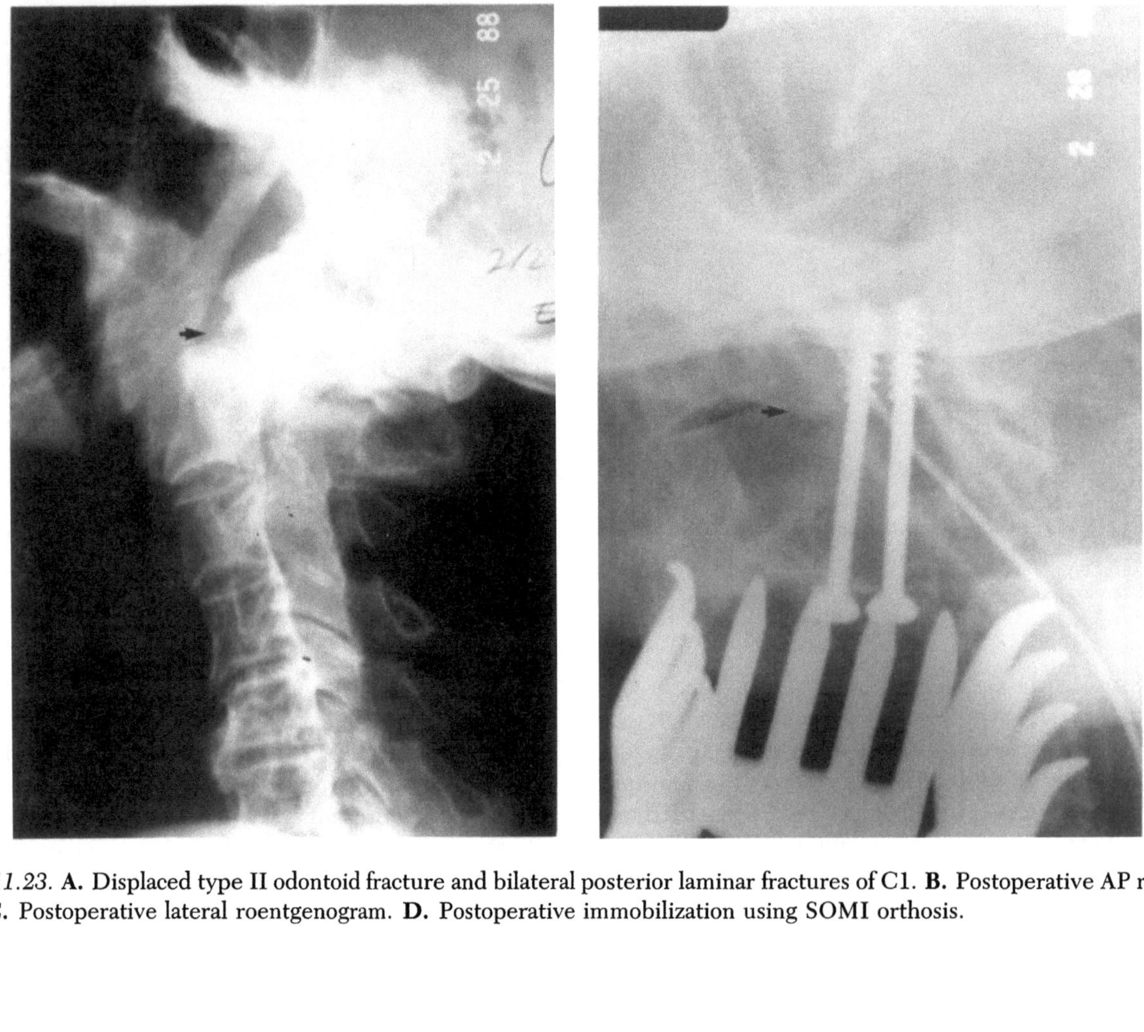

A B

Figure 11.23. **A.** Displaced type II odontoid fracture and bilateral posterior laminar fractures of C1. **B.** Postoperative AP roentgenogram. **C.** Postoperative lateral roentgenogram. **D.** Postoperative immobilization using SOMI orthosis.

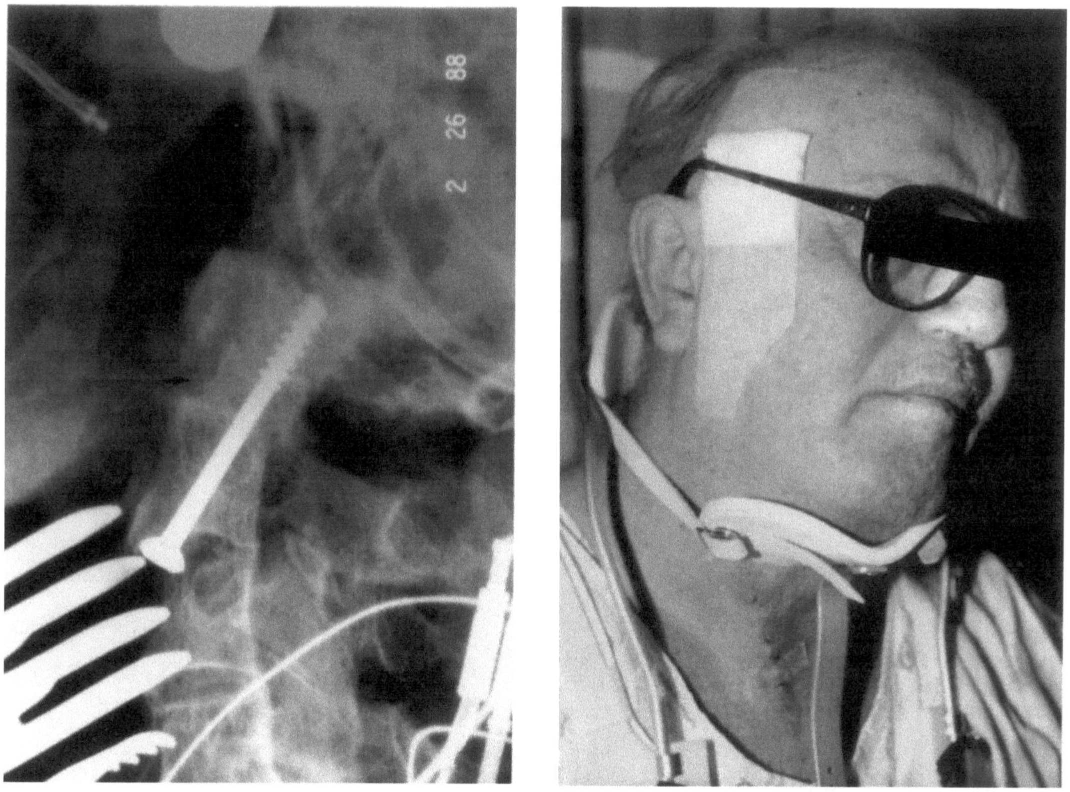

C D

Figure 11.23

arising at the junction of the primary bilateral ossification centers of the dens and the singularly present secondary ossification center at the tip.[24] A type II fracture occurs at the junction of the waist (or neck) of the odontoid or close to the body of C2 (Fig. 11.24A). A type III fracture of the odontoid is a fracture extending through or into the cancellous portion of the body of C2 (Figs. 11.25A–11.25C). This fracture frequently extends laterally into the superior facet of C2.

The nonunion rate of odontoid fractures varies between 5% and 64%.[83–85] The primary causes of this pathological process include (1) failure to gain initial fracture stability, (2) the fracture type, (3) the patient's age, and (4) the method of initial management. Because of the possibility of complications related to the presence of an odontoid fracture nonunion (i.e., spinal cord myelopathy or secondary spinal cord injury), it is important to ensure union. Type I fractures, by virtue of their nature, should be managed conservatively using some form of restrictive immobilization (halo) for 12 weeks. Nondisplaced type II fractures with good reduction can be managed by cervical traction for a period of 6 weeks followed by a SOMI orthosis or a halo vest. In those instances where fracture instability exists (identified by repeated loss of reduction, as with prone and supine positioning), posterior stabilization (between C1 and C2) is recommended (Figs. 11.24B and 11.24C). Of the three fracture types, the type II fracture is most frequently associated with nonunion. The anatomical rationale for stabilization is the attachment of the transverse ligament to the posterior dens (or odontoid process), which in turn is attached to the foramen magnum, and the remainder of C2 articulation with C3 and the lower cervical spine. Other indications for the operative management of type II fractures include older patients, patients with significant neurological injury and on ventilators, or those with fractures that demonstrate nonunion at 3 months. Type III fractures in the pediatric patient (less than 2 years old) generally represent an epiphyseal injury. This epiphyseal line does not completely close until early in the second decade and therefore can be managed conservatively. Type III fractures in the adult, if induced by flexion, result in involvement of the anterior aspect of the body of C2 and can be managed in extension in traction for 6 weeks followed by a light orthosis or a halo vest. Extension injuries, on the other hand, initially should be managed conservatively; but by virtue of their instability in extension frequently require surgical stabilization. Otherwise, they too are managed initially in traction (4 to 6 weeks), followed by either a halo or SOMI orthosis.

Numerous operative procedures are suggested for the stabilization of the C1–C2 complex. These include the

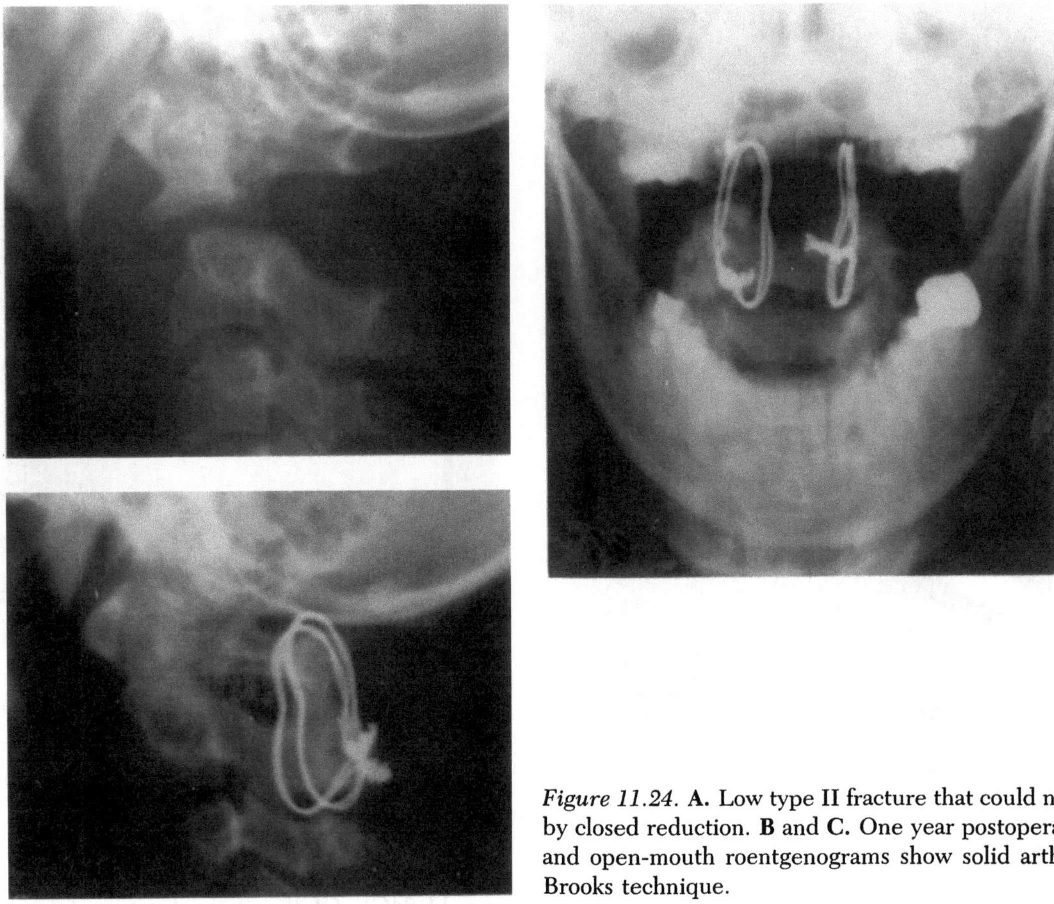

A

B

C

Figure 11.24. **A.** Low type II fracture that could not be reduced by closed reduction. **B** and **C.** One year postoperatively, lateral and open-mouth roentgenograms show solid arthrodesis using Brooks technique.

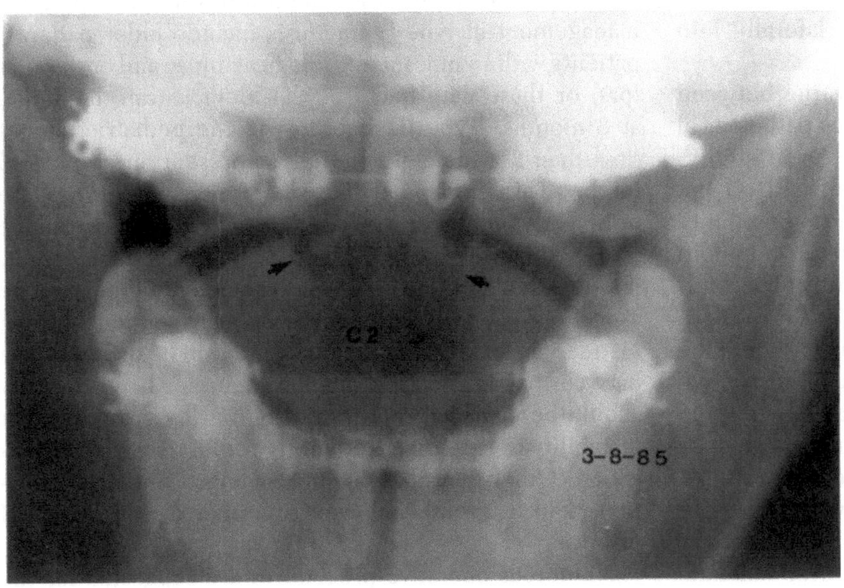

A

Figure 11.25. Type III odontoid fracture. **A.** Open-mouth view. **B.** Lateral roentgenogram. Note additional fractures (*arrows*). **C.** CAT scan shows fracture extending laterally into superior facets of C2.

B 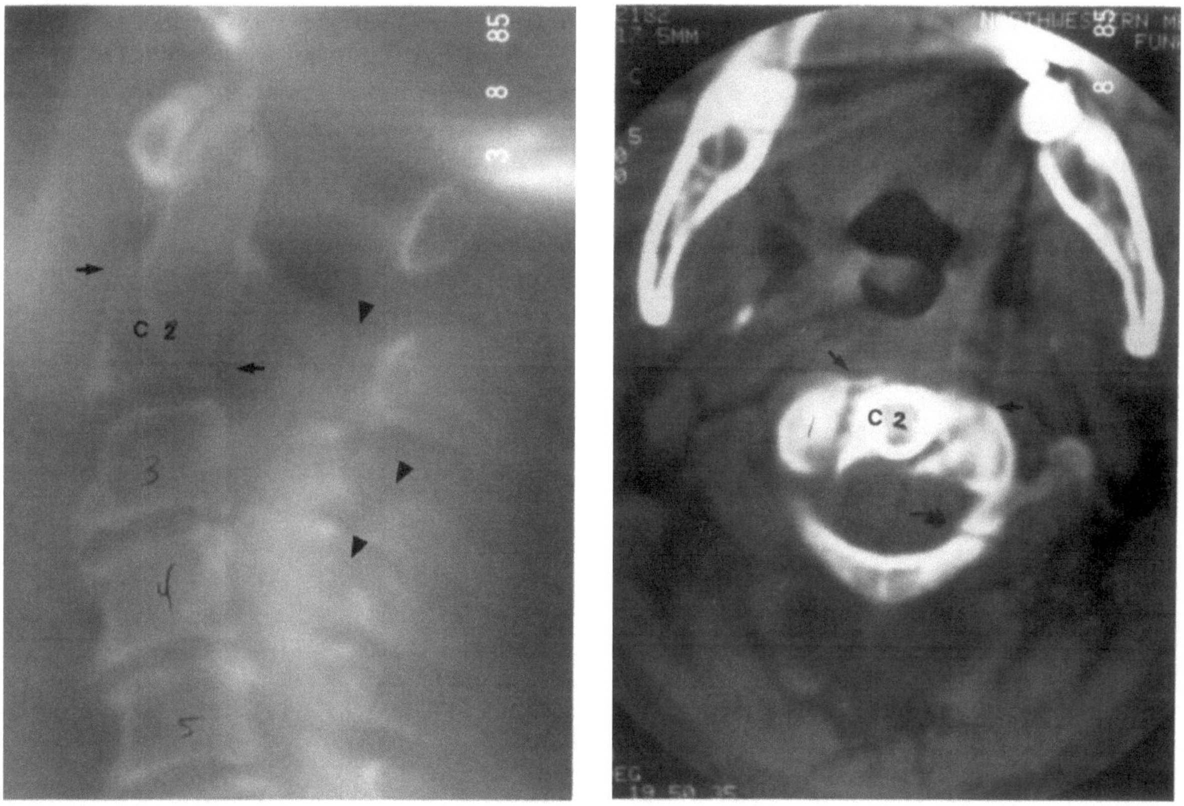 C

Figure 11.25

Gallie procedure,[86] the modified Gallie procedure[24] (Fig. 11.26), the Fielding modification,[87] the Brooks[88] (Figs. 11.27A–11.27E), the modified Brooks,[89] the bone block,[90] and the posterior procedure suggested by Meyer.[24] Each technique varies slightly but all are directed toward the establishment of stability of the C1–C2 complex. Some variation of the modified Brooks procedure is most often used.

The patient is placed in a prone position on the wedge Stryker frame with the cervical spine maintained in longitudinal Gardner–Wells tong traction. With the patient prone on the frame, careful attention is paid to the position of the odontoid fracture by obtaining a preoperative lateral radiograph of the upper cervical spine. It is appropriate to monitor the patient's neurological function using the SSEP unit. A posterior midline incision is carried down through the skin and subcutaneous tissue extending from the inion process (external occipital protuberance) to the level of the posterior spinous process of C3 (7 cm). Careful attention is directed toward the midline posterior subperiosteal dissection and exposure of the C1 and C2 laminae. At the level of C1 lamina, the use of subperiosteal dissection from midline to lateral prevents the surgeon from inadvertently encountering the vertebral artery as it passes over and around the superior lateral surface of the posterior ring of C1. By sharp dissection, if it is not already torn, an incision of the ligamentum flavum between C1 and the occiput and C1 and C2 is carried out. Using a curved ligature holder (aneurysm needle), a #1 dermalon suture is passed beneath the posterior element of C1 and C2 in a staggered manner.[24] This is followed by the tying of the ligature as it exists beneath posterior element C2 onto an appropriately fashioned strand of 18-gauge wire. This wire is then pulled proximally under the posterior elements of C2 and C1. This technique is performed bilaterally, or simultaneously, if the strand of wire being pulled through is a loop of wire. Having pulled the loop through, it is cut in two at its proximal end and careful attention is directed toward keeping the wire separated so as not to cross beneath the laminae. Shaping the bone graft obtained from the iliac crest into two rectangular corticocancellous grafts measuring approximately 1 by 2.5 cm in length, a hole is placed at each end of the graft so that the end of the wire exiting between the occiput and C1, and the other end between C2 and C3, can be passed through the bone graft cancellous side down. This procedure is performed bilaterally simultaneously and the wires are twisted and tightened simultaneously.

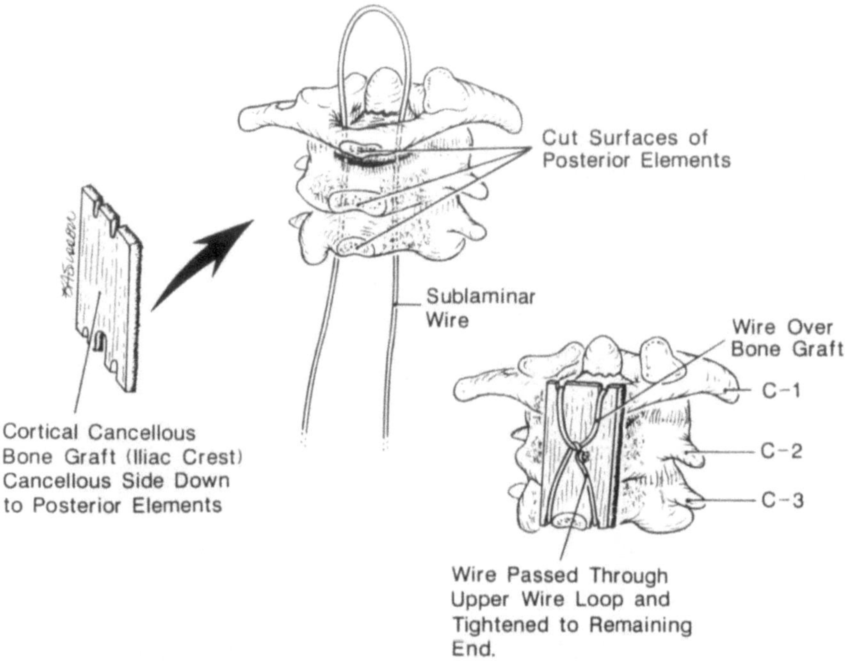

Figure 11.26. Modified Gallie fusion technique for three-level stabilization. (Reprinted with permission from Meyer PR Jr, ed. Surgery of Spine Trauma. New York: Churchill Livingstone, 1989:497, Fig. 15–58.)

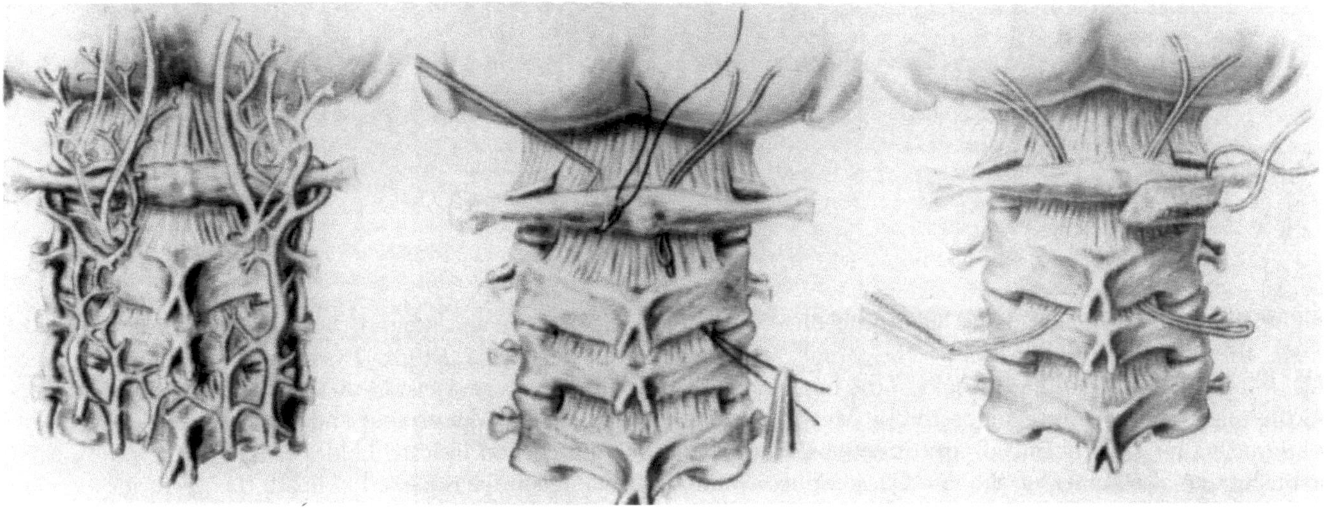

A,B

C

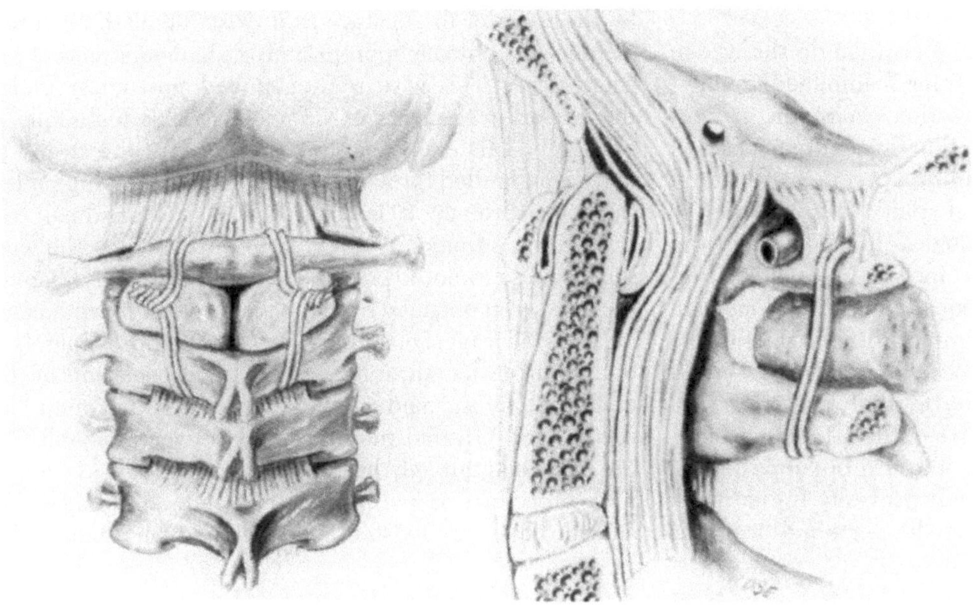

D,E

Figure 11.27. Brooks fusion technique. **A.** Through midline approach, occipital nerves, which emerge from C1–C2 interlaminar space, and vertebral arteries are well protected by neck muscles. **B.** Sutures are passed under posterior arches of C1 and C2. Sutures are then used to guide wire under laminae of C1 and C2. **C.** After wires are passed, bone wedges are placed. **D** and **E.** Wires are tightened to secure bone graft and provide immediate stability. (Reprinted with permission from Brooks AL, Jenkins EB. Atlanto-axial arthrodesis by the wedge compression method. J Bone Joint Surg 1978;60A(3): 279–284.)

Compression of the posterior elements of C1 and C2 can be obtained by appropriately positioning the holes in the bone graft as the wires are tightened. The Brooks modification includes the placement of a small segment of bone graft between the posterior elements of C1 and C2 and only using the sublaminar wire for fixation. This variation can be used at any time depending on the surgeon's preference. Additional cancellous bone is placed laterally and in the midline to supplement the longitudinal bone graft. A diamond-tip burr can be used to shorten the length of the bone graft beneath the occiput if the graft is found to be too long.

A word of caution: Before placement of the sublaminar wires beneath C1 and C2 and before insertion of the bone graft, a right-angle nerve root hook should be used to pull the sublaminar wires against the posterior lamina at the interspace of C1 and C2. This eliminates the problem of forward looping of the wire and reduces the chances of posterior compression of the dura and its contents by the wire. Also, before insertion of the bone graft, the posterior cortices of C1 and C2 laminae should be roughened with a high-speed burr to freshen these bony surfaces and enhance the fusion.

Ring of C2 Fractures (Hangman's Fracture)

Like fractures of the odontoid, fractures of the posterior element or the pars interarticular region of C2 also vary in position and, therefore, can be classified into three types.[24] Generally, this fracture follows an axial loading-extension injury to the head–neck junction. Anatomically, because the spinal canal opposite the posterior border of the body of C2 out to the sublaminar surface of C2 is wide (1.95 cm), the spinal cord (measuring 1 cm in thickness) seldom is injured. If so, the injury that results is usually a central cord type with an excellent prognosis for neurological recovery. In the author's series of 59 hangman's fractures, 48 (81%) were intact, 10 (17%) incomplete, and 1 (1.7%) complete. Type I fractures through the pedicle of C2 generally do not significantly distort the relationship between the body of C2 and its posterior elements. For this reason, this fracture can be managed conservatively in a halo vest orthosis for 10 to 12 weeks, or in cervical traction for 3 to 4 weeks followed by a light orthosis for the remainder of the 3 months required for fracture healing. Type II fractures, on the other hand, have several variations (A-B-C), each indicating increasing amounts of instability between the vertebral body of C2 and its posterior element. Because this fracture so often involves areas of posterior elements and the body of C2, large surfaces of cancellous bone are involved. Consequently, fracture healing is more often the rule than not. Type III fractures demonstrating significant displacement are thought to represent a flexion-compression rather than an extension injury.[91,92] Where there is gross displacement between the anterior and posterior elements, as in type III fractures, or there is subluxation or dislocation of the anterior C1–C2 complex from the posterior element of C2, fusion may be indicated using a procedure similar to the management of odontoid fractures.

It should be noted, when considering the management options available for hangman's fractures, that such fractures are frequently accompanied by other fractures involving the upper cervical spine. Examples include fractures of the ring of C1 with associated pedicle fractures of C2, type II odontoid fractures, or pedicle fractures, etc. The management scheme suggested by the authors, as in all other areas of the vertebral column, is as follows. Multiple-level fractures should, unless grossly unstable, be managed conservatively. As noted in the discussion of fractures of the posterior ring of C1, when the posterior ring of C1 is unilateral, the use of sublaminar wires for fixation is not contraindicated for posterior element fixation. Of the 59 cases referred to, 52 (88%) were managed conservatively and 7 (12%) required some variation of facet-spinous process wiring.

Surgery of C1–C3 Complex

As a rule, the use of sublaminar wires below C2 in the neurologically intact patient is contraindicated. The rationale for the statement is evidence of neurological deterioration or injury in patients having had surgical fusion with the use of sublaminar wires below the level of C3. The recommended technique is as follows (Figs. 11.28A–11.28C): one wire is placed beneath the lamina of C1 in a routine fashion, and a second 20-gauge wire is placed transversely through a hole in the base of the spinous process at C3. Rather than the loop of wire being cut in two as it passes out from under the superior aspect of the posterior ring of C1, this loop is pulled intact, inferiorly, and "hooked" beneath the inferior border of the spinous process of C3. Longitudinally, a rectangular bone graft is then applied over the posterior surface between C1 and C3. The inferior ends of the wire lying beneath the ring of C1, on each side, are placed through an appropriately placed hole in the rectangular bone graft, allowing the free ends to be passed through the holes from the cancellous side of the graft to the cortical side. The wires are tightened after the inferior wires are similarly placed through the inferior holes near the end of the bone graft. This allows for fixation of the bone graft at both of the levels of C1 and C3, and bypasses any fracture that might be present and involving the posterior element of C2 (i.e., hangman's fracture).

Dislocation of the Cervical Spine

Neurological injury following facet joint dislocation varies with the extent of injury. In the Northwestern University series of 1484 cervical spine injuries, unilateral facet dislo-

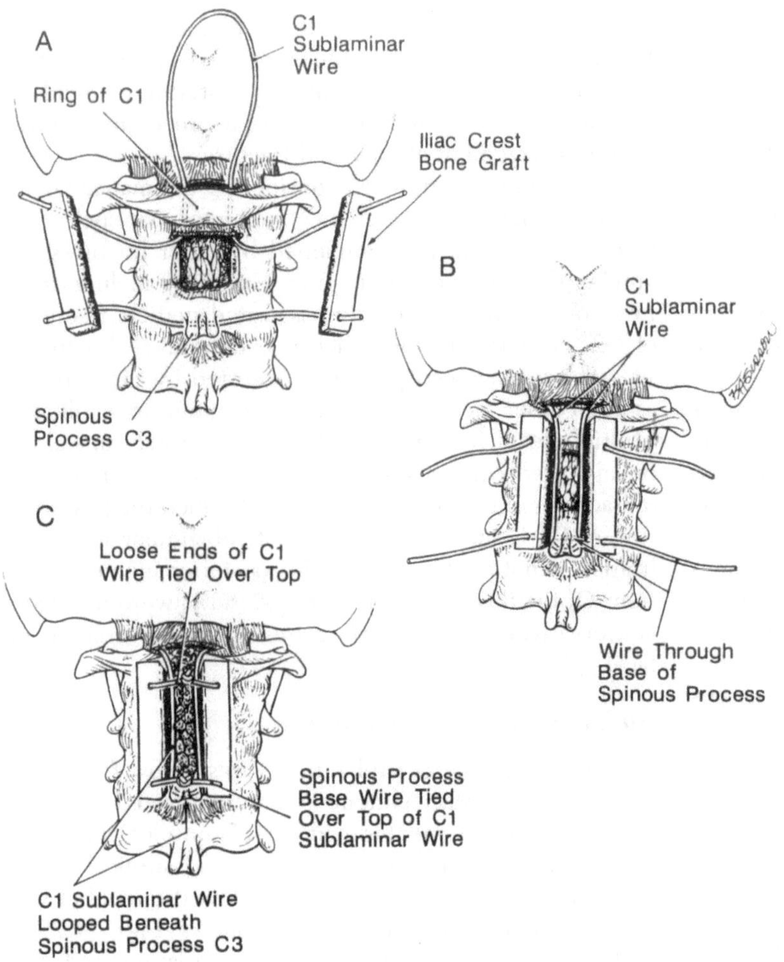

Figure 11.28. **A–C.** C1–C3 fusion technique.

cation resulted in 31% complete injury, 39% incomplete injury, and 30% intact. Of those bilateral facet dislocations, 47% were complete, 45% incomplete, and only 8% intact.[24] Neural canal compromise resulting from the presence of facet subluxation, unilateral facet dislocation, or bilateral facet dislocation varies from 25 to 100%. Bedbrook[93] stated that the dura and the contents of the spinal canal can withstand a 50% narrowing without demonstrating neurological deficit. Thus, immediate closed reduction (or open reduction if the patient demonstrates an irreducible bony injury in the presence of an incomplete neurological injury) is required. This is accomplished by the use of incremental cervical tong traction and, when indicated, in the consciously alert patient, manipulation.[3] The attempt here is to bring about immediate relief of bone or soft-tissue compromise of the spinal cord and its nerve roots.[3,24] Following closed reduction, radiographic examination is indicated. Once a reduction has been achieved, and before an anticipated posterior cervical spine fusion, a myelogram or MRI should be obtained to rule out the presence of anterior compromise to the neural canal or the presence of a ruptured intervertebral disc. Should this latter pathology be identified, an anterior cervical spine approach, with disc excision accompanied by a bone graft fusion and internal fixation using a plate and screws, is indicated.[3,94a,b] (Figs. 11.29A and 11.29B).

There are reports[6,95] suggesting that facet joint dislocations, once reduced and maintained in appropriate alignment, undergo autofusion, often with an associated anterior interbody fusion at the level of injury. This has not been found to be the general rule. Reduced facet dislocations, in the absence of fracture, fail to undergo sufficient capsular healing so as to instill cervical spine stability. Recurrent subluxations or dislocations have been reported.[6,96,97]

Posterior fusion and stabilization techniques used for dislocations of the cervical spine are based primarily on variations of the Rogers,[98,99] Robinson–Southwick,[100] or Garber–Meyer[24] procedures. Each has modifications that include the use of multiple-level wires (Figs. 11.30A–11.30C). The preoperative radiographic assessment plays a major role in determining the number of levels of the cervical spine requiring surgical stabilization. In the absence of laminae or facet fractures, the Rogers fusion is most often indicated. The multiple-wire procedure is indicated for cervical spine dislocations in the absence of facet

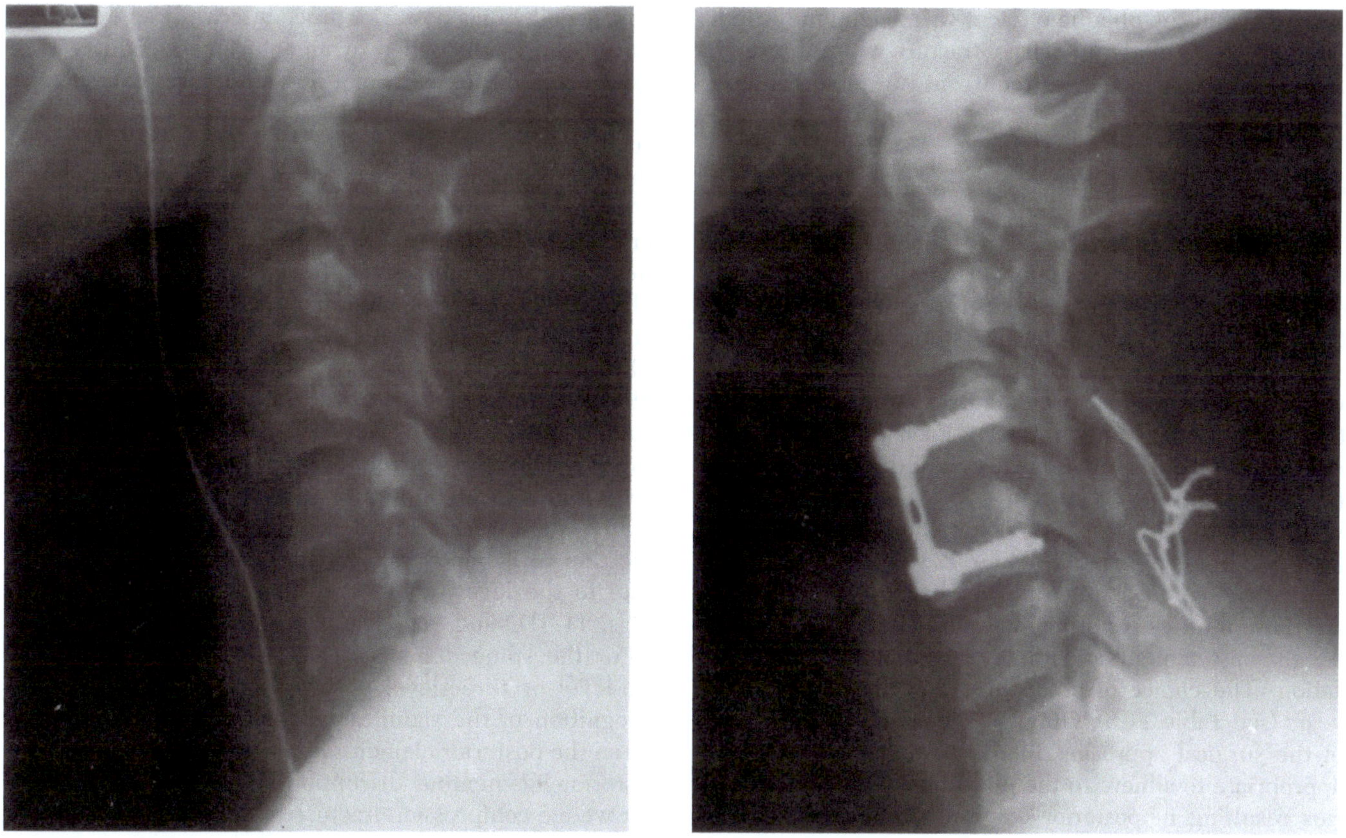

A B

Figure 11.29. **A.** C4–C5 unilateral facet dislocation in patient with incomplete quadriplegia. MRI demonstrated herniated disc. **B.** Anterior discectomy. Smith–Robinson fusion and stabilization followed by posterior open reduction and fusion using triple-wire technique.

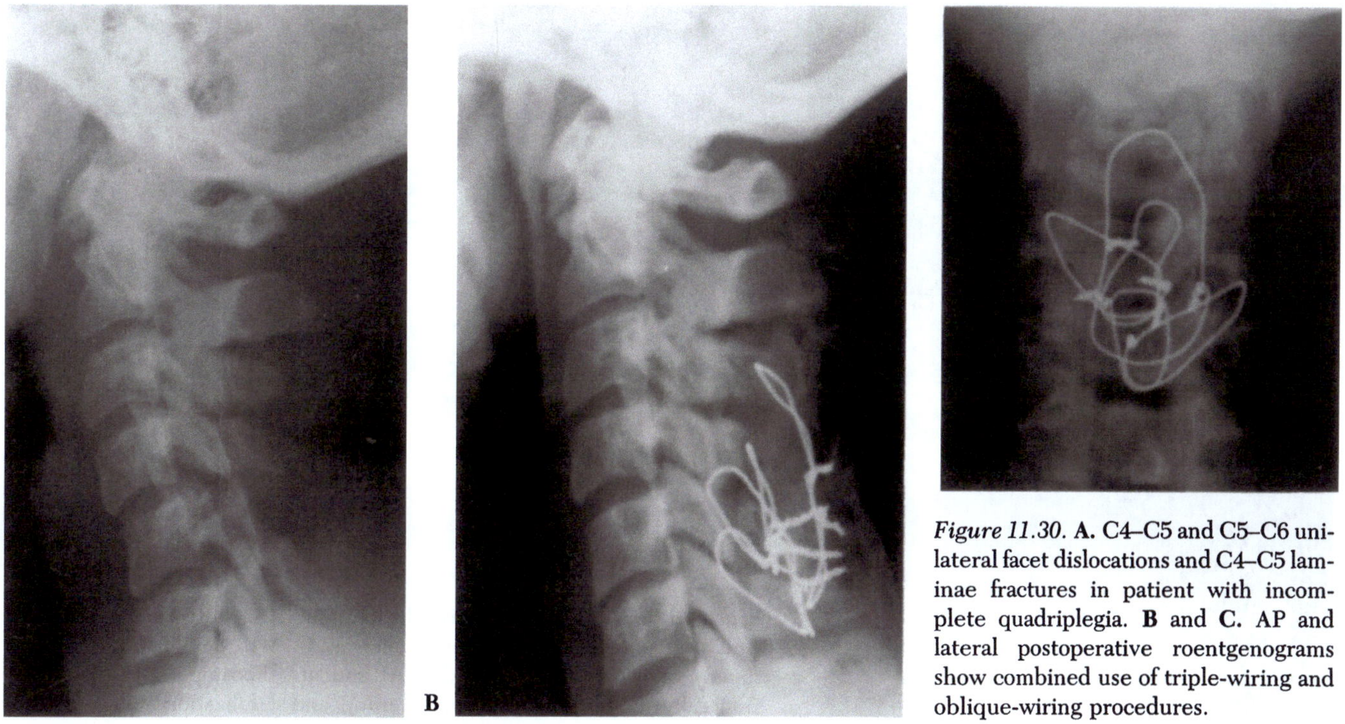

A B C

Figure 11.30. **A.** C4–C5 and C5–C6 unilateral facet dislocations and C4–C5 laminae fractures in patient with incomplete quadriplegia. **B** and **C.** AP and lateral postoperative roentgenograms show combined use of triple-wiring and oblique-wiring procedures.

fractures, and the oblique or facet wire technique is indicated if there is evidence of facet fracture with subluxation or of facet dislocation with recurrent (unstable) subluxation.

Fractures of the Cervical Spine

Stable cervical spine injuries are defined as (a) injuries to the cervical spine resulting in no abnormal (>3 mm) displacement between vertebral elements on flexion-extension films, (b) multiple-level posterior and anterior element fractures in good alignment, or (c) nonweight-bearing vertebral element fractures (anterior wedge fracture of the vertebral body up to 25%). Each of these can be managed by conservative means, including cervical traction using Gardner–Wells tongs for 4 to 6 weeks, a halo vest for 10 to 12 weeks, or a combination of traction and light cervical orthosis (SOMI) for 12 weeks.

Unstable cervical spine injuries below the level of C2 are those injuries resulting in abnormal displacement between bony elements and usually requiring surgical stabilization. The choice of procedures has changed over the years (see Table 11.6). Of note is the change in direction of the surgical approach. In the past, it has been most appropriate to adhere to the philosophy that flexion injuries resulting in posterior column stability should best be managed with a posterior procedure while an extension injury is best approached by an anterior procedure. This has changed on the basis of a single fracture that is found to represent a most unstable flexion injury. This injury usually occurs at the C5 level, and is an axial load flexion injury resulting in retrolisthesis of the superior vertebra on the next inferior vertebra, a triangular anterior inferior vertebral body fracture of the superior vertebra, and, most often, on tomography or CAT scan evaluation, evidence of bilateral posterior element fracture at the level of injury (Figs. 11.31A and 11.31B).

Frequently, the use of a posterior surgical fusion alone will fail. Because of the retrolisthesis of the superior vertebra and anterior spinal cord compression (Fig. 11.31C), neurological injury is frequently present. In the incomplete neurologically injured patient, the appropriate procedure is always anterior decompression followed by the insertion of a bone graft and either fixation of an A-O plate to the levels above and below the level of injury (Figs. 11.31D and 11.31E), or posterior stabilization.

For the spine demonstrating facet joint instability, a two-level or three-level posterior fusion is indicated in recognition of the significant widening of the space between the posterior elements at the level of injury. Where posterior ligamentous disruption is associated with anterior wedge compression fracture of the vertebra, a three-

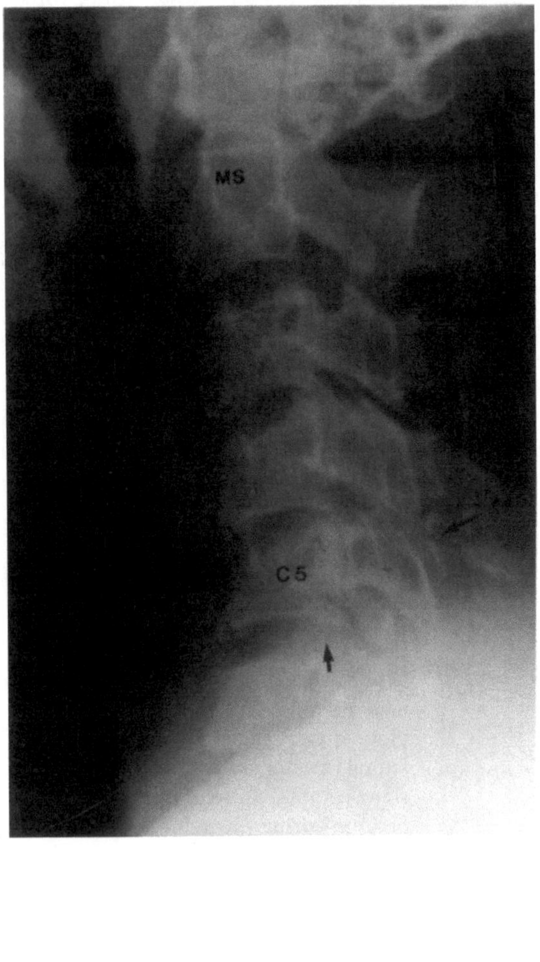

A

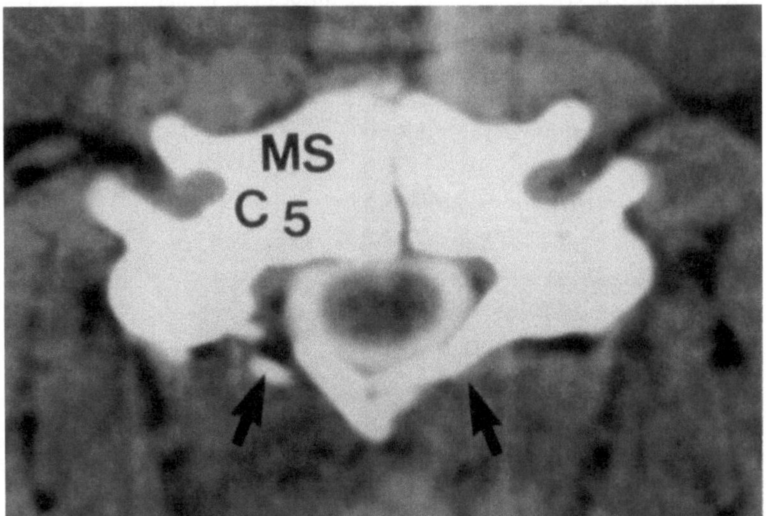

B

Figure 11.31. **A.** C5 compressive flexion injury. **B.** Metrizamide-enhanced CAT scan shows bilateral lamina fractures. **C.** MRI demonstrates anterior spinal cord compression. **D** and **E.** AP and lateral postoperative roentgenograms after C5 corpectomy, bone grafting, and stabilization with A-O plate.

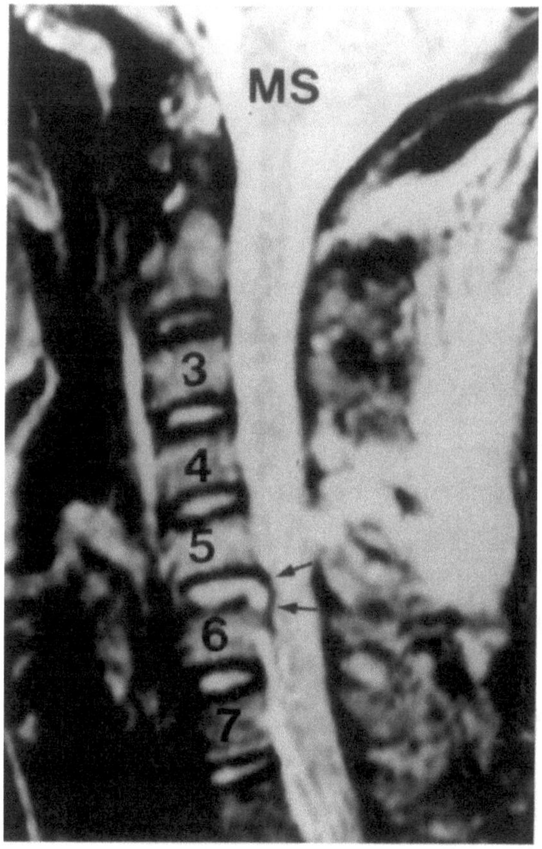

C

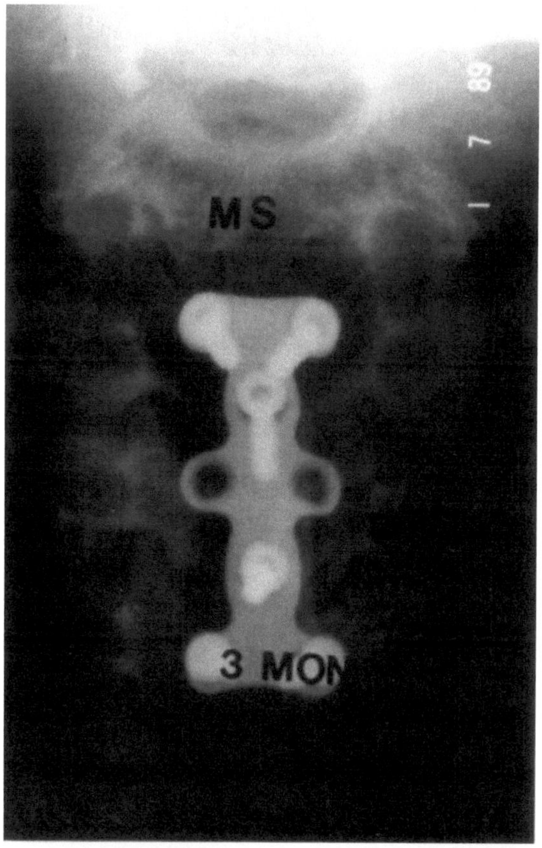

D

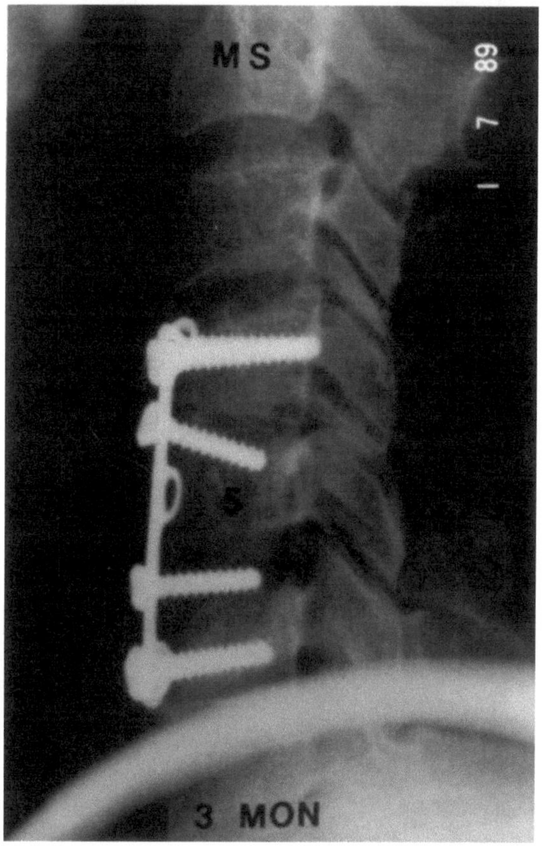

E

level posterior fusion or an anterior plate and screw procedure is indicated. When in the presence of stable posterior elements at each level, a triple-wire technique is often used (Figs. 11.32A–11.32C).

Again, the only exception to fusion of an unstable cervical spine, either anterior or posterior, is in the patient who has multiple-level fractures and where a fusion procedure would significantly alter or eliminate cervical motion of multiple levels and result in increasing disability.

Posterior Cervical Fusion Technique

As noted, there are numerous modifications of the Rogers technique. Initially, the patient is placed supine on a Stryker frame, is intubated either naso- or endotracheally with the assistance of a fiberoptic bronchoscope, and once stabilized, turned prone. The patient is always managed in Gardner–Wells cervical tong traction, which reduces the chance of forward displacement of the head and neck during either supine or prone positioning and assists in maintaining linear or straightaway cervical spine alignment. Once the patient is in the prone position, roentgenograms should be obtained to ensure the maintenance of the spinal reduction and to verify that an unsafe situation does not exist. This latter technique may not be required if spinal cord function is being monitored continuously

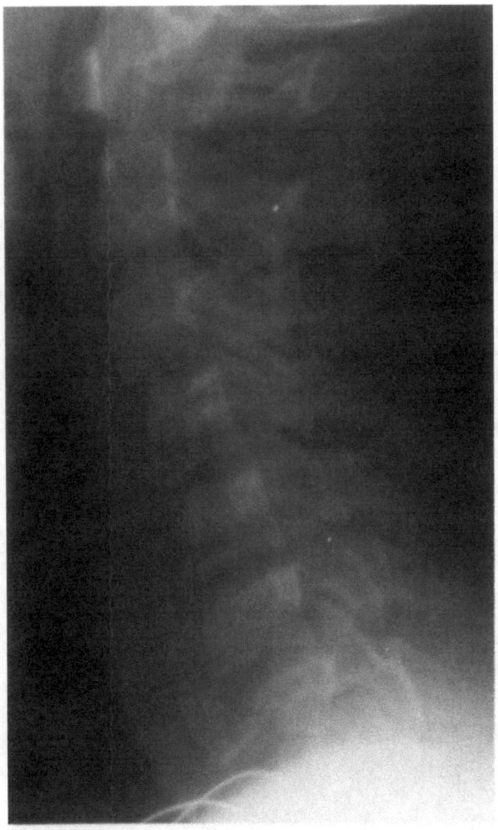
A

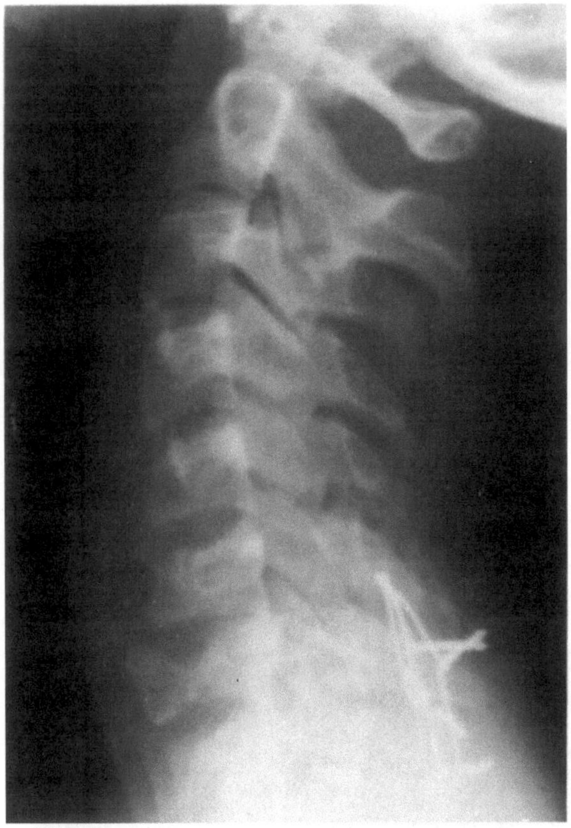
B

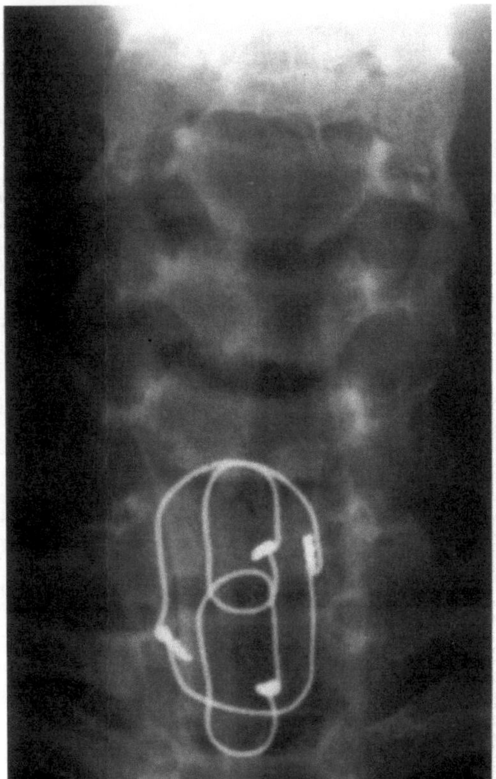
C

by SSEP. A midline posterior incision (Fig. 11.33A) is made over the levels of the cervical spine intended to be fused, and the paraspinal muscles are dissected subperiosteally by means of electrocautery or periosteal elevator dissection assisted by Metzenbaum scissors. Hemostasis is maintained using bipolar electrocautery. The posterior elements (spinous processes, laminae, and facets) at each level to be fused are decorticated superficially using a high-speed carbide burr. In the absence of either lamina or facet fractures, drill holes are made at the base of the spinous process at the level above and below the injury site using the right-angle burr (Fig. 11.33B). The drill holes are enlarged using a towel clip. An 18-gauge stainless steel wire is passed through the base of the spinous process at the upper and lower limits of the intended fusion. A bone graft harvested from either the posterior iliac crest or the proximal medial tibial metaphysis is fashioned into two strips of corticocancellous graft (Figs. 11.33C and 11.33D). Additional cancellous bone graft is obtained from

Figure 11.32. **A.** C7 burst fracture in a neurologically intact patient. **B.** Lateral roentgenogram shows modified triple-wiring technique. **C.** AP roentgenogram shows addition of wire through base of superior spinous process to complement triple-wiring technique.

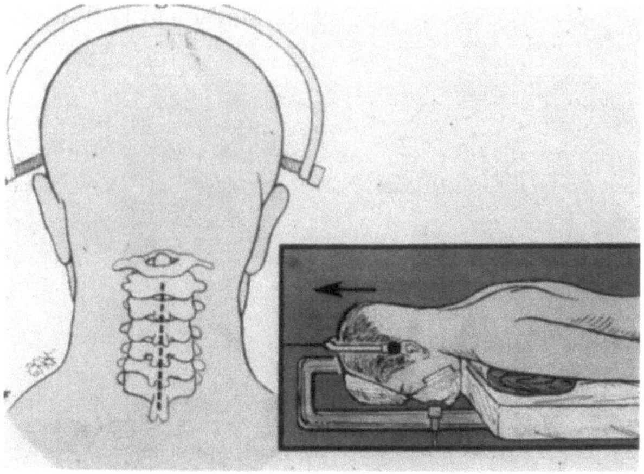

A

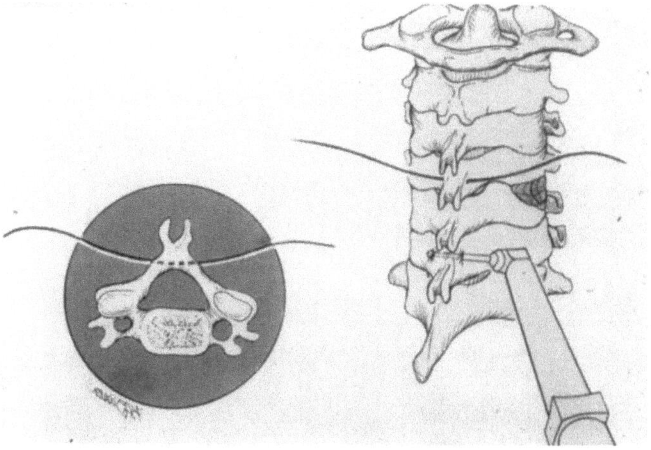

B

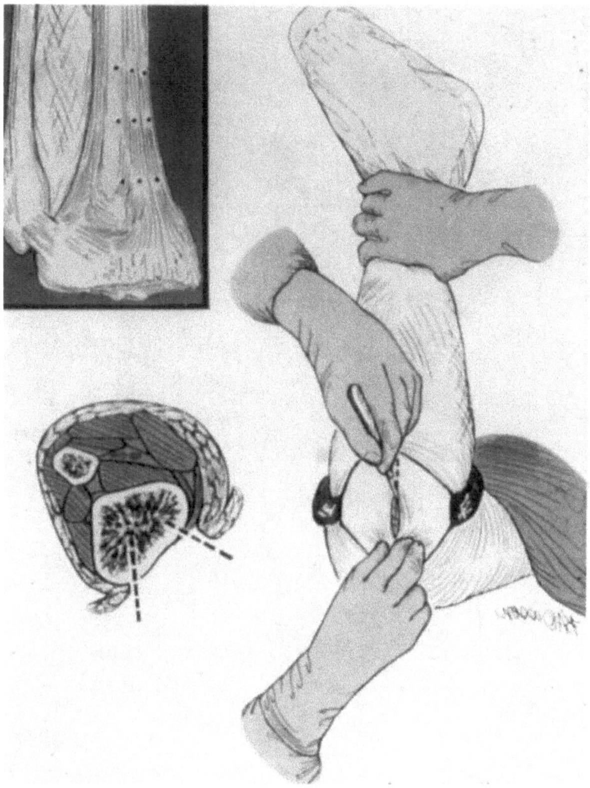

C

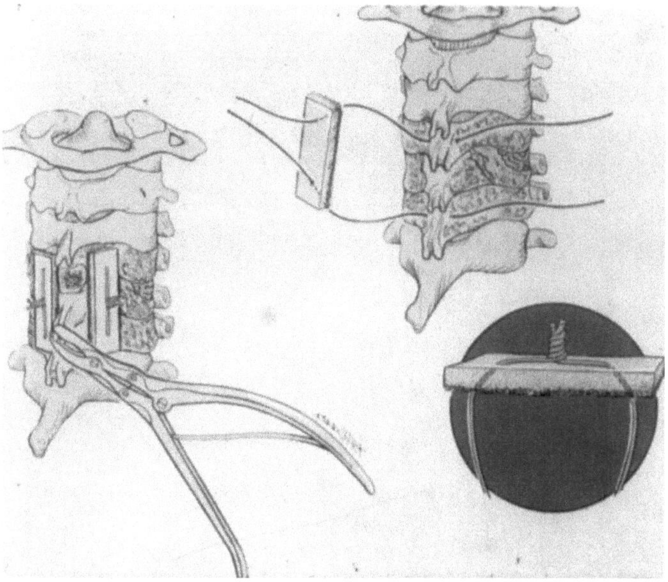

D

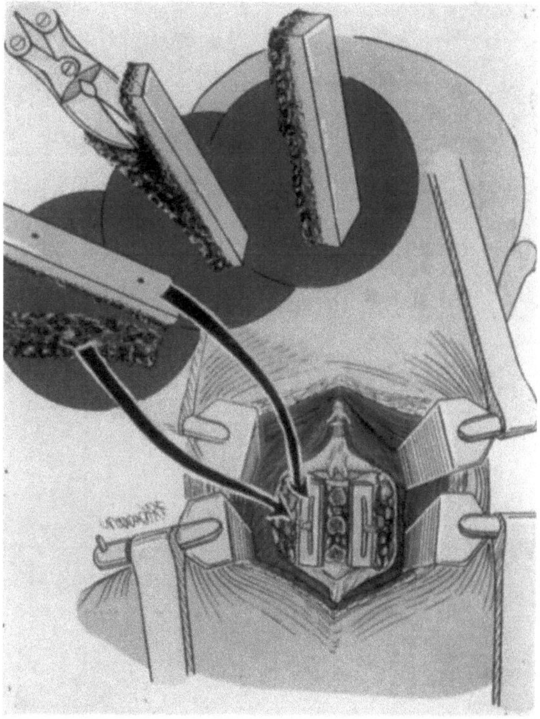

E

Figure 11.33. Modified Rogers technique. **A.** Patient is positioned prone on wedge turning frame; midline posterior exposure is made. **B.** Drill holes are made in bases of spinous processes one level above and below injury level using right-angle burr. **C.** Technique for harvesting medial proximal tibial metaphyseal graft. **D.** Wire is passed through bases of spinous processes. Oblique drill holes are made; wires are placed through bone plates and tightened. **E.** After wiring bone plates, graft is placed over posterior elements. (*Continued.*)

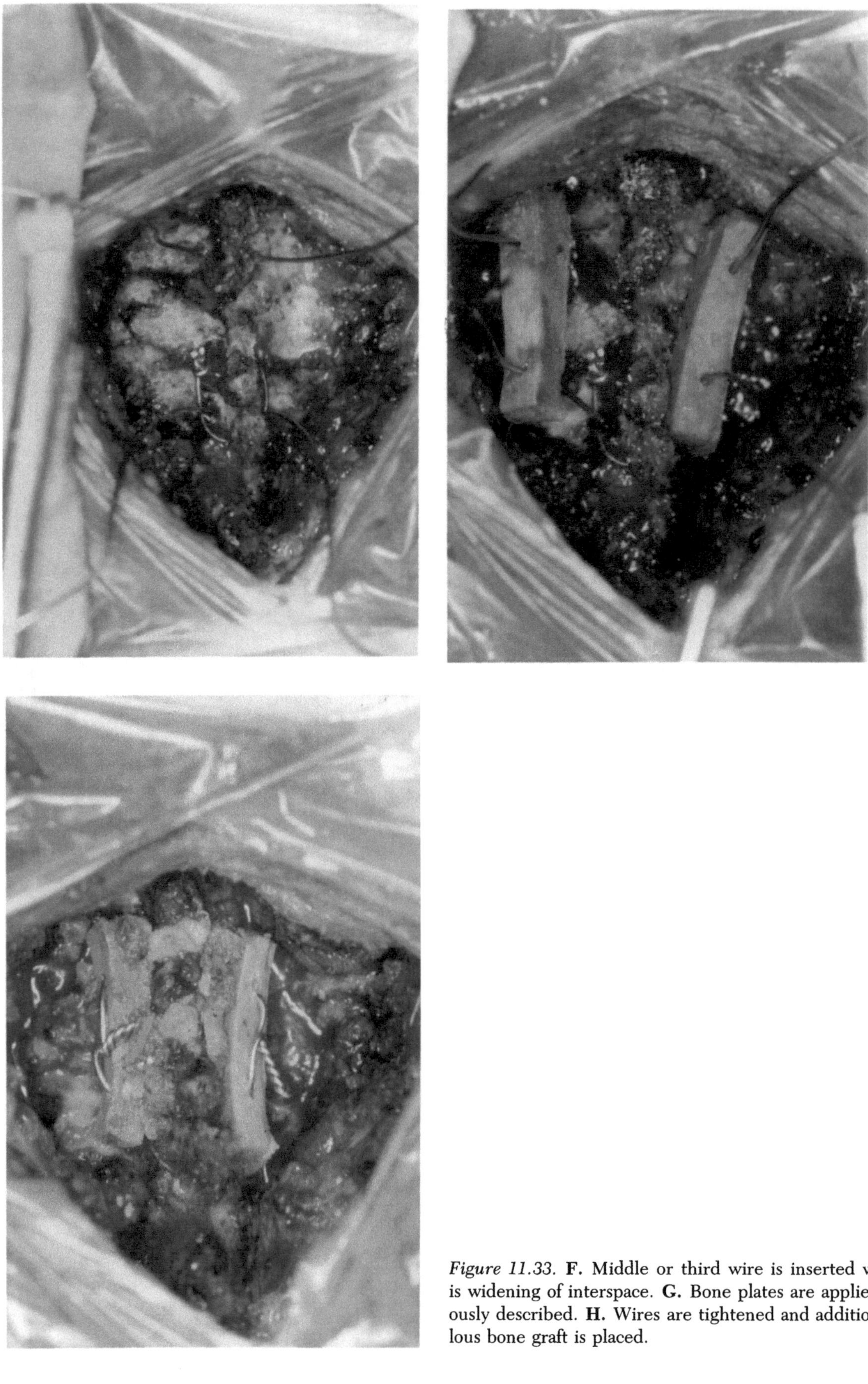

F G H

Figure 11.33. **F.** Middle or third wire is inserted when there is widening of interspace. **G.** Bone plates are applied as previously described. **H.** Wires are tightened and additional cancellous bone graft is placed.

either the proximal tibial metaphysis or the iliac crest as an adjunct to the corticocancellous bone graft. The secondary bone graft sites are closed in a routine manner.

After sizing the bone graft, oblique drill (outward, 45°) holes are placed through each end of the bone graft so that the wires will converge over the center of the cortical surface of the bone graft (Fig. 11.33E). The superior and inferior wires bilaterally are tightened simultaneously. Restoration of cervical extension should occur with the tightening of these wires.

Occasionally, if a posterior fusion is performed where there is an obvious widening of the interspace between two of the posterior elements at the center of the proposed fusion, the insertion of a third wire is indicated. In this variation, the wire is placed through the base of the spinous process of the middle posterior element (the level of the anterior fracture), wrapped on one side beneath the next inferior spinous process, and then tightened (Fig. 11.33F). This portion of the fusion is performed before the insertion of the corticocancellous grafts just described. After the bone grafts have been appropriately tightened in place (Fig. 11.33G), a check roentgenogram should demonstrate acceptable cervical spine alignment. Additional cancellous bone graft is placed in the lateral gutters of the proposed fusion site (Fig. 11.33H) and the wound is closed in layers.

In the presence of single level-injury, such as a bilateral facet joint dislocation, often only a two-level posterior fusion is required. In this case, a similar procedure is used: two wires are placed through the base of the adjacent spinous processes, passed through the corticocancellous bone grafts, and tightened to produce compression between the two adjacent posterior elements. In every case, as the wires are tightened, cervical spine traction weights should be removed.

In those instances where instability of the facet joints remains, an additional wiring procedure has been used with great success. Using a Penfield dissector placed between the inferior and superior facets at the level of instability, a drill hole is made in the center of the inferior facet using a right-angle drill. A 20-gauge stainless steel wire is passed through this hole, brought out through the facet joint using a nerve hook, and tightened around the next inferior intact spinous process. This procedure is carried out bilaterally for bilateral facet instability. This oblique wiring technique is not used alone, but as a supplement to the modified Rogers or triple-wire fusion as described.

Anterior Cervical Fusion Technique

The use of the anterior approach to the cervical spine, in association with an anterior fusion technique, is the approach of choice for surgical decompression of the anterior spinal cord when the structure is compromised. The rationale is self-explanatory. The principal vascular supply to the spinal cord is the anterior spinal artery. This structure, when singularly compromised, is capable of producing irreversible "infarct" injury to the spinal cord, resulting in significant motor and sensory damage. Prolonged or insidious compromise of this important anterior structure in the incomplete neurologically injured patient can be relieved, and the neurological injury often improved or reversed, by means of an anterior decompression.

A procedure popularized in the 1970s was the Cloward[101] anterior dowel procedure. This procedure and the Robinson–Southwick anterior intervertebral body fusion technique are both contraindicated in the presence of two-column instability with resulting significant cervical spine instability. This is particularly true when there is evidence of existing posterior column instability. With an anterior dowel fusion procedure, further cervical spine instability results. The consequence is the displacement of the inserted anterior bone graft, requiring a second anterior procedure.

Vertebral Body Reconstruction and Fusion Technique

Patients undergoing anterior fusion are usually in cervical skeletal traction in the supine position on a wedge Stryker frame. The standard approach is the anterolateral horizontal or oblique approach on the surgeon's side of preference (Fig. 11.34A). Following incision of the skin and subcutaneous tissue and separation of the platysma muscle in line with its fibers, the cervical spine is exposed by blunt dissection. The recurrent laryngeal nerve lies just posterior to the trachea, therefore great care must be taken during the dissection to remain lateral and posterior to the esophageal tracheal interval. As the esophagus and trachea are carefully retracted towards the midline, the carotid sheath and its contents are carefully retracted laterally. To avoid carotid artery compromise during the surgical procedure, the anesthesiologist monitors the presence of temporal artery pulse. During the operative procedure when either self-retaining or individual retractor pressure is suspected of producing excessive carotid artery compression, the anesthesiologist should be requested to determine the presence of the temporal artery pulse.

When the anterior cervical spine has been exposed, a needle is placed in an appropriate intervertebral space and a lateral radiograph of the cervical spine obtained to accurately determine the level of the surgical procedure. The site having been selected, the cephalad and caudad intervertebral discs are surgically removed in toto by sharp dissection using a rongeur or pituitary forceps. The dissection is carried posteriorly to expose the posterior longitudinal ligament. If preoperative CAT scans have demonstrated the presence or suggestion of a posteriorly

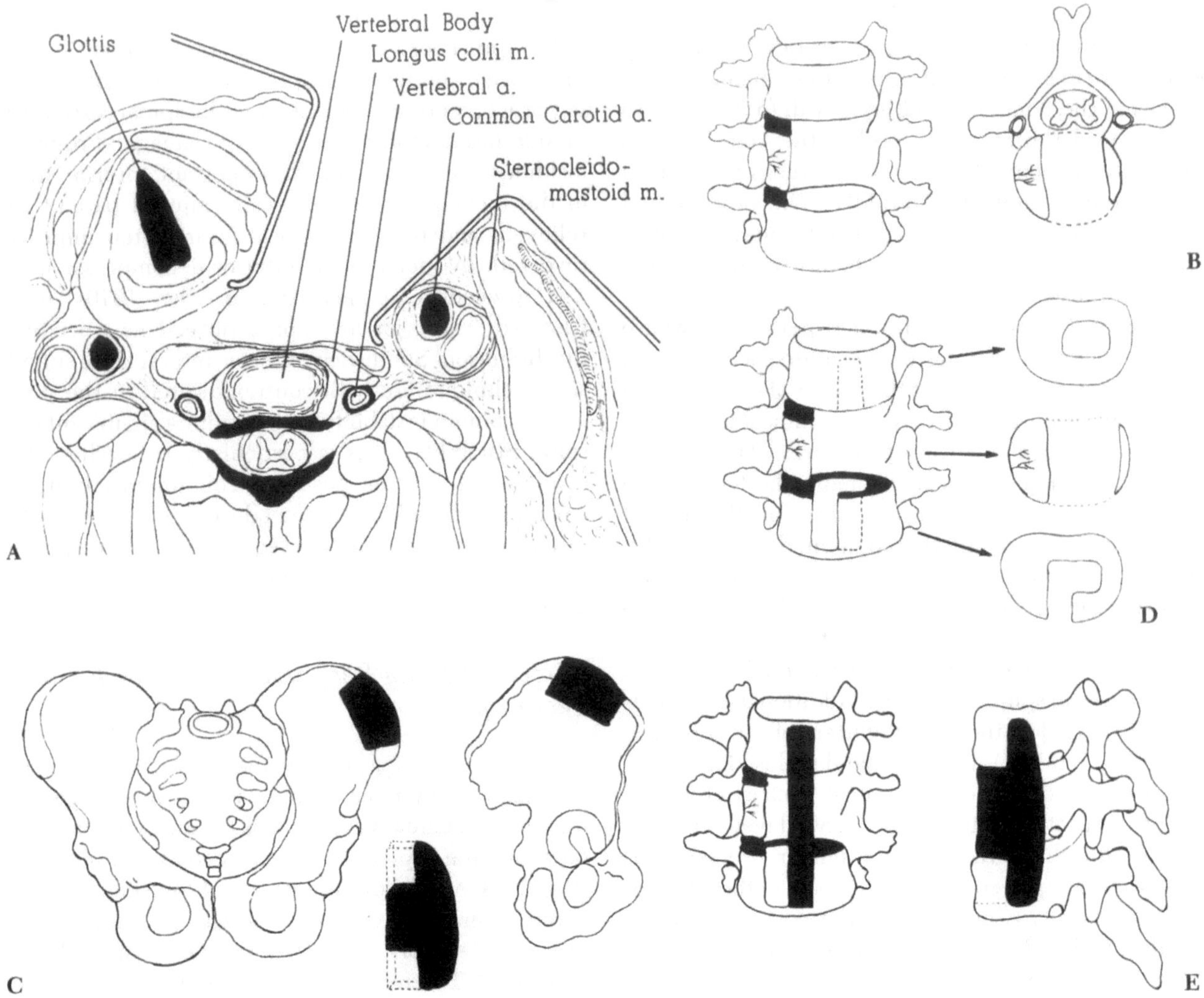

Figure 11.34. Anterior cervical vertebral body reconstruction and fusion. **A.** Anterolateral approach is made. **B.** AP and axial views of decompression. **C.** Harvesting and fashioning of tricortical graft. **D.** Preparation of vertebral bodies for graft insertion. **E.** Final position of tricortical graft.

herniated disc, careful attention must be directed proximally and distally for loose fragments of extruded disc material. Where the intervening vertebral body is either significantly involved with fracture or retropulsed posteriorly into the spinal canal, this vertebra is removed completely in its anterior midportion using a pituitary rongeur, a Leksell rongeur, or pituitary forceps (Fig. 11.34B). The endplates both superiorly and inferiorly are superficially denuded of their cartilaginous surface using either a high-speed burr or a curette (Fig. 11.34C).

When performing an anterior three-level fusion with corpectomy of the center vertebra, the space between the superior and inferior vertebrae is spanned by an appropriately shaped anterior iliac crest tricortical bone graft (Fig. 11.34D). The bed into which this graft will be placed is prepared by placing a horizontal groove across and through the superior surface of the inferior vertebra, taking care to leave the anterior vertebral border intact. A similar horizontal groove is made on the inferior surface of the superior vertebra. Normally, the vertebral body in the cervical spine measures 18 mm from anterior to posterior; therefore, with the insertion of a bone graft that will be invaginated superiorly and inferiorly, additional traction or a cervical distractor may be used during the insertion of the graft but removed on insertion of the bone graft. Care must be taken that the depth of the bone graft is such that it will not produce pressure posteriorly on the anterior dura (Fig. 11.34E). If the cervical spine is stable posteriorly, the patient may be supported postoperatively either in a halo vest or a SOMI orthosis. If there is any question of instability, a halo vest should be used postoperatively for 10 to 12 weeks.

In those instances where spinal instability along with spinal canal compromise has existed, requiring corpectomy and insertion of a bone graft, cervical spine stability can be enhanced by insertion of an anterior A-O plate and screws extending from the level above to the level below the corpectomy site. The screw length again varies from 18 to 22 mm, and must be monitored by intraoperative radiographs. In the osteoarthritic cervical spine, areas of spondylosis at the ends of the vertebrae endplates require "paring down" for the plate to fit flushly against the anterior vertebral bodies to which the plate is applied. A single 16-mm screw is used in the intervening space to fix the bone graft to the plate and maintain its relationship with the vertebral bodies above and below. Again, attention is directed to the need for removal of all cervical traction prior to the insertion of a plate and screws. Postoperative stability is maintained by means of a SOMI orthosis if spinal stability does exist, or a halo vest if there is continued concern.

"Tricortical" Intervertebral Arthrodesis

As noted earlier, the insertion of a tricortical iliac bone graft into the interspace between adjacent vertebral bodies as described by Smith–Robinson[102] is a procedure that is indicated in the degenerative cervical spine which has not undergone trauma and does not demonstrate evidence of instability. This arthrodesis technique is reserved for those cervical spines requiring excision of either posterior spondylitic spurs producing encroachment upon the anterior dural column or radiographic myelographic evidence of a herniated disc (Figs. 11.35A–11.35D). Horseshoe-shaped bone grafts from the anterior iliac crest, which measure 1 cm in depth and approximately 5 to 6 mm in width, are inserted into the interspace between the two adjacent vertebrae and are gently tapped posteriorly to allow at least 1 or 2 mm of anterior vertebral body cortex to extend outward over the tricortical graft. This serves as a deterrent to bone graft extrusion, following further excision of the pathological intervertebral disc and freshening of the vertebral endplates down to cortical bone.

Intraoperative lateral radiographs of the cervical spine are obtained to ascertain the correct depth of the bone graft. The cervical traction, which was by tong traction and/or the cervical distractor to maintain linear alignment of the head and neck during the initial portion of the procedure and to facilitate the insertion of the bone graft respectively, is removed at the end of the procedure. A

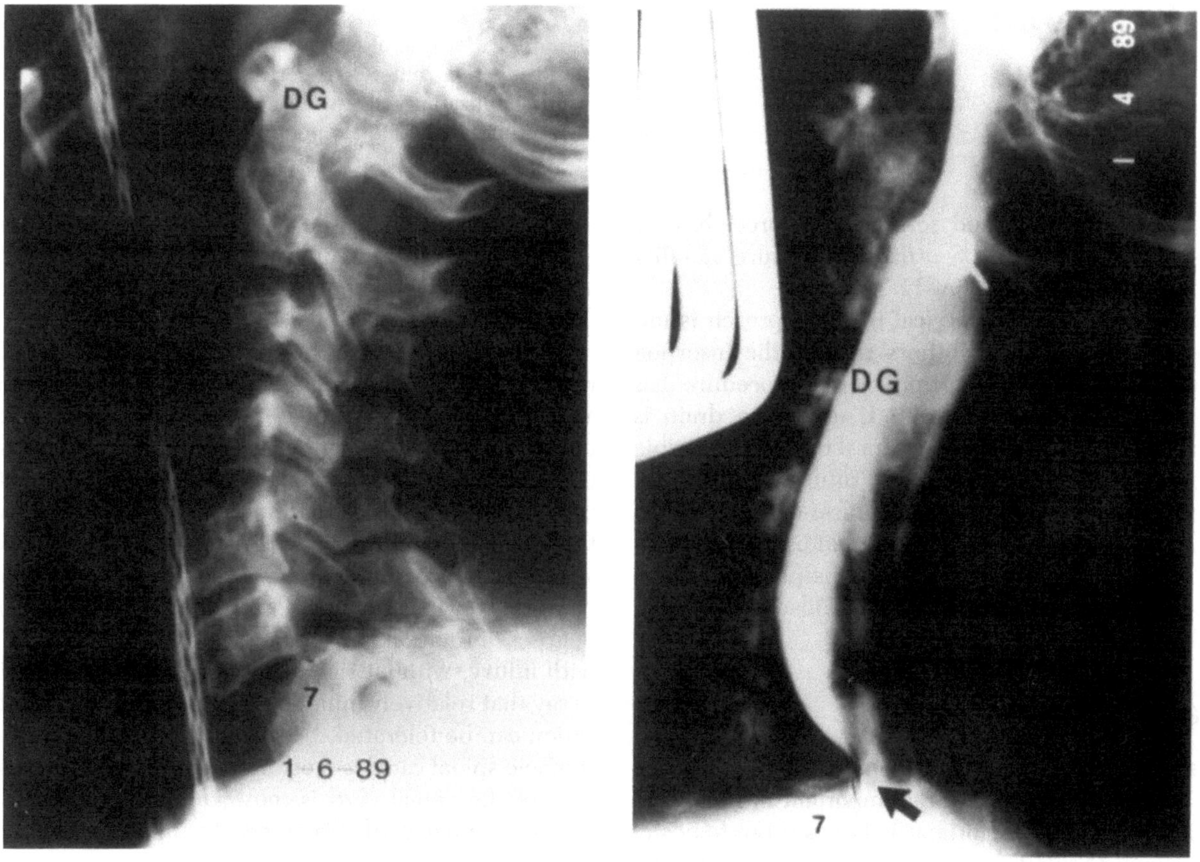

A B

Figure 11.35. **A.** Six-month-old unrecognized C6–C7 fracture-dislocation case that had two chiropractic manipulations for neck pain. **B.** Lateral myelogram shows C6–C7 herniated disc and narrow spinal canal. (*Continued.*)

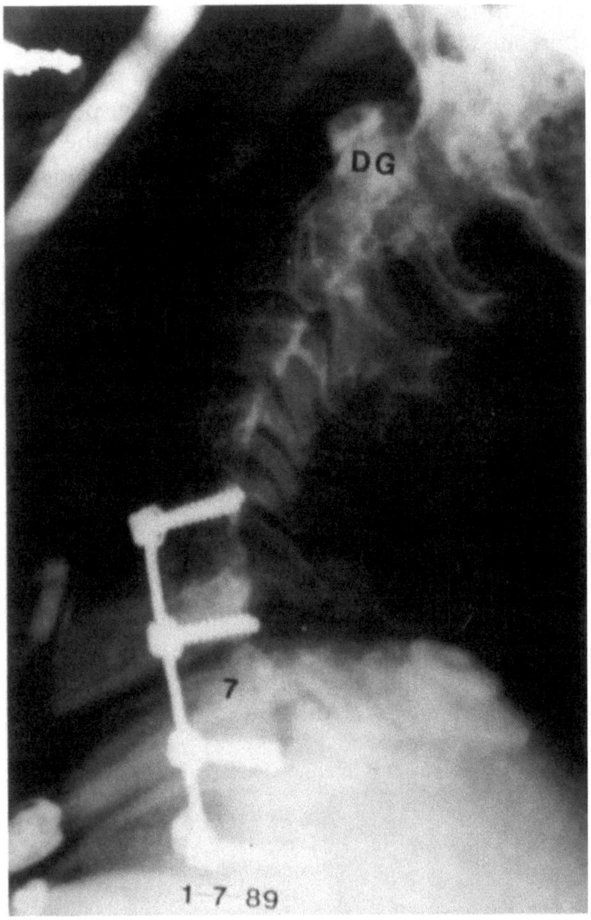

C

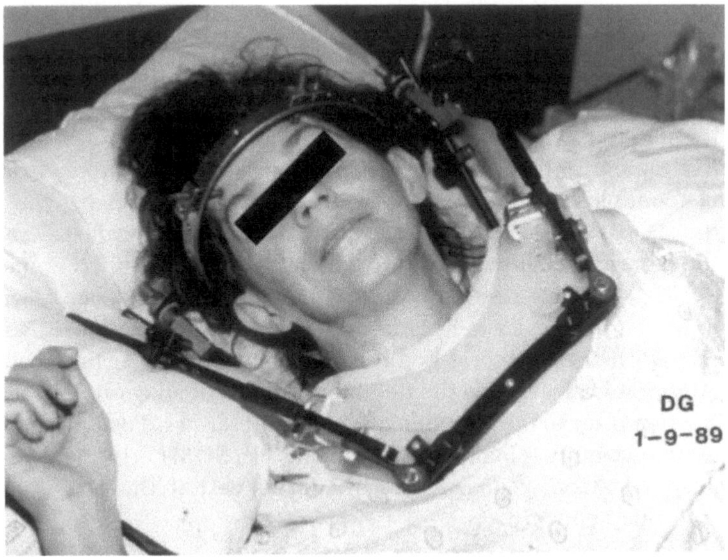

D

Figure 11.35. **C.** Because of incomplete quadriplegia, C6–7–T1 laminectomies, reduction, anterior tricortical fusions at C5–C6, C6–C7, C7–T1, and stabilization with plate and screws were performed. **D.** Patient was immobilized in halo postoperatively.

two-level anterior plate and screw fusion procedure as described previously can be utilized to ensure stability of the bone graft (Fig. 11.36A–11.36C).

Closure of the anterior cervical fusion approach is uncomplicated. While some authors suggest the insertion of a retained drain, this portion of the procedure has not been used or found helpful. If used, the drain is removed in the first 24 to 48 hours, or if there is negligible drainage, postoperatively. The only sutures required for the closure include approximation sutures of the platysma muscle, subcutaneous tissue sutures, and usually a subcuticular suture in the skin. The patient is protected for 8 to 10 weeks in a SOMI orthosis or Philadelphia collar depending on the surgeon's choice.

Thoracic and Lumbar Spine

Injuries to the thoracic and lumbar spine vary from injuries to the cervical spine in several important ways. Facet joints of the cervical spine primarily face anterior to posterior allowing for a significant range of flexion and extension. Because of the anatomical relationship of C1 and C2, 70% of all rotations of the cervical spine exist at this interval, the atlas (C1) around the axis (C2). When there are no restraining structures, injuries resulting from significant abnormal ranges of motion (axial load, flexion, rotation) frequently result in irreversible neurological injury.

In the thoracic spine, the area from T1–T12, a significant restriction of motion exists as a result of the confinement and fixation of the spine bilaterally secondary to the attachment of the ribs to both the transverse processes and the vertebral bodies at each level. Because of this anatomical relationship, little free motion exists anywhere in the thoracic spine. White and Panjabi[18] call attention to the anatomical variation of the facet joints down to the level of T6 to T9 whereby, because of facet architecture, minor degrees of rotation, flexion, and extension can occur, even with injury, without significant bony fracture. That is not to say that relatively minor degrees of subluxation or dislocation can be tolerated, because the contrary is true. The thoracic spinal canal is most narrow at T6 and the vasculature of the spinal cord is most vulnerable in the upper thoracic spinal cord. Tolerance to injury in this area is low.

Attention is directed to the type of fracture frequently identified at the vertebral interval T12–L1 (Fig. 11.37).

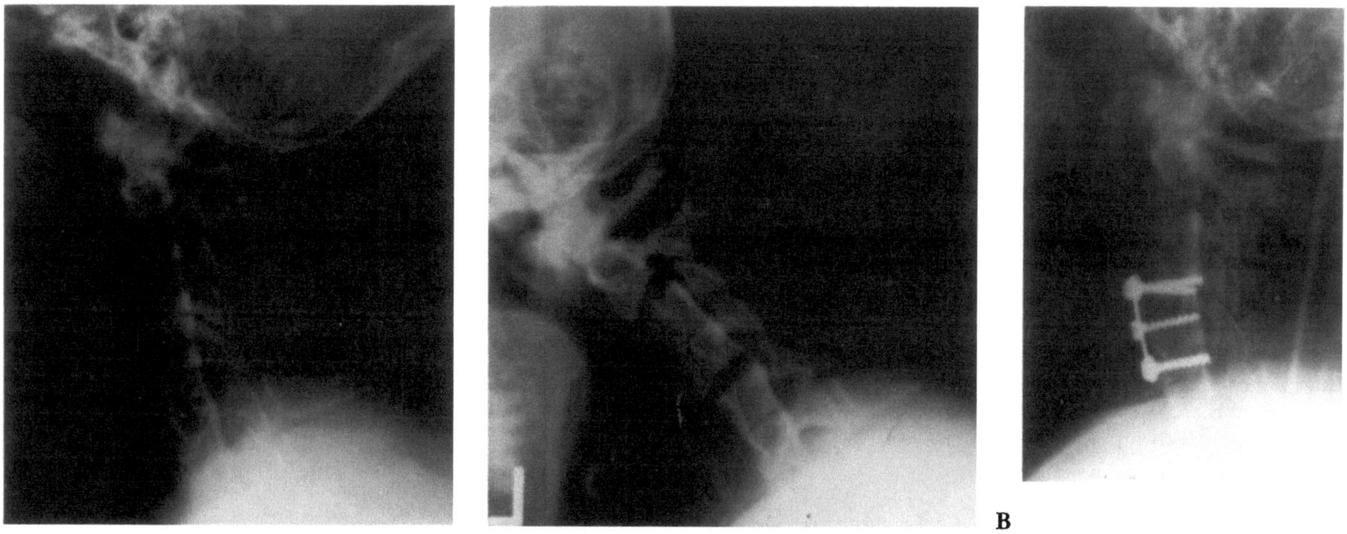

Figure 11.36. **A.** Lateral roentgenogram of patient with Klippel–Feil syndrome and incomplete quadriplegia after fall. MR imaging showed herniated C4–C5 disc. **B.** Lateral flexion roentgenogram shows C4–C5 subluxation. **C.** Smith–Robinson arthrodesis and stabilization with internal fixation were performed.

Injury at this level is typified by the inward/outward-facing facet joints at the T12–L1–L4 levels. This anatomical relationship is responsible for the frequency by which fractures of the pedicle occur as a result of rotational injuries. Rotation, particularly at T12–L1–L2, is not well tolerated because of facet joint "entrapment." The most frequent injuries found to occur in the thoracic region of the spine (T1 through T9) are wedge compression fractures (Figs. 11.38A and 11.38B). Unless the injury is associated with a horizontal-type (translatory) injury, displacement of one vertebral element from its adjacent member is rare. Again, this is the case because of the relationship of the ribs to the thoracic vertebrae. Fractures at T12–L1–L2 generally have combined components producing compression fractures of the vertebral body in association with vertical or split fractures of the vertebral body that result from both axial loading and rotation. In the presence of compressive flexion and in combination with rotation, a unilateral

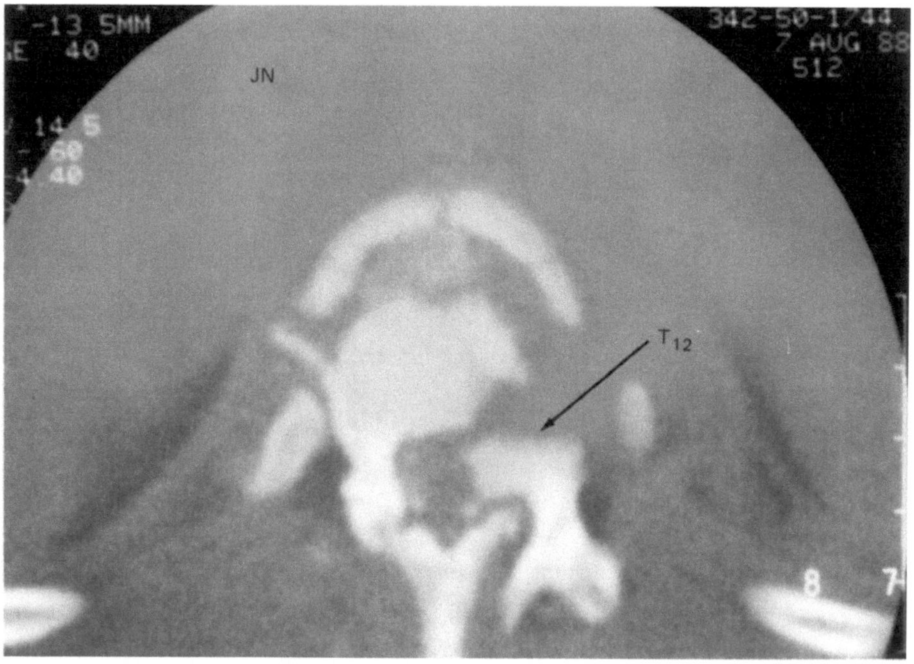

Figure 11.37. CAT scan of T12 burst fracture demonstrates displaced pedicle fracture from rotation and facet joint "entrapment."

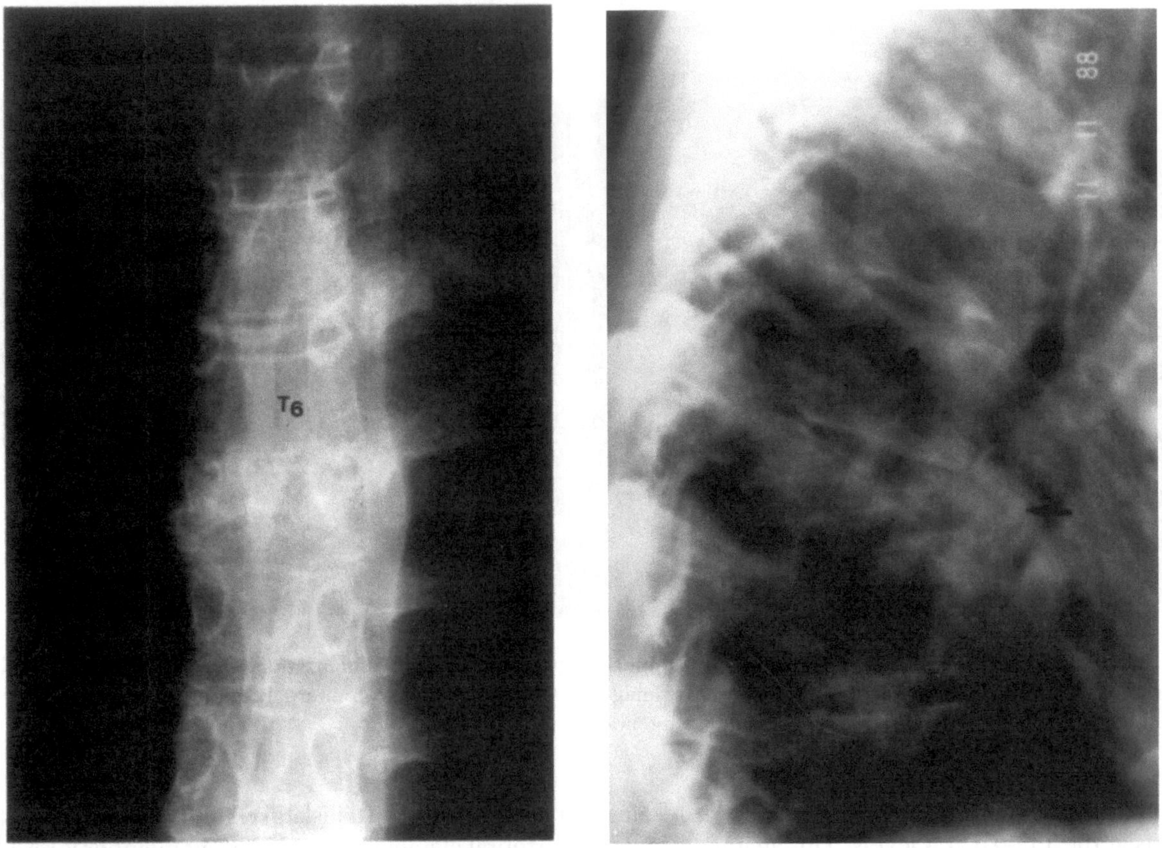

A

B

Figure 11.38. AP (**A**) and lateral (**B**) roentgenograms of T7 vertical compression fracture. Patient was managed conservatively by Knight–Taylor orthosis without complications.

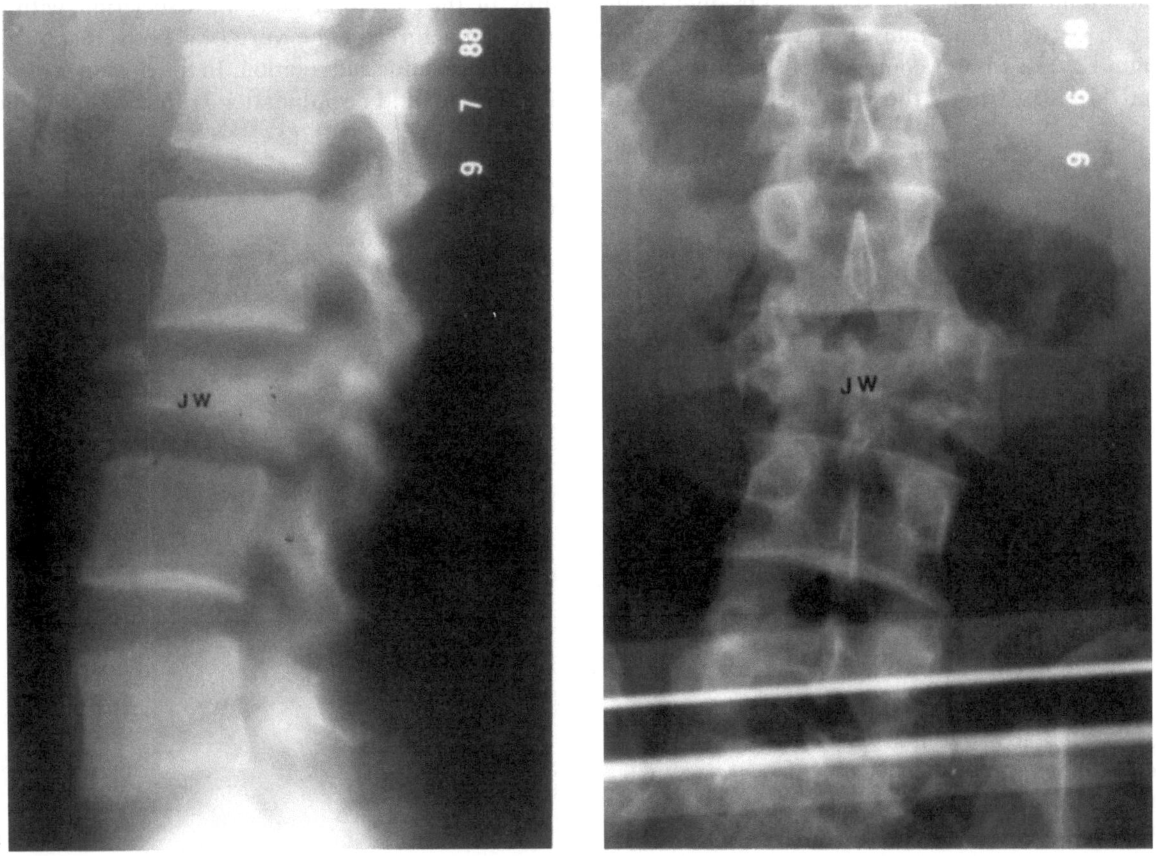

A

B

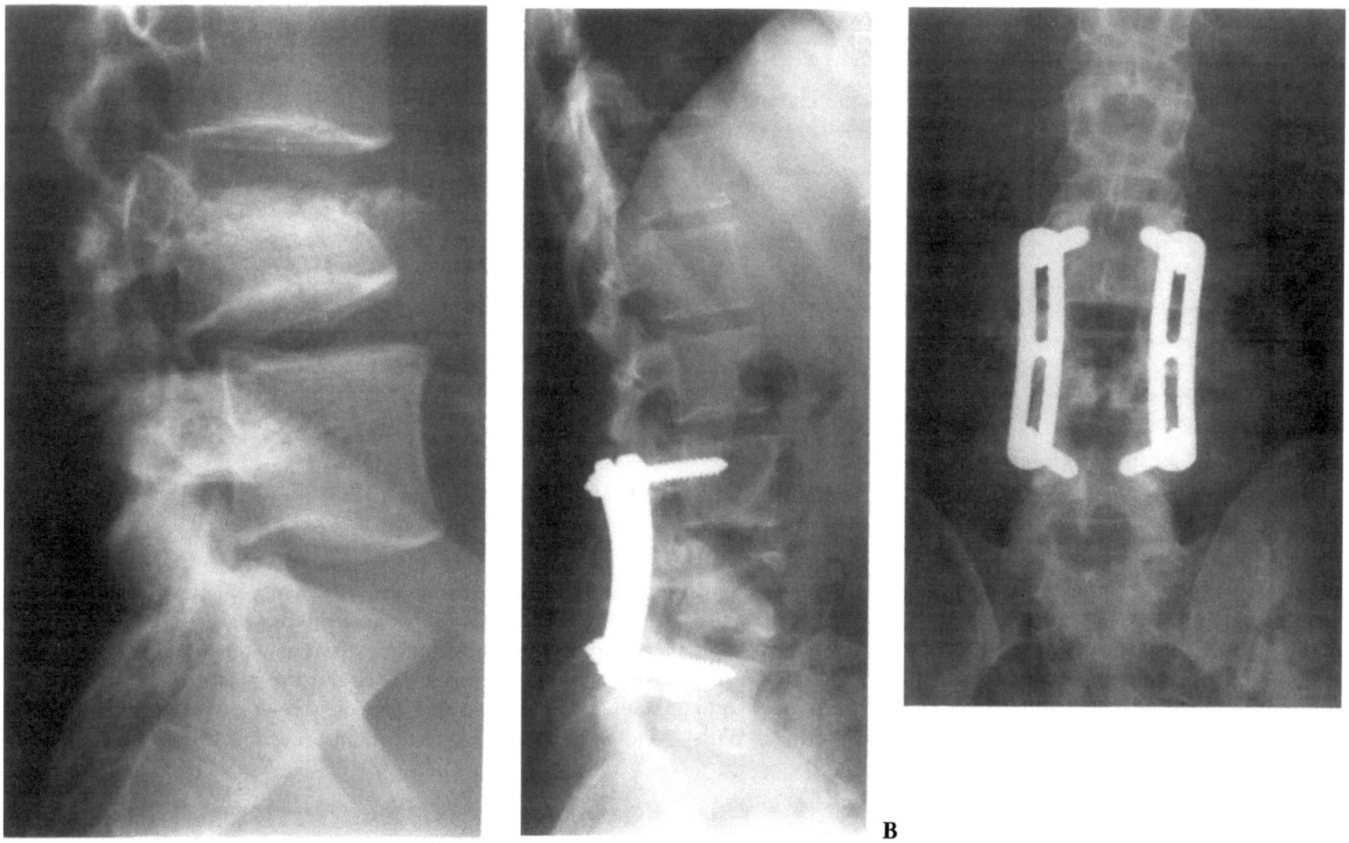

Figure 11.40. **A.** L4 burst fracture in patient with incomplete paraplegia. **B** and **C.** Posterior decompression stabilization with Steffee plates and fusion with posterolateral iliac grafting.

depression of the vertebral body with lateral displacement of one pedicle and facet is the injury most commonly identified (Figs. 11.39A and 11.39B).

Because of the inward-outward facet anatomical relationship that exists from T12 to L4, a great deal of lumbar spine flexion and extension motion is available. Gross axial loading of the lumbar spine frequently results in burst compression fractures at the L2, L3, or L4 level (Figs. 11.40A–11.40C). The result is injury to the cauda equina by virtue of bone extrusion from the posterior wall of the involved vertebra posteriorly.

The question of stability of the thoracolumbar spine is defined as an angular deformity of less than 30% of kyphosis, less than 30% loss of vertebral body height with no injury to the middle column, and less than 10% of scoliosis.[18,103,104] Fractures of the upper thoracic spine can generally be treated conservatively (see Fig. 11.9). Unstable fractures (defined as two-column injuries resulting in specific degrees of angular or horizontal displacement) require surgical intervention (Fig. 11.41). The unstable spine frequently requires surgical intervention by one of several means: Harrington rods,[19a,34,36] the addition of Edwards sleeves to Harrington rods,[35] Jacobs rods (a variation of the Harrington rod theme),[13,105] Luque rods,[28] the Keene Wisconsin compression systems,[106] Roy-Camille[107,108] or Steffee[109] plates and pedicle screws, Cotrel–Dubousset (C–D) pedicle screws,[24] and A-O pedicle screw internal fixator.[56] Each of these procedures has its primary function as the restoration of spine stability, more rapid mobilization, and rehabilitation. Some authors are of the opinion that early restoration of spinal stability prevents the occurrence of such complications as adult respiratory distress syndrome (ARDS), multiple organ system failure (MOSF), deep venous thrombosis (DVT), and pulmonary embolism.[34,110,111]

Figure 11.39. **A.** L3 compressive flexion or burst fracture. **B.** AP roentgenogram demonstrates rotational component.

Surgical Approach to the Thoracic, Thoracolumbar and Lumbar Spine

Stability of the thoracic or lumbar spine can be achieved either through the posterior approach using internal fixation (Figs. 11.42A and 11.42B) or anteriorly using either plates and screws,[112] Kostuik screws with Harrington rods,[113] the Zielke,[114] or the Dwyer[115] device when anterior neural canal decompression is required.

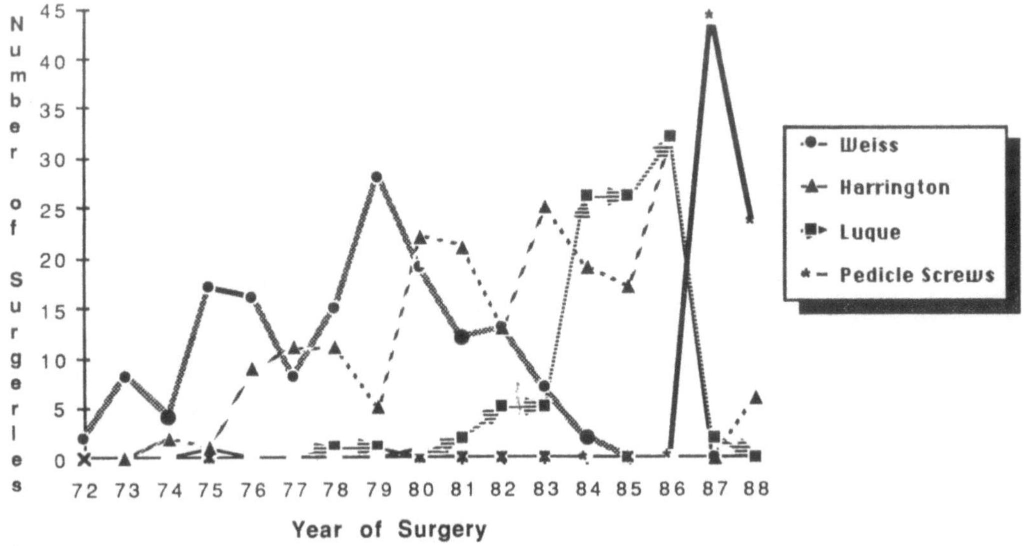

Figure 11.41. Trends in fusion and internal fixation techniques for thoracolumbar spine fractures, Northwestern University Acute Spine Injury Center, June 1972–October 1988. Evolution in spine fracture instrumentation procedures. Operative intervention of fractured spine came into vogue. Introduced into the United States (1972) were the Polish Weiss springs. With experience gained from scoliosis management, Harrington rod instrumentation (1973) became the most acceptable and consistent spine fixation technique. Two new techniques: Luque rods with sublaminar wires (1981) and the most direct approach to stabilization of the spine, pedicle screws (1986). Internal fixation and spine fusion are companion procedures.

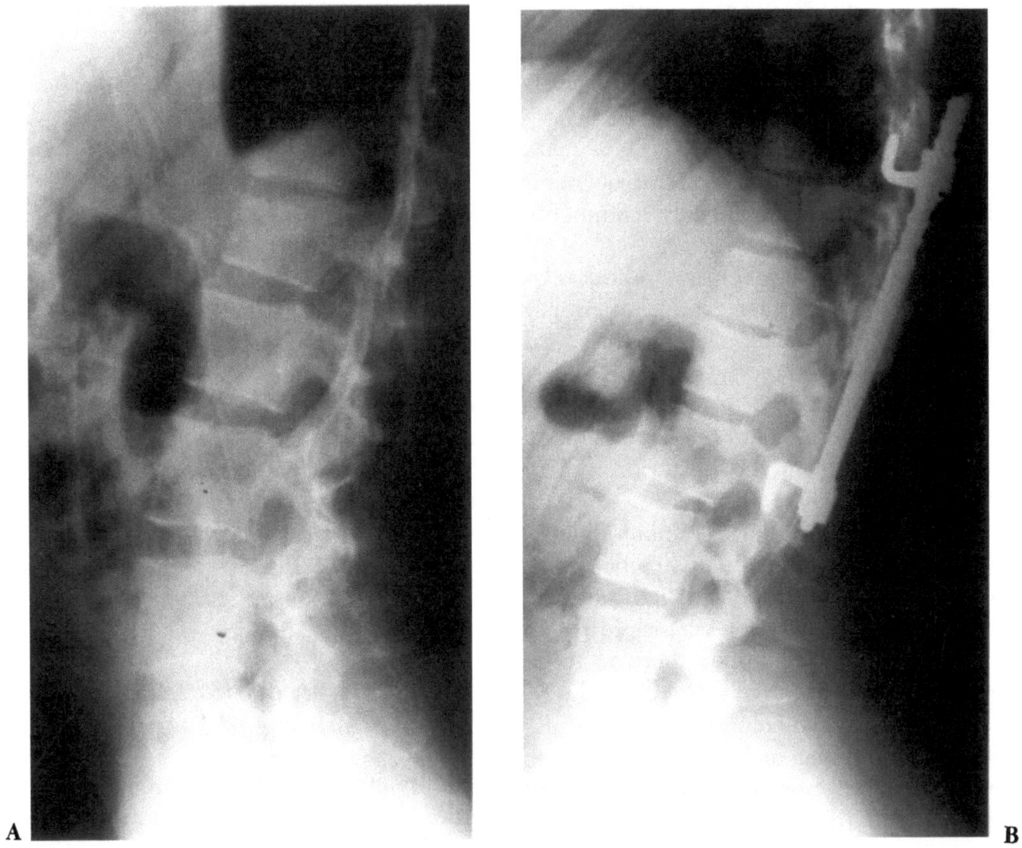

Figure 11.42. **A.** L1 burst fracture in neurologically intact patient with 30% canal compromise. **B.** Posterior stabilization and fusion performed with Harrington rods, Edwards sleeves, and iliac crest bone graft.

Table 11.7. Surgical approaches to thoracic and lumbar spine, June 1972–October 1988[a]

	Cervical (C1–C7)	Thoracic (T1–T9)	Thoracolumbar (T10–L2)	Lumbar (L3–L5)	Thoracolumbar Total	Thoracolumbar %
Posterior	532	118	250	36	404	—
Combined	7	9	46 (13%)	2	57	14
Anterior	140	4	16	4	24	—
Staged	6	3	15 (4%)	1	19	5
Missing	26	8	18	4	30	—
Total	711	142	345	47	534	—

[a] The more frequent surgical approach to either the cervical or thoracolumbar spine is the posterior approach. As noted in Fig. 11.15, the increased use of the A-O plate fixation for fractures of the cervical spine has resulted in a comparable increase in the number of anterior approaches. Of note in the thoracolumbar region is the rather high frequency with which the combined (simultaneous) anterior-posterior approach versus the staged anterior-posterior approach was used. The rationale was a need for posterior stabilization of the vertebral column, followed immediately by anterior neural canal (dural) decompression, and either vertebral column bone grafting and/or internal fixation.

Where significant vertebral column instability exists in combination with intact or incompletely injured neurological tissue and is compromised anteriorly, a combined (either simultaneous or staged) approach (Table 11.7) is preferred. In those cases where anterior fracture decompression of the neural canal is indicated, a vertebral body corpectomy (Figs. 11.43A and 11.43B) with bone grafting is performed. Stability is not gained by this procedure alone but in combination with a posterior procedure (Figs. 11.44A and 11.44B). It is the surgeon's choice as to whether the procedure is performed either first, posteriorly followed by anteriorly, together, or vice versa. Between 1972 and October 1988, 534 thoracolumbar spinal injuries were operated upon at Northwestern University (Table

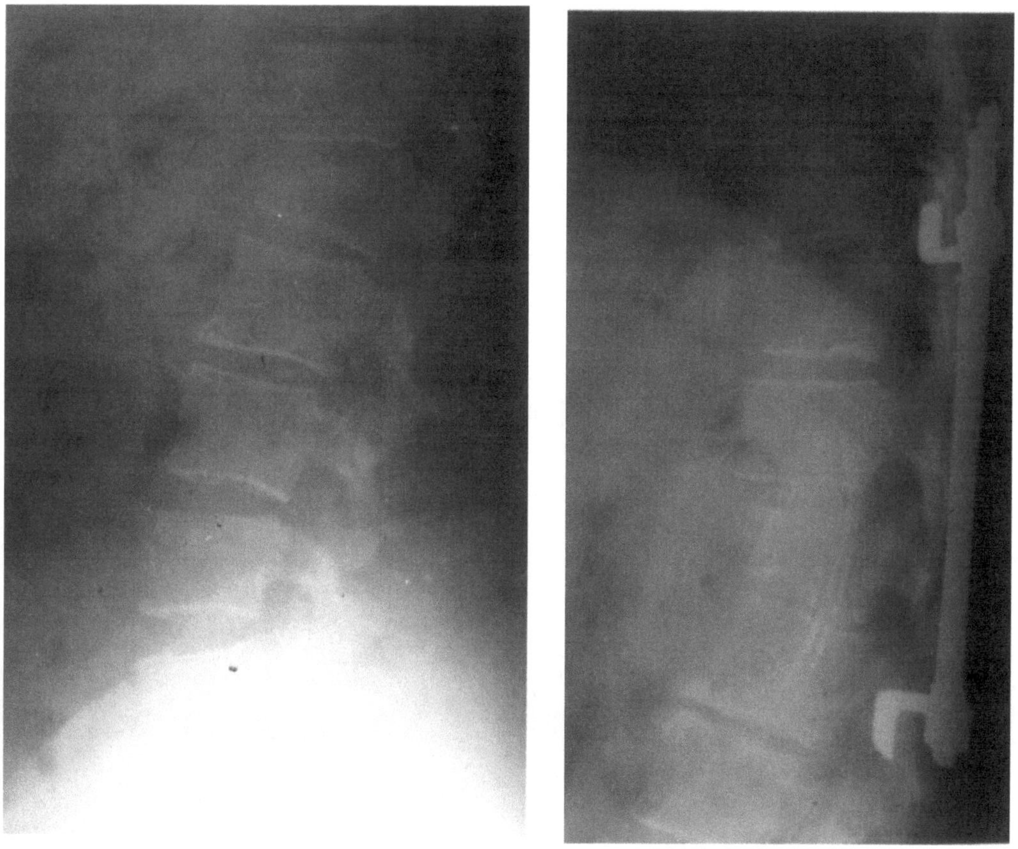

A B

Figure 11.43. **A.** T12 burst fracture in patient with 50% canal compromise and incomplete paraplegia. **B.** Anterior corpectomy and fusion with rib autografts and simultaneous posterior stabilization with Harrington rods and iliac crest autograft. Note fatigue fractures of rib grafts.

Table 11.8. Surgical deaths from cervical-thoracic-lumbar spine procedures, June 1972 to October 1988

	Cervical (C1–C7)	Thoracic (T1–T9)	Thoracolumbar (T10–L2)	Lumbar (L3–L5)	Missing thoracolumbar	Thoracolumbar	
						Total	%
Posterior	18	6	2	0	1	9/404	2
Combined	1	0	1	0	0	1/57	2
Anterior	6	1	0	0	1	2/24	8
Staged	1	1	0	0	0	1/19	5
Missing	1	1	0	0	0	1/30	3
Total	30	9	3	0	2	14/534	2.6

11.8). There were 14 deaths in the series (2.6%). In the patients who underwent posterior surgery alone (404), there were 9 deaths (2%). In the 100 patients who had anterior spinal surgery, there were 2 deaths in the anterior alone group (8%), 1 death in the staged group (5%), and 1 death in the combined group (2%). Although the patient numbers are small, the mortality rates are lowest, but still not statistically significant, for the combined group when evaluating the anterior spinal surgery patients.

There is seldom an indication for the performance of the laminectomy procedure in the thoracic or lumbar spine in association with trauma. If utilized, the laminectomy must be accompanied by an arthrodesis with internal fixation[12,77,116] (Figs. 11.45A–11.45D). There is controversy over whether it has any beneficial effects in trauma.[5,75,76]

Axial Load Compression or Burst Fractures

Axial load burst fractures of the vertebral column occur most frequently at the thoracolumbar junction (T10–L2) and the midlumbar spine (L2–L4). These are the result of excessive compression and/or flexion forces and frequently produce failure of all three "Denis" columns.[4,51] In the presence of this combination of forces in which the anterior and posterior columns fail and the middle

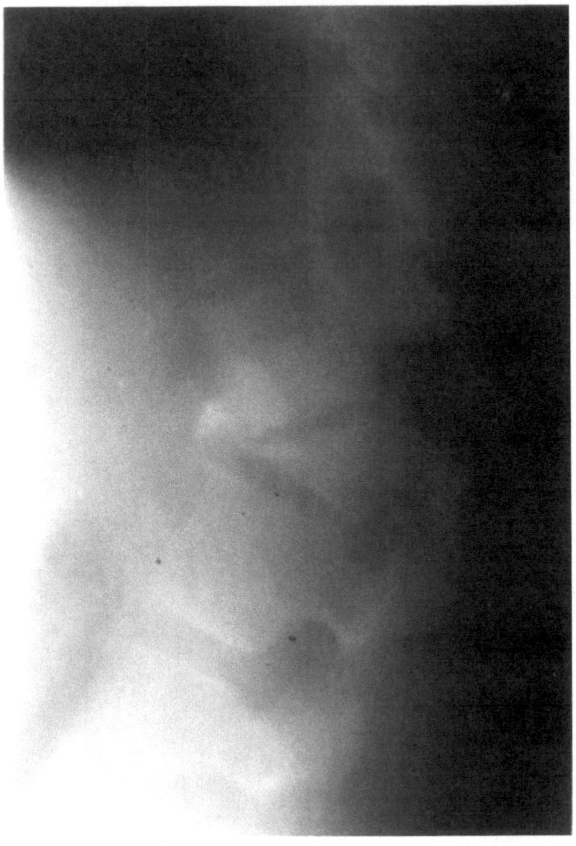

A

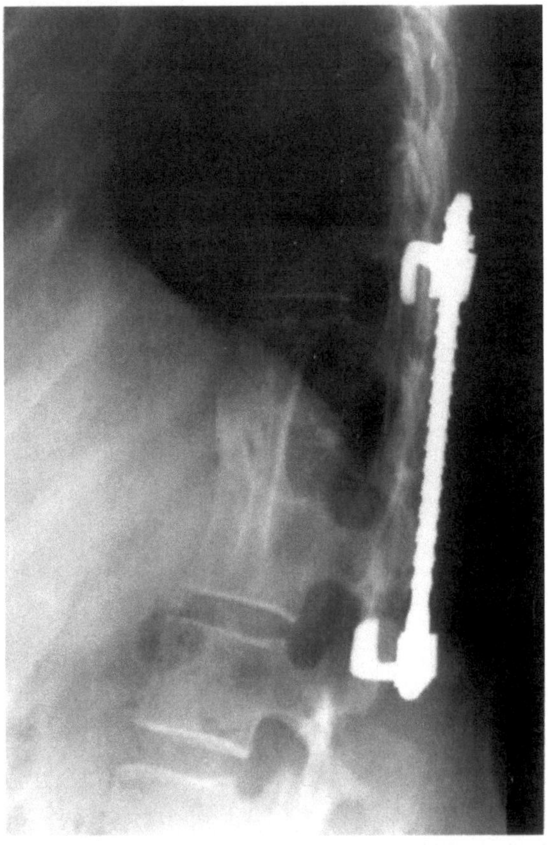

B

Figure 11.44. **A.** Lateral tomogram of L1 burst fracture in patient with complete paraplegia who was treated nonoperatively. Pain and deformity were reasons for referral. **B.** Anterior corpectomy and fusion with tricortical iliac graft and posterior stabilization with Edwards compression rods and fusion with iliac crest graft.

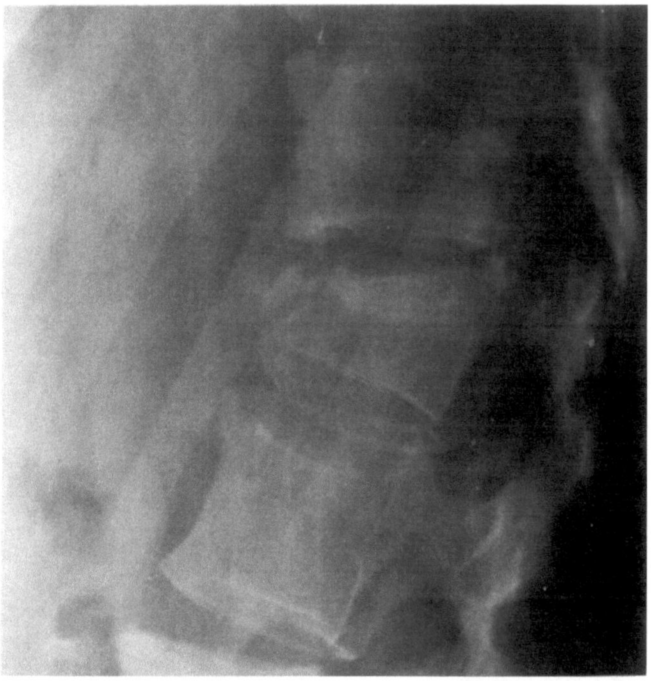
A

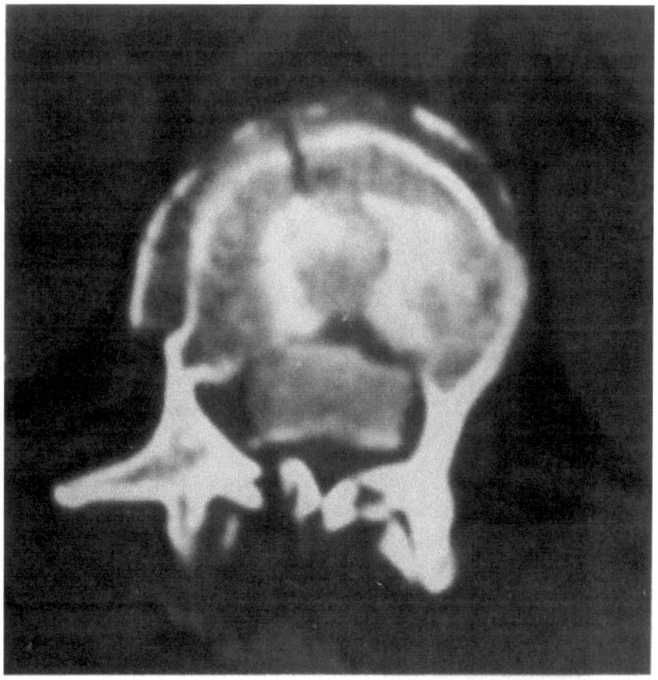
B

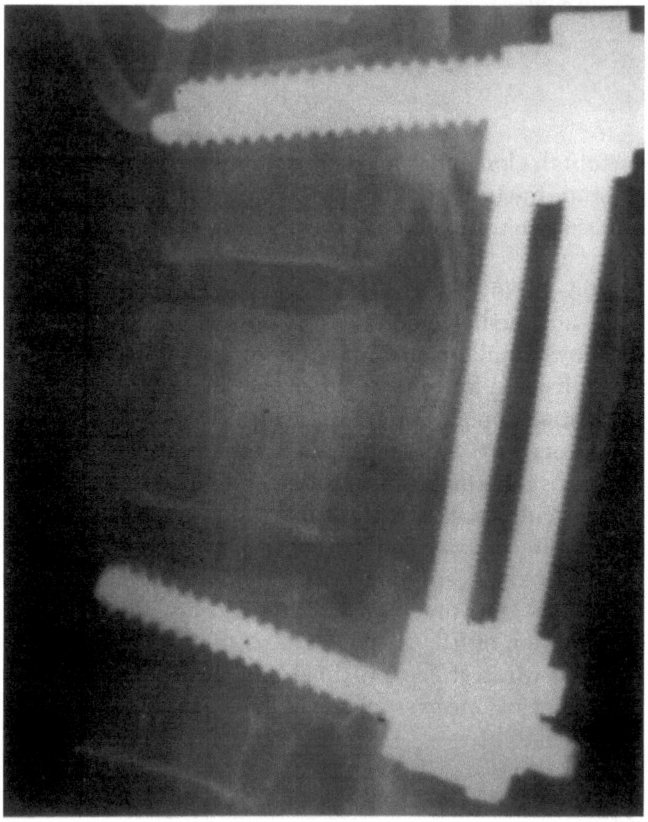
C

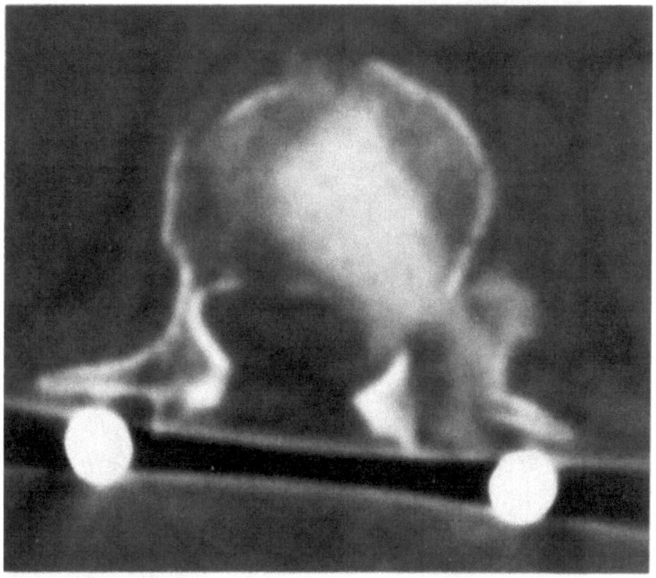
D

Figure 11.45. **A.** L2 burst fracture in patient who fell and had incomplete paraplegia. **B.** Axial CAT scan shows 90% canal compromise. **C.** Reduction, fixation using posterior spinal fixator (PSF), and posterolateral arthrodesis with iliac crest bone graft were performed 6 months previously. **D.** Axial CAT scan shows laminectomy defect for canal compression and intravertebral body bone grafting (iliac crest) via the pedicle. (Courtesy of Professor Sven Olerud, Uppsala, Sweden.)

column remains intact,[7] Harrington distraction or compression rods,[13,19a,34,36] pedicle screws and plates,[107–109] internal spinal fixators,[56] or Luque rods[28] represent the methods of fixation most appropriate. The Magerl "external spinal fixator"[117] has not yet reached a state of use or acceptance to be adequately discussed. On the other hand, the Luque rod system is now recognized as not being indicated as a means of internal stabilization when axial loading has resulted in a gross bursting of the vertebral body and lateral translation between the two adjacent

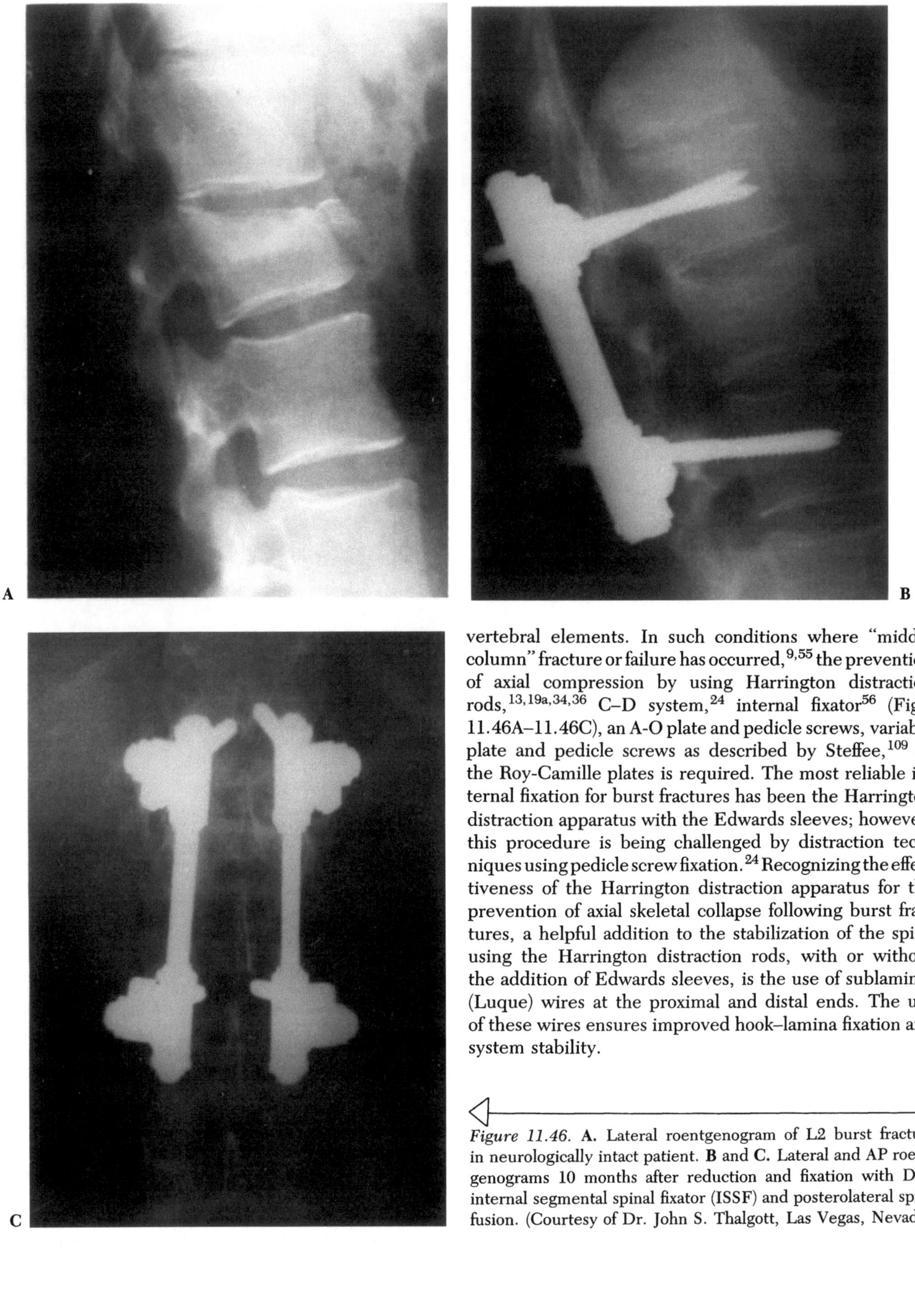

vertebral elements. In such conditions where "middle column" fracture or failure has occurred,[9,55] the prevention of axial compression by using Harrington distraction rods,[13,19a,34,36] C–D system,[24] internal fixator[56] (Figs. 11.46A–11.46C), an A-O plate and pedicle screws, variable plate and pedicle screws as described by Steffee,[109] or the Roy-Camille plates is required. The most reliable internal fixation for burst fractures has been the Harrington distraction apparatus with the Edwards sleeves; however, this procedure is being challenged by distraction techniques using pedicle screw fixation.[24] Recognizing the effectiveness of the Harrington distraction apparatus for the prevention of axial skeletal collapse following burst fractures, a helpful addition to the stabilization of the spine using the Harrington distraction rods, with or without the addition of Edwards sleeves, is the use of sublaminar (Luque) wires at the proximal and distal ends. The use of these wires ensures improved hook–lamina fixation and system stability.

Figure 11.46. **A.** Lateral roentgenogram of L2 burst fracture in neurologically intact patient. **B** and **C.** Lateral and AP roentgenograms 10 months after reduction and fixation with Dick internal segmental spinal fixator (ISSF) and posterolateral spine fusion. (Courtesy of Dr. John S. Thalgott, Las Vegas, Nevada.)

In the presence of bony compression into the neural canal in the patient with incomplete neurological injury, anterior decompression as noted previously is frequently required in conjunction with posterior stabilization. The anterior approaches most frequently utilized are the eleventh rib thoracotomy approach,[24] and the transpleural, retroperitoneal, and thoracolumbar approaches.[2,24,117,118,119]

Chance Fractures

The Chance or seatbelt fracture[120–122] is a flexion distraction injury to the vertebral column. Chance fractures vary in type and stability.[123] Because these fractures are often pure bony fractures, that is, injuries that horizontally split the transverse process and posterior elements (Figs. 11.47A–11.47D), they can be managed in extension by postural reduction and body casting. Associated with Chance fractures is a high incidence of intraabdominal injuries (20%).[24] Because of the mechanism of injury, preference is given to the use of compressive devices (Figs. 11.48A–11.48E), which might include Weiss springs,[24] Harrington compression rods, C–D system, or A–O internal fixator devices in addition to spine fusion. Compression of the diastased posterior elements is particularly required when a ligamentous injury is associated with a Chance fracture or Chance-type injury.

Facet Dislocations

Facet dislocations are frequently flexion distraction injuries of the upper and midportion of the lumbar spine. A unilateral facet dislocation is often associated with a torsional flexion force (Figs. 11.49A and 11.49B) while the bilateral facet dislocation (Figs. 11.50A and 11.50B) is usually one of flexion and distraction.[7] During the resuscitation phase, patients sustaining this type of injury in the presence of a complete neurological injury are treated by closed reduction,[24] or, in the presence of an incomplete neurological injury, require postural reduction and subsequent internal fixation with spine fusion. When a dislocation of facets exists in the presence of an intact or incomplete neurological system, immediate open reduction should be undertaken if there is evidence of increasing neurological compromise, or early open reduction (within 24 to 36 hours) if the neurological examination reveals the nervous system to be intact or stable.

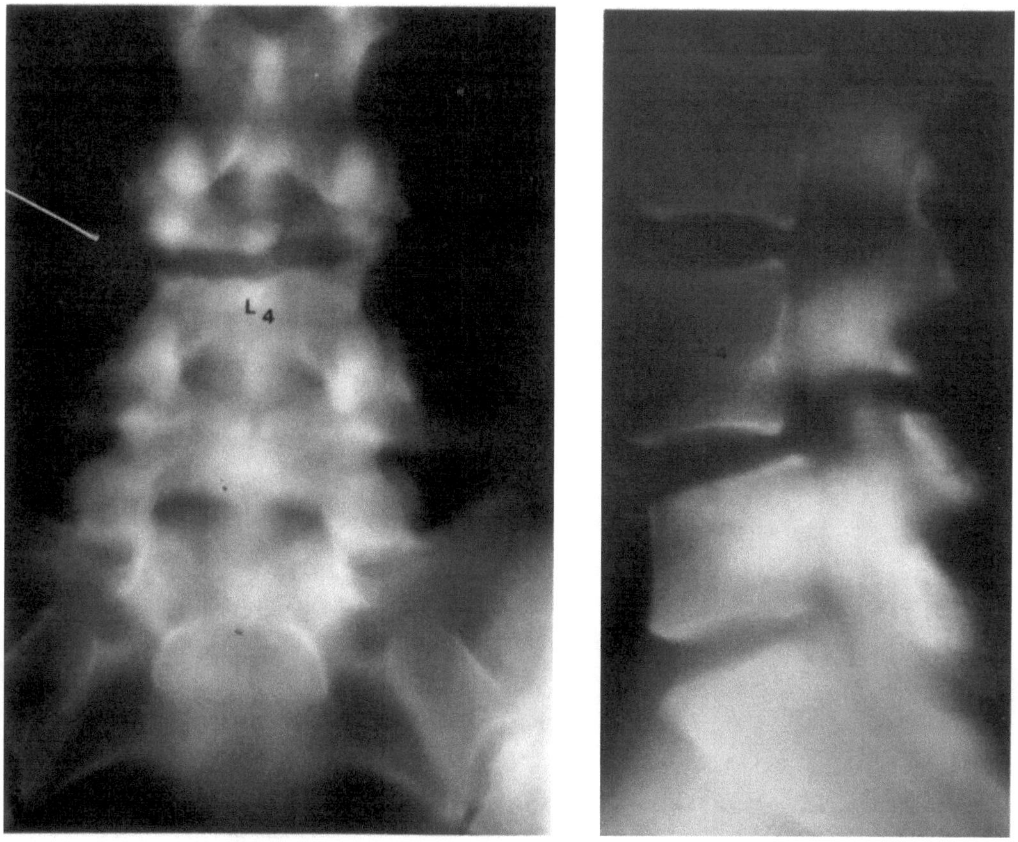

A B

Figure 11.47. L4 Chance fracture. **A.** AP tomogram. **B.** Lateral tomogram. **C** and **D.** Postoperative views after stabilization with Cotrel–Dubousset pedicle screw fixation and posterolateral iliac fusion (*see next p.*).

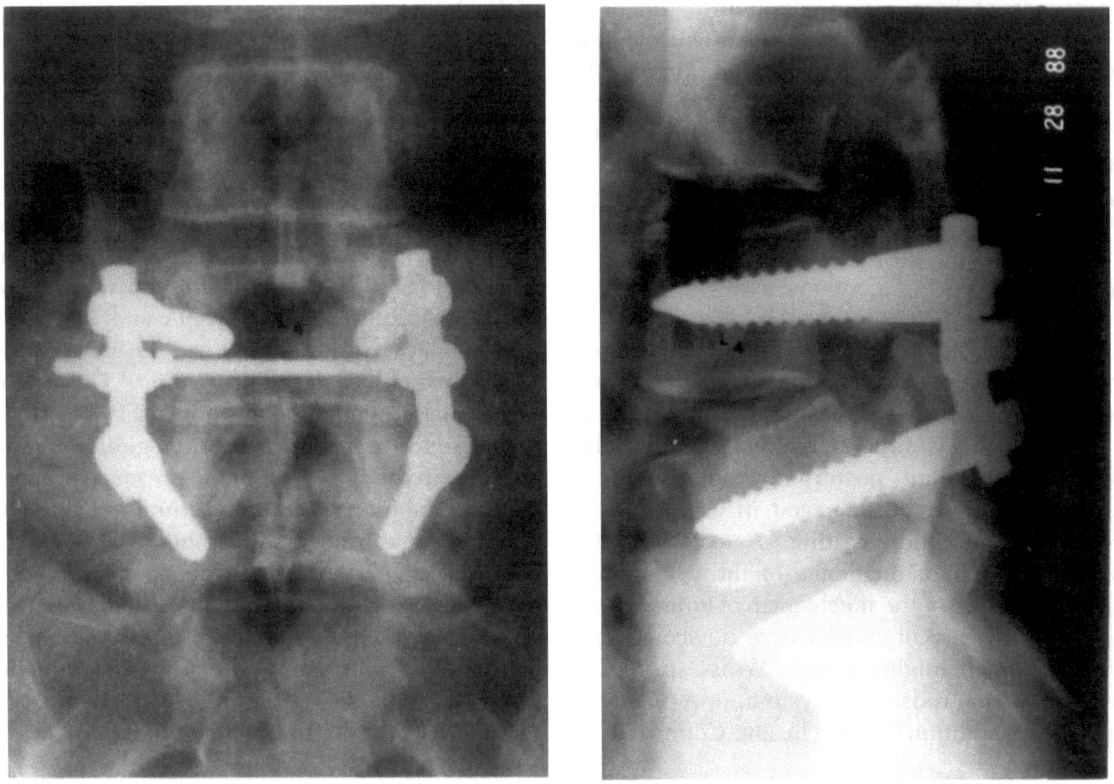

C D

Figure 11.47

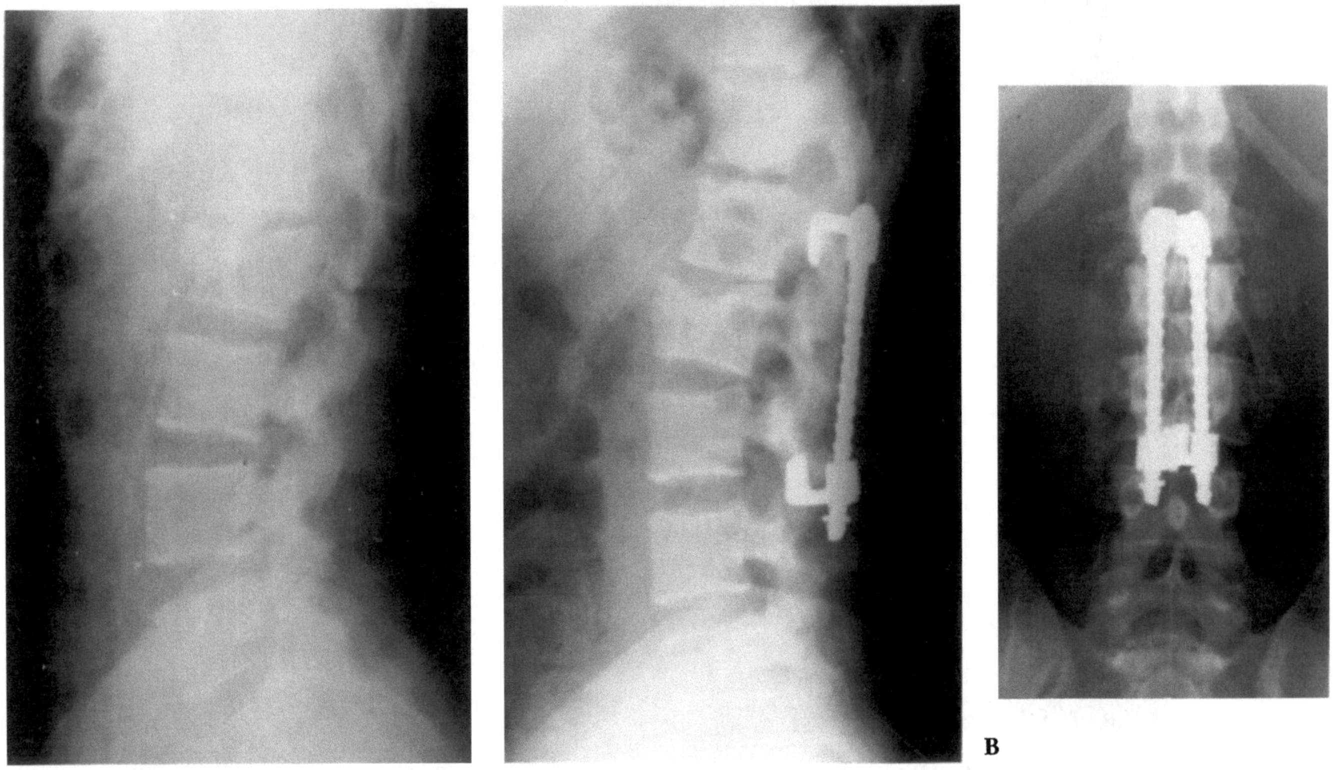

A B C

Figure 11.48. **A.** L2 Chance fracture **B** and **C.** AP and lateral roentgenograms of Chance fracture treated with Edwards compression rods and posterolateral iliac graft.

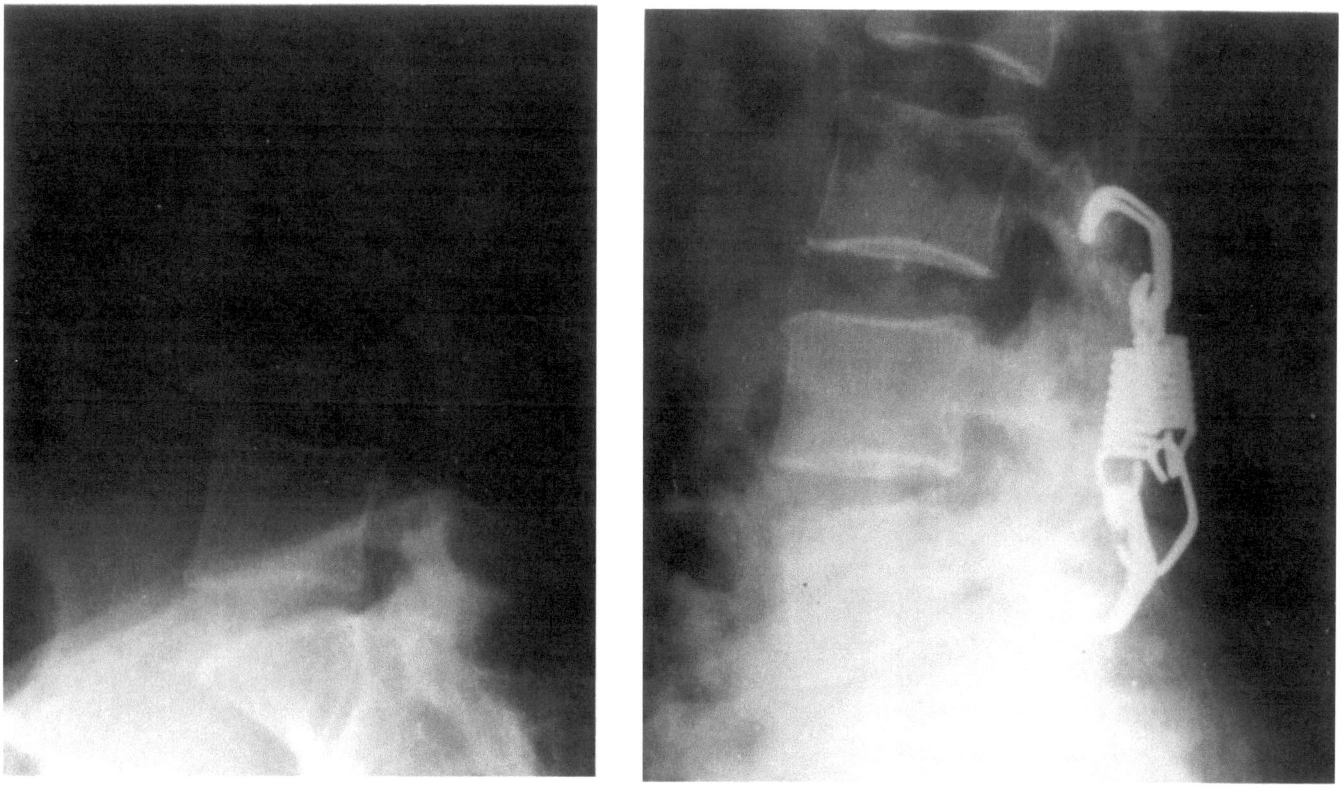

A B

Figure 11.49. **A.** L4–L5 unilateral facet dislocation. **B.** Injury was treated by Weiss springs and posterolateral fusion with iliac crest graft.

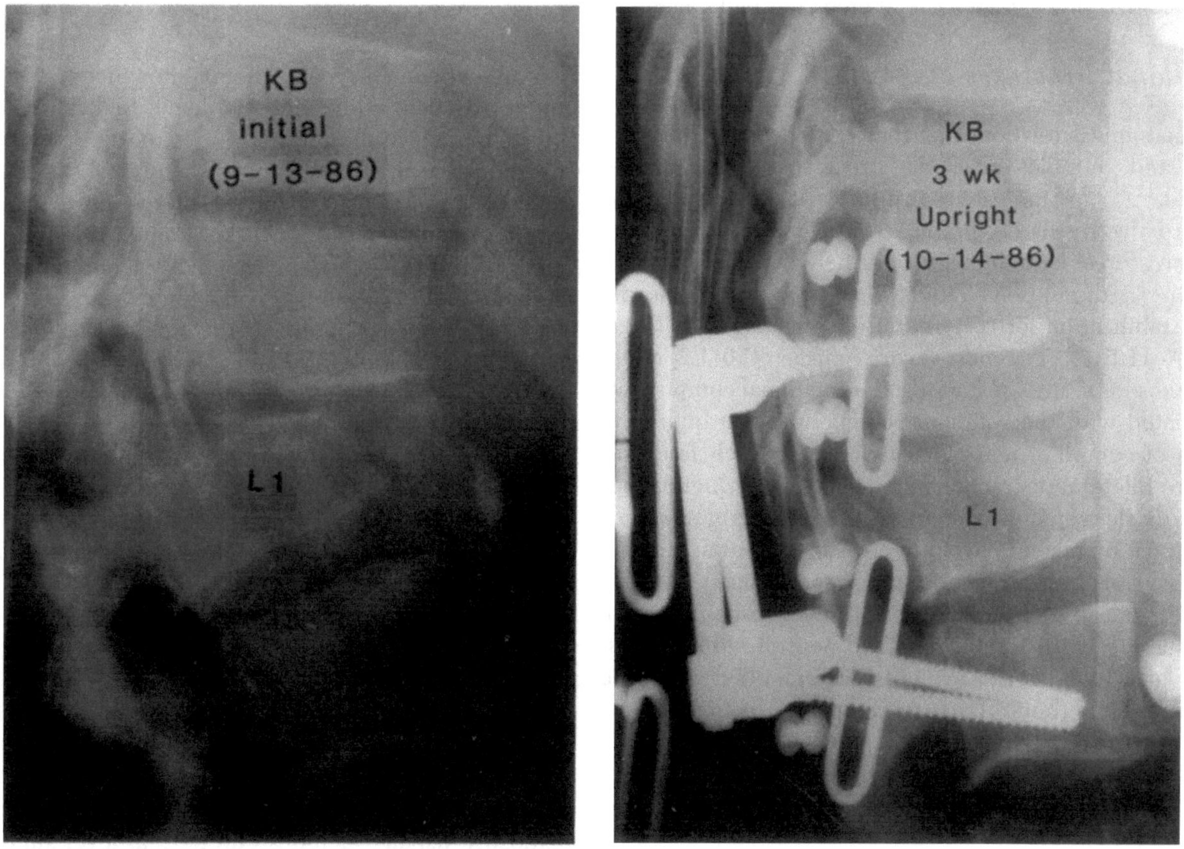

A B

Figure 11.50. **A.** T12–L1 bilateral facet dislocation with complete paraplegia treated by (**B**) open reduction, stabilization with Vermont spinal fixator (VSF), and posterolateral fusion. (Courtesy of Dr. Martin Krag, Burlington, Vermont.)

A,B

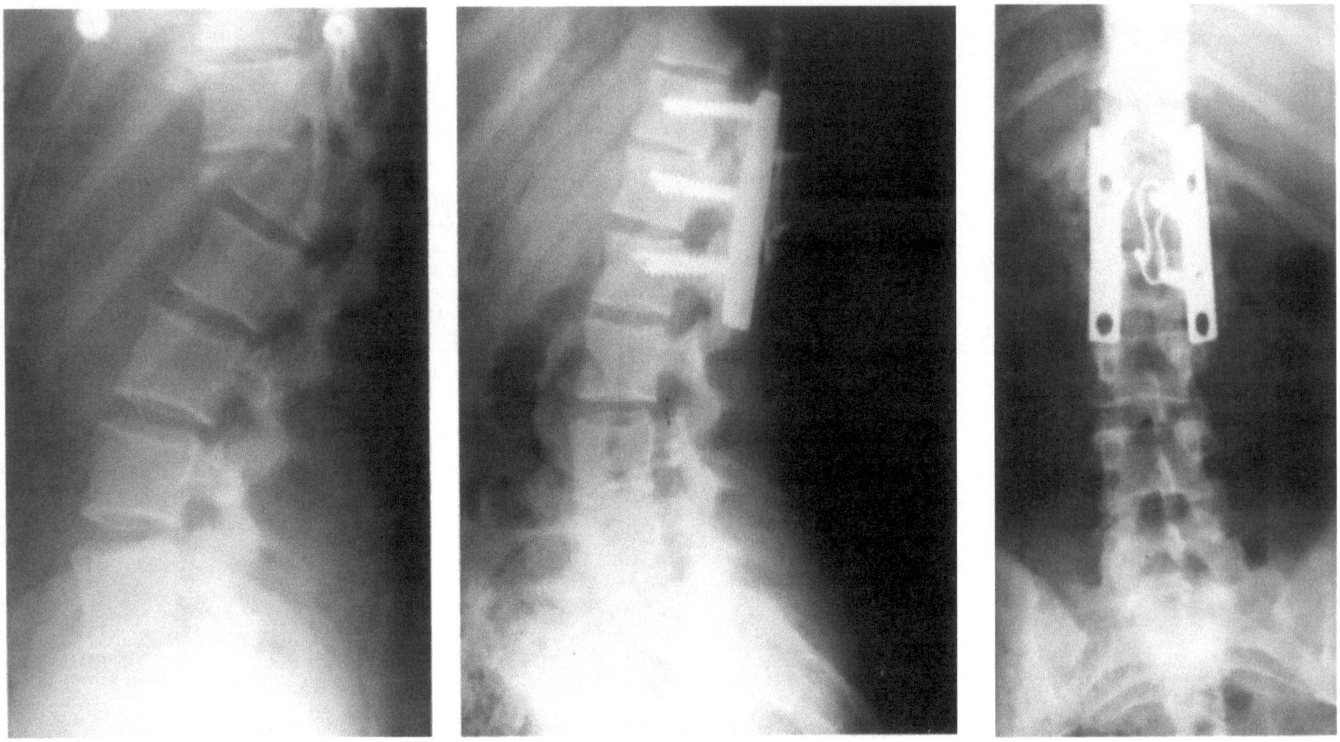

C

Figure 11.51. **A.** T12–L1 Holdsworth fracture. **B** and **C.** After open reduction, reduction was maintained with interspinous wires and A-O plates; posterolateral fusion was performed.

Rotational Fractures

The anatomical relationships that exist between the thoracic and lumbar articular processes, as just described,[12,18,24,52] indicate that injuries at this level generally are the result of combined axial load, flexion, and rotation forces producing a grossly unstable three-column[4,51] disruption (Holdsworth fracture) requiring early stabilization for restoration of spinal stability (Figs. 11.51A–11.51C). The most severe injuries (T10–L2) result from those fractures sustaining the rotational component. Associated with the rotational component is a high incidence of complete neurological injury.[24] Such fractures require bilateral distraction stabilization (Harrington rod, Edwards sleeve, C–D system, and A–O internal fixator). Care must be taken to avoid overdistraction from circumferential soft-tissue envelope disruption in many of these injuries. Because of the failure to provide sustaining axial load stability with Luque rods and neutralization plates, these latter two devices are not recommended when the vertebral body (burst) fracture component is present.

Thoracolumbar Spine Fusion Techniques: Posterior Approach

The patient sustaining fracture to the thoracolumbar spine is most often managed on a wedge Stryker frame or a RotoRest bed. The goal is the maintenance of spinal alignment by means of the most stable method. The placement of the patient in the prone position on the operating table for the performance of a posterior surgical stabilizing procedure is most easily achieved by having the patient already placed on a wedge Stryker frame. A midline incision centered at the level of the most prominent posterior spinous process (gibbus) is carried down through the skin and subcutaneous tissue to the tips of the spinous processes. By Cobb elevator and electrocautery subperiosteal dissection, the posterior elements are exposed out to and including the facet joints. Exposing the tranverse process at the affected level (Fig. 11.52A) is included in the exposure when a costotransversectomy approach to the spinal canal is anticipated, a posterior lateral fusion is to be incorporated, or anatomical identification of the levels of the pedicles (where pedicle screws are to be used) is required. The normal extent of the required exposure depends on the procedure for posterior fixation. If Harrington distraction rods (with or without Edwards sleeves) or Luque rods are to be used, normal exposure includes posterior elements two normal levels above and two normal levels below the level of injury. For the patients in whom pedicle screw fixation is the treatment of choice, exposure usually includes one normal level superior and inferior to the level of injury. In the presence of what is described as a "ligamentous Chance" flexion distraction

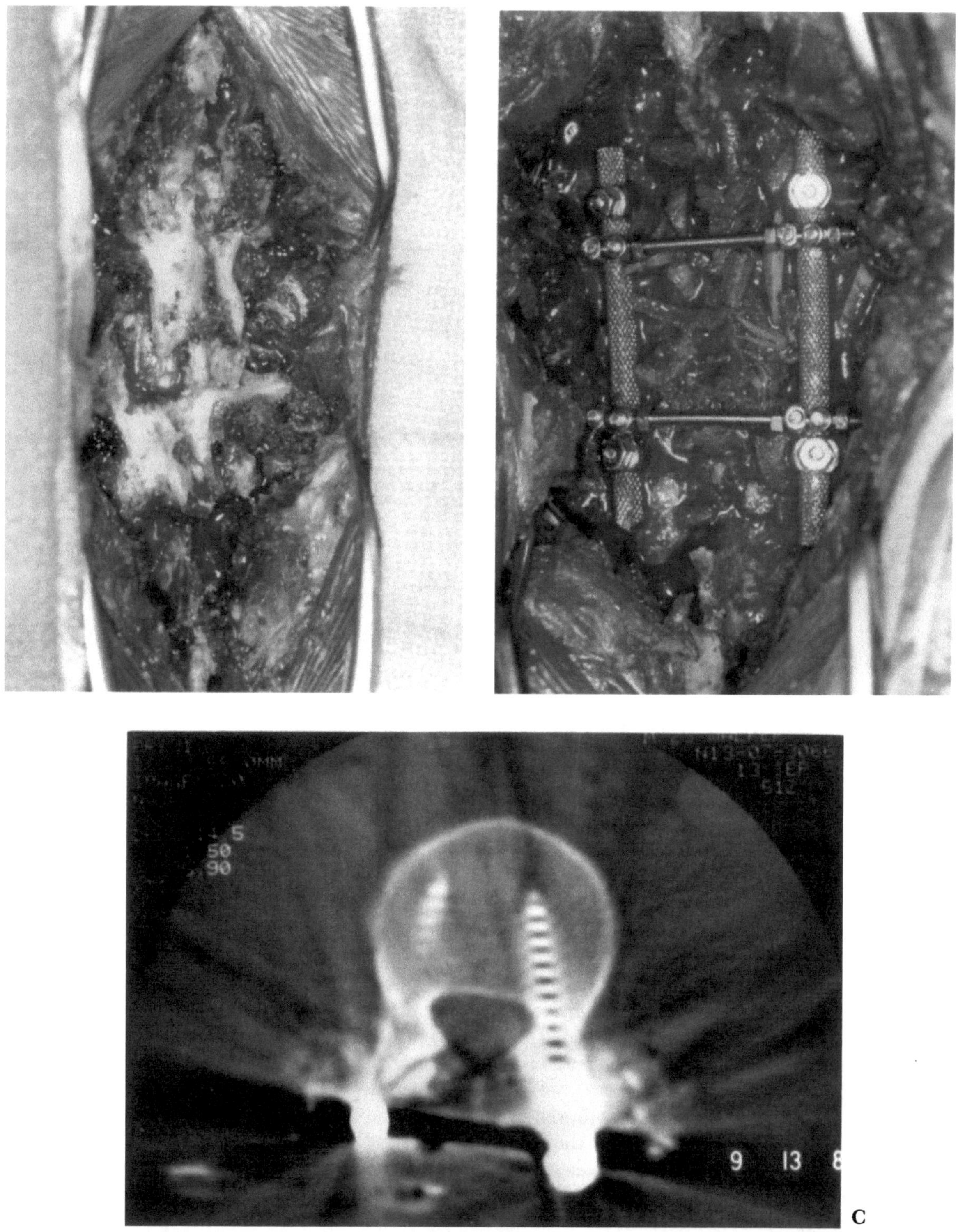

A B C

Figure 11.52. Posterior thoracolumbar spine fusion techniques. **A.** Exposure of posterior elements. **B.** Bone graft placement. **C.** Postoperative CAT scan displays ideal placement of pedicle screws. (*Continued.*)

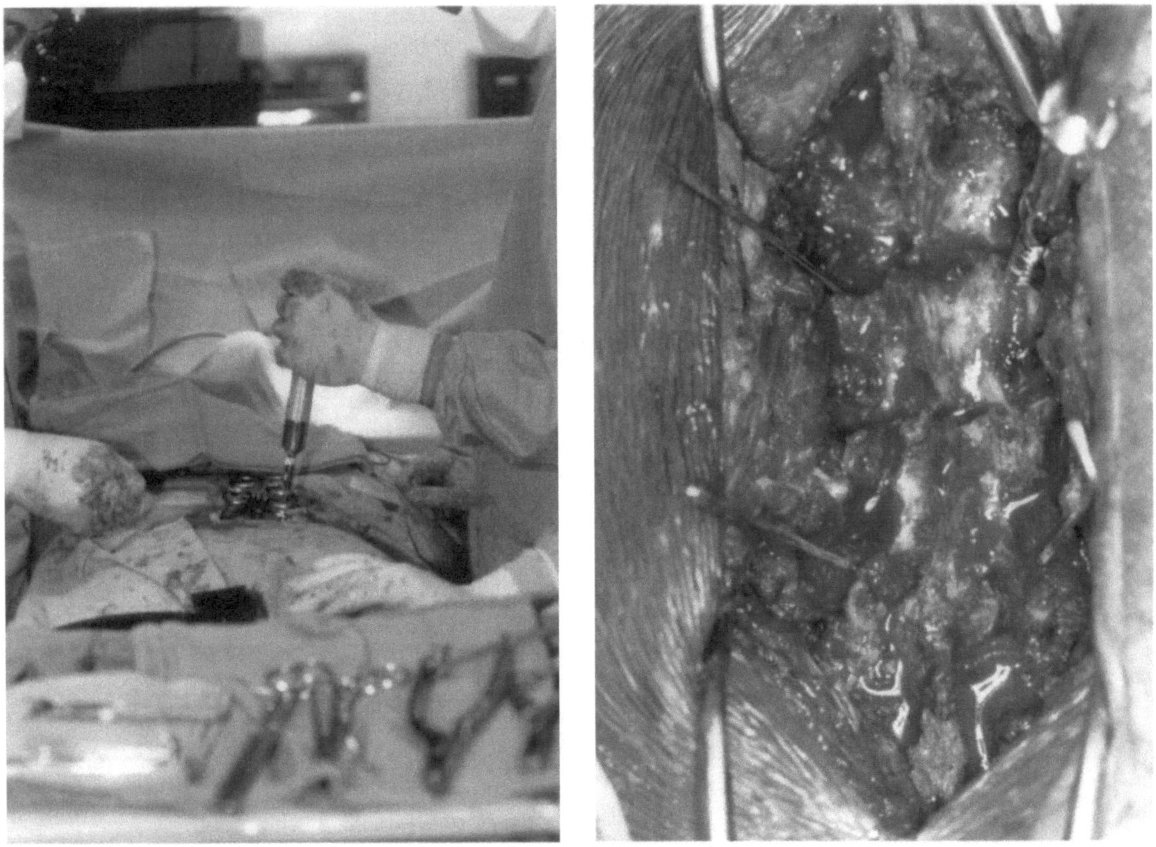

Figure 11.52. **D.** Sounding pedicle. **E.** 2-mm pins mark pedicles before insertion of pedicle screws (upper right).

injury, only the adjacent posterior elements at the level of the injury, if remaining intact, need to be stabilized. This implies the use of a cerclage wire around the spinous process,[24] neutralization plate and screws, or similar procedure.[109]

Soft tissue is removed from the posterior elements with a pituitary rongeur, Leksell rongeur, curette, and a high-speed carbide burr. This latter method of soft-tissue debridement is very effective for cleansing the external surface of the posterior bony elements. A high-speed diamond-tip burr is used when there is either concern for slippage of the burr or when working close to nervous tissue while using the burr. It is always appropriate to obtain an intraoperative lateral radiograph of the spine to document the appropriate level of the injury segment.

The posterior elements, including the spinous processes and laminae, and the appropriate facet joints are denuded of their external cortical surfaces with a high-speed carbide burr. This allows for exposure of a bleeding cancellous bone surface. As noted, the articular cartilage within the facet joints can either be removed using an appropriate size high-speed burr or a leksell rongeur. The instrumentation of choice is implanted based on the pathology and the requirements as described previously. When Harrington distraction hooks are used, very careful attention must be directed toward the notching (using a right-angle Kerrison rongeur) of the posterior laminae superiorly and inferiorly adjacent to the spinous processes so that the hook adequately enters the sublaminar space during insertion. Where enhanced stability of the distraction device is required, sublaminar wires at either one or two levels above and below the injury site can improve rod stability to the posterior lamina. Transverse wires between the two upright structures (one proximally and one distally) further enhance instrumentation stability.[24] After insertion of the appropriate internal fixation device, bone graft obtained from some additional source is inserted posteriorly and laterally. The spinous processes in the midline are frequently rongeured using the Leksell or Adson rongeur to expose bleeding bone to the bone graft. Cancellous bone is placed between the spinous processes, in the area of the facet joints, across the posterior laminae and out laterally between the transverse processes if these structures have been exposed (Fig. 11.52B).

In those instances where pedicle screws (Fig. 11.52C) are recommended, a 2-mm drill inserted through the pedicle into the vertebral body is directed internally in the thoracolumbar junction and the lumbar spine area 5° to

10° and perpendicular to the table top (Fig. 11.52D). Adjustment in the perpendicular (superior or inferior) orientation of the drill is achieved by intraoperative roentgenograms. After all drill holes and pedicles have been made and 2-mm pins have been inserted as markers, insertion of the pedicle screw of choice can then take place (Fig. 11.52E).

Bone Graft Site

Bone grafts can be obtained from one of two sources: the patient (autograft) or external donors (allograft). Where autogenous bone from the same patient is preferred, bone graft is normally obtained through a separate incision over the posterior lateral iliac crest. The incision follows the crest line to approximately the level of the sacroiliac joint with the ilium and external table exposed by careful subperiosteal and submuscular dissection. Depending on the type of graft desired, a segment of ilium to include both inner and outer tables may be removed, but more frequently external cortical "curls" and copious cancellous bone curls are obtained. These corticocancellous and cancellous strips are obained with a sharp gouge and mallet or curette. Bone harvested should be kept covered in blood-soaked sponges in a protective basin until used.

Commercial allografts are becoming available.[124] The allografts most frequently used are those obtained by the joint arthroplasty surgeon who, under sterile conditions, harvests the excised femoral head of the patient with severe coxa magna as a consequence of degenerative osteoarthritis of the hip. This latter bone graft, if adequate in size, is an excellent source of cancellous bone.

A third area from which bone is frequently obtained is from the rib excised during the thoracotomy approach. Every effort should be made to excise as much of the length of the rib as possible. This allows the rib to be split longitudinally and transversely, generally sufficient for four 6-cm "matchstick" grafts.

An additional source of bone graft for spanning an area of an excised vertebral body is the fibular graft (Fig. 11.53A). A section of fibula is removed through a separate incision over the lateral aspect of the midcalf. By careful subperiosteal dissection along the anterior border of the peroneal muscles between tissue planes, an area of fibula approximately 10 to 15 cm in length can be excised. This graft, once harvested, can either be inserted in toto after

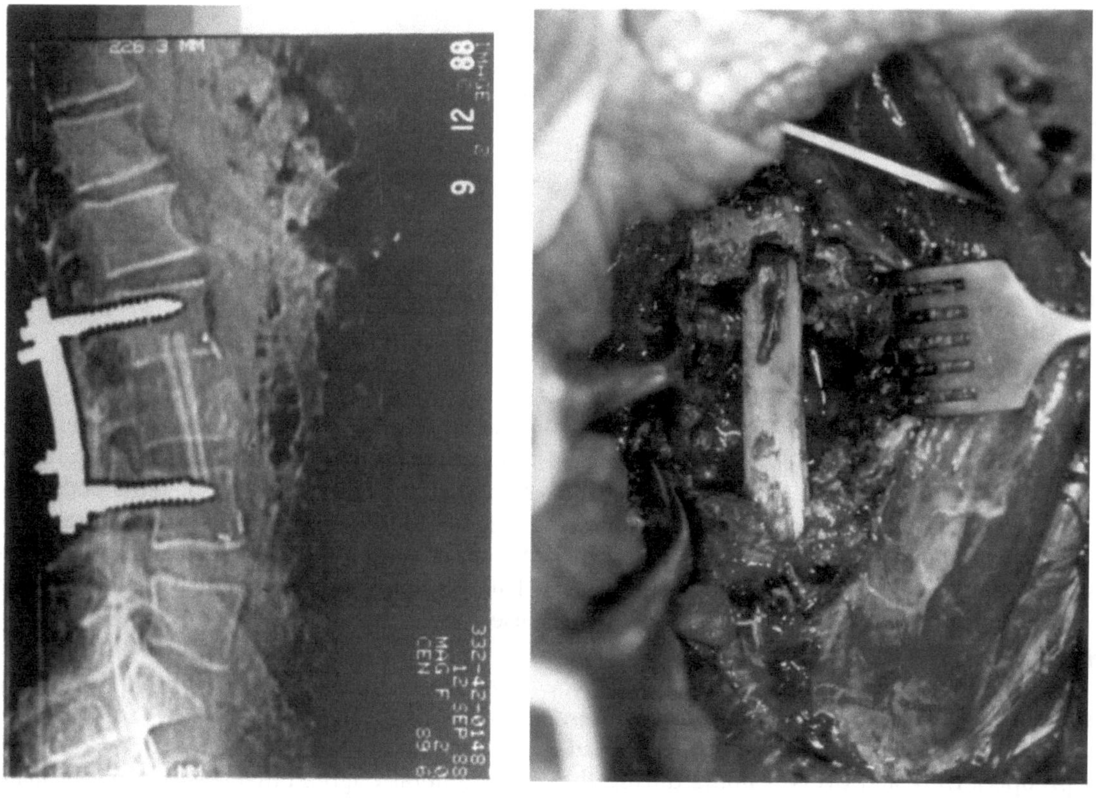

A B

Figure 11.53. **A.** Fibular graft spans L3 vertebral body after L3 corpectomy. **B.** Whole fibular graft inserted after corpectomy. (*Continued.*)

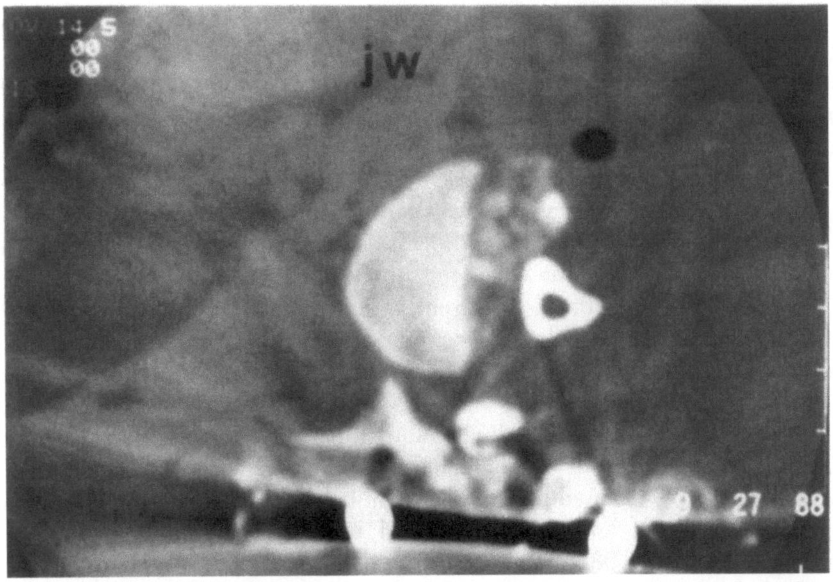

C

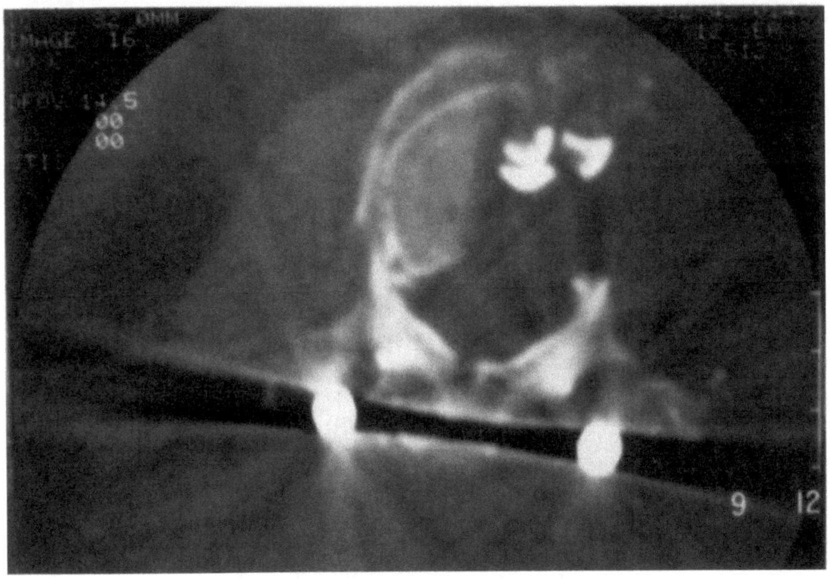

D

Figure 11.53. **C.** Postoperative CAT scan shows decompression and whole fibular graft. **D.** Postoperative CAT scan displays decompression and split fibular grafts.

being cut to an appropriate length (Figs. 11.53B and 11.53C) or split longitudinally and inserted as "matchstick" fibular grafts. The split fibular graft is thought to be the more appropriate technique, one that simultaneously exposes both the cortical and the cancellous surfaces of the fibula to surrounding new blood supply (Fig. 11.53D).

Antibiotic Coverage

Antibiotics are used during all major spine procedures. Normally, a gram of first-generation cephalosporin is administered preoperatively and every 4 hours during the operative procedure. This antibiotic administration is maintained every 6 hours parenterally for 48 hours. Likewise, the wound is irrigated throughout the operative procedure with an orthopaedic antibiotic irrigation solution that includes 1000 ml of 0.9% sodium chloride to which is added, under sterile conditions in the pharmacy, 80 mg of gentamycin and 10 meq of sodium bicarbonate. This solution is only for wound irrigation, not for parenteral use.

Thoracolumbar Spine Fusion Technique: Anterior Approach

It is generally agreed that, because of the anatomical relationship of the aorta and vena cava to the thoracic and thoracolumbar spine, the appropriate direction to the spine is via the left thoracotomy or flank approach. The level of the surgical approach obviously relates to the level of pathology. The most utilitarian approach to the thoracolumbar spine for lesions lying between T10 and L2 is that made by an approach through the chest at the T11 level with excision of the eleventh rib and the use of this rib as a "matchstick" graft.[24] The performance of this approach when involving the chest is transpleural. To facilitate this exposure, the diaphragm, which takes its origin from the rib cage (the crux of the diaphragm) between T10 and T12, is incised from posterior to anterior.

For lesions involving the thoracic spine between T1 and T6, the most appropriate approach is through the right chest or through an extended right sternocleidomastoid incision carried inferiorly through the sternoclavicular joint and the first and second ribs. The right approach to the upper thoracic spine is preferred as it is easier mobilizing the azygos vein than the aortic arch.

Utilizing the left flank approach, the internal oblique muscles and transversalis muscle are incised and the dissection is carried posteriorly and retroperitoneally via the interval between the psoas muscle and the posterior peritoneal. Careful attention must be paid to identifying the ureter, which is taken anteriorly with the reflected peritoneum and those nerve roots that exit through the iliopsoas from the upper lumbar spine (ilioinguinal, iliofemoral, and femoral nerves).

The positioning of the patient on the operating table that most easily facilitates the thoracotomy or flank approach is the right lateral decubitus position. The patient is so placed on the table with the right side down and the patient perpendicular to the table top. The patient's pelvis and shoulders are fixed to the table with sandbags, kidney rests, bean bag, or adhesive tape. Changes in the patient's position can be made by lateral rotation of the operating table if required.

Upon entering the chest or the retroperitoneal area, the vertebral column is identified, a needle marker inserted into an easily identified disc space, and a lateral roentgenogram of the spine obtained for proper level identification. Using electrocautery dissection of the reflective pleura and subperiosteal dissection overlying the vertebral bodies, the anterior longitudinal ligament, which is firmly adherent at each level to the annulus fibrosis, is incised. Segmental vessels passing from the area of the neuroforamen posteriorly to anteriorly, identified during the dissection, are either ligated by vascular clips or cauterized using electrocautery and then cut in two by cautery or sharp dissection. To present, no documented neurological injury has followed or been associated with the unilateral anterior transection of segmental vessels.

With the development of the subperiosteal anterior longitudinal ligament plane, Chandler or Bennett retractors are inserted to further establish and protect the anterior structures from the vertebral column surgical dissection.[24,118,119] Following accurate identification of the level of injury (Figs. 11.54A–11.54E), the intervertebral disc proximal and distal to the affected area is excised by sharp dissection and the use of a leksell rongeur. Dissection should always be directed away from the anteriorly placed retractors. The excision of the affected vertebral body and eventual posterior neural canal decompression is accomplished by removal of major segments of the fractured vertebral body using a Leksell rongeur. Small loose fragments of comminuted vertebral body and/or cancellous bone can be removed with a pituitary rongeur. Compacted bone is easily removed using the high-speed carbide burr (two-hand technique). When approaching and working in close proximity to the dura, a diamond-tip burr is used.

The extent of vertebral body corpectomy depends in large part on the pathology. Normally, the right anterior and lateral aspects of the vertebral body need not be removed, only a sufficient amount of vertebral body to allow visualization and decompression of the dural column anteriorly. The cartilaginous endplates of the superior endplate of the inferior vertebral body and the inferior endplate of the superior body are cleansed by sharp dissection curettage and a high-speed carbide burr. Because of the presence of epidural veins, dissection in the area of the dura may be tedious, and blood loss, while appearing to be modest, in time may be significant. Bipolar cauterization of all epidural bleeders is indicated if possible.

When cleansing of the vertebral endplates is complete, the graft bed is prepared. Using a high-speed carbide burr, a groove is made in the anterior lateral surface of the superior aspect of the inferior vertebral body and a similar groove is made in the anterolateral inferior aspect of the superior vertebra. This groove extends back from the endplate approximately 1 cm and enters the vertebral body in depth by approximately 1 to 2 cm. The width of this groove should not exceed 1 cm on its external cortical surface, but may be undercut into a hollow cave to accept the longitudinal "matchstick" grafts as they are impacted into the grooves superiorly and inferiorly.[24] If a tricortical iliac crest graft has been selected rather than a matchstick graft, this graft can likewise be inserted into the grooved area with appropriate shaping of the graft. When inserting the primary intervertebral body graft, additional cancellous bone is applied anteriorly to the graft, filling the space out to the anterior longitudinal ligament. To prevent inadvertent dural compression, no additional bone graft is placed posteriorly. The reflected pleura periosteal cuff incised during the approach is closed with a running #0 chromic suture. The diaphragm is closed with a #2-0 interrupted dexon suture.

Several important considerations: The surgical approach to the chest and the abdomen is routinely made with appropriate surgical consultants; decompression of the

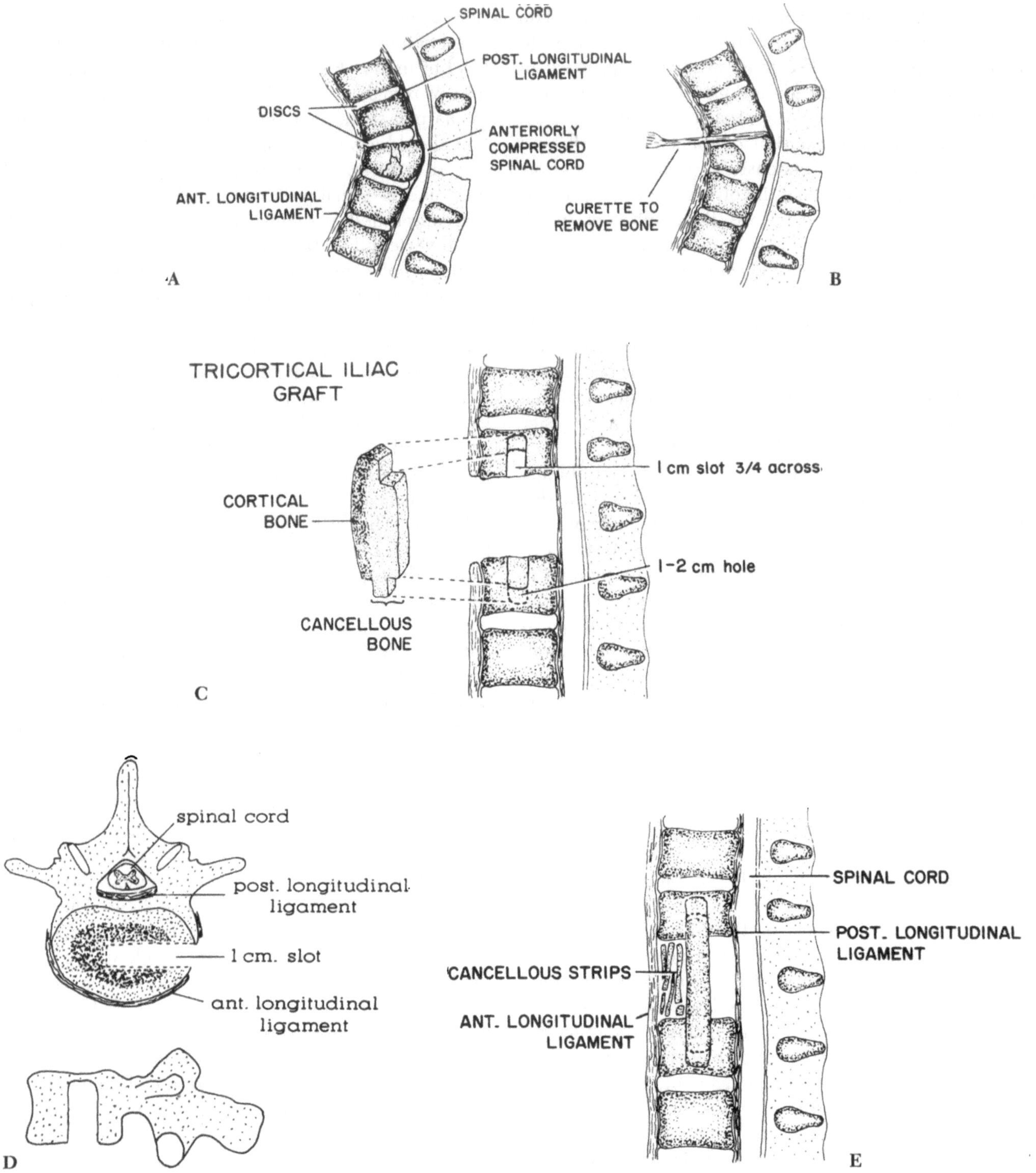

Figure 11.54. Anterior thoracic and lumbar spinal fusion techniques. **A.** Involved vertebra is identified. **B** and **C.** Sufficient bone with proximal and distal intervertebral disc is removed to decompress neural canal. Tricortical iliac crest graft is sculpted to fill void. **D** and **E.** Proximal and distal troughs are developed in vertebral bodies adjacent to junction of anterior two-thirds and posterior one-third of adjacent vertebral bodies to be closest to their axis of rotation. (Reprinted with permission from Cotler HB, Cotler JM, Stoloff A. The use of autografts for vertebral body replacement of the thoracic and lumbar spine. Spine 1985;10(8):752.)

dura is often done with a neurosurgeon. Attention to the retraction of the iliopsoas muscle at its origin (L1–L3) is important because of the exiting nerve roots, which provide function to the quadriceps (femoral nerve, L2–L4) and sensation over the anterior inferior abdomen and upper thigh. Blood loss must be carefully monitored. The use of the cell saver is of invaluable assistance in capturing and resupplying autogenous blood, but the use of captured cells with this system reduces the presence of available blood coagulation components (platelets and fibrinogen). These latter substances must be replaced, depending on the extent of blood loss. For thoracotomy approaches, a #28 or 32 chest tube is inserted before chest closure. Hemovac suctions are used in the areas from which bone grafts are obtained and, where indicated, retroperitoneal closed drainage tubes may be used.

Despite the use of an anterior tricortical iliac or rib graft spanning an area of vertebral body corpectomy for dural decompression purposes, unless posterior vertebral column stability exists, the presence of an anterior graft is insufficient to prevent vertebral column kyphosis with axial loading. Generally speaking, the anterior approach is used in the presence of the stable spine for excision of anterior spinal pathology (tumor, infection, etc.) or in chronic anterior dural compression. For acute trauma, posterior stabilization will support axial loading following anterior decompression and bone grafting with the use of an external orthotic device. This latter support will be required for 3 to 4 months.

Sacral Fractures

Isolated sacral fractures are very rare, but when present are associated with major fractures involving the pelvic ring. Careful visualization of an anteroposterior roentgenogram of the sacrum will often signal the presence of a sacral fracture. The physician should direct his attention to the smooth cortical lines circumscribing the second and third sacral foramen. Any break in the continuity of that sacral foramen heralds the presence of pathology or fracture. Most helpful in the recognition and diagnosis of sacral fractures are biplane tomograms and CAT scans.

The most common type of sacral fracture is the vertical transforamenal fracture associated with ipsilateral upper and lower sacral segments. The lower sacral fracture is the most common of the two, and is usually the result of a direct horizontal-type injury resulting in a stable horizontal fracture. It is not uncommon for root neurological injury to occur with such a fracture. Controversy exists as to whether there are beneficial effects of surgical decompression of sacral fractures in the presence of neurological injury.[8,24,125] The authors have not found surgical exploration to be a successful means of restoring lost sacral root function. In the presence of sacroiliac joint separations often associated with a fracture of the anterior ring of the pelvis, surgical stabilization both anteriorly and posteriorly has been effectively utilized.

Conclusion

Fractures of the cervical, thoracic, and lumbar spine result from violent injury. In approximately 50% of all spine-injured patients, additional multiple trauma or multiple organ system injuries also exist.[24] Management of the acute spine-injured patient, therefore, requires patient assessment and management by a multidisciplinary team. The orthopaedic surgeon may be in the leadership role or may be a consultant providing diagnostic and surgical skill in the area of spine stability assessment, internal stabilization, orthotic external application, and postinjury rehabilitation. Stable injuries to the vertebral column and fractures at multiple levels of the vertebral column are best managed by nonoperative conservative management. Unstable injuries of the spine, as described in this chapter, are best managed by early spine reduction and operative stabilization.

Better patient outcome, both surgical and rehabilitative, is anticipated in an environment where a multidisciplinary spine trauma team exists and in which there is direct and continuous rehabilitative interaction. This environment is available in regional trauma and spinal cord injury centers.

References

1. Bedbrook GM, Sir. Fracture dislocations of the spine with and without paralysis. A case for conservatism and against operative techniques. In: Leach RE, Hoaglund FT, Riseborough EJ, eds. Controversies in Orthopaedic Surgery. Philadelphia: Saunders, 1982:423–445.
2. Cotler HB, Cotler JM, Stoloff A, et al. The use of autografts for vertebral body replacement of the thoracic and lumbar spine. Spine 1985;10:748.
3. Cotler HB, Miller LS, DeLucia FA, et al. Closed reduction of cervical spine dislocations. Clin Orthop 1987;214:185.
4. Denis F: The three-column spine and its significance in the classification of acute thoraco-lumbar spinal injuries. Spine 1983;8:817.
5. Doppman JL, Girton M. Angiographic study of the effect of laminectomy in the presence of acute anterior epidural masses. J Neurosurg 1976;45:487.
6. Evans DK. Anterior cervical subluxation. J Bone Joint Surg 1976;58B:318.
7. Ferguson RL, Allen BL, Jr. A mechanistic classification of thoracolumbar spine fractures. Clin Orthop 1984;189:77.
8. Fountain SS. Transverse fractures of the sacrum: a report of six cases. J Bone Joint Surg 1977;59A:486.
9. Frankel HL, Hancock DO, Hyslop G, et al. The value of postural reduction in the initial management of closed inju-

ries of the spine with paraplegia and tetraplegia, Part I. Paraplegia 1969;7:179.
10. Guttman L, Sir. Spinal deformities in traumatic paraplegics and tetraplegics following surgical procedures. Paraplegia 1969;7:38.
11. Guttman L, Sir. Surgical aspects of the treatment of traumatic paraplegia. J Bone Joint Surg 1949;31B:399.
12. Holdsworth F, Sir. Fractures, dislocations and fracture-dislocations of the spine. Review article. J Bone Joint Surg 1970;52A:1534.
13. Jacobs RR, Nordwall A, Nachemson A. Reduction, stability, and strength provided by internal fixation for thoracolumbar spinal injuries. Clin Orthop 1982;171:300.
14. Leidholt JD, Young JJ, Hahn DR, et al. Evaluations of late spinal deformities and fracture-dislocations of the dorsal and lumbar spine in paraplegics. Paraplegia 1969;7:16.
15. Pierce DS, Barr JS, Jr. Fractures and dislocations at the base of the skull and upper cervical spine. In: The Cervical Spine. Philadelphia: Lippincott, 1983:196–206.
16. Stauffer ES. Open reduction and internal fixation of unstable thoracolumbar fractures and dislocations. In: Leach RE, Hoaglund FT, Riseborough EJ, eds. Controversies in Orthopaedic Surgery. Philadelphia: Saunders, 1982:446–454.
17. Watson-Jones R, Sir. Injuries of the spine. In: Wilson JN, ed. Fractures and Joint Injuries. Ed. 5. Edinburgh: Churchill Livingstone, 1976:798–849.
18. White AA, Panjabi MM. Clinical Biomechanics of the Spine. Philadelphia: Lippincott, 1978.
19a. Yosipovitch Z, Robin GC, Makin M. Open reduction of unstable thoracolumbar spinal injuries and fixation with Harrington rods. J Bone Joint Surg 1977;59A:1003.
19b. Bradford DS, Thompson RC. Fractures and dislocations of the spine. Indications for surgical intervention. Minn Med 1976;7:711.
19c. Davies WE, Morris JH, Hill V. An analysis of conservative (non-surgical) management of thoraco-lumbar fractures and fracture-dislocations with neurological damage. J Bone Joint Surg 1980;62A:1324.
19d. Donovan WH, Dwyer AP. An update on the early management of traumatic paraplegia (nonoperative and operative management). Clin Orthop 1984;189:12.
20. Bedbrook GM, Sir. Treatment of thoracolumbar dislocation and fractures with paraplegia. Clin Orthop 1975;112:27.
21. Burke DC, Murray DD. The management of thoracic and thoraco-lumbar injuries of the spine with neurological involvement. J Bone Joint Surg 1976;58B:72.
22. Stranger JK. Fracture-dislocations of the thoraco-lumbar spine with special references to reduction by open and closed operations. J Bone Joint Surg 1947;29:107.
23. Young JS, Dexter WR. Neurological recovery distal to the zone of injury in 172 cases of closed traumatic spinal cord injury. Paraplegia 1978;16:39.
24. Meyer PR, Jr, ed. Surgery of Spine Trauma. New York: Churchill Livingstone, 1988.
25. Dorr LD, Harvey JP, Jr, Nickel VL. Clinical review of the early stability of spine injuries. Spine 1982;7:545.
26. Gertzbein SD. Assessment of cervical spine instability. In: Tator CH, ed. Early Management of Spinal Cord Injury. New York: Raven Press, 1982:41–52.
27. Lewis J, Kibben B. The treatment of unstable fracture-dislocations of the thoracolumbar spine accompanied by paraplegia. J Bone Joint Surg 1974;56B:603.
28. Luque ER, Cassis M, Ramirez-Wiella G. Segmental spinal instrumentation in the treatment of fractures of the thoracolumbar spine. Spine 1982;7:312.
29. McSweeney T. Deformities of the spine following injuries to the cord. In: Hand Neurol 1976;26:159.
30. Nicoll EA. Fractures of the dorso-lumbar spine. J Bone Joint Surg 1949;31B:376.
31. Osebod WE, Weinstein SL, Sprague BL. Thoracolumbar spine fractures; results and treatment. Spine 1981;6:13.
32. Roberts JB, Curtis PH. Stability of the thoracic and lumbar spine in traumatic paraplegia following fracture or fracture-dislocation. J Bone Joint Surg 1970;52A:115.
33. Sareff J. Assessment of the late results of traumatic compression fractures of the thoracolumbar vertebral bodies. Stockholm: Karalinska Hospital, 1977:1–88.
34. Dickson JH, Harrington TR, Erwin WD. Results of reduction and stabilization of the severely fractured thoracic and lumbar spine. J Bone Joint Surg 1978;60A:799.
35. Edwards CC, Levine AM. Early rod-sleeve stabilization of the injured thoracic and lumbar spine. Orthop Clin North Am 1986;17:121.
36. Flesch JR, Leider LL, Erickson DL, et al. Harrington instrumentation and spine fusion for unstable fracture and fracture-dislocations of the thoracic and lumbar spine. J Bone Joint Surg 1977;59A:143.
37. Hannon K. Harrington instrumentation in fractures and dislocations of the thoracic and lumbar spine. South Med J 1976;69:1269.
38. Jacobs RR, Asher MA, Snider RK. Thoracolumbar spinal injuries. A comparative study of recumbent and operative treatment in 100 patients. Spine 1980;5:463.
39. Wharton GW. Stabilization of spinal injuries for early mobilization. Orthop Clin North Am 1978;9:271.
40. Hospital resources for optimal care of the injured patient. Bulletin of the American College of Surgeons, August 1979.
41. National Academy of Sciences, National Research Council Committee on Trauma and Committee on Shock. Accidental death and disability: the neglected disease of modern society. Washington, DC: NAS-NRC, 1966.
42. Optimal hospital resources for care of the seriously injured. Bulletin of the American College of Surgeons, September 1976.
43. Recommendations of the conference on the guidelines for the categorization of hospital emergency capabilities. Chicago: American Medical Association, 1971.
44. Trauma Appendices to Hospital Resources for Optimal Care of the Injured Patient Report; Bulletin of the American College of Surgeons, February 1980.
45. Trauma Systems Development Manual for Emergency Medical Services (Burn and Spinal Cord Injury) Systems; Contract #232-78-0170; Health, Education and Welfare, October 1979.
46. American Spinal Injury Association and American Spinal Injury Association Foundation, Guidelines for Facility Cat-

egorization and Standards of Care. Chicago: Spinal Cord Injury, 1987:7.
47. Meyer PR, Jr, Raffensperger JG. Special centers for the care of the injured. J Trauma 1973;13:308.
48. Bedbrook GM, Sir. Lifetime Care of the Paraplegic Patient. New York: Churchill Livingstone, 1985.
49. Meyer PR, Jr. Complications of treatment of fractures and dislocations of the dorsolumbar spine. In: Epps CH, Jr, ed. Complications in Orthopaedic Surgery. 2d Ed. Philadelphia: Lippincott, 1986:713–794.
50. Annual Progress Report of the Midwest Regional Spinal Cord Injury Care Systems, Northwestern University. Chicago: U.S. Depart. of Education, 1987.
51. Denis F. Spinal instability as defined by the three-column spine concept in acute spinal trauma. Clin Orthop 1984;198:65.
52. Holdsworth F, Sir. Fractures, dislocations and fracture-dislocations of the spine. J Bone Joint Surg 1963;45B:6.
53. Kelly RP, Whitesides TE. Treatment of lumbo-dorsal fracture-dislocations. Ann Surg 1968;167:705.
54. Whitesides TE. Traumatic kyphosis of the thoracolumbar spine. Clin Orthop 1977;128:78.
55. McAfee PC, Yuan HA, Fredrickson BE, et al. The value of computed tomography in thoracolumbar fractures. An analysis of 100 consecutive cases and a new classification. J Bone Joint Surg 1983;65A:461.
56. Aebi M, Etter C, Kehl T, Thalgott J. Stabilization of the lower thoracic and lumbar spine with the internal spinal skeletal fixation system: indications, techniques and first results of treatment. Spine 1987;12:544.
57. Louis R. Surgery of the Spine: Surgical Anatomy and Operative Approaches. Berlin: Springer-Verlag, 1983.
58a. Louis R. Spinal stability as defined by the three-column spine concept. Anat Clin 1985;7:33.
58b. Louis R. Fusion of the lumbar and sacral spine by internal fixation with screw plates. Clin Orthop, 203:18, 1986.
59. Apley AG. Fractures of the spine. Ann R Coll Surg Engl 1970;46:210.
60. Babcock JL. Cervical spine injuries: diagnosis and classification. Ann Surg 1976;111:646.
61. Beatson TR. Fractures and dislocations of the cervical spine. J Bone Joint Surg 1963;45B:21.
62. Bedbrook GM, Sir. Spinal injuries with tetraplegia and paraplegia. J Bone Joint Surg 1979;61B:267.
63. Bohler L. The Treatment of Fractures. 5th Ed. New York: Grune and Stratton, 1956:323.
64. Gehwiler JA, Jr, Clark MA, Schaaf RE, et al. Cervical spine trauma: the common combined conditions. Radiology 1979;130:77.
65. Harris JH, Jr, Edeiken-Monroe B, Kopaniky DR. A practical classification of acute cervical spine injuries. Orthop Clinics North Am 1986;17:15.
66. Jacobs B. Cervical fractures and dislocations of (C3–7). Clin Orthop 1975;109:18.
67. King DM. Fractures and dislocations of the cervical part of the spine. Aust NZ J Surg 1967;37:57.
68. Roaf R. A study of the mechanics of spinal injuries. J Bone Joint Surg 1960;42B:810.
69. Selecki BR, Williams HBL. Injuries to the cervical spine and cord in man. Australian Medical Association. Mervyn Archdall Medical Monograph No. 7, New South Wales: Australian Medical Publishing, 1970.
70. Weir DC. Roentgenographic signs of cervical injury. Clin Orthop 1975;109:9.
71a. Whitley JE, Forsyth HF. The classification of cervical spine injuries. AJR, 1960;83:633.
71b. Brookman R, Penning, L: Injuries of the cervical spine. Amsterdam, Excerpta Medica, 1971.
72. Stauffer ES. Diagnosis and prognosis of acute cervical spinal cord injury. Clin Orthop 1975;112:9.
73. Kulkarni MV, McArdle CB, Kopaniky DR, Miner ME, Cotler HB, Lee KF, Harris JH, Jr. Acute spinal cord injury: MR imaging at 1.5T. Radiology 1987;164:837.
74. Cotler HB, Kulkarni MV, Bondurant FJ. Magnetic resonance imaging of acute spinal cord: Preliminary report. J Orthop Trauma 1988;2:1.
75. Comarr AE, Kaufman AA. A survey of the neurological results of 858 spinal cord injuries. A comparison of patients treated with and without laminectomy. J Neurosurg 1956;13:95.
76. Morgan R, Brown JC, Bonnett C. The effect of laminectomy on the pediatric spinal cord injured patient. J Bone Joint Surg 1974;56A:1767.
77. Morgan TH, Wharton GW, Austin GM. The results of laminectomy in patients with incomplete spinal cord injuries. Paraplegia 1971;9:14.
78. Romanick PC, Smith TK, Kopaniky DR, et al. Infection about the spine associated with low-velocity missile injury to the abdomen. J Bone Joint Surg 1985;67A:1195.
79. Alker GJ, Oh YS, Leslie EV. High cervical spine and craniocervical junction injuries in fatal traffic accidents: A radiological study. North Am Orthop Clin 1978;9(4):1003.
80. Wertheim SB, Bohlman HH. Occipitocervical fusion. J Bone Joint Surg 1987;69A:833.
81. Georgopoulous G, Pizzutillo PD, Lee ML. Occipito-atlantal instability in children. J Bone Joint Surg 1987;69A:424.
82. Anderson LD, D'Alonzo RT. Fractures of the odontoid process of the axis. J Bone Joint Surg 1974;56A:1663.
83. Aymes EW, Anderson FM. Fractures of the odontoid process. Arch Surg 1956;72:377.
84. Ekong CU, Schwartz ML, Tator CH, et al. Odontoid fracture: Management with early mobilization using the halo device. Neurosurgery 1981;9:631.
85. Schatzker J, Rorabeck CH, Waddell SP. Fractures of the dens (odontoid process). An analysis of 37 cases. J Bone Joint Surg 1971;53B:392.
86. Gallie WE. Fractures and dislocations of the cervical spine. Am J Surg 1939;46:495.
87. Fielding JW, Hawkins RJ, Ratzan SA. Spine fusion for atlanto-axial instability. J Bone Joint Surg 1976;58A:400.
88. Brooks AL, Jenkins EB: Atlanto-axial arthrodesis by the wedge compression method. J Bone Joint Surg 1978;60A:279.
89. Griswold DM, Albright JA, Schiffman E, et al. Atlanto-axial fusion for instability. J Bone Joint Surg 1978;60A:285.
90. Edwards CC, Levine AM, Murphy J, et al. New techniques in spine stabilization. Warsaw, Indiana: Zimmer, 1982.
91. Effendi B, Roy D, Cornish B, et al. Fractures of the ring

of the axis. A classification based on the analysis of 131 cases. J Bone Joint Surg 1981;63B:319.
92. Levine AM, Edwards CC. The management of traumatic spondylolisthesis of the axis. J Bone Joint Surg 1985; 67A:217.
93. Bedbrook GM, Sir, Edibam RC. The study of spinal deformity in traumatic spinal paralysis. Paraplegia 1973; 10:321.
94a. Raynor RB. Discography and myelography in acute injuries of the cervical spine. J Neurosurg 1971;35:529.
94b. McKenzie K. Fracture, dislocations and fracture-dislocations of the cervical spine. Can Med Assoc J, 1935;32:263.
95. Burke DC, Berryman D. The place of closed manipulation in the management of flexion-rotation dislocations of the cervical spine. J Bone Joint Surg 1971;53B(2):165.
96. Bohlman HH, Boada E. Fractures and dislocations of the lower cervical spine. In: The Cervical Spine Research Society, eds. The Cervical Spine. Philadelphia: Lippincott, 1983:232–267.
97. Stauffer ES. Management of spine fractures C3–7. Orthop Clin North Am 1986;17:45.
98. Rogers WA. Treatment of fracture-dislocation of the cervical spine. J Bone Joint Surg 1942;24:245.
99. Rogers WA. Fractures and dislocations of the cervical spine. J Bone Joint Surg 1957;39A:341.
100. Robinson RA, Southwick WO. Indications and techniques for early stabilization of the neck in some fracture dislocations of the cervical spine. South Med J 1960;53:565.
101. Cloward R. Surgical treatment of dislocations and compression fractures of the cervical spine by the anterior approach. In: Proceedings of the 17th Veterans Administration Spinal Cord Injury Conference, New York, Veterans Administration, Washington DC 1969:26–35
102. Smith GW, Robinson RA. The treatment of certain cervical spine disorders by the anterior removal of the intervertebral disc and interbody fusion. J Bone Joint Surg 1958;40A:607.
103. Gertzbein SD. Orthopaedic management of the injured spine. In: Block RF, Basbaum M, eds. Management of Spinal Cord Injuries. Baltimore: Williams & Wilkins, 1986:65.
104. Malcolm B. Spinal deformities secondary to spinal injuries. Orthop Clin North Am 1979;4:943.
105. Jacobs RR, Casey MP. Surgical management of thoracolumbar spinal injuries. Clin Orthop 1984;189:22.
106. Keene JS, Drummond DS. Wisconsin compression system surgical technique. Warsaw, Indiana: Zimmer 1981.
107. Roy-Camille R, Saillant G, Mazel C. Internal fixation of the lumbar spine with pedicle screw plating. Clin Orthop 1986;203:7.
108. Roy-Camille R, Saillant G, Mazel C. Plating of thoracic, thoracolumbar and lumbar injuries with pedicle screw plates. Orthop Clin North Am 1986;17:147.
109. Steffee AD, Sitkowski OAC, Topham LS. Total vertebral body and pedicle arthroplasty. Clin Orthop 1986;203:203.
110. Johnson KD, Cadambi A, Seibert GB. Incidence of adult respiratory distress syndrome in patients with multiple musculoskeletal injuries: effect of early operative stabilization of fractures. J Trauma 1985;25:375.
111. Green D, Lee MY, Ito T, Cohn T, et al. Fixed vs. adjusted-dose heparin in the prophylaxis of thromboembolism in spinal cord injury. JAMA, 1988;260:1255.
112. Bone LB, Johnston CE, Ashman RB, Roach JW. Mechanical comparison of anterior spinal instrumentation in a burst fracture model. J Orthop Trauma 1988;2:195.
113. Kostuik JP. Anterior fixation for fractures of the thoracic and lumbar spine with or without neurologic involvement. Clin Orthop 1984;189:103.
114. Zielke K, Strempel AV. Posterior lateral distraction spondylodesis using the twofold sacral bar. Clin Orthop 1986;203:131.
115. Dwyer AF, Schafer MF. Anterior approach to scoliosis. J Bone Joint Surg 1974;56B:218.
116. Tencer AF, Allen BL Jr, Ferguson RL: A biomechanical study of thoracolumbar spinal fractures with bone in the canal, Part I: The effect of laminectomy. Spine 1985;10: 580.
117. Magerl FP. Stabilization of the lower thoracic and lumbar spine with external skeletal fixation. Clin Orthop 1984;189:125.
118. Bohlman HH. Acute fractures and dislocations of the cervical spine: an analysis of 300 hospitalized patients and a review of the literature. J Bone Joint Surg 1979;61A: 1119.
119. Bohlman MK, Eismont FJ. Surgical techniques of anterior decompression and fusion for spinal cord injuries. Clin Orthop 1981;154:57.
120. Chance GQ. Note on a type of flexion fracture of the spine. Br J Radiol 1948;21:452.
121. Kaufer H, Hays JT. Lumbar fracture-dislocations. J Bone Joint Surg 1966;48A:712.
122. Smith WS, Kaufer H. Patterns and mechanisms of lumbar injuries associated with lap seat belts. J Bone Joint Surg 1969;51A:239.
123. Gertzbein SD, Court-Brown CM. Flexion-distraction injuries of the lumbar spine. Clin Orthop 1988;227:52.
124. Musculoskeletal allograft tissue, Musculoskeletal Transplant Foundation. Little Silver, New Jersey.
125. Sabiston CP, Wing PC. Sacral fractures: classification and neurologic indications. J Trauma 1971;26:1113.

12

Fusion Techniques for Pediatric Disorders

G. Dean MacEwen, Andrew G. S. King, Frank Bonnarens, and *Stephen D. Heinrich*

"I will prescribe regimen for the good of my patients according to my ability and judgment. I will never do harm to anyone."

Hippocrates of Cos

Congenital Anomalies of the Craniovertebral Junction

This group of lesions includes occipitalization of the atlas and basilar impression. Also discussed in this section are the Klippel–Feil deformity, which has a common association with craniovertebral junction anomalies, and atlanto-occipital hypermobility, which is being reported with increasing frequency.

These conditions share many clinical features. Attention may be drawn to the clinical features typical of the associated Klippel–Feil deformity, namely, short neck, low hairline, and decreased range of neck motion.[1] Associated anomalies may be found in the skull and face, and children may first present to an oral surgeon or ear, nose, and throat surgeon.[2] The anatomical variations seen with these conditions place abnormal stresses on the functioning articulations of the cervical spine that may lead to dangerous instability. The role of the orthopaedic surgeon is to define the abnormality in anatomical terms and to recognize the possibilities for dangerous instability and neurological compression. Occipitocervical fusion may be required.

Although the condition may be diagnosed in childhood, symptoms from neurological compression often become manifest in the second or third decade of life or later.[3–9] Reasons for the delay in onset of neurological symptoms may include gradually increasing ligamentous laxity and instability at levels adjacent to fused segments, the earlier onset of cervical osteoarthritis with associated osteophytes and ligmentous thickening, and the decreasing tolerance of the aging brain stem and cervical spinal cord to compression.

If late instability is a factor in the onset of neurological symptoms, then early fusion might be expected to delay the onset or retard the progression of those symptoms already present.[10] The importance of intervention to avoid the onset of neurological symptoms is underlined by the fact that decompression of the craniovertebral spine for relief of an existing neurological deficit carries considerable risks and is unlikely to restore the patient to normal function.[7,9–12]

Neurological symptoms, if they occur, may originate from all structures traversing the occipitoatlantal motion segment. These include the cerebellar tonsils, alone or in the presence of an Arnold-Chiari malformation, which may be seen in as many as 60% of patients.[3,13,14] The cord itself may be widened by the presence of a syrinx. The vertebral arteries may become compressed in the region of the foramen magnum and cause symptoms of vertebrobasilar insufficiency, and there also may be dysfunction of the cranial nerves that traverse the foramen magnum. Anteriorly the medulla oblongata or spinal cord may be compressed by an odontoid process that has migrated cranially in basilar impression or is too large or angled posteriorly in antlantooccipital assimilation.[3] Posteriorly, the neural structures may be constricted by dural thickening, forming a tight band. In short, neurological compression may be caused by an impingement from bony and ligamentous structures anteriorly and posteriorly, with excessive crowding of the neurological structures in the middle. Added to this static picture is the dynamic problem caused by occipitoatlantal or atlantoaxial instability. The abnormal motion may lead to intermittent bruising and irritation of the spinal cord.[10]

Symptoms caused by the neurological deficit, especially in the early stages, are extremely vague and nonspecific and will depend on which neurological structure is primarily affected. Symptoms can include ataxia, upper extremity or lower extremity paresis, diplopia, nystagmus, papilledema, tinnitis, earache, dysphasia, poor phonation, and others. For this reason, the diagnosis is often delayed and attributed to diffuse neurological conditions such as multiple sclerosis or amyotrophic lateral sclerosis.[3,4,6,13]

Exciting new developments have occurred in the last 10 years for evaluating these conditions. Previously, one had to rely on plain radiographs and computed tomography (CT). Much emphasis was placed on the drawing of lines between bony landmarks to establish the diagnosis. Gas myelography was used to help confirm or exclude the presence of Arnold-Chiari malformation and syringomyelia. CT scanning with transaxial slices, and sagittal and coronal reconstructions, can dramatically demonstrate abnormal bony configuration, especially in basilar impression, and should now be regarded as the primary method of diagnosing this condition. Magnetic resonance imaging (MRI) has displaced the need for gas or dye myelography to demonstrate the Arnold-Chiari malformation or syringomyelia. Thus, CT best demonstrates the bony abnormalities, and MRI assesses the neurological tissue. We recommend cineroentgenography as the most reliable method of demonstrating the third component of neurological compression, namely the instability.

The development of improved anesthetic protocols and techniques coupled with usage of intraoperative corticospinal-evoked potentials has greatly improved the margin of safety for the patient undergoing surgical correction, while the development of new techniques of surgical stabilization of the occipitocervical region has significantly improved the technical success of the surgical procedures.

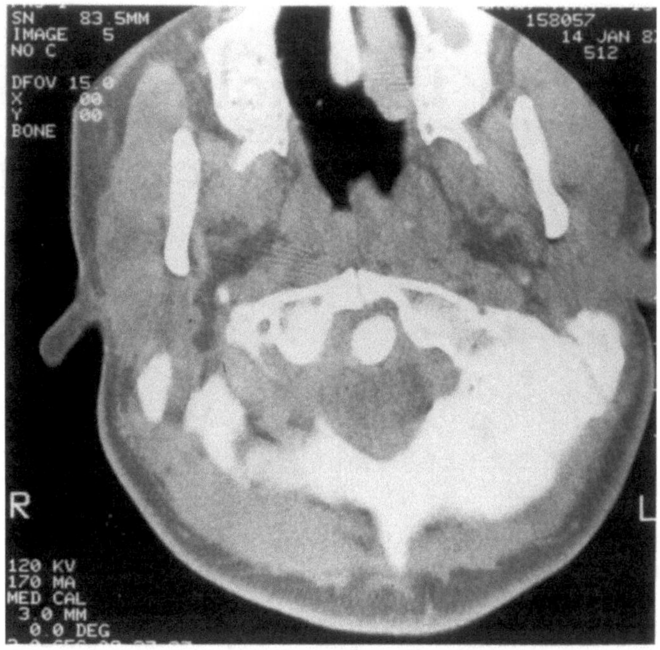

Figure 12.1. CT scan of occipitocranial junction in 15-year-old female. Patient has Klippel–Feil deformity involving all cervical segments except one, Sprengel's deformity, and pulmonary stenosis. CT scan shows bony continuation between occipital bone and anterior arch of atlas, confirming diagnosis of occipitalization of atlas. Spinal canal and cord can be visualized and show no stenosis. Patient is neurologically intact.

Occipitalization of the Atlas

Atlantooccipital fusion and assimilation of the atlas are synonyms for occipitalization of the atlas. This condition consists of some degree of bony union between the skull and the atlas. Any or all parts of the atlas may be fused. For example, one lateral half of the atlas may be completely assimilated and the other not.[3] There is a strong association between this condition and Klippel–Feil deformity, with congenital fusion of the second and third cervical vertebrae seen in 17 of 25 cases in McRae's series[14] (Fig. 12.1). Seven of the 12 cases that had flexion and extension films showed an associated atlantoaxial instability. The atlantoaxial instability is thought to be significant in the production of neurological compression, along with an excessively long or large odontoid process, an odontoid process angled posteriorly at the level of the transverse ligament, or an anteroposterior (AP) diameter of the spinal canal behind the odontoid process of 19 mm or less.[4]

Compression of the neural structures may also be caused by the presence of a dural band pressing against the back of the cord at the level of the foramen magnum. Herniation of the cerebellar tonsils or Arnold-Chiari malformation is not uncommon, and again will be more commonly associated with neurological symptoms.[13]

Patients with occipitalization of the atlas will often show a characteristic short-necked appearance with a low hair line, torticollis, and a decreased range of motion of the cervical spine. There is a 20% incidence of associated anomalies including cleavage of the mandible, maxilla, palate, or nasal cartilage. Hypospadias and other genitourinary anomalies may also be associated.[5]

The average age at which neurological symptoms appear is in the third decade, often after a head or neck injury in the absence of a fracture. Interestingly, the most common symptom is weakness or incoordination of the legs. Other symptoms include numbness or pain in the extremities, more commonly, the arms, and a dull aching pain in the upper neck. Less common complaints include diplopia, tinnitis, earache, dysphasia, and poor phonation, all of which may result from cranial nerve or bulbar irritation. Nystagmus is a prominent finding, and when present generally indicates herniation of the cerebellar tonsils. Cases have been reported of visual disturbances associated with papilledema, again usually in cases with Arnold-Chiari malformation.[6] The precise neurological picture manifests compression of the anterior column of the spinal cord that appears to predominate over pressure on the posterior columns, which are more often spared. This tends to implicate the odontoid, rather than any posterior dural constriction band, as the primary cause of neurological compression. Few pathological specimens have been examined, but all have shown grooving of the medulla oblongata by the odontoid.

The subjective symptoms and neurological signs are often vague and diffuse. In McRae's series, the neurological picture was commonly ascribed to multiple sclerosis before the neck condition was diagnosed.[3,14]

Standard plain lateral roentgenograms may suggest the presence of atlantooccipital fusion, but confirmation is best accomplished by tomograms. In addition, tomograms often show an unusual shape to the foramen magnum and malformations of the odontoid process, including posterior tilting.

CT scanning using thin overlapping transaxial sections combined with sagittal reconstructions will give more precise delineations of the bony anatomy and may often show compression of the cord if present. The neurological structures, including any herniated cerebellar tonsils or Arnold-Chiari malformation, will be best shown with MRI scanning. Cineroentgenography may be especially helpful in showing atlantoaxial instability, which is often seen in those patients who have progressed to overt neurological symptoms.

No treatment is advocated in children and young adults who are asymptomatic and in whom atlantooccipital fusion is discovered on an incidental radiograph. Patients with a neurlogical deficit may be managed with different methods. If intermittent cord compression from an associated atlantoaxial instability segment is thought to be the main cause of the neurological deficit, then posterior fusion alone will suffice.[10] If static bony compression of the neural structures is thought to be the main cause, then a decompression of the bony structures is required. This may include surgical enlargement of the foramen magnum and removal of fibrous bands, or a posterior laminectomy. This operation, however, should always be accompanied by a fusion. Posterior decompression of the occiput-C1 level should be approached with great caution because there are reports of respiratory arrest and death at the time of surgery.[7,15]

In cases of long-standing atlantoaxial instability associated with atlantooccipital fusion, the odontoid may be fixated in a posterior position with respect to the arch of the atlas. A period of preliminary halo gravity traction should first be employed. If the odontoid does not reduce, an in situ fusion should be carried out because operative reduction has resulted in neurological deficits.[6,7]

Basilar Impression

Basilar impression is a deformity characterized by upward bulging of the margins of the foramen magnum to the extent that the occipital condyles are seen at or above the line of the forament magnum.[3] Thus the cervical spine appears to indent into the base of the skull. The tip of the odontoid protrudes upward into the foramen magnum and may cause pressure on the brain stem. The condition is rare. The clinical signs are often vague in the early stages, and the natural history and treatment recommendations are poorly defined.

The first description of this condition was by Chamberlain, who used the terms platybasia and basilar impression interchangeably.[16] Authors since have taken pains to point out that they are separate conditions and rarely occur together.[3,14] Platybasia indicates a flattening of the basal angle of the skull, which is determined by the angle between a line drawn along the plane of the anterior fossa with a line drawn along the plane of the clivus.

There are two types of basilar impression, primary and secondary. Primary basilar impression is a congenital malformation, and is sometimes seen in conjunction with other craniovertebral abnormalities. Hensinger and MacEwen[8] noted a common association with atlantooccipital fusion, hypoplasia of the atlas, deficient posterior arch of the atlas, odontoid abnormalities, and Klippel–Feil syndrome (Fig. 12.2). McRae, however, found no association with occipitalization of the atlas in his patients and only one with fusion of the second and third cervical vertebrae.[3] There is a frequent association between basilar impression and Arnold-Chiari malformation, especially the Chiari type I and II malformations. In type I, the cerebellar tonsils and medial part of the inferior lobe are below the foramen magnum without displacement of the fourth ventricle. In type II, the candal migration of the lower part of the cerebellum is more pronounced and is associated with downward displacement of the fourth ventricle with its foramen opening into the spinal subarachnoid space. A third type of Arnold-Chiari malformation, consisting of the cerebellum and medulla displaced into the cervical spinal canal within a meningocele, has not yet been reported in association with basilar impression.[13]

Secondary basilar impression is a developmental condition caused by softening of the bone at the base of the skull with upward invagination of the cervical spine. It may be seen in osteomalacia, rickets, Paget's disease, and osteogenesis imperfecta.

An entity termed pseudobasilar impression has been recognized with increased frequency in severe deforming rheumatoid arthritis. In this condition, erosion of the occipitoatlantal joints or, more commonly, atlantoaxial joints leads to a relative vertical movement of the odontoid to

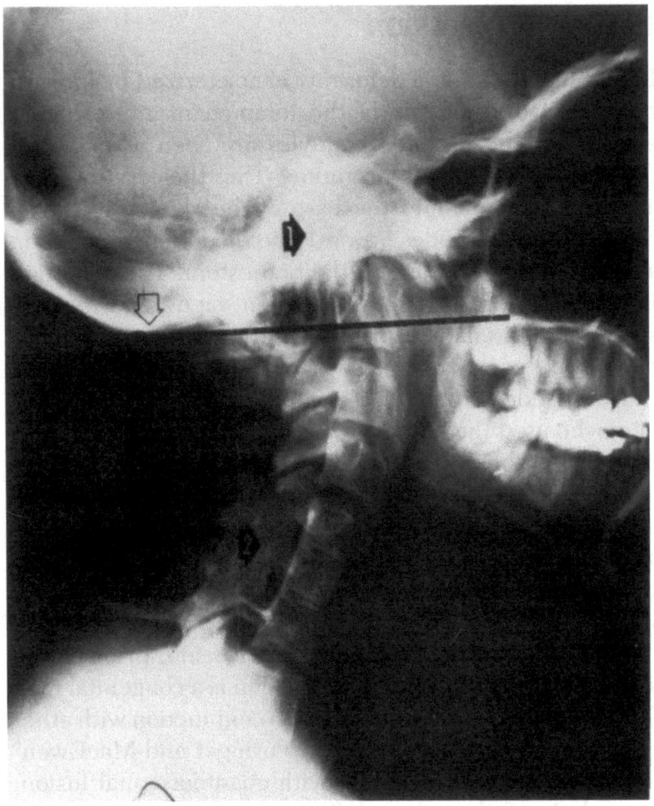

Figure 12.2. Fifteen-year-old male evaluated for headaches and dizziness. *Open arrow* depicts McGregor's line passing from posterior tip of hard palate to inferior border of occiput. *Dark arrow* (1) shows tip of odontoid process more than 4.5 mm above McGregor's line. Dark arrow (2) shows Klippel–Feil deformity of fifth, sixth, and seventh cervical vertebrae. Patient also has only one kidney.

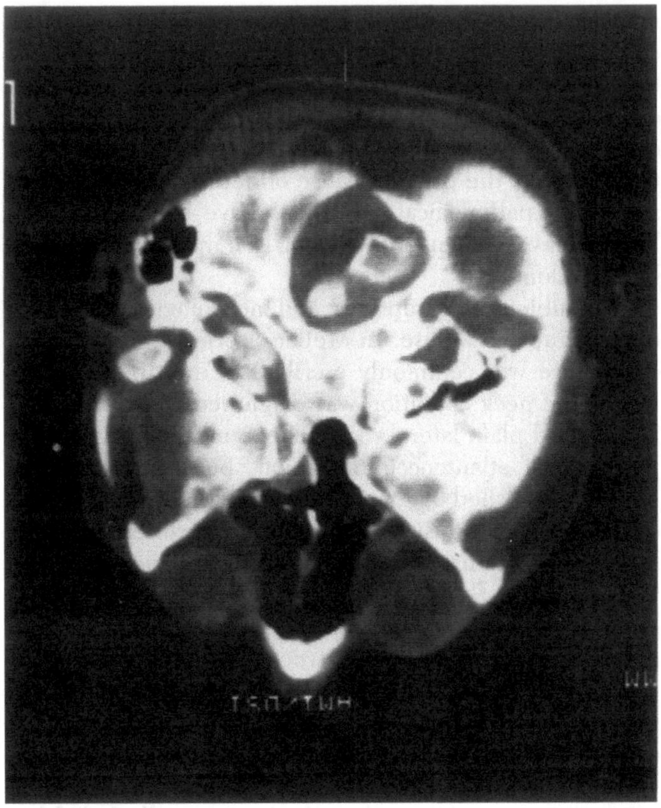

Figure 12.3. CT scan of base of skull. Tip of odontoid can clearly be seen anteriorly at level of foramen magnum. In addition, patient had unusual bony abnormality of occiput, C1–C2 region with intrusion of bone from lateral mass of C1 into foramen magnum. Canal is narrowed with obvious neurological impingement.

the point where it may encroach on the foramen magnum.[17]

Much has been written on the conventional roentgenography of this condition.* Many of the bony points of reference were difficult to define on plain films, and thus AP and lateral tomograms were often advocated to add accuracy in drawing lines to make the diagnosis. Conventional radiography may now be regarded as an initial screening test; CT and MRI scanning will confirm the diagnosis with accuracy. McRae[3] observed that if the tip of the odontoid lies below the foramen magnum, the patient will probably be asymptomatic, whereas if it lies above the foramen magnum symptoms can be expected. The presence of the odontoid at or above the foramen magnum can be easily defined by CT scanning. The information may be gained from the transaxial slices or from sagittal reconstructions. To ensure good quality of the CT scans and reconstruction, slices of 3 mm or less should be taken (Fig. 12.3).

The most common line drawn on plain films was the McGregor line, a line drawn from a point on the upper surface of the posterior edge of the hard palate to the most caudal point of the occipital bone in a true lateral roentgenogram.[18] This was an improvement on Chamberlain's line in which the line from the posterior edge of the hard palate was drawn to the posterior lip of the foramen magnum, a point of reference that was difficult to define. If the tip of the odontoid was more than 4.5 mm above McGregor's line, the diagnosis of basilar impression could be made.[18] Fischgold et al.[20] drew lines taken from AP tomograms. They showed that in a normal skull the line passing through the digastric grooves should pass well above the odontoid process, and a line passing along the bottom of the mastoid processes should pass through the tip of the odontoid (Fig. 12.4).

MRI will outline the presence or absence of Arnold-

* 3, 16, 9, 18, 19.

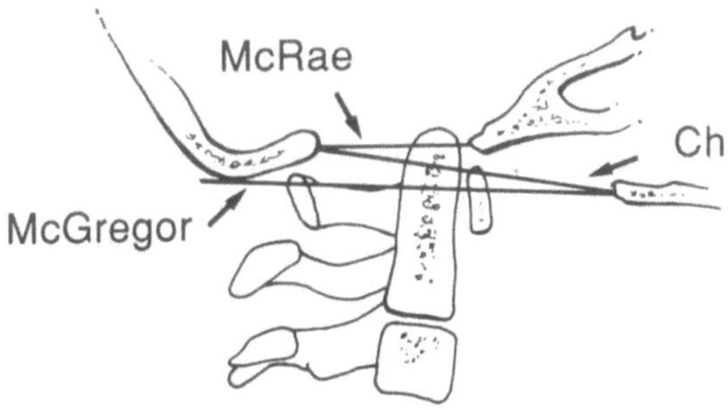

Figure 12.4. Representation of lateral section of craniovertebral junction shows conventional lines drawn for diagnosis of basilar impression. McRae's line is drawn between margins of foramen magnum. This can usually only be defined on lateral tomograms. Any protrusion of odontoid process cephalic to this line is abnormal. Chamberlain's line passes from posterior lip of hard palate to posterior lip of foramen magnum. A more useful line is the McGregor line, passing from posterior lip of hard palate to most inferior part of occiput. If tip of odontoid lies more than 4.5 mm above this line, basilar impression can be diagnosed with confidence. CT scanning has rendered these lines useful for screening purposes only.

Chiari malformation and syringomyelia if present. Before the advent of MRI, gas myelography had been used, but rarely is now.

The clinical symptoms have been best described by Caetano de Barros,[9] who studied 66 patients from Brazil. A short neck is seen in 78% of cases, and asymmetry of the skull and/or face in 68% of cases. Clinical symptoms in most cases become apparent in the second and third decades, 10 years earlier than are seen with occipitoatlantal fusion. Some cases may have symptoms that can be predominantly related to the Arnold-Chiari malformation. Here the clinical picture will be characterized by motor incoordination and unsteadiness of gait, vestibular signs, and involvement of the ninth and tenth cranial nerves. Others may have symptoms attributable to pressure on the neurological structures anteriorly by the odontoid process. Here one will see a pyramidal syndrome with weakness and paresthesias in the limbs. Posterior impingement of the neurological structures may be caused by fibrous bands from thickening of the meninges. Crowding of the foramen leads to a relative stenosis, and compression of the vertebral arteries may cause symptoms such as dizziness, seizures, and mental deterioration and syncopy.[8,18] The neurological picture may be complicated by the association of syringomyelia and syringobulbia. With all this considered, it is not surprising that many of these patients are first diagnosed as having tumors, multiple sclerosis, or amyotrophic lateral sclerosis.[3]

When basilar impression is recognized in an otherwise asymptomatic individual, no treatment is required apart from close and careful observation. The patient should be advised against sports and other activities that could cause neck sprains. Surgery is generally recommended for patients who have a neurological deficit, particularly if it is progressive.[5,9,13]

Most reports from the neurological literature stress posterior decompression accomplished by laminectomy of C1 and C2 and a suboccipital craniectomy, especially if an Arnold-Chiari malformation or a syrinx is present. Most of these authors suggest opening the dura and removing any tight posterior dural bands. In Caeteno de Barros's series of 32 cases undergoing operations, postoperatively 2 patients had no complaints and a normal neurological examination, 19 were much better than before the operation, 4 were unchanged, and 7 patients died. Some authors add an occipitospinal fusion to the decompression.[4]

Anterior cord compression by the odontoid process occurs less frequently in this condition than with occipitalization of the atlas, and transoral resection is less commonly advocated.[11]

Hensinger and MacEwen[8] speculated as to the reasons that the symptoms of basilar impression are delayed to the second or third decade. They thought that this may result from a gradually increasing ligamentous laxity and instability with aging, similar to the delayed myelopathies reported after atlantoaxial dislocation or the increasing instability at C1–C2 in patients who have odontoid agenesis or hypoplasia. They also believed these patients were more prone to the early development of cervical osteoarthritis, with a decreasing tolerance of the aging brain and spinal cord to compression. If this late instability is indeed a major factor, then early fusion might be expected to delay the onset of neurological symptoms or retard the progression of those already present. This, however, has never been documented in the literature, and prophylactic fusion cannot be recommended at this stage.

Occipitoatlantal Hypermobility

Weisel and Rothman reported two patients who presented with translational instability of the occiput on C1. One presented at age 23, the other at age 17. One had increasing dizziness and occipital headaches, the other intermittent weakness in the arms and legs. Radiographs in flexion and extension showed horizontal translation of 20 and 5 mm, respectively, of the occiput on C1. Both patients underwent posterior occiput to C2 fusion with resolution of the symptoms. Both patients had congenital fusions below the atlas, and it was postulated that the symptoms were caused by irritation of the brain stem or upper cord from the abnormal range of motion. There was no evidence of actual impingement of the cord either in flexion or extension. This indicates that at this level, dynamic factors in the absence of static compression may be sufficient to cause neurological symptoms. The same authors studied 20 normal subjects and found the normal range of horizontal translation in flexion/extension to be no more than 1 mm.[21,22]

Congenital fusions below the atlas can be expected to place more strain on the occipitoatlantal motion segment leading over time to attrition of the ligaments at this level. Wiesel proposed a method for measuring this abnormal motion from the lateral radiograph in flexion and extension. It is possible that atlantooccipital instability may accompany other conditions such as basilar impression, Klippel–Feil syndrome, and atlantoaxial instability, but be overlooked because of the subtle findings on plain radiographs.

Georgopoulos[23] reported on a further five cases of occipitoatlantal instability in children with two cases of a nontraumatic etiology. Neither case had a congenital fusion of the upper cervical spine, and a review of 150 patients with Klippel–Feil deformity failed to show any evidence of occipitoatlantal instability. They postulated that the etiology was a congenital abnormality of the cervicocranial junction.

Diagnosis can be made on plain radiographs by the method of Powers or Wiesel, but poor definition of the bony landmarks makes CT scanning in flexion and extension more reliable. Measurements are made from the sagittal reconstruction. Cineradiography may also be helpful. Both patients in the series of Georgopoulos et al had a successful arthrodesis from the occiput to C1 with complete resolution of symptoms.

Klippel–Feil Deformity

This syndrome includes all patients with a congenital fusion of cervical vertebrae. This may be limited to two segments, to an isolated congenital cervical blocked vertebra, or may involve the entire cervical spine.[24]

The original description by Klippel and Feil outlined the classical clinical triad of low posterior hairline, short neck, and limitation of neck motion.[1] Some authors believe isolated block vertebrae below the second cervical vertebra is a condition distinct from Klippel–Feil syndrome because it is rarely associated with the typical clinical features.[25] However, MacEwen showed that the classic clinical picture was seen in less than half of their cases with Klippel–Feil syndrome, and in addition relatively normal motion of the cervical spine could be seen clinically in children with extensive fusions with the development of hypermobility at the few remaining open interspaces.[24]

While fusion of the cervical spine in children may be seen in acquired conditions such as rhematoid arthritis, Klippel–Feil syndrome appears to be the result of a failure of normal segmentation of the cervical somites during the third to eighth week of embryonic life. There is a high rate of associated congenital anomalies involving numerous systems. The occurrence of these associated anomalies is stressed, as they may be much more important for the physical well-being of the patient than any problems associated with the neck condition.[24] One anomaly is scoliosis, which is seen in 60% of patients. It may be congenital and caused by vertebral anomalies or compensatory scoliosis below the area of cervical fusion. Children with congenital scoliosis may require spinal fusion for progressive deformity.[26] Winter[26] retrospectively studied the cervical spine radiographs of 1,215 patients with congenital scoliosis and discovered 25% had segmentation defects in the cervical spine, most of which had been unappreciated at the time of evaluation of their scoliosis, 35% had renal abnormalities of significance, which may be asymptomatic in a young child, but result in pyelonephritis and kidney failure in the adult. Therefore, all patients with Klippel–Feil should have a renal ultrasound to exclude significant abnormalities. Other abnormalities include Sprengel's deformity in 30%, deafness in 30%, synkinesis, which consists of involuntary paired movements of the hand and occasionally the arms, cardiovascular anomalies, and less commonly ptosis, lateral rectus palsy, facial nerve palsy, syndactyly, hypoplastic thumb, and upper extremity hypoplasia.[24]

The majority of patients with Klippel–Fiel are asymptomatic. When symptoms do supervene, they often do so in the second or third decade and are associated with the increased mechanical stresses concentrated at levels of retained motion adjacent to fused segments. Spinal stenosis may occur from hypertrophic spurring at a mobile level and may cause radiculopathy or myelopathy. Disabling mechanical cervical spine pain may occur from developing instability caused by increasing ligamentous laxity. With trauma, the injurious forces will again tend to localize at a level of retained motion. Lee and Weiss[25] described two cases of quadriparesis seen in patients with cervical block vertebra after relatively minor injuries.

The roentgenologic assessment should start with plain films, but these may be difficult to interpret in young children in whom ossification of the vertebral body is not complete. Elucidation of more complex deformity may require tomograms. CT scan and MRI will outline the relationship of the cord to the bony abnormality. They may also help exclude the presence of associated conditions such as syringomyelia, hydromyelia, or Arnold-Chiari malformation.

There are recognized patterns of fusion of the lower cervical vertebrae that expose the patient to a higher than normal risk of cervical instability. First fusion of C2–C3 with occipitalization of the atlas was first reported in 1953 by McRae.[3] This pattern was described more fully earlier under occipitoatlantal fusion. Second, a single open interspace between two long fused segments will cause all motion to become concentrated at the one open segment with the development of degenerative changes, osteophytic spurring, and ligamentous laxity (Fig. 12.5) A long fusion of the cervical spine with normal occiput-C1 and C1–C2 articulations is usually compatible with normal life expectancy.[24]

Treatment directed toward the cervical spine is not commonly required in Klippel–Feil syndrome. However, it is prudent to advise patients against activities that have the potential for putting large stresses on the cervical spine, particularly in those cases with high-risk patterns of fusion.[26] The role of prophylactic surgical fusion in asymptomatic patients with high-risk patterns is undefined. Extension of the spine during a posterior wiring procedure led to neurological deterioration in one case described by Lee.[25] It seems reasonable, therefore, to limit surgery to those patients with gross instability or neurological compromise. Because the early symptoms and signs of this may be subtle, it is important that the patients be well educated, and periodic clinic visits including a thorough neurological examination should be recommended.

In the presence of a neurological deficit, decompression combined with fusion should be carried out. The best technique to accomplish this is a lateral interfacet fusion, wiring either rib or split-thickness iliac bone graft to the facet joints. This is followed by immobilization in a halo until fusion is complete.[12]

Occipitocervical Fusion

Occipitoatlantal fusion may be required for a variety of clinical conditions including congenital anomalies, acquired instabilities, and trauma. Certain generalized skeletal dysplasias, particularly patients with Morquio's syndrome, have a high incidence of congenital anomalies of the odontoid and atlantoaxial instability. It is now believed that patients with this syndrome are at risk for acute quadriparesis and possible sudden death, as well as rapidly progressive myelopathy.[27] In these cases, a localized atlantoaxial fusion is usually not feasible, and occipitocervical fusion is recommended.[28]

Some cases of long-standing atlantoaxial rotatory fixation have developed counter occipitoatlantal subluxation.[29,30] If this is present, an in situ occipitocervical fusion without attempt at reducing the atlantoaxial fixation is recommended on the neurologically intact patient.[29]

Cervical fractures and dislocations are uncommon in children, but when they do occur, the craniocervical region predominates.[31] The fulcrum of normal cervical spine motion in children under 8 years old is C3 as compared to C5–C6 in the adult. Nonfatal traumatic occipitoatlantal instability can occur, with occipitoatlantal fusion required for stabilization.[32,33]

Extension of an atlantoaxial fusion to the occiput has been advocated in cases in which an isolated atlantoaxial fusion using traditional wiring technique cannot be carried out because of a bifid posterior arch of the atlas. However, Lipson[34] described a posterior wiring procedure that can be carried out in this situation. Alternatively, lateral and

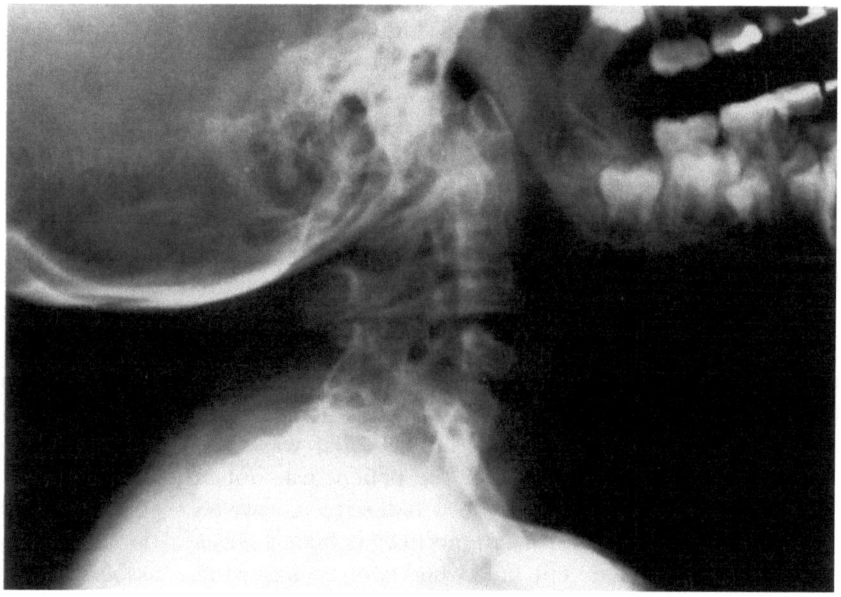

Figure 12.5. Lateral radiograph of cervical spine of 5-year-old child. Note extensive Klippel–Feil deformity with fusion of second through fourth, and fifth through seventh, vertebrae. Lone mobile segment is C4–C5. In addition, patient has left Sprengel's deformity and congenital lumbar scoliosis. Patient is neurologically intact and asymptomatic. Patient is being observed with yearly radiographs of lateral cervical spine in flexion and extension.

anterior methods may be used as options to avoid extension of the arthrodesis to include the occiput.[35–37]

A more common indication for occipitocervical fusion in children is progressive deformity following a wide posterior decompression for tumors such as neurofibromas, ependymomas, or astrocytomas which arise in the posterior fossa and extend through the foramen magnum into the upper cervical spine.[38] Wertheim[39] reported on two patients requiring occipitoatlantal fusion in whom the occipitoatlantal joint had been destroyed by infection, leading to occipitocervical dislocation with gross instability and quadriparesis.

Cases of basilar impression, congenital occipitoatlantal fusion, and other craniovertebral anomalies with a neurological deficit may be first approached with a posterior fusion rather than a decompression. Posterior decompression may be dangerous because hematomyelia may develop from decompression of compressed arteries. If necessary, an anterior or posterior decompression may be done later, after the fusion is established. Anterior decompression in the presence of a solid posterior fusion will not cause increasing instability.

Operations that have been described for occipitocervical fusion fit into three broad categories: (1) simple onlay grafts; (2) wire fixation, in which bone graft is wired into the spine to serve the dual function of arthrodesis and conferring a degree of postoperative stability; and (3) rod or plate fixation, in which onlay bone graft is used, but rigid fixation is gained through the use of screws, plates, or rods with minimal or no need for external immobilization.

Onlay cancellous bone grafts were used by Perry and Nickel[40] in 1959. Most of the patients had instability resulting from poliomyelitis. Postoperatively, they were immobilized in a halo cast. Newman and Sweetnam[41] described an onlay graft that they stated was "simple, safe and reliable." The patient was placed prone with the head in skeletal traction. A midline incision was made, and the lamina and spinous processes of the axis and central part of the arch of the axis were cleared of soft tissue. Similarly, muscle was detached from the occiput and the margin of the foramen magnum. The most cephalic portion of the incision was a point near the superior nuchal line. Decortication was carried out, followed by packing the area from the occiput to the axis with a mass of finely chipped cancellous bone removed from the outer table of the ilium. The patient was then transferred to a Stryker frame with continuous skeletal traction, where he remained for 6 weeks. A molded plastic collar was then applied that was worn whenever the patient was out of bed for a further 6 weeks or until radiographs showed consolidation of the graft. All patients in Sweetnam's series developed a fusion except one who required a second graft after a pseudarthrosis developed.[41] The author believes that this technique is useful for children, who will have a higher rate of fusion from a simple onlay technique than adults. A well-molded halo body jacket may be substituted for the 6 weeks of traction in the Stryker frame. This method cannot be used if there has been a wide laminectomy between the occiput and C2.

Numerous authors have described operations in which bone graft is wired into place from the occiput to the cervical spine. This improves the biomechanical stability and allows less reliance on external immobilization.[42] Robinson and Southwick[43] wired in bone grafts with facet wires below C1, sublaminar wires around the posterior arch of C1, and wires passing through burr holes and out the foramen magnum for attachment to the occiput. The placing of wires through burr holes in the occiput involves the risk of bleeding from the occipital sinuses. More recent constructs have passed the occipital wires through the outer table of the cranium only, usually under a ridge in the midline, thus avoiding penetrating of the inner table and the problem of bleeding from the occipital sinus.[39,44,45] A burr is used to create a ridge in the midline adjacent to the external occipital protuberance, and a hole is then made through the ridge. Wires passed through the bony ridge may then be used to anchor the grafts in a trough on either side. We believe the Wisconsin wires with buttons attached may be helpful in this area (Fig. 12.6).

Heywood has mapped out the average thickness of the skull in the basiocciput. The midline ridge above the foramen magnum is between 9 and 16 mm deep and is the most suitable area for wiring. The thinnest bone is laterally on either side of the foramen magnum, being only 3–5 mm deep.[45] If there has been a decompression of the basiocciput in the midline for a tumor, the grafts must be seated more laterally. Often the depth will be insufficient to allow passage of a wire through one cortex only, and full-thickness burr holes may be required.

Wiesel and Rothman[46] favored autogenous rib grafts because they found that the natural curve of the rib fitted the graft site best when the occiput was in the neutral position relative to C1. Wertheim[39] used the natural curve of the iliac crest from front to back to give a graft with an appropriate contour. Grantham also used autogenous iliac crest bone and warned against the use of bank bone; in one case in which it was used, there was complete graft resorption.[44] Some authors have advocated encasing the wire construct in methylmethacrylate to avoid using bone graft.[47] This is not recommended in children. Bone graft is weakest at the time of insertion and becomes progressively stronger with time. Methylmethacrylate is strongest at insertion and progressively weakens. In addition, there are reports that use of methylmethacrylate is associated with a higher incidence of deep infection and loss of reduction.[48]

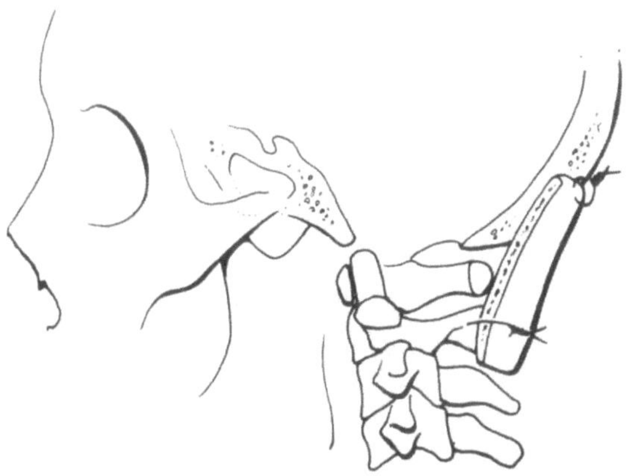

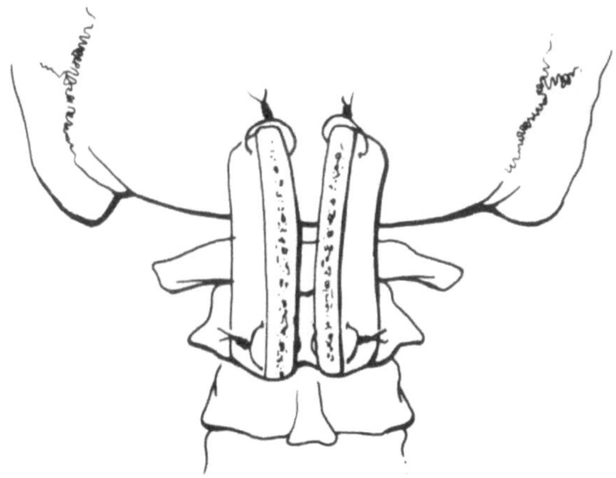

Figure 12.6. Representation of occipitocervical fusion. This construct uses paired slabs of corticocancellous bone. Proximally slabs are placed in trough formed with burr on either side of ridge of bone in midline adjacent to external occipital protuberance. Wire is placed through graft and through ridge, avoiding penetration of inner table of cranium. Wires beneath are passed through spinous process of C2. For additional stability, graft may be fixed with sublaminar wires passed beneath arch of C1. Construct is not sufficiently secure to avoid need for postoperative halo immobilization.

Rigid internal fixation with screws, plates, or rods was reported as early as 1966.[49] Ransford et al.[50] recommended a molded Luque rod wired to the spine and attached to the skull through burr holes. They described three patients, of whom the youngest was a 21-year-old man with severe basilar impression secondary to osteogenesis imperfecta. Ransford stated that the internal fixation was developed to allow anterior decompressive surgery to be undertaken in patients who, despite posterior decompression, have progressive cervicomedullary compression leading to tetraparesis. Roy-Camille[51] has described premolded occipitocervical plates for occipitocervical fixation and fusion. At the cervical level, the fixation is achieved with screws into the articular masses of the vertebra. Fixation to the occiput is with 13-mm screws. More recently, Heywood used a small T-plate in 14 patients. This plate screwed into the occiput in the midline and the spinous process of C2. This internal fixation requires an intact posterior arch of C2.[45]

Internal fixation with plates and screws will rarely be required in a pediatric population. Their use has been mainly in patients with rheumatoid arthritis or instability secondary to resections for tumors.[52,53]

Atlantoaxial Instability

Atlantoaxial instability (AAI) in children is seen in association with a wide variety of clinical syndromes, conditions, and traumatic events. It is seen in mucopolysaccharidoses, in particular Morquio's syndrome,[54,55] bone dysplasias such as spondyloepiphyseal displasia,[56], chondrodystrophia calcificans congenita,[57], Down's syndrome,[58] and neurofibromatosis.[59] Atlantoaxial instability may develop from attrition of the transverse ligament in occipitoatlantal fusion[60] and in Klippel–Feil syndrome, particularly in cases with congenital fusion between C2 and C3.[61]

The preceeding list is diverse, and as knowledge accumulates, it seems certain that other less common syndromes will be added. Therefore, it is prudent for the orthopaedic surgeon treating a patient with any genetic condition to routinely assess the upper cervical spine with a lateral radiograph in flexion and extension. This is particularly important if the patient is to undergo general anesthesia.

The clinical significance of AAI in many conditions has not been fully defined. Lipson[54] has cited AAI as a common cause of quadriparesis, quadriplegia, and death in Morquio's syndrome. However, for many of the other conditions associated with AAI, the true incidence of morbidity or death may still be unrecognized. The traumatic event triggers the symptoms, if present at all, may be trivial, and attention may be directed to other problems associated with the condition. With a poorly defined natural history, few authors have recommended prophylactic atlantoaxial fusion in asymptomatic children. An exception is Morquio's syndrome, in which AAI has been cited as the most common cause of death; prophylactic atlantoaxial fusion has been advocated by some authors[54,62] (Fig. 12.7).

Other authors have emphasized the risks of surgery and halo fixation in children, and because of these concerns, the place for prophylactic fusion, especially in an asymptomatic patient, has not been clearly defined.

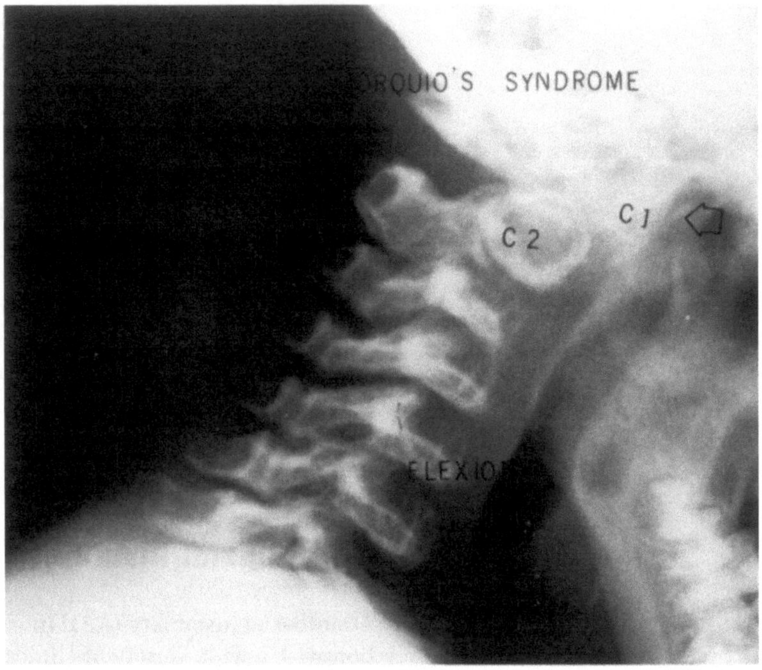

A

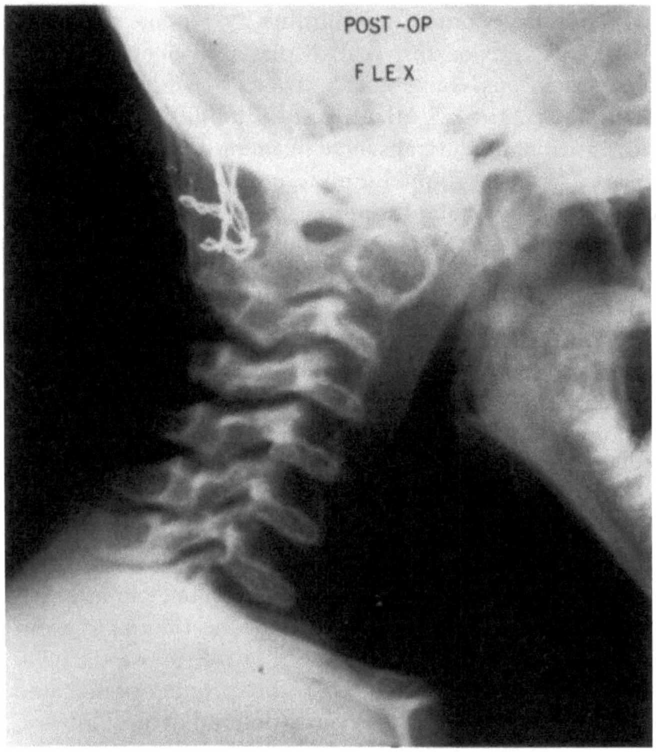

B

Figure 12.7. **A.** Six-year-old child with type A Morquio's syndrome (keratan sulfatase deficiency). Lateral cervical spine radiograph in flexion shows generalized platyspondyly and aplastic odontoid with enlarged C2 vertebral body. There is 4-mm translational shift of C1 on C2 with flexion and extension. *Open arrow* indicates anterior arch of C1. **B.** Same patient after occiput-to-C2 fusion with wire fixation. Patient had dysplasia of lateral aspect of both proximal tibial epiphyses, resulting in severe bilateral genu valgus. Occipitocervical fusion was elected early in anticipation of further general anesthesia procedures for correction of lower extremity deformities.

Anatomy and Kinematics

Knowledge of the complex anatomy and kinematics of the atlantoaxial joint is helpful in understanding the pathogenesis of disorders of the articulation as well as for planning rational, conservative, and operative treatments.

It was believed that the occiput-C1 articulation was limited to flexion and extension and the C1–C2 joint to rotation. Several authors recently have shown that flexion and extension occur at both the occiput-C1 level and at the C1–C2 level to almost equal degrees, giving a combined range of motion averaging 23.4°.[63] Rotation is, however, still thought to occur primarily at the atlantoaxial joint. The complex sloping configuration of the atlantoaxial joint gives rise to an interesting coupled motion. Coupling has been defined as mandatory motion along two axes occurring simultaneously. At C1–C2, axial rotation is coupled to vertical translation.[64] The atlas is at its zenith at zero degrees of rotation and at its lowest position when fully rotated to either side.

During forced flexion of the head, the anterior surface of the odontoid process abuts against the anterior arch of the atlas. Excessive displacement of the atlas on the occiput is restricted only by the tectorial membrane, the alar ligaments, and the capsular ligaments.[65] Despite this, there is little translational movement of the atlas on the occiput, and if significant movement is detected it may be considered pathological. During extension, the odontoid process acts as a buttress preventing posterior sliding of the axis. Posteriorly, extension is limited by abutment of the posterior margin of the foramen magnum, the posterior arch of the atlas, and the spinous process of the axis. While there is no translational movement forward and back during flexion and extension at the occiput-C1 articulation, significant movement may be seen in the normal spine at C1–C2. Jackson's studies, which involve adults and children, showed a maximum of 2.5 mm in adults and 4 mm in children.[66] Fielding found that a force of 84 kg was required to rupture the transverse ligament and allow 3 to 5 mm of anterior shift of C1 on C2 in adults. After the transverse ligament ruptures, a similar amount of force is required to allow further displacement of C1 on C2, as much as 12 mm. This occurs by stretching of the accessory ligaments, particularly the paired alar ligaments.

Fielding thus thought that 3 to 5 mm of atlantoaxial instability in an adult implied disruption of the transverse ligament and that displacement exceeding 5 mm implied increasing stretch to all remaining ligaments.[67]

Steel[68] proposed a system of primary and secondary restraints. The primary restraint to translation is the transverse atlantal ligament. If this has ruptured acutely, as in trauma, a degree of instability will be present, but this instability will worsen slowly because of attrition and stretching of the secondary restraints, namely the alar ligaments.

While most lateral bending of the cervical spine occurs below the atlantoaxial joint, some motion is permitted at the occipitoatlantal joint, but none at the atlantoaxial joint. Lateral translation at C1–C2 is controversial. Certainly apparent translation is seen during anteroposterior (AP) cineradiography with rotation of the head to the right and left. Narrowing of the gap between the lateral mass and the dens, first on one side then the other, is clearly seen and is used in making the diagnosis of atlantoaxial rotatory fixation. This movement, however, may simply be from radiographic distortions.[63,65] Vertical displacement of the atlas on the axis is limited by tension in the capsules of the articular facets and by the anatomical fact that the odontoid is thicker above the transverse ligament than below, giving a buttonhole effect.[69]

Radiology

The most important information is gained from the lateral radiograph in neutral, full flexion, and extension. Attention should be paid to the atlanto-dens interval which in children should be no greater than 4 mm in flexion.[66] Measurement of the atlanto-dens interval (ADI) is of clinical significance only if the odontoid process is intact and attached to the body of the axis. In the case of a fracture of the odontoid or an os odontoideum, the odontoid fragment may remain attached in a normal anatomical configuration to the anterior arch of the atlas and slide forward in flexion with it. This may markedly narrow the canal without any change in the atlanto-dens interval. For this reason, McRae focused attention on the space available for the cord (SAC). This is the distance between the posterior aspect of the odontoid or in the case of os odontoideum or fracture, the posterior body of the axis, and the nearest posterior structure, usually the posterior ring of the atlas. McRae[70] thought that neurological symptoms would always be present if this space was 19 mm or less.

Subsequent work by Greenberg[71] showed that a cord compression was always present when this space was 14 mm or less; compression was sometimes present between 15 and 17 mm, and never occurred with more than 18 mm (Fig. 12.8). While a widened atlanto-dens interval and a decreased SAC in the presence of an intact odontoid would normally appear together, isolated congenital narrowing of the canal has been recorded.[72] Steel's rule of thirds simplifies and restates the facts uncovered by canal measurements. He defined the area enclosed within the arch of the atlas as being divided into three. One-third is taken up by the odontoid, and this should include the transverse ligament, which usually measures at least 3 mm. One-third is represented by the cord, and one-third represents free space, through which displacement can occur without neurological impingement.[61,68]

Although most attention is focused on bony encroachment of the canal, it must be remembered that a neurological deficit may occur if the amount of neural tissue is increased, for example, in the presence of cerebellar herniation in the Arnold-Chiari malformation, or if the free space is encroached on by tissue, such as granulation tissue in rheumatoid arthritis. More advanced radiological techniques have allowed us to clearly define these soft-tissue components. Roach[73] showed that high-resolution CT scanning of this area in children with the neck sequentially in flexion and extension can nearly always clearly visualize

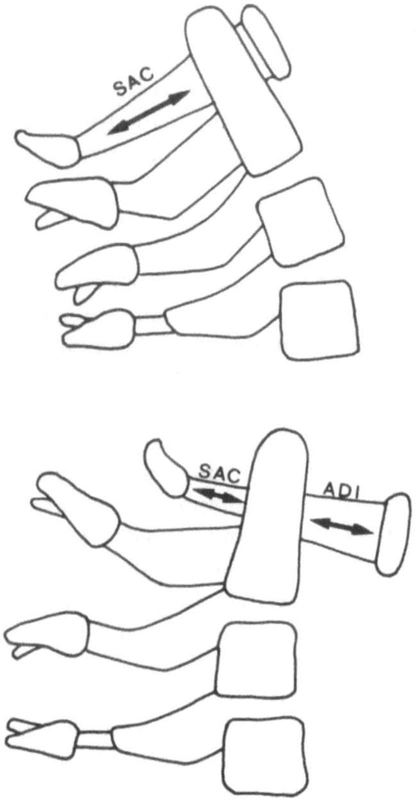

Figure 12.8. Graphical representation of relationship between atlanto-dens interval (ADI) and space available for cord (SAC). With intact odontoid process, space available for cord will be decreased as atlanto-dens interval increases. In cases of instability associated with os odontoideum where os remains attached to anterior arch of atlas and moves with it, space available for cord may be severely decreased without any change in atlanto-dens interval.

the cord and show compression at the stage before clinical symptoms may be present. MRI dramatically outlines the cord as it traverses the atlantooccipital area, and should be considered a standard diagnostic procedure in cases with pathology at this level. The only disadvantage is that current scanning times may require sedation or even general anesthesia for young or uncooperative children. Future improvements will include much shorter scanning times and improved surface coils for greater resolution of pathology in this area. The advent of MRI has meant that myelography is now virtually never required in the craniocervical region in children.

In practice, atlantoaxial instability is most commonly seen in association with os odontoideum, with other anomalies of the odontoid, and in children with Down's syndrome. These conditions are now considered in more detail.

Anomalies of the Odontoid

The most common anomaly of the odontoid is os odontoideum, but complete absence of the odontoid (aplasia) and partial absence (hypoplasia) have also been described.[74,75] The body of the odontoid process is embryologically derived from the mesenchyme of the sclerotome of the first cervical vertebra. It separates from the centrum of the first cervical vertebra, moves caudally, and fuses with the axis to become the odontoid process. Ossification of the odontoid occurs from three centers, two on either side, forming vertical pillars that fuse by the time of birth and are separated from the body of the axis by a cartilaginous growth plate, the neurocentral synchondrosis. The neurocentral synchondrosis is dovetailed into the body of the axis; thus, a considerable portion of the embryological odontoid process forms part of the body of the axis and lies below the anatomical neck, which is at the level of the most cephalic and medial portion of the C1–C2 articular facets. The neurocentral synchondrosis fuses to the body of the axis before the age of 7 years. The apex of the odontoid process is derived from the mesenchyme of the fourth occipital sclerotome and is not ossified at birth; thus a small V-shaped dip may be seen in the odontoid. A separate center of ossification may appear at age 3 years and fuse with the body of the odontoid process by the age of 12. This separate center, before fusion, may be called an ossiculum terminale.

In recent years evidence has accumulated to support the theory that the majority of conditions that were previously termed congenital anomalies of the odontoid, especially the os odontoideum, are the result of trauma. Often patients with an os odontoideum have a history of a significant episode of trauma occurring during childhood.[76] Fielding[67] documented four patients in whom an os odontoideum developed after a normal odontoid process had previously been documented to have been present. Support for this theory also comes from both clinical data, in that the condition is more common in boys, and morphological data, in that absence of that portion of the embryological odontoid that incorporates into the body of C2 is virtually never seen.[67]

Os odontoideum is rarely seen in association with other congenital spinal abnormalities such as diastematomyelia. Fielding et al. had the opportunity of examining the case report of a child with an os odontoideum who died. They showed that the alar ligaments attaching the occiput to the tip of the odontoid process had pulled the tip of the odontoid fragment cranially. They therefore contended that after the odontoid process had been traumatically disrupted at its anatomical base, contracture of the alar ligaments exerted a distraction force on the proximal fragment encouraging nonunion. An intact transverse atlantoaxial ligament maintained the fragment adjacent to the ring of the atlas. Blood supply to the odontoid fragment is precarious, because a large portion of the odontoid is covered with articular cartilage, and blood vessels passing cephalically from the body of C2 may be disrupted by the fracture.[77] These factors predispose to nonunion, while variations in the final morphology of the os can be explained by the age at which the fracture occurred, some occurring as early as birth.

Patients frequently come to medical attention following an episode of minor trauma that leads to a radiograph. Further symptoms may be mechanical such as spasm, neck pain, and torticollis.[78] A second cause of symptoms may be obstruction of the vertebral arteries, and in these patients there may be symptoms and signs of cerebral and brain stem ischemia. Third, patients may present with a neurological deficit. This may take the form of a slow and insidious onset of quadriparesis or an acute onset of quadriparesis following trauma. In the former, as is seen in craniovertebral anomalies, clinical symptoms and physical examination may be confusing, and these patients may be initially diagnosed as having demyelinating conditions or hereditary ataxias.

An os odontoideum is a small round or oval ossicle separate and cranial to a hypoplastic odontoid process. The ossicle may be in the normal position adjacent to the tip of the odontoid process or may exist more cephalad near the basion or even fuse to the basion.[79]

Atlantoaxial instability is commonly seen in association with os odontoideum. This may be demonstrated on lateral radiographs in flexion and extension. Narrowing of the space available for the cord can be calculated by measurements of the lateral radiographs. If the bony landmarks are imprecise, lateral tomograms are required (Fig. 12.9). Ideally, once the clearest cut is seen on the tomogram, flexion and extension views should be made at that level. This, however, can sometimes be difficult to achieve. We have used the method of Roach in taking CT scans of this area with the head in flexion and extension. A high-resolution transaxial scan of small thickness can usually demonstrate the cord and show any flattening or impingment.[73]

It is important to remember that instability can be anterior (most common) but also posterior. In Fielding's series,[76] a significant number had *both* anterior and posterior instability. In the presence of a neurological deficit, an MRI scan should be employed to assess impingement of the neurological structures and exclude associated conditions such as syringomyelia.

The indications for fusion in patients with os odontoideum with or without atlantoaxial instability are controversial. Sheppard believes that all patients should have elective stabilization to eliminate the possibility of an acute neurological catastrophe with minimal trauma.[80]

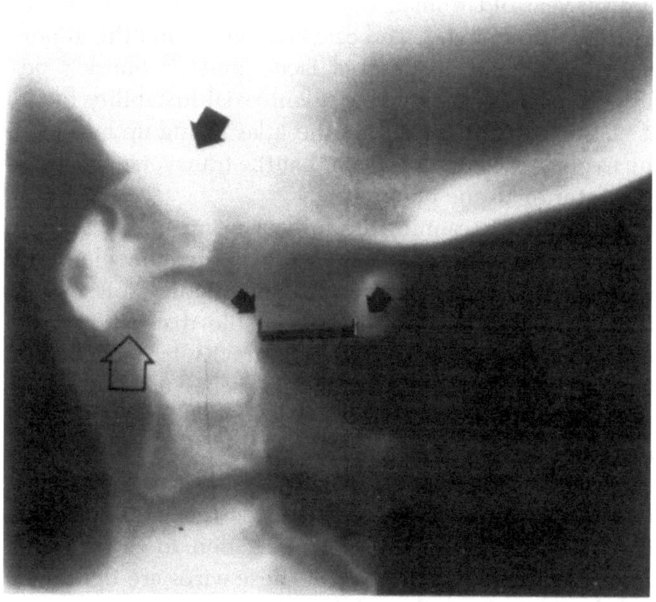

Figure 12.9. Lateral tomogram of 8-year-old child with os odontoideum and atlantoaxial instability. Os (*large black arrow*) maintains its relationship with anterior arch of atlas. Atlanto-dens interval measures 6 mm (*open arrow*). Space available for cord (between *small black arrows*) is narrowed to 14 mm. Etiology of odontoid pathology is probably traumatic because significant portion of body of C2 remains projecting upward beyond neurocentral synchondrosis.

Hensinger[76,81] stated that ". . . there is general agreement that surgical stabilization is indicated in the event of neurological involvement, even if transient; instability of greater than 5 mm anterior or posterior; or progressive instability or persistent neck complaints." Some authors, however, believe that the risk of surgery outweighs risks associated with the natural history. Isolated reports of neurological catastrophes after fusion have been described. In Fielding's series, however, 26 of 35 patients studied underwent a Gallie fusion between C1 and C2. In none of the patients who were operated on was the neurological deficit increased, and all of the patients with neurological deficits had resolved following the operations, with the exception of two patients with quadriparesis, both of whom were improved.[76]

Special caution is advised for those patients with os odontoideum and irreducible C1–C2 dislocation with or without a neurological deficit. Posterior decompression may worsen the C1–C2 instability, and there is a definite danger of neurological impairment if an attempt is made to reduce an irreducible subluxation at the time of surgery for fusion. Irreducibility is probably related to the length of time the atlantoaxial complex has been in the subluxed position. Nagashima described a case of an os odontoideum in a 50-year-old woman that was irreducible because of arthritis, osteophytes, and calcification around the abnormally positioned atlantoaxial facet joints.[82] Sherk[83] described a case of irreducible atlantoaxial instability found at necropsy to be caused by the atlas riding up and over the hypoplastic odontoid such that the transverse ligament was anterior to the odontoid.

CT and MRI scanning are important in the assessment of irreducible dislocations, CT to show the bony elements and MRI to show the neural elements and soft tissue. The initial treatment of an irreducible dislocation is to attempt slow reduction with halo gravity traction before any surgery. If reduction cannot be achieved, passage of sublaminar wires beneath the posterior arch of the atlas and axis, as in a Brooks' fusion, will be hazardous. Less encroachment of the canal will be gained by passing a sublaminar wire only around the posterior arch of the atlas and extending this to gain fixation to the spinous process of the axis. However, if these wires are tightened and the posterior arches of the atlas and axis approximate in a spine that cannot be anatomically reduced, the canal will be narrowed and a neurlogical deficit may supervene. For this reason, we believe that most patients with an irreducible C1–C2 dislocation should be treated with an in situ posterior fusion from the occipit to C2 with postoperative immobilization in a halo body jacket. The technique of this fusion is discussed in the section on occipitocervical fusion.

Because os odontoideum appears to result from an unrecognized or ununited fracture of the odontoid in a child, a short word shall be said regarding these fractures. Odontoid fractures are an uncommon cause of atlantoaxial instability in children. The fracture occurs most commonly at the level of the synchondrosis and less commonly at the waist.[84] In Sherk's series, the majority were able to be treated conservatively by postural or manipulative reduction and immobilization for at least 6 weeks. Recently authors have stressed that if reduction is attempted through recumbency and hyperextension, allowance must be made for the relatively larger head of a child as compared to an adult. If a child is placed on a flat spine board or bed, the cervical spine will be held in flexion. Therefore, divided mattresses are required to allow the head to fall back into extension.[85]

Atlantoaxial Instability in Down's Syndrome

Atlantoaxial instability in children with Down's syndrome was first reported by Spitzer in 1961.[58] Since that time, it has become a world-recognized entity. Many children and adults with Down's syndrome enjoy sporting activities and participation in the Special Olympics. In 1983, the Committee of the Special Olympics, in response to concern that catastrophic neurological injury may occur in a Down's syndrome child with unrecognized atlantoaxial instability during events such as tumbling, put forward guidelines for people with Down's syndrome who wish to compete. All prospective participants with Down's syndrome were required to have a lateral radiograph of the cervical spine in flexion and extension. An atlanto-dens interval of 4.5 mm or greater was used as the criterion to restrict participation.[86]

The incidence of atlantoaxial instability in Down's children has been quoted at betweeen 10% and 25%.[87–90] Miller[91] noted a preponderance in men with a 24% incidence compared to 15% in women. Pueschel[88] noted a 1:2.3 ratio in favor of females, and 6 of 7 patients with neurological symptoms were female. The only difference in the series was that 40% of Miller's cases were over the age of 37 years whereas in Pueschel's study most cases were under the age of 15 years.

The cause of atlantoaxial subluxation in Down's syndrome patients is not known. Some authors believe it is a local manifestation of the generalized ligamentous laxity seen in these patients. Various other radiological anomalies have been reported in the cervical spine of Down's syndrome patients including flattening of the vertebral bodies.[87,91] Miller demonstrated areas of nonaeration of the sinuses that he believed to be a maturation defect of the basicranium. In addition, various congenital anomalies of the odontoid have been well described, including os odontoideum ossiculum terminale[92] and divided odontoids.[93] Odontoid hypoplasia in Down's syndrome probably represents a developmental anomaly similar to that which causes the well-known platyspondyly in the remainder of the spine. However, a large number of the remaining defects including the ossicles may be explained by trauma occurring during the very early stages of ossification, with a fracture occurring even as early as delivery.[93] French thought the most rational hypothesis for the ossicle superior to the odontoid was an ununited avulsion fracture of the tip of the dens. His argument for this centered on the fact that his cases with this anomaly often still had a dens of normal length.[92]

There appears to be an association between Down's syndrome and juvenile rheumatoid arthritis.[94–97] The cervical spine manifestations of juvenile rheumatoiid arthritis may be additive to those of Down's syndrome, leading to serious clinical problems. Rosenbaum[94] described two such patients who developed atlantooccipital instability of a marked degree. This is not as obvious roentgenographically as atlantoaxial instability but can have serious neurological consequences of its own. It has been speculated that Down's syndrome patients who have an atlantoaxial fusion may later develop occipitoatlantal instability. For this reason, some authors advocate fusion to the occiput in Down's syndrome. There is no body of information at this time, however, to support that position.

There is some evidence that the incidence of atlantoaxial instability in Down's syndrome increases with age.[90] However, the natural history is largely unknown. Prospective studies that were begun in the last 10 years, initiated by screening for the Special Olympics, need to be carried forward to establish whether patients without atlantoaxial instability as children develop the condition as adults. Also, information needs to be gathered to establish whether existing atlantoaxial instability improves or worsens with age. At present the recommendation of the Committee on Sports Medicine of the American Academy of Pediatrics advocates a single radiographic series. Perhaps serial radiographs every 5 years would be more appropriate, particularly in those children engaged in active sports.

It has been estimated that only approximately 2% of children identified as having atlantoaxial instability will have a symptomatic neurological condition.[87,88] The onset of neurological symptoms may be sudden and dramatic following a fall,[98] or, more commonly, have a slow and insidious onset. These children may be unable to accurately describe their symptomatology. Increasing hypotonia and physical deterioration may be mistaken as a generalized manifestation of Down's syndrome. The result is that the neurological impairment may be advanced by the time of diagnosis. The surgeon should be aware that children who develop difficulty walking, with a characteristic "rag doll" picture, may well be manifesting quadriparesis.[97]

There is no consensus on the management of asymptomatic atlantoaxial instability in Down's syndrome. In general, the marked disparity between the percentage of children with instability and the much smaller percentage who are neurologically symptomatic indicates that a prophylactic fusion for instability alone is not recommended.[99] However, these children should be followed on a regular basis. Clinical examination alone is often inadequate to detect an early neurological syndrome. Pueschel[88] has shown abnormal somatosensory-evoked potentials (SSEPs) in patients with atlantoaxial instability who appear otherwise normal. Roach[73] showed that CT examination of the craniocervical region could be carried out with the spine in flexion and extension, and could show early flattening of the spinal cord. We believe that instability with an atlanto-dens interval of 6 mm or greater, with one of the foregoing two investigations positive, would be best served with an atlantoaxial fusion. Pueschel et al. stated that all their patients with an atlanto-dens interval of greater than 7 mm displayed neurological symptoms. Once neurological symptoms have appeared the outcome of fusion is less satisfactory. Of 35 patients who underwent surgery, only 8 made a complete neurologic recovery; 14 showed some improvement, 7 did not improve, 4 died, and the outcome for 2 was unknown.[88]

The condition of atlantoaxial subluxation should be kept in mind with all Down's children who are undergoing surgery for other conditions, for example, congenital heart defects, as intubation during anesthesia may precipitate an acute neurological defect.[100]

Patients with irreducible deformity should undergo a period of halo gravity traction in an attempt to reduce subluxation and effectively decompress the canal. In neurologically intact patients with reducible deformity, we advocate Griswold's modification of Brook's fusion, which will be described in detail.[101] Patients with irreducible deformity or any degree of neurological abnormality should not have sublaminar wires passed under C2; a Gallie-type fusion, with an H-graft as described by Fielding, is safer.[102] Lipson[103] described a modification of this technique and has shown it to be as stable as the fusion techniques in which wires are passed under the arch of C2 on both sides. However, we would recommend restriction in a halo in the postoperative period after a standard Gallie fusion.

Patients with occipitoatlantal instability or those patients with associated rheumatoid arthritis and proximal odontoid migration should be fused to the occiput.[94,96]

Atlantoaxial Rotatory Subluxation

Pathological rotation of the atlas on the axis may be seen in a wide variety of conditions. The etiology ranges from ligamentous laxity associated with viral pharyngitis to minimal trauma or severe trauma from motor vehicle accidents. The clinical picture of a wry neck may be transitory and self-resolving, or may become chronic and fixed, requiring operative reduction or fusion. Acute traumatic bilateral atlantoaxial rotatory dislocation has been described on a number of occasions.[104–106] At the other end of the spectrum, cases of torticollis are not uncommon in childhood, being either of spontaneous origin or related to a bacterial or viral pharyngitis. The majority of these usually respond to nonspecific conservative measures such as heat, massage, or a soft surgical collar.

Torticollis, however, may be the presenting symptom of a number of more serious conditions. Ineffective initial treatment may allow a relatively simple case of atlantoaxial rotation to become fixed, increasing the problems of treatment. It is important, therefore, to evaluate at the initial presentation each case of a child with torticollis. This examination should exclude congenital anomalies of the cervical spine such as Klippel–Feil, atlantooccipital fusion, and basilar impression. Torticollis may be the presenting symptom for spinal cord and cerebellar tumors, or afflictions of the cord such as syringomyelia. Infectious and inflammatory conditions include tuberculosis and rheumatoid arthritis.

Atlantoaxial Rotatory Fixation

This syndrome was first described by Wortzman and Dewar in 1968.[107] Fielding and Hawkins[108] reviewed 17 cases of irreducible atlantoaxial rotatory fixation and classified them into four types. The first type, the most common, occurred in patients in whom the fixed rotation was within the normal range of atlantoaxial rotation. The transverse and alar ligaments were intact and no increased atlantoaxial interval was seen on the lateral radiograph. In the second type, the atlas moved forward and into rotation at one atlantoaxial joint, the other remaining intact as a pivot. In these cases, an increased atlanto-dens interval is seen, but measuring less than 5 mm. It is postulated that in this type the transverse ligament is plastically deformed. In the third type, there was a deficiency in both the transverse and secondary ligaments so that both lateral masses were displaced anteriorly and into rotation. Here the transverse ligament is incompetent, as are the secondary restraining ligaments, and the atlanto-dens interval may be increased greater than 5 mm. The final type is that of rotatory fixation with posterior displacement, which is rare, and was described in one adult patient with rheumatoid arthritis.

In Fielding's series the cause of fixation was spontaneous in four patients, upper respiratory tract infection in five, minor trauma in three, and major trauma in two. Most important, there was an average of 11.6 months before the condition was diagnosed. Clinically, the patients may develop plagiocephaly. Pain is usually mild. The condition can be differentiated clinically from congenital torticollis by the fact that the sternomastoid, which is tight or in spasm, is on the side to which the head is cocked in congenital torticollis, but on the opposite side in atlantoaxial rotatory fixation, as if the tight sternomastoid was attempting to correct the deformity.

The condition of atlantoaxial rotatory fixation can be suggested but not proven by the plain films. The AP open-mouth odontoid film will show that the odontoid is closer to one lateral mass of the atlas than the other. This, however, is a normal finding when the atlas is rotated on the axis. When rotating the head back to the opposite side, it should reverse so that the odontoid is now closer to the contralateral mass. In atlantoaxial rotatory fixation, the lateral mass on one side remains fixed in its proximity to the odontoid despite attempts at rotation of the head to the opposite side. For this reason, the diagnosis can often be made best with cineroentgenograms where the immobility of the atlantoaxial joint can be graphically demonstrated. (Fig. 12.10). The lateral plane film will show an increased atlantoaxial interval in types II and III. Computerized tomography may also show the asymmetric position of the odontoid and will document the change in the axis of rotation between the atlas and the axis.

Johnson and Ferguson[109] described two cases of acute atlantoaxial rotatory fixation following moderate trauma in children. Both resolved after a period of halter traction and wearing a soft collar for a number of weeks. The authors emphasized that if this diagnosis is confirmed radiologically early in the course, simple methods of treatment may be applied, as opposed to the series of Fielding[108] in whom the condition was detected late and fusion was the usual outcome. Long-term atlantoaxial rotatory fixation may develop a compensatory counter occipitoatlantal sub-

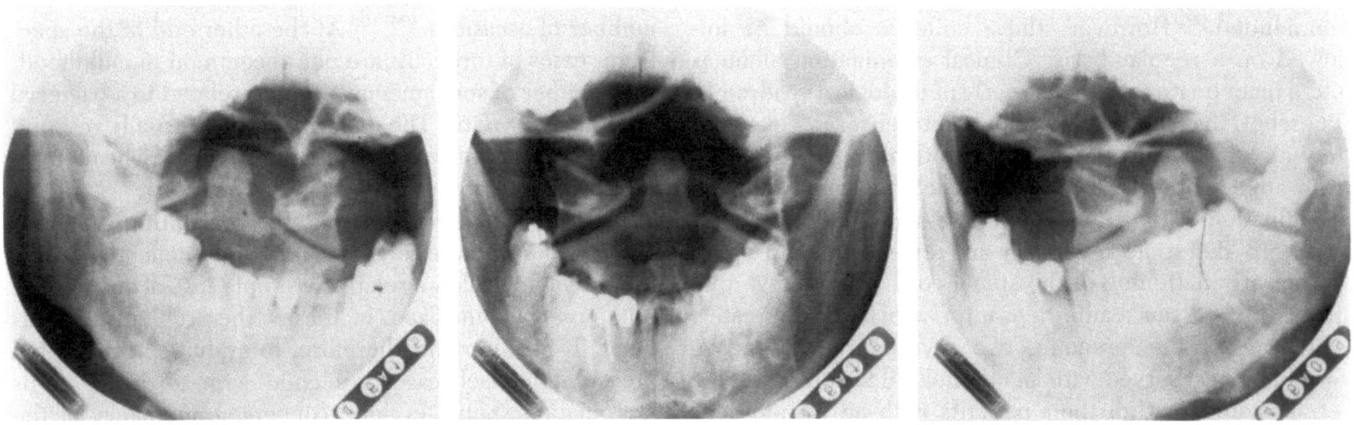

Figure 12.10. Anteroposterior cineroentgenograms of 20-year-old patient with atlantoaxial rotatory fixation. Central picture with head in neutral position shows right lateral mass of C1 in closer proximity to odontoid than contralateral mass. This proximity remains fixed despite rotation of head to either side, as can be seen by noting direction of jaw and teeth on films on right and left.

luxation. Many patients in Fielding's series presented with mild clinical deformity, and this may have been on the basis of some compensatory subluxation at adjacent levels such as the occipitoatlantal level. The importance of this finding is underlined by the fact that a fusion confined to the atlantoaxial joint may exacerbate the occipitoatlantal subluxation. An in situ fusion from the occiput to C2 is recommended in these cases.

In patients with long-standing fixation (more than 3 months), Fielding recommended fusion, with preoperative traction for 2 to 3 weeks to achieve as much correction of the deformity as possible. This will usually allow the head to be corrected to the neutral position. The fusion is confined to the atlantoaxial joint. Fielding et al. reported that loss of rotation was not a significant clinical problem to their patients at follow-up

Technique of Atlantoaxial Arthrodesis In Children

In 1910, Mixter and Osgood[110] described a technique for atlantoaxial arthrodesis using onlay bone graft and a strip of fascia lata passed under the posterior arch of C1 and behind the spinous process of C2. Gallie[111] described a similar operation, but used wire instead of a fascial graft. Since that time, many and varied procedures have been advocated. The operations vary in three major areas; first, in the use of bone graft, which may be used in the form of an onlay graft either as chips or a slab, or may be wedged between the vertebrae, becoming integral to the stability of the fusion construct. The second variation is in the use of internal fixation. While wire has been used most commonly, newer methods using clamps and screws have been described. Finally, variation exists in the levels chosen to be incorporated in the fusion. Extension to the occiput will lose motion at the occipitoatlantal joint as well as at the atlantoaxial, and the moments generated by the weight of the head will be added to the fusion. Similarly, extension into the lower cervical spine may improve the strength of the fixation at a cost of reduced normal movemnt.

A fusion construct must be planned that accomplishes as many as possible of the following goals: (1) Eliminate motion at the C1–C2 motion segment, which will enhance incorporation of bone graft and decrease the rate of pseudarthrosis. (2) Provide immediate secure fixation to a point where postoperative external support may be minimal or eliminated. Many of the complications associated with atlantoaxial fusion in children have been caused by the halo fixation. (3) Limit the fusion to C1 and C2 and thus preserve motion at the occipitoatlantal and lower cervical spine levels. (4) Ideally, no part of the fusion construct should enter the spinal canal, decreasing the possibility of neurological damage from the fixation.

The primary motion at the atlantoaxial joint is rotation, averaging 47°. There is no lateral bend but there is significant flexion and extension. White and Panjabi have analyzed the various constructs from a biomechanical point of view to see which best counteracts these motions.[63]

A midline wire used alone, as used in a Gallie fusion, is biomechanically unsatisfactory. This wire is poorly situated to resist rotation. It will resist extension only if tightened to the point where the posterior arch of C1 is approximated to the posterior arch of C2. This will give an unphysiological degree of extension, and may cause posterior protrusion of an odontoid fragment into the canal. Some series document a high rate of failure of fusion employing this technique.[112] McGraw and Rusch[113] attempted to improve the operation biomechanically by fashioning an iliac crest H-graft notched to accommodate the spinous process of the axis and the wires. They achieved fusion in 14 of 15 patients using their technique. Similar techniques have been advocated by Fielding[102] and Lipson.[103]

Brooks and Jenkins[114] in 1978 described a wedge-compression method of arthrodesis. In their technique doubled wires are passed under the posterior arch of the atlas and the posterior arch of the axis on both sides. A wedge of corticocancellous bone is then placed in the gap between the atlas and the axis and the wire is tightened over it. The lateral placement of the graft restricts rotation by effectively becoming a friction block.[63] Vertical displacement of the axis is eliminated. Flexion and extension are also blocked, but with preservation of a normal atlantoaxial distance, leaving any odontoid fragment in a more physiologic position. Griswold[101] reported on 30 such cases and compared them with 11 treated by single midline wiring and 19 treated by plaster jacket and brace. Although direct comparison of the results of treatment in the three groups was not possible because of the many variables that may have influenced the results, the incidence of solid fusion was distinctly higher after the Brooks fusion despite less postoperatively immobilization.

There is one distinct disadvantage with this technique. Passage of wire under the posterior arch of C2 may be difficult and is indeed dangerous in irreducible dislocations. To obviate the need for passage of sublaminar wires, Mitsui[115] devised a quadrilateral clamp with hooks that pass over the cephalic aspect of the arch of C1 and caudal to the lamina of C2 but not to the point of canal intrusion. He described its use in patients with rheumatoid arthritis but not in children. While the device appears to satisfy the biomechanical requirements of a wedged compression arthrodesis, it appears bulky and possibly unsuitable for children. Similar clamps using two Cotrel–Dubousset (C–D) rods and hooks on either side of the arch of C1 and C2 have been used.[116] A further clamp device has been described by Roosen,[117] who used it in three patients, one of whom had an os odontoideum.

The fusion currently used by the authors is the modification of the fusion originated by Brooks and Jenkins, as described by Griswold.[101] This operation is used in children with atlantoaxial instability that is fully reducible and in whom CT and MRI scans have confirmed adequate canal dimensions and no neurological compression. Awake nasotracheal intubation is obtained by an anesthesiologist experienced in the technique. A surgeon ensures that no excessive neck movement occurs during intubation. Confirmation of normal neurological status is obtained after intubation and before induction. Cortico-spinal evoked potential monitoring is used. In older children and young adults, a Gardner pin-vise head holder is attached to the patient's head. Gentle traction is maintained as the patient is rolled onto chest rolls. The pin-vise holder is then attached to the table after placing the head with the chin tucked in the position of a "soldier at attention." This position will ensure that the atlantoaxial joint will remain in the reduced position and there will be a satisfactory degree of clearance between the occiput and the posterior arch of C1. A lateral radiograph is then taken to check this position, and if necessary further adjustments of the head position are carefully and gently made before draping. Great care must be taken to firmly anchor the nasotracheal tube. The head must be positioned sufficiently over the end of the bed such that the chin is not resting against a hard surface. Eye protection is essential. The patient's arms are placed at the side.

With younger children we prefer to use a padded horseshoe head holder rather than the pin-vise holder. The head is firmly attached to this holder with tape. After suitable skin preparation and draping, the landmarks of the craniovertebral junction are palpated. The most prominent anatomical landmark is the spinous process of C2. A vertical incision is made and carried down in the midline. Bleeding is controlled with bipolar diathermy. The small muscles attached laterally to the bifid tip of C2 are divided sharply, but the interspinous ligament and the soft tissues between C2 and C3 are left intact. A small curved periosteal elevator is then used to gently expose the lamina of C2. Small cotton packs soaked in thrombin solution are placed to maintain this dissection. The posterior arch of C1 is then identified.

Sharp dissection is carried out laterally on both sides for only 1 cm cephalically and 1.5 cm caudally. The vertebral artery and vein pass over the lateral and cephalic aspect of the posterior arch of the axis. Blunt dissection allows retraction of the suboccipital musculature between C1 and C2, 2 cm lateral from the midline, exposing the thin membrane linking C1 and C2. A large vein is often seen in this interval and should be avoided as it may cause profuse bleeding that may be hard to control. An elevator is then used to dissect subperiosteally circumferentially around the posterior arch of the atlas in the midline to the point where a number 3 Penfield instrument can be easily placed around the posterior arch. Similarly, the soft tissues are dissected off the cephalic and caudal aspects of the lamina of C2.

We agree with Griswold that braided 24-gauge stainless wire has preferable working properties to larger smooth wires. A 60-cm length of wire is bent back on itself. One end is held with a hemostat; the other is placed in a Lovejoy drill and twisted until there are three turns per centimeter. The rounded end is then passed in the midline along the undersurfaces of the atlas and axis from cephalic to caudal. Gentle pressure is exerted on the wire end, and the tip is guided by a needle holder. The most difficult part of the procedure is passage under the arch of C2. We have tried passing an aneurysm needle attached to a silk suture and then attaching the silk suture to the end of the wire. We have abandoned this technique because it lacks control. A small fine Moynihan forcep is passed from the caudal aspect of the lamina of C2 so its tip is just visible at the cephalic border. The sharp curve of the Moynihan more closely resembles the curve of the posterior arch of C2 than a circular aneurysm needle. The wire is placed in its jaws, and the forcep is gradually retracted While the wire is fed caudally with a needle holder. The first two wires on each side are then gently moved laterally approximately 1.5 cm to allow room for the remaining right and left midline wires.

Bone grafts are obtained from the ilium in the usual manner and bone grafts should be approximately 1.5 cm long, 1.2 cm wide, and, if possible, 1 cm deep. The cancellous bone is sculptured until the graft fits like a wedge in the gap between the atlas and axis. Small notches are placed in the upper and lower ends of the graft to accommodate the wires and prevent medial or lateral shifting. The length of the grafts are adjusted so they extend from the cephalic aspect of the posterior arch of C1 to the caudal aspect of the lamina of C2. The wires are then tightened into position using a Bowen wire tightener. Before final tightening of the wires, the exposed bony surfaces of the atlas and axis are lightly decorticated with a fine burr. A lateral radiograph is taken on the table to check wire positions and adequacy of reduction. The wound is closed in layers with interrupted sutures. The pin-vise holder is detached from the operating table and used to control the head of the patient while being rolled prone onto a bed. It is then removed, and a Philadelphia collar is applied. As soon as possible, the patient is encouraged to sit and ambulate. So long as the fixation appears solid at the time of surgery, the only postoperative immobilization is a Philadelphia collar, which is worn for 3 months. Other surgeons have advocated the use of a collar with a thoracic extension (Fig. 12.11).

We have used the foregoing technique in 16 patients since 1981 with no fusion failures. The fusion described

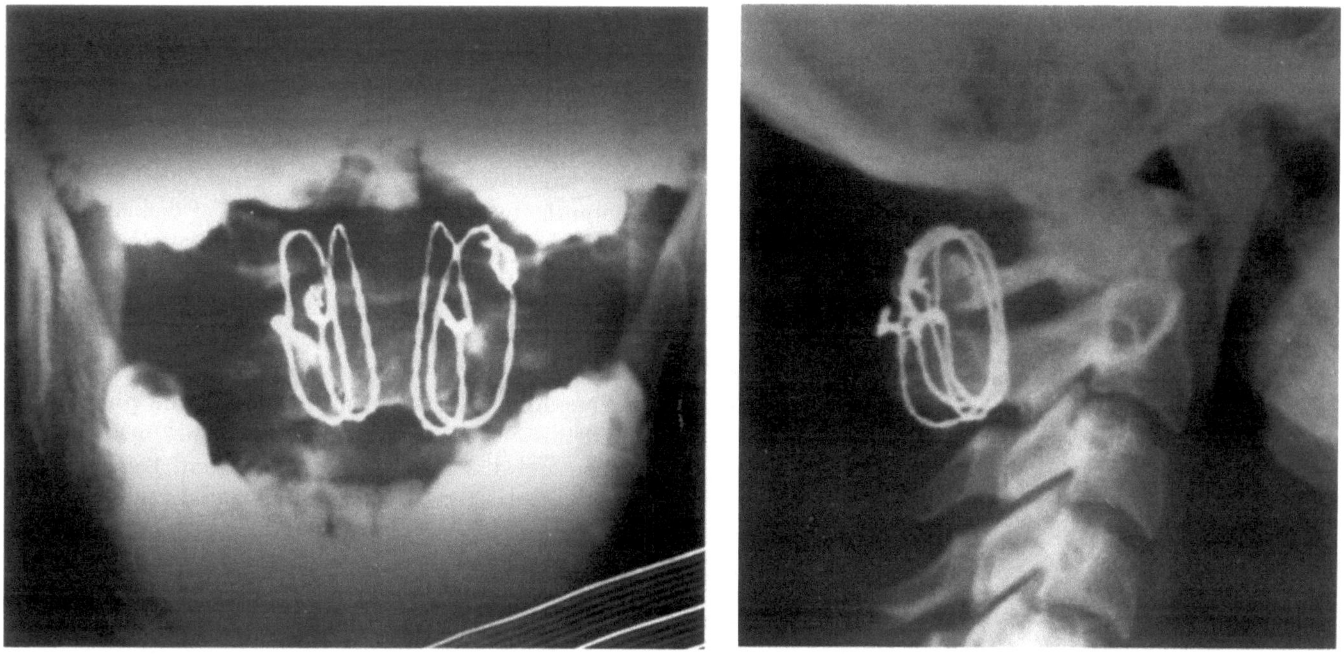

A B

Figure 12.11. (**A**) AP and (**B**) lateral radiograph shows atlantoaxial fusion using Griswold's modification of Brook's fusion. In this case the indication was odontoid fracture.

by Brooks and Jenkins was essentially similar to this, the only difference being that a double stainless steel wire was inserted on both sides. This had the advantage that there are only two wire passages instead of four with less chance for error. We believe, however, that their method gives somewhat less firm fixation of the bone graft. A very similar operation was described by Sorensen.[118]

The clamps described by Mitsui and the use of the pediatric C–D instrumentation as described by Guyotat have appeal in that no sublaminar wires are passed. The sublaminar wires do have a function in preventing anterior migration of the graft locked between C1 and C2. The interlaminar ligament here is thin and tenuous and sometimes nonexistent. Although no neurological complications were reported by Mitsui, the possibility remains for anterior migration of the graft when the clamps are tightened.

When the canal is narrow, passage of wire under the posterior arch of C2 should be avoided. We *then* use the wiring technique described by Fielding[102] and McGraw and Rusch.[113] They describe a 20-gauge wire that is folded upon itself and fashioned into the shape of a hook. It is passed anterior to the posterior arch of the atlas from caudal to cephalic and then drawn distally to loop around the spinous process of the axis. A square bone graft is then placed between the posterior arch of C1 and the spinous process of C2, and notched to hold the wires in place. The wire is then tightened over the top. Lipson[103] described a similar technique which he believed allowed a wedge-compression arthrodesis in the presence of a bifid posterior arch of the atlas. A bifid arch of C1 is commonly regarded as a contraindication to C1–C2 wiring and a reason for extension to the occiput. By appropriately notching the rectangular graft, the wires could be kept lateral and a satisfactory construct was made.

The most important complication is the possibility of neurological impairment, which was frequently reported in the older literature. More recent articles, which include atlantoaxial fusion for atlantoaxial instability and odontoid fractures, have shown low morbidity and mortality in experienced hands. Anderson[119] has reviewed nine series involving 189 fusions; 175 united, giving a percentage success rate of 93%. No neurological complications and no deaths were attributable to the operation. Spinal cord monitoring by either somatosensory-evoked potentials or motor-evoked potentials should be used routinely.

In children, great care must be taken with the dissection to avoid the possibility of extension of the fusion mass to the occiput and below C2. Inclusion of the occiput in the posterior fusion will be required for congenital anomalies of the occipitocervical junction, cases in which a posterior decompression of the posterior arch of C1 or the foramen magnum is required and where there is marked irreducible anterior shift of C1 on C2. It must be stressed again that it is dangerous at surgery to attempt reduction of forward shift that was not reducible before surgery by conservative means. In these cases, we recommend a posterior fusion from the occiput to C2, which may be followed by a decompression operation either anterior or posterior if necessary after the fusion is solid.

Anterior Approaches

Introduction

There are few absolute indications for an anterior approach to the upper cervical spine in children. The goal of an anterior procedure may be fusion for instability, anterior decompression of the spinal cord and medulla, excision of a tumor, or drainage of an abscess or vertebral osteomyelitis. In most cases, fusion will be carried out from the posterior approach. Resort to an anterior approach will be for persistent pressure on the anterior aspect of the cord or medulla oblongata. The anterior approach may be required for fusion after an extensive decompression posteriorly with a resulting instability or deformity. In addition, in children, this approach may be necessary for the biopsy and curettage of tumors or vertebral osteomyelitis involving the body of C2.

There are three basic approaches to the upper anterior cervical spine First, the transpharyngeal approach which can be extended to the lower cervical spine by splitting the mandible and tongue. Second, the anterior retropharyngeal approach which is a superior extension of the anterior approach to the lower cervical spine of Robinson and Smith. The third approach is the lateral retropharyngeal approach of Whitesides. Each approach has its best application in certain clinical situations, so there does not appear to be a universal anterior approach. Most series are small and have few pediatric patients, the majority of operations being carried out for adult complications of rheumatoid arthritis.

Transoral Approach

This approach was popularized by Fang and Ong[120] in 1962. They described transoral surgery for the reduction and fusion of a chronic atlantoaxial dislocation. The body of C2 and the C2–C3 disc lie in the immediate field of the transoral approach. The anterior arch of C1 lies above the soft palate, and to gain access to it and the basiocciput, incision and retraction of the soft palate and occasionally the hard palate must be carried out.

To gain access below C2, Hall[121] described an operation in which the mandible and tongue are split and the lower incisor removed. The transoral approach has a risk of infection, that can be decreased by preoperatively taking a throat culture and covering the patient perioperatively with an appropriate antibiotic intravenously.[120,122] In addition, meticulous repair of the posterior pharynx is advised, and a nasogastric or nasopharyngeal tube should be avoided, as it may cause irritation and breakdown of the posterior wall of the pharynx. If infection occurs in the pharyngeal wound, meningoencephalitis may ensue, particularly if the dura has been inadvertently opened. Dissection laterally in an attempt to gain access for fusion of the antlantoaxial joint runs the risk of damage to the vertebral artery. Hemorrhage from the vertebral artery also appears to increase the risk of infection.

The advisability of bone grafting through a transoral approach is open to question. The bone graft may dislodge or cause prominence of the posterior pharyngeal soft tissues, resulting in a failure of healing of the pharyngeal wall. If this occurs, there is a much higher incidence of infection and dissolution of the bone graft. Despite this, Bonney[122] reported 16 cases of transoral bone grafting that included a case of os odontoideum and a case of basilar impression. In 13 cases, the pharyngeal wound healed by first intention, and in 12 cases, the graft became well incorporated and stabilization was achieved, thus avoiding the necessity for a posterior fusion. In most cases, a peg of iliac crest bone graft was used with a notch at its cephalic end to fit either the anterior arch of the atlas or, if this was missing, the base of the occiput. A tracheostomy was used in all cases. Sakou[123] also advocated bone grafting at the time of anterior decompression.

In conclusion, we believe a transoral approach is most suited for lesions of the body of C2, and for resection of the odontoid in cases of basilar impression or chronic atlantoaxial subluxation where the odontoid is causing significant pressure on the anterior neural structures. Fusion can be obtained by a posterior occiput to C2 or C3 fusion either before or after the decompression. Because of the increased risk of infection with bone grafting, we advocate that anterior operations primarily for fusion should be carried out by a retropharyngeal approach.

Anterolateral Approach

This retropharyngeal approach was first described by DeAndrade and Macnab.[124] It is an extension of the commonly used anterior approach to the lower cervical spine described by Robinson.[125] In that approach, the cephalic limitation is the superior thyroid artery and vein and the external branch of the superior laryngeal nerve. While the artery and vein can be ligated, the superior laryngeal nerve will run across the field and may need to be divided. This may lead to persistent postoperative hoarseness and laryngeal fatigue.[126] In the cephalic part of the incision, the hypoglossal nerve is prone to damage.

McAfee[127] reported the accumulated experience from Johns Hopkins University School of Medicine with this approach. One case of basilar impression required a C2 corpectomy and an odontoid excision and arthrodesis; most cases had an adjuvant posterior fusion. The approach has considerable anatomical complexity, but is suitable for both anterior decompression, for example, for basilar impression, as well as bone grafting from the basiocciput to C3. McAfee mentioned one case of permanent injury to the hypoglossal nerve and two other cases of neuropraxia, as well as a neuropraxia of the mandibular branch of the facial nerve. There were no infections and no nonunions.

Lateral Retropharyngeal Approach

This approach was first described by Henry,[128] but Whitesides and Kelley first reported on its clinical use in 1966.[129,130] The approach passes anterior to the sternomastoid muscle but behind the carotid sheath. The approach therefore is retropharyngeal and avoids the risk of infection from contamination with organisms from the pharynx. There is less anatomical complexity than the anteromedial approach, and it avoids damage to the superior laryngeal nerve. It gives exposure as high as the ring of C1, and can be easily extended into the lower cervical spine. It is probably safer to use in children than in adults because of the greater elasticity of the soft tissues.

The disadvantages are twofold. First, cephalic extension is limited and the basiocciput is not accessible. This is because the carotid sheath and the nervous structures are anchored by their exit from the base of the skull and excessive anterior retraction may lead to avulsion. This is less likely in a child than in an adult. Second, fusion of both lateral C1–C2 articulations is possible as is strut grafting, but decompression is more difficult because the vertebral bodies are being approached more from one side than from directly in front as is allowed by the anteromedial approach. With both retropharyngeal approaches, extensive dissection may cause retropharyngeal edema with a possible need for tracheostomy.

Congenital Kyphosis

The first description of this condition is credited to von Rokitansky who described a case report in 1844. Further case reports appeared mainly in the European literature up until 1932, when van Schrick[131] was the first to clearly delineate the two major types of congenital kyphosis: group I (failure of segmentation) and group II (absence of one or more vertebral bodies).

The largest and most comprehensive series to date, was published by Winter.[132]

It consisted of 84 patients from the author's personal experience and a further 46 patients contributed to the series by members of the Scoliosis Research Society. Winter modified van Schrick's classification such that van Schrick's group II became type I: failure of formation, and his group I became type II, failure of segmentation. Winter also added a type III: mixed deformities (Fig. 12.12).

The embryological development of the spine is divided into three stages. The first is the mesenchymal stage, which continues until 4 to 5 weeks of gestation. Next is the chondrification stage, from 5 to 9 weeks, and then the ossification stage, which begins at 9 weeks. Tsou[133] believes that the insult to the embryo that causes congenital kyphosis occurs during the late chondrification stage. The nature of the insult is uncertain, but some authors believe that a disturbance in the vascularization of the vertebral bodies leads to the lack of development.[134] The posterior elements develop from separate ossification centers and are usually not affected. This, therefore, differs from the classical hemivertebra in which there is an ipsilateral absence of half of the centrum and the neural arch and which, therefore, is thought to be developmentally of an earlier origin.

Failure of segmentation is caused by partial osseous metaplasia of the annulus fibrosis. To appreciate the full extent of this metaplasia and therefore the full extent of the anterior bar that is the cause of the kyphosis in type II lesions, one must await full ossification. Some patients in their teenaged years may show evidence of spontaneous anterior interbody fusion from one to three levels above or below a previously obvious anterior bony bar. In addition, there are some in whom the vertebral growth potential seemed quite normal in early life yet subsequently form an anterior interbody fusion and kyphotic deformity.[135] Congenital kyphosis, in particular type I deformities, is associated with congenital anomalies else-

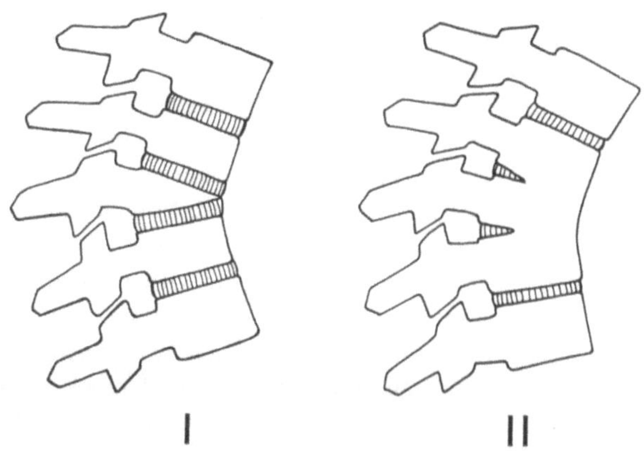

Figure 12.12. Schematic representation of congenital kyphosis classification of Winter. Type I represents failure of formation resulting in a posterior hemivertebra. Type II represents failure of segmentation. In addition, Winter added type III, mixed deformities.

where in the body but to a lesser extent than that seen with other congenital spine deformities such as Klippel–Feil and congenital scoliosis, presumably because of their genesis at a later stage of embryological development. There are sporadic reports of familial involvement.

Using the classification of Winter, type I is the most common deformity. In Montgomery's series[136] it was three times more common than type II. In Winter's series,[132] of 130 cases, 86 were type I, 19 type II, and 18 type III; 7 could not be accurately classified.

The type I deformity has a much sharper angulation, with the cord angled over the residual vertebral body. Type II curves have a more rounded angulation and generally are of lesser severity. The most serious complication from congenital kyphosis is paraplegia. Congenital kyphosis is second only to tuberculosis in the cause of paralysis from spinal deformity. It is seen almost exclusively in the type I lesion, and tends to occur during the period of rapid growth in the preadolescent years. Neurological changes were seen in 32% of type I deformities in Montgomery's series and 16 of 86 patients in Winter's series. It was most common with high thoracic curves. The onset of paralysis may be spontaneous, or in relation to a minor trauma.[132,136,137,138]

Untreated, congenital kyphosis undergoes relentless progression, measuring on average 7° per year for type I deformities and 5° per year for type II.[137,138] Although a neurologic deficit could be expected more commonly in more severe cases, Williams[139] documented a case of transient paraparesis with a congenital kyphosis measuring only 25°. The measurement of kyphosis may be deceptive. A compensatory lordosis exists above and below the kyphotic segment, and if measurements are taken from endplates of vertebrae in the compensatory lordosis, a much more benign measurement of the degree of kyphosis is obtained. This may also give the erroneous impression that the kyphosis is not progressing. Plain radiographs may be deceptive, and may give a picture similar to the spine deformity seen in bone dysplasias. Similarly, in countries where tuberculosis is common, the spine deformity is often attributed to late changes seen in this disease. The deformity is best elucidated by lateral tomograms, which will give a better delineation of the bony defect than CT scanning.[140] In patients with a neurological deficit, MRI scanning or a myelogram may be used; MRI scanning may be preferable, because a myelogram with the patient prone may show up as a total block. These tests may also be useful in ruling out an associated diastematomyelia or tethered cord, particularly if surgery is contemplated.

Complaints of back pain are more common in type II deformities. The pain occurs in the low back in the region of the compensatory lumbar hyper-lordosis. Pain is most frequent in thoracolumbar lesions. Pulmonary function is also affected but to a lesser extent than with scoliotic deformities.

Associated congenital anomalies are less common than with congenital scoliosis. More congenital anomalies are associated with type I deformities than with type II. Renal anomalies were only seen in 4 of 150 cases in Winter's study, much less than the 20%–30% seen with congenital scoliosis.[132] However, all patients with congenital kyphosis should undergo a renal ultrasound or intravenous pyelogram (IVP) to exclude those congenital anomalies that may predispose to renal failure. Other congenital anomalies may be found in the heart, chest wall, abdominal wall, upper extremities, and lower extremities, including clubfoot.[141] Diastematomyelia, tethered cord, and butterfly vertebra can also occur, but in Winter's series, were present in only 4 of 130 cases.

Conservative treatment includes bracing and controlled observation. The natural history of this condition has been sufficiently delineated to allow the physician to predict, with reasonable certainty, the likelihood of progression. Brace treatment has been reported for a small group of type II lesions. Of 6 patients so treated, only 1 showed significant progression of the deformity, but no patient had notable improvement in the major kyphosis at the end of brace treatment. Therefore, it was not recommended.[135] Type I deformities may retain some mobility in the very young years but soon become rigid and uncorrectable, making brace treatment of little value.

Both type I and type II lesions, if detected at an early age, may be successfully treated with a posterior fusion. This will arrest any further deformity at the level of the lesion, and if the fusion extends one or two levels above the anomalous segment, some spontaneous correction may occur with time by the production of lordosis from a posterior bony tether. Winter and Moe[142] reviewed 49 patients thus treated. They found a minimum of bending of the fusion mass into increased kyphosis, and only 1 patient had the creation of an unsightly lordosis. In that patient, the fusion had been erroneously extended too many levels above and below the kyphosis.

A posterior fusion alone gives best results if the patient is less than 3 years old and with less than 50° of kyphosis at the time of surgery. The patient may need exploration and refusion at 6 months. The thicker the posterior fusion mass, the less likely it is to bend. If the patient is older than 3 years and the curve greater than 50°, then combined anterior and posterior fusions are usually required. Although anterior and posterior surgery will stop progression of the disorder, it will not allow for spontaneous correction with growth as is seen in posterior fusions alone, because of elimination of the existing anterior growth plate.[142] Following an in situ posterior fusion, the patient should be immobilized in a cast for at least 6 months. In Winters' series, patients were kept 6 months nonambulatory, followed by a further 6 months ambulatory, for a total of 12 months in a cast.

In the older patient, consideration must be given to both correction of the deformity and, if necessary, decompression of the cord in the presence of paraplegia or paraparesis. Surgical treatment of a rigid kyphotic deformity with a type I congenital defect is fraught with danger. Mobility is often retained only in the compensatory lordotic segments above and below. Attempts to correct the kyphosis, particularly using methods that involve distraction, will cause straightening and elongation in spinal segments of the compensatory curves while the rigid kyphotic segment remains unchanged. This has the effect of drawing the cord anteriorly and more tightly across the kyphotic segment, with the possibility of causing a neurological deficit. For this reason, halo-femoral or even halo-gravity traction should be avoided preoperatively if bending radiographs show no flexibility through the kyphotic segment.

Posterior fusion using Harrington distraction instrumentation must also be avoided for the same reason. If the deformity is severe enough to require correction, an anterior procedure must be performed: All discs are removed. Some correction may be gained by posterior pressure on the kyphos, and this degree of correction may be maintained with an anterior strut graft. We still prefer to use autogenous fibular strut grafts in this situation. A rib taken during the anterior approach may be used to help fill in the remaining space anteriorly, but rib alone is usually not strong enough to withstand the axial pressure from the correction.

If the spine is inflexible on bending films, we advocate the use of tomograms preoperatively to check for any spontaneous ankylosis of the posterior elements. We have noted this to occur in a number of cases of kyphosis of varying etiologies, and if present will make it impossible to get any correction whatsoever from the anterior proce-

A
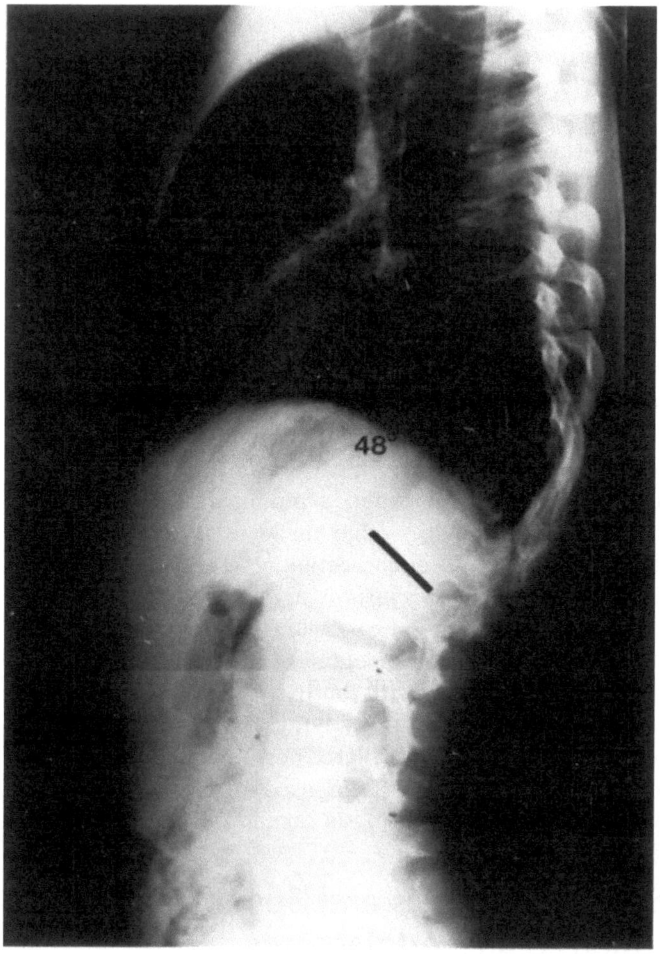

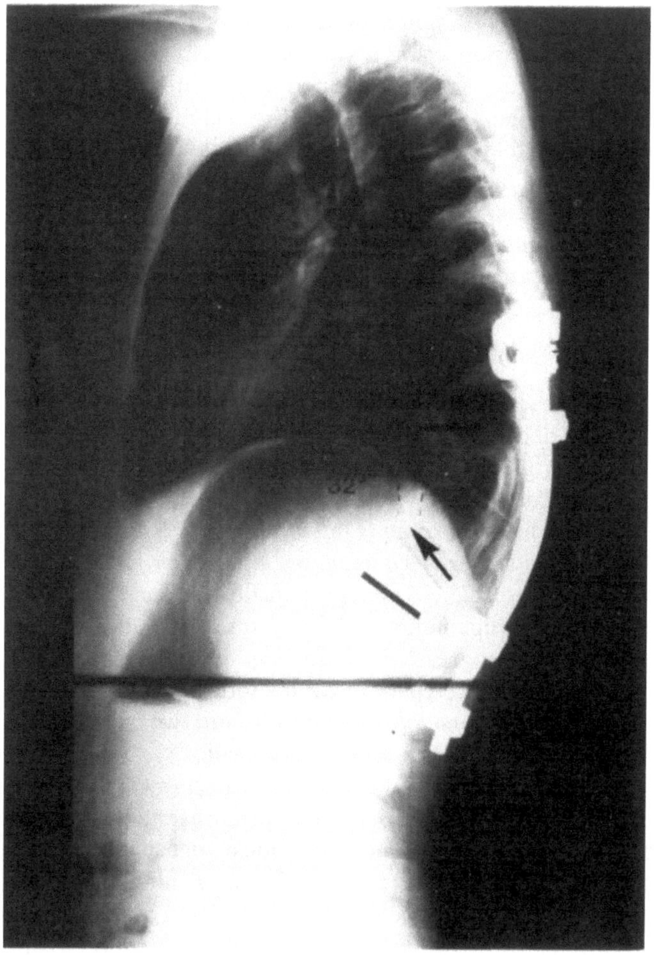
B

Figure 12.13. **A.** Fourteen-year-old boy with type I congenital kyphosis at T11. There had been an 8° progression in previous 6 months, and local kyphosis measured 48°. MRI scan was normal and patient was neurologically intact. **B.** Same patient 6 months after anterior fusion with vascularized rib pedicle graft and posterior fixation and fusion using C–D instrumentation. Moderate correction of kyphosis was gained, to 32°. Rib graft (*small arrow*) shows complete radiologic incorporation.

dure. The ankylosis, however, is unable to prevent continuing progression of the kyphosis in the absence of an anterior fusion. At posterior surgery, it will be noticed that the posterior elements, under tensile forces, tend to flatten and elongate. The spinous processes become flattened to be almost parallel with the vertebra and the facet joints lose all motion. Even if there is still some movement at the facet joints, the elongation of the posterior bony column will block any significant correction even after anterior releases. In this situation, the surgical treatment is further complicated, because the patient will require posterior osteotomies followed by anterior releases or osteotomies, and often a third stage for posterior instrumentation, to gain significant correction. A three-stage procedure such as this has the potential for considerable morbidity in the hands of surgeons without great experience in these cases.

In most cases, the magnitude of the kyphosis is of a lesser degree and the need for correction is not important. The patient, however, is often too old to be able to rely on posterior fusion alone. In this situation, we prefer anterior in situ fusion using a vascularized rib pedicle graft. This technique is well described in the literature. It requires a surgeon well versed in the technique and takes more time than autogenous graft or fibular strut graft, but has the advantage of rapid incorporation and less pseudarthrosis.[143,144] This is followed by a second stage either during the same anesthetic or a week to 10 days later, using in situ posterior instrumentation. At the present time, we prefer C–D instrumentation, which allows rigid fixation without compression or distraction (Fig. 12.13).

The presence of a neurological deficit will require an anterior decompression in addition to the anterior and posterior fusions. There is now abundant evidence in the literature that a laminectomy will not decompress the cord when the spine is in kyphosis.[145,146] In addition, it decreases the area available for a posterior fusion, thus increasing the chances for a pseudarthrosis, and by removing posterior ligaments and bony restraints adds to the chances for progression of the kyphosis. Winter[132] reported that all three patients in his series treated by laminectomy were worse postoperatively, and two were partial paraplegics, becoming totally paraplegic.

Anterior decompression can be carried out by a costotransversectomy or through a transthoracic approach. A costotransversectomy may seem ideal, because it avoids opening the pleura and the use of a chest tube postoperatively in patients whose pulmonary function may be compromised. However, in our hands the transthoracic approach allows better visualization and a more complete decompression. In the thoracolumbar region, this may need to be combined with an extraperitoneal dissection of the lumbar spine and detachment of the diaphragm. The technique of anterior decompression is similar to that advocated by Hodgson for cord compression in TB[147] and by Bohlman for spinal fractures.[148] The posterior portion of the apical vertebra is excised allowing the cord to move anteriorly into the void. Decompression must be extended in a cephalic and caudal direction until the cord lies quite loose with no further tendency to move forward. Pulsation should be seen at the end of an adequate decompression, and on some occasions we have noted immediate improvement in the latency of the somatosensory-evoked responses. Following decompression, a vascularized rib pedicle graft or a fibular strut graft may be inserted. A posterior instrumentation should be carried out as a second stage, using C–D instrumentation.

Much less radical surgery is usually required for type II deformities, especially if treatment is instituted earlier before severe deformity has occurred. In a young child with considerable growth potential, a posterior fusion alone should be carried out. The posterior fusion should be extended one segment above and one below those joined by the anterior bar.[135] This may allow some correction from continued growth through the open endplates anteriorly. The posterior fusion may be reinforced with instrumentation. We prefer either Harrington compression rods or C–D instrumentation.

If at the time of initial evaluation the curvature is already severe producing low back pain from the lumbar hyperlordosis or an unsightly cosmetic deformity, then a corrective operation is required. This may take the form of anterior and posterior osteotomies and fusion in either a two- or three-stage operation. However, we feel this condition is ideal for a spinal osteotomy carried out solely from the posterior approach using the transpedicular (eggshell) method outlined by Heinig[149] (Fig. 12.14). This operation has the advantage of being carried out in a single stage, and the spine is shortened avoiding distraction on the spinal cord. A single wedge made in this manner may give as much as 50° of correction.[149] The vertebral body at the apex of the kyphosis is approached through both pedicles and a wedge of cancellous bone is curetted out. A wedge of the posterior elements of appropriate size is then removed along with both pedicles. The posterior cortex of the vertebral body lying anterior to the cord is involuted into the decancellated vertebral body. Compression instrumentation is then used to close the wedge, and posterior bone grafting is carried out (Fig. 12.15).

Spondylolisthesis and Spondylolysis in Children and Adolescents

The goal in treating spondylolysis and spondylolisthesis in children and adolescents is to safely augment stability while minimizing the deformity. Herbineaux[150] recorded

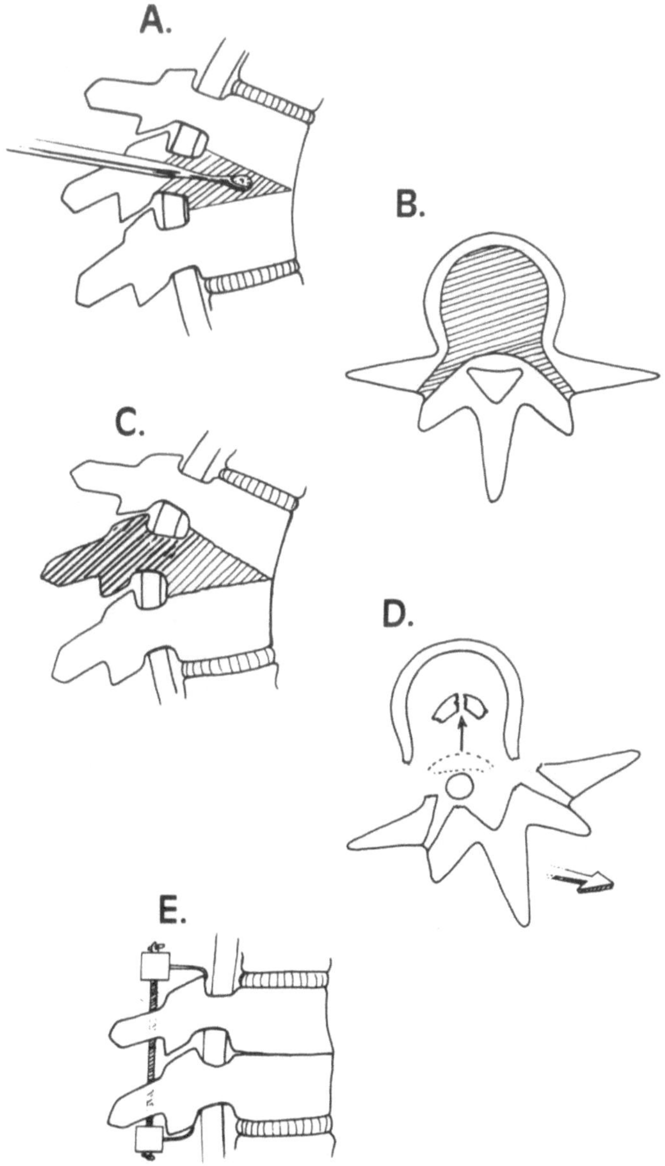

Figure 12.14. Graphical representation of correction of type II congenital kyphosis using transpedicular vertebral enucleation and posterior wedge osteotomy as described by Heinig.[149] **A** and **B.** Medullary cavity of pedicles on both sides are enucleated to give access to vertebral body and allow decancellation in form of wedge. Spinal cord and nerve roots are protected during this stage by cortical bone, which forms boundary of medullary cavity of pedicle. **C.** Appropriately sized wedge of posterior elements is then removed exposing spinal cord and nerve roots. Pedicles are excised down to their bases. Before this stage, hook sites for instrumentation have been prepared. **D.** Rim of cortical bone lying anterior to cord is impacted into decancellated vertebral body by gently passing "joker" anterior to spinal cord. This prevents retropulsion of this bone back into canal during correction phase. **E.** Compression instrumentation, either Harrington compression rods or C–D, are used to close the osteotomy and give correction. Approximately 40° of correction of kyphosis can be reliably gained with this method.

the earliest description of the forward displacement of one vertebra on another. Neugebauer[151] was the first to describe the two different defects that could lead to slippage: (1) a break in the continuity of the neural arch (i.e., spondylolysis) or (2) elongation of the pars interarticularis. Unfortunately, his work was overlooked until recently.

The classification in general usage is that of Wiltse, Newman, and MacNab,[152] who divided the patients into five major groups.

I. Dysplastic: a congenital deficiency of the facet joints of the upper sacrum or L5 arch leads to a gradual slipping of the vertebrae relative to each other.
II. Isthmic: the defect exists in the pars interarticularis. This category is subdivided into three types.
    a. lytic: the pars is separated by a fatigue fracture
    b. attenuation or elongation of the intact pars interarticularis
    c. acute fracture of the pars
III. Degenerative: long-standing intersegmental instability leads to degeneration of the joints, allowing displacement.
IV. Traumatic: acute injury to the bony elements other than the pars, permitting anterior translation of the superior segment.
V. Pathologic: generalized or local disease leads to attenuation or lysis of the pars, pedicle, or facets.

This chapter will consider exclusively types I and II, which are seen in children and are a form of instability. They differ markedly from the other types, which are usually seen in adults and represent degenerative changes.

Etiology

The term spondylolisthesis was coined by Killian[153] in 1854 who realized that the displacement occurred gradually. In 1855, Robert[154] demonstrated that displacement could not occur until a defect was made in the posterior neural arch. Many experimenters have felt that trauma is the cause of the arch defects. It has been shown that only extreme force in an abnormally flexed position could produce the need changes in the arch. However, the changes usually occur gradually during growth. To date, there has been no embryologic or anatomic evidence to support the hypothesis that spondylolysis and spondylolisthesis represent congenital anomalies of the spine.[155] Only one child with an age less than 12 months has been found to have a lesion;[156] however, the incidence in adults is approximately 5%. It is rare in children less than 5 years old, but by 8 years the incidence approaches that of the general population.

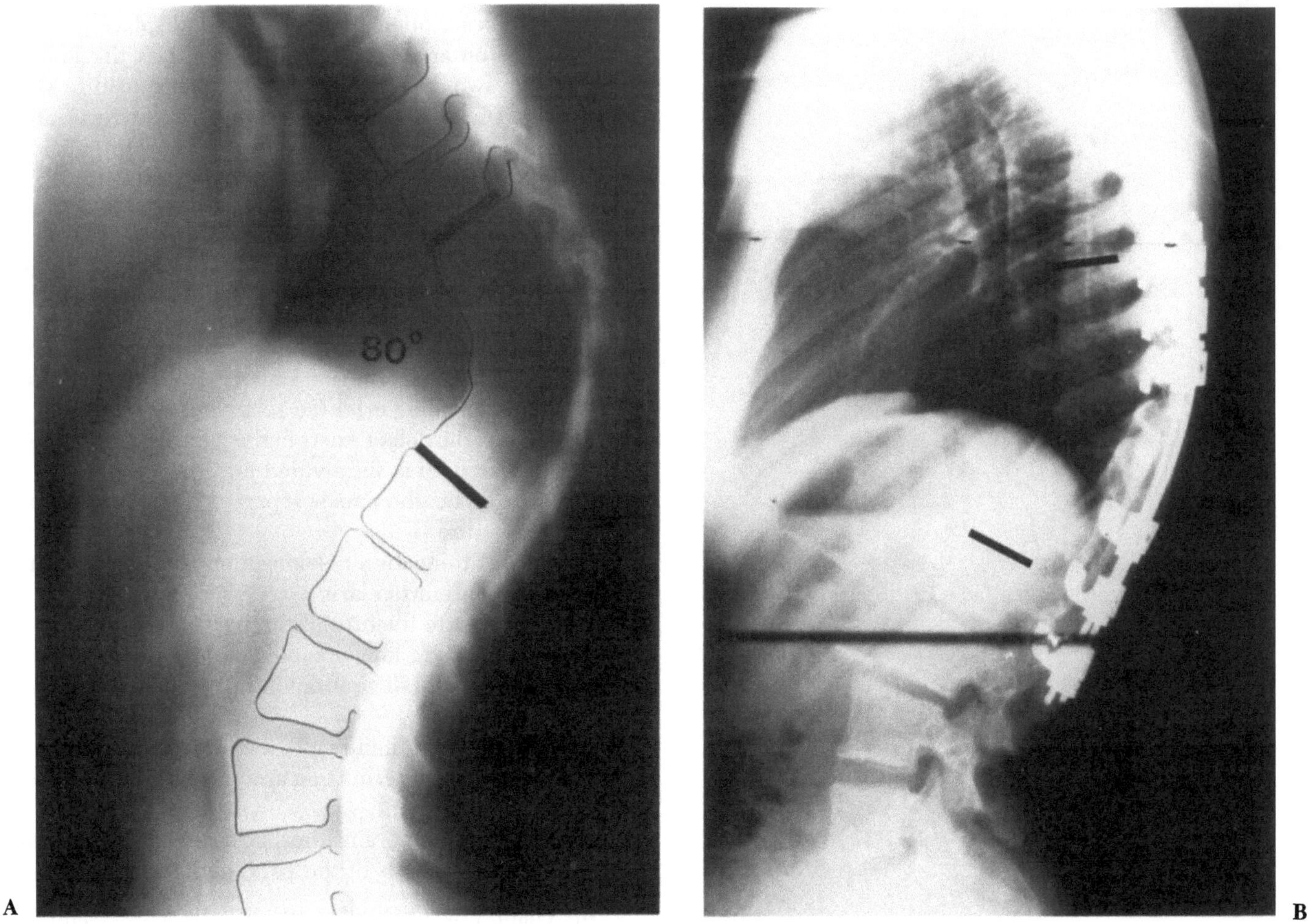

Figure 12.15. **A.** Lateral tomogram of 11-year-old girl with type II congenital kyphosis (failure of segmentation) measuring 80°. Myelogram was normal and patient was neurologically intact. **B.** Roentgenogram taken 2 years postoperatively after single-stage posterior wedge osteotomy using transpedicular vertebral body decancellation. Kyphosis is corrected to 37°. The patient is asymptomatic and has a normal-appearing sagittal contour.

The defect occurs roughly twice as frequently in whites compared to blacks, and 2.5 times more frequently in males compared to females in the same racial groups.[155] The highest incidence, 6.4%, is in white males. Isolated communities may have a very high incidence, and certain Eskimo groups have an incidence approaching 34%.[157] A study of the first-degree relatives of 70 index patients with type I and II spondylolysis and spondylolisthesis, done at the Alfred I. duPont Institute,[158] found an overall incidence of 22% in first-degree relatives. The incidence in dysplastic patients was 29%, and in those with the isthmic form, 21%. The dysplastic form was most common in the relatives regardless of the form in the index patients. There was a high incidence, 61%, of spina bifida occulta in the patients, with no difference between the lytic or elongated groups. Other investigators[159] have found a familial incidence ranging from 27% to 69% with a similar frequency of spina bifida occulta. In spite of the increased incidence of spina bifida and congenital lack of development of the proximal sacrum, there has been no evidence that spondylolysis or spondylolisthesis develops as a failure of fusion between two separate centers of ossification.

Several researchers subsequently hypothesized that upright gait played a role in the development of this condition. A population of people who had never walked were examined radiographically.[160] The incidence of spina bifida and transitional vertebrae was similar to that found in the general population. Not one patient was shown to have spondylolysis or spondylolisthesis. An increased incidence is found in athletes who routinely hyperextend their spines. In female gymnasts, the defect occurs at four times the expected frequency.[161] Development in football linemen, weight lifters, and soldiers made to carry heavy packs while performing exercises during early training is well documented.[162–164] The conclusion drawn from these studies was that spondylolysis and spondylolisthesis represent the result of stress fracturing, with or without attenuation of the bone during its attempt to heal.[162,164] The forward translation of the superior vertebra is permitted by the weakened support of the pars at this time.

The data currently available support a combined theory in which repetitive stresses may lead to formation of a spondylolysis in susceptible individuals. If healing occurs during a subsequent forward displacement, spondylolisthesis will be present; if healing is incomplete, then a spondylolysis will exist. There is a hereditary predisposition toward the condition, but unless the necessary forces are applied the defect will not form.

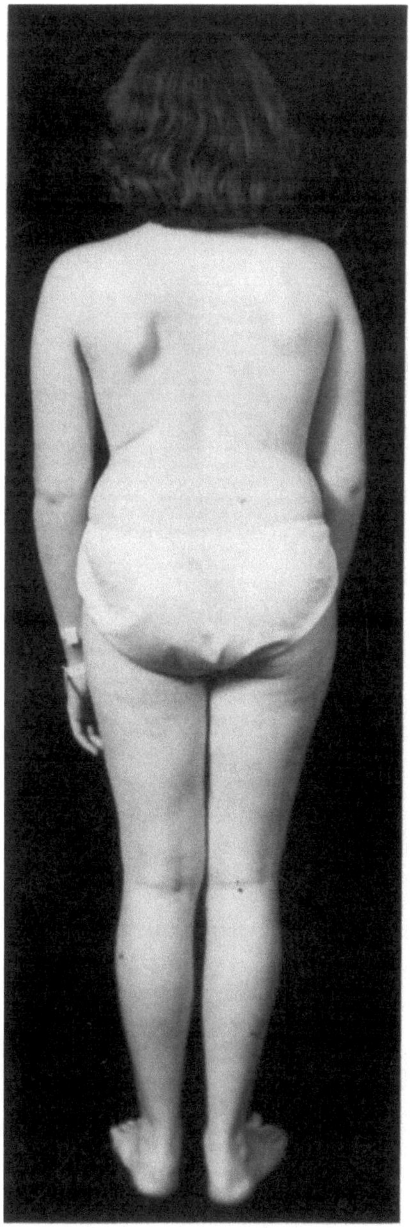

Figure 12.16. Eleven-year-old girl with grade I spondylolisthesis, hamstring tightness, and characteristic flattened buttocks.

Clinical Findings

For a condition with an incidence of 5%, symptomatic patients are surprisingly rare. A group of 500 unselected first-grade schoolchildren were followed longitudinally.[165] The incidence of spondylolisthesis and spondylolysis was 4.4% in 6-year-olds and increased to 6% in adulthood. Advancement of the slip was unusual, occurring only at the time when the slip was first discovered. Progression was seen during the adolescent growth spurt but was of small degree. It was unusual for the children to complain of pain. The investigators' conclusion was that pain and the olisthesis occur concomitantly with the development of the pars interarticularis defect. They believed that the asymptomatic patient did not warrant treatment.

Children who become symptomatic usually do so during the adolescent growth spurt.[165] The pain they develop is usually in the lower back, and may extend into the buttock and thighs. Radicular symptoms below the knee are unusual, and should spur investigation for another cause of the pain. The neurological exam is usually normal. The most common sign is that of tight hamstrings, which are not pathognomonic (Figs. 12.16 and 12.17). It is important for the neurological exam to be done carefully because hamstring tightness can also be a sign of neurological compression secondary to conditions such as cauda equina syndrome, tethered cord, herniated lumbar disc, and spinal cord tumors—all of which are rare. The tightness may be minimal or it may be so extreme that the patient is unable to flex the hips with the knees extended. Severe hamstring tightness produces a characteristic gait de-

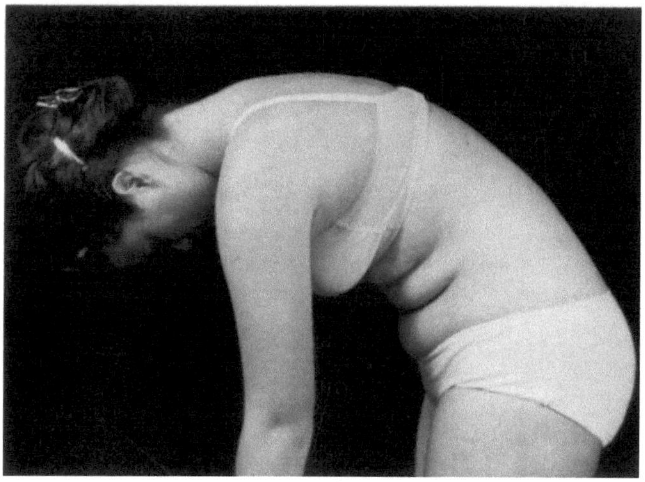

Figure 12.17. Limited maximum forward flexion secondary to hamstring tightness in 11-year-old girl with grade I spondylolisthesis.

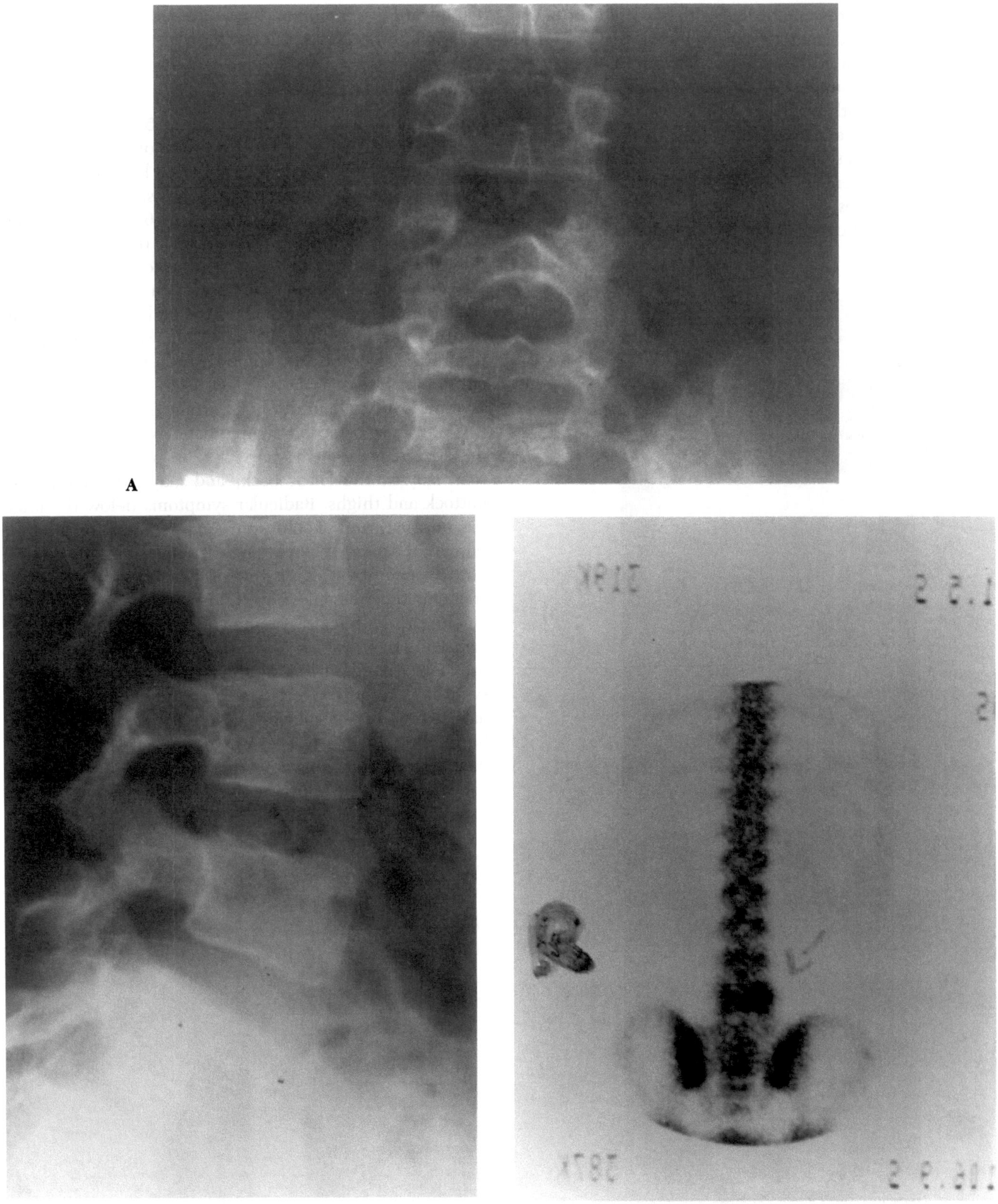

Figure 12.18

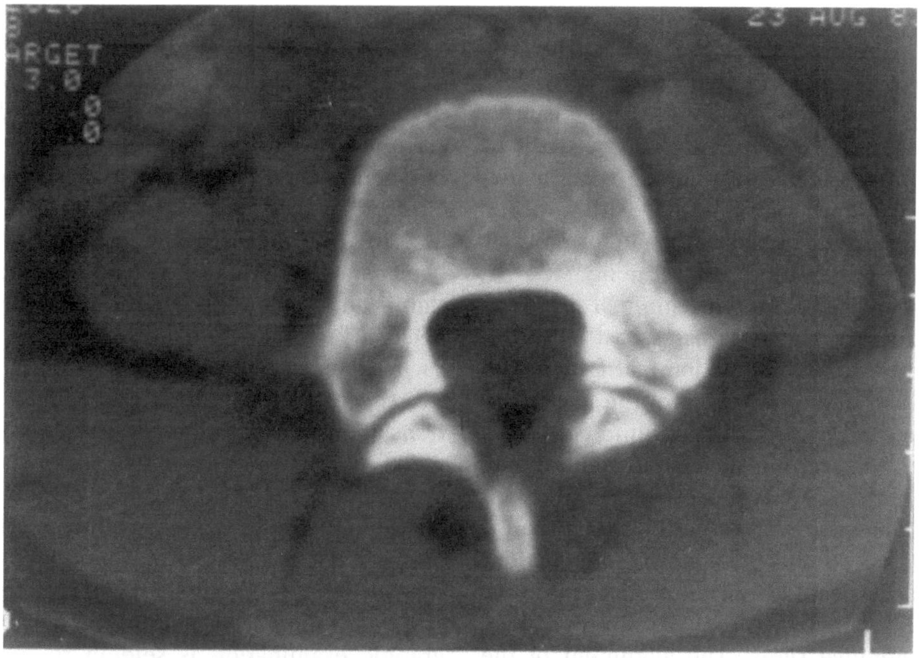

D

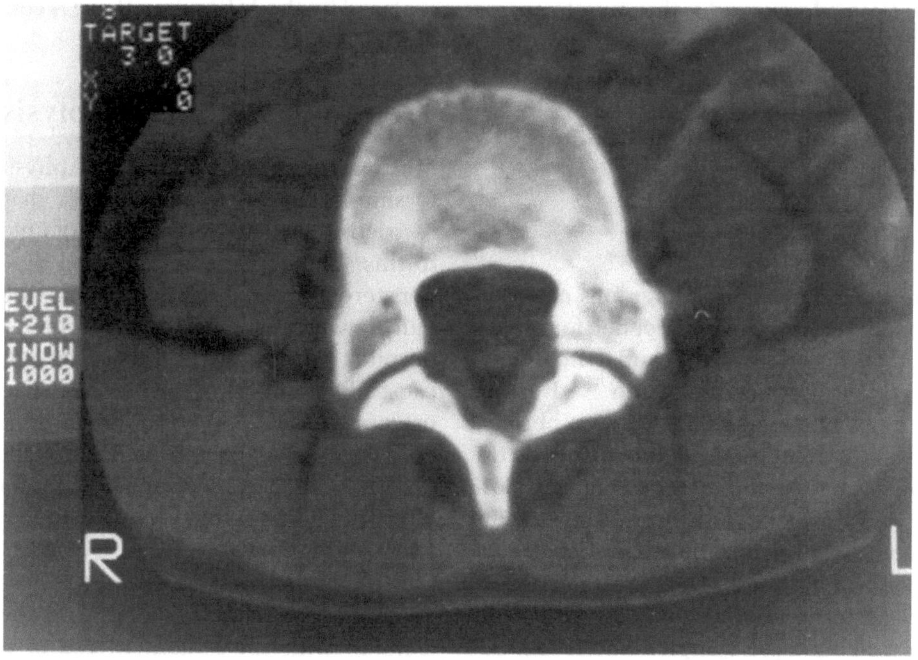

E

Figure 12.18. **A.** Anteroposterior radiograph of lumbar spine in 9-year-old girl with 7-month history of low back pain. Patient's pain failed to respond to 2-month course of activity modification and aspirin. Sclerosis in region of left L5 pedicle is present. **B.** Lateral radiograph of lumbar spine demonstrates sclerosis of L5 pars interarticularis. **C.** Increased bone scan activity is noted in region of left L5 pedicle, consistent with unilateral spondylolysis. **D.** CT scan of L5 vertebra through defect in pars interarticularis. **E.** CT scan after 2 months of Risser cast immobilization reveals early healing of spondylolysis. Patient remained free of pain after cast removal.

scribed as a pelvic waddle. The gait abnormality may be the reason for the patient's visit to the office. The gait pattern is that of a short stiff stride with excessive pelvic rotation that improves with increased speed. This is caused by the tight hamstrings, which force a backward tilt of the pelvis and its prevention of hip flexion with an extended knee. The gait may not improve with time or conservative treatment. On occasion the abnormal gait may be the major reason for surgical treatment.[162]

Physical examination of patients with minimal slips may be entirely normal. As the slip progresses past 50%, the patient may develop a transverse abdominal fold in the region of the umbilicus and a flattening of the back. The buttocks will flatten, and as the lumbar spine continues its forward march on the sacrum, a palpable step-off may be felt at the level of the spinous process of the involved vertebrae. These changes are more easily understood if the slip is viewed as a localized kyphosis. The patient may look better than expected from the radiographic appearance; conversely, patients with severe slips may have no symptoms and minimal signs. The alignment of the patient's body may be made worse by the muscle spasm and tightness. Scoliosis may be seen in association with spondylolisthesis. Most investigators believe that the scoliosis is often secondary to the olisthesis and that with treatment of the slip the scoliosis will resolve or be greatly reduced in degree.[167,168]

Roentgenographic Findings

Generally, AP, lateral, and oblique radiographs are sufficient. Special radiographic views may be needed for identification of the defect. On occasion, a 20% caudal tilt oblique will be needed for identification of a lesion.[169] Further clarification can often be obtained with a CT scan because the plane of the lysis is transverse to the plane of the CT scan.[170] The defect may be unilateral as much as 20% of the time (Fig. 12.18). Spondylolisthesis can develop without a recognized defect in the bone, particularly in the form with dysplasia of the joints. The dysplastic patient in whom the intact posterior elements slip forward is the one who is the most likely to be symptomatic. With this particular defect, a cauda equina paralysis may result even if the slip is as small as 25%, in contrast to the total displacement that can be seen if the pars is broken. The paralysis is caused by the intact arch decreasing the space available for the cord. If the arch is broken, the space available for the cord increases with the forward progression of the slip. In spondylolysis, neurological compromise is unlikely because the posterior elements are left in place. There may be increased stress on the intact pedicle when a unilateral defect exists that can lead to sclerosis of the intact side.[171] This may be confused with an osteoid osteoma because the bone scan will show that the area of increased uptake is on the sclerotic side. The defect on the opposite oblique radiograph will help distinguish between the two problems, as can the use of a CT scan.

Classically, the degree of spondylolisthesis has been classified according to Meyerding,[172,173] who grouped them based on the percent of displacement of one vertebra on another: 0% to 25%, type I; 26% to 50%, type II; 51% to 75%, type III; and 76% to 100%, type IV. It has been established that the position of the spine will change significantly when the patient is standing. It is, therefore, necessary to take the radiographs in the same position each time, and the standing position is preferred. The two types of slippage that can occur can be grouped into translations and rotations. Translation is most easily measured using the method of Talliard by showing the percentage of slip. Sagittal rotation shows the angular relationship between the body of the vertebra and the posterior aspect of the first sacral vertebra. Rounding of the anterior superior border of the first sacral vertebra is thought to demonstrate an increased possibility of progression. Myelographic examination is seldom required, and has been replaced by the MRI when there is concern about a coexistent lesion.

Treatment of Spondylolysis

Most patients who present to the physician's office respond to simple conservative measures that initially consist of restricting vigorous activity. If symptoms do not respond to this, bed rest, immobilization in a cast or brace, and nonsteroidal analgesics will usually suffice. Those rare individuals who continue to be symptomatic in adolescence, despite the conservative measures and elimination of other causes for symptoms such as disc space infection, osteoid osteoma, spinal cord tumor, diastematomyelia, tethered cord, etc., may require surgical stabilization. When the defect is at L4, surgical stabilization is required more often than when the lesion is at the more common L5 site[174] (Fig. 12.19).

We use the surgical technique described by Nicol and Scott.[175] The patient is placed in the prone position on a frame with the abdomen free of pressure. A midline vertical incision is made stripping the muscles off the spinous process, being careful in the exposure because of the increased incidence of spina bifida. The laminae and transverse processes of the affected vertebrae are cleared subperiosteally and the articular facets are also cleared leaving the capsule intact. The affected segment is identified by its mobility and confirmed with roentgenograms. The surface of the defect, along with the dorsal surface of the lamina and transverse processes of the involved segment, are stripped to the bleeding bone. A loop of 20-gauge stainless steel wire is passed around the transverse process adjacent to the pedicle of the involved

A 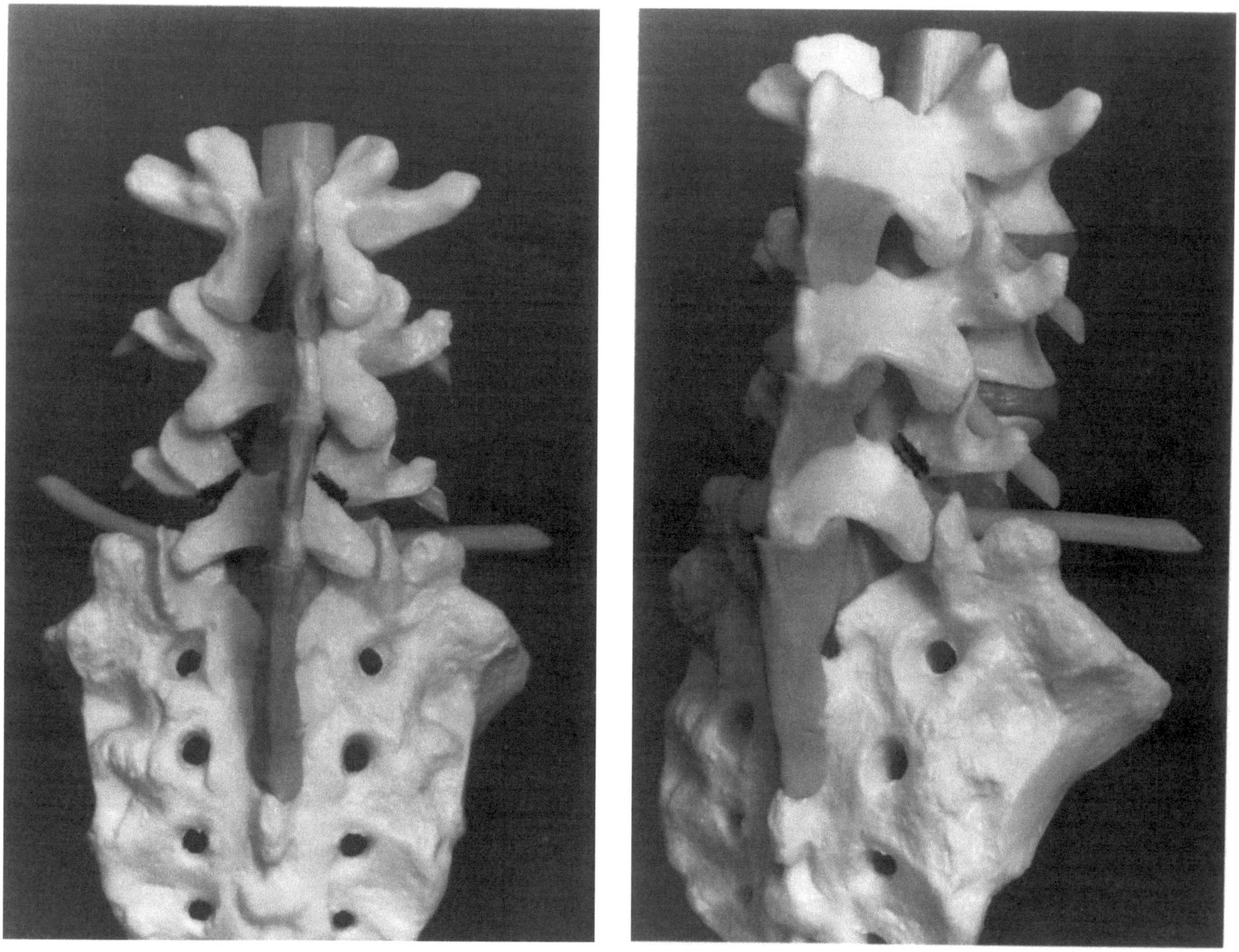 B

Figure 12.19. **A.** Model of lumbosacral junction demonstrates spondylolysis of L5 pars interarticularis. **B.** Oblique view of L5 pars defect. This projection demonstrates "Scottie dog" that is formed from posterior to anterior by spinous process, lamina, inferior articular facet, pars interarticularis, superior articular facet, and transverse process of affected vertebra.

vertebra. The wire is looped around the spinous process of the involved vertebra and the procedure is repeated on the other side with a second wire. Cancellous bone chips are packed onto the surface and a strip of cancellous bone is laid across the defect in such a way as to be trapped by the wires as they are tightened. The spine is then extended from its flexed position. A wire tightener is applied tightening the pairs of wires to each other. The wound is closed in the standard fashion and a pressure dressing is applied.

The patient is placed at bed rest. A double-leg pantaloon spica cast may be applied for 6 weeks if there is any concern. This is followed by bracing for a total of 3 months. No significant heavy lifting or work is permitted for the following 3 months or until signs of solid fusion are present.

The other techniques are more complicated, so we think that the Scott technique is the best in most surgeons' hands. Other techniques have been suggested, including that of Buck,[176] who proposed direct fixation of the pars using a screw and bone grafting. It is important to emphasize that the Gill procedure or laminectomy is not indicated in these patients. Removal of the posterior element will increase the instability and chances of increasing spondylolisthesis postoperatively. The Scott technique has proven to be both simple and reliable.

Treatment of Spondylolisthesis

Asymptomatic spondylolisthesis of less than 50% displacement in the immature individual requires no therapy other than periodic roentgenograms. The patients and their parents should be informed of the nature of the defect, and

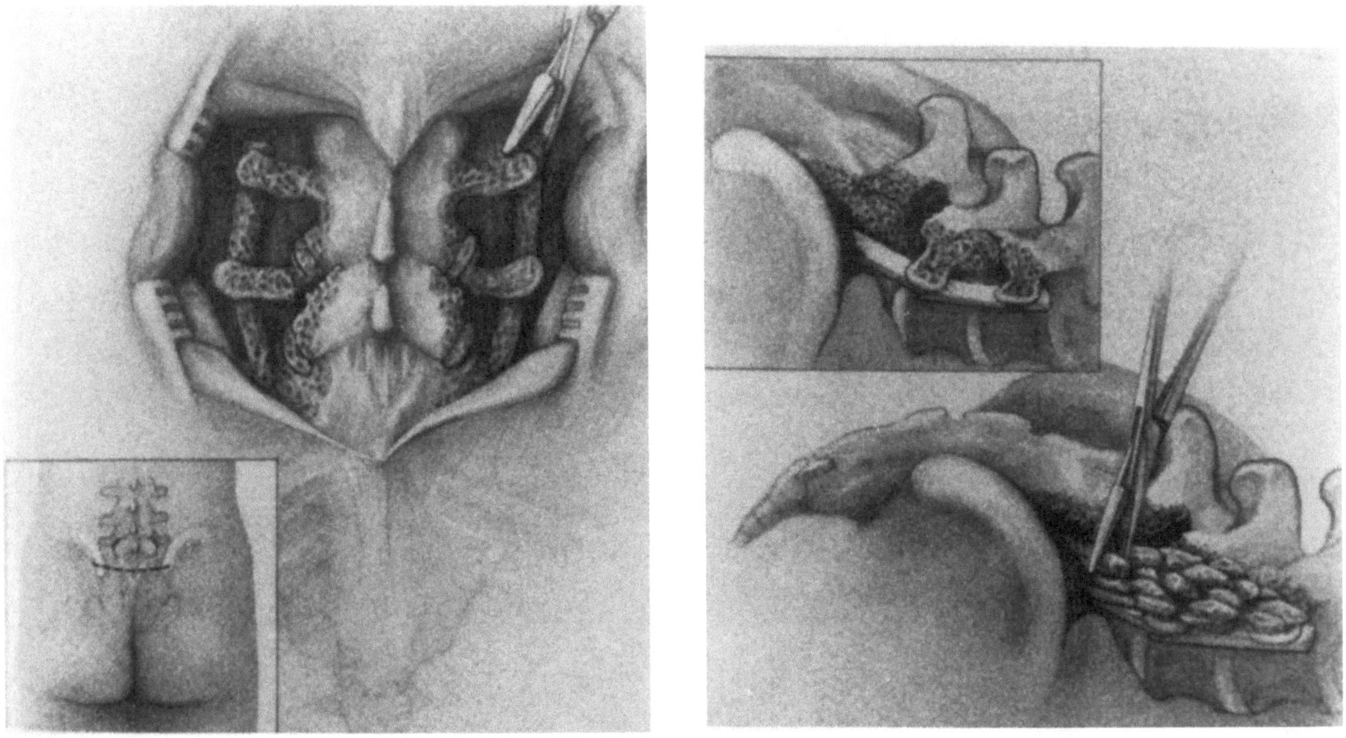

A

B

Figure 12.20. **A** and Insert: A gently curved transverse skin incision is centered on the S1 spinous process and directed toward each iliac wing. Corticocancellous bone graft is positioned anterior to the tip of the transverse process of L4 and L5. **B** and Insert: The bone graft bridging from the sacral notch to the anterior border of the transverse process tip serves as a stable base for a large amount of cancellous bone graft. Reprinted with permission.[180]

patients should be checked during their adolescent growth spurt. Of 155 patients with spondylolysis and spondylolisthesis, it was shown that the only factors correlating radiographic pathology with progression were slippage of greater than 25%, low lumbar index (i.e., height of the anterior portion of the vertebra being less than 75% of the height of the posterior portion of the vertebra), and spondylolysis at the L4 level.[174,177,178] Those patients who do not have these risk signs can usually be permitted to carry out activities of daily living without fear of progression. Children having these risk signs should be observed more closely. If any doubt exists, flexion and extension lateral roentgenograms of the area can be obtained. If there is no translational movement, the child should be treated as normal. For the patient who becomes symptomatic and does not respond to the conservative measures used for patients with a spondylolysis, surgery should be considered.

The indications for surgery are pain unrelieved by conservative measures, progression of subluxation or spondylolisthesis to more than 50% in still immature patients, postural deformity, or significant gait abnormalities from tight hamstrings.[166,179–181] The cosmetic deformity is produced by the sagittal rotation, which produces a localized kyphosis. If reduction is planned, it is to reduce the kyphosis (rotation) not the forward translation. Two questions then arise: whether or not to reduce the spondylolisthesis, and, if reduction is planned, how will it be done. It is important to remember that most studies show that with an in situ fusion the majority of the symptoms will disappear.[166,182,183] The rate of fusion is equal with or without reduction. Additionally, open reductions, particularly those that combine anterior and posterior procedures, tend to have a significant rate of neurological complication.[184–187] With this in mind, we strongly prefer the following regimen to produce an in situ fusion.

It is our belief that the results of the posterior lateral bone grafting procedure for spondylolisthesis and spondyloptosis are reproducible and reliable for all degrees of slippage.[179–182] The procedure is performed with the patient prone on a frame that permits the abdomen to hang free. Both lumbar and sacral regions are visualized. Identification of the level of the defect is made by a roentgenogram taken with a marker before making the incision. A gently curved transverse incision is made centered over the S1 spinous process and directed toward each iliac crest (Fig. 12.20). Significant curvature of the skin incision should be avoided to decrease the risk of skin necrosis. The incision is carried down through the subcutaneous tissue to the fascia. A single incision is then made through the lumbosacral fascia. The spinous process of each vertebra to be fused is exposed. It is necessary to emphasize the high incidence of spina bifida, and care must be taken in making the exposure. The posterior elements of L5 are exposed subperiosteally along the spinous processes. The facet joints and transverse processes are also exposed. The fusion is extended to L4 if the slip exceeds 50% and that vertebra is similarly exposed. The posterior two-thirds of the iliac crest is then exposed to obtain bone graft. Bone wax is applied to the bleeding bone at the graft donor site to help obtain hemostasis and the wound is closed tightly.

The dorsal surfaces of the transverse processes and their tips are then exposed subperiosteally. The lateral surface of the pars interarticularis, the lateral surface of the superior facets, and the superior surface of the sacrum are also decorticated. A notch is then made in the superior surface of each sacral ala to receive bone graft. Care is taken to avoid going medially during decortication, when making the alar notch, or in placing the graft, to prevent pressure on the peripheral nerves as they leave the foramen. The notch functions as a trough for the corticocancellous strips so that they can be placed in a horizontal position to function as struts that extend from the ala to the anterior border of the tips of the transverse processes of L5 and L4. The struts also create a floor for the cancellous bone grafts. No graft is placed posteriorly over the lamina. Watertight closure of each layer is then made and a pressure dressing is applied.

The patient is then placed at bed rest for 1 week. An extension double-leg pantaloon spica with pressure over the sacrum is then applied. The cast is for stability during the postoperative period because the soft-tissue stripping during surgery increases the instability. The cast also has the benefit of reducing the local kyphosis. The patient is kept in this cast for 3 months, at which point ambulation is permitted in an orthoplast jacket for the next 3 months. Once flexibility and strength are regained, the brace is discontinued and full activity is resumed. The Gill procedure is rarely if ever indicated because exposure of the dura increases the potential for scar formation and the symptoms that can accompany the scar.

In the rare patient that has both a severe absolute displacement and angular deformity, reduction of the slip may be contemplated, but again risks of neurological complication must be considered. Reduction can be carried out by isolated posterior or combined anterior and posterior procedures. We have had no personal experience with these techniques; the reader is referred to the literature to form their own conclusions regarding the risks to benefit ratios.[185–191]

We found a high incidence of small-degree scoliosis in patients with spondylolisthesis.[192] It does not appear to be structural when it is associated with spondylolisthesis. The experience of most researchers is that the scoliosis resolves or does not progress further when the spondylolisthesis has been treated successfully.[168] If a true scoliosis exists, the treatment should be separate and directed to it as specifically indicated.

Acknowledgments. We would like to thank Dr. Joseph Nadell for all his advice and use of his cases. Thanks are also due to Dr. Robert Peinert for his assistance.

References

1. Klippel M, Feil A. Un cas d'absence des vertebres cervicales avec cage thoracique remontant jusqua's la base du craine. Nouv Icon Salpetriere, 1912;25:223.
2. Hensinger, RN: Osseous anomalies of the craniovertebral function. Spine 11(4):323, 1986.
3. McRae DI. Bony abnormalities in the region of the foramen magnum: correlation of the anatomic and neurologic findings. Acta Radiol 1953;40:335.
4. List CF. Neurologic syndromes accompanying developmental anomalies of the occipital bone atlas and axis. Arch Neurol Psychiatry 1941;45:577.
5. Zimbler S, Belkin S. Birth defects involving the spine. In: Symposia on birth defects and the orthopaedic surgeon. Orthop Clin North Am 1976;7:303.
6. Hensinger RN. Atlanto-occipital fusion. In: The Cervical Spine. The Cervical Spine Research Society. Philadelphia: Lippincott, 1983:161–163.
7. Wadia NH. Myelopathy complicating congenital atlanto-axial dislocation. Brain 1967;90:449.
8. Hensinger RN, MacEwen GD. Congenital anomalies of the spine. In: Rothman RH and Simeone F, eds. The Spine. Philadelphia: Saunders, 1982, 2nd ed. Vol. I, 188.
9. Caetano de Barros M, Farias W, Ataide L, Lins S. Basilar impression and Arnold–Chiari malformation. A study of 66 cases. J Neurol Neurosurg Psychiatry, 1968;31:596.
10. Nicholson JT, Sherk HH. Anomalies of the occipitocervical articulation. J Bone Joint Surg 1968;50A:295.
11. Pasztor VJ, Piffko P, Horvath M. Transoral surgery for basilar impression. Surg Neurol 1980;14:473.
12. Van Gilder JC, Menezes AH, Doland KD. The Craniovertebral Junction and its Anomalies. New York: Futura, 1987:235–236.
13. Raynor RB. Congenital malformations at the base of the skull. In: The Cervical Spine. The Cervical Spine Research Society. Philadelphia: Lippincott, 1983:147.
14. McRae DL, Barnum AS. Occipitalization of the atlas. Am J Radiol 1953;70:23.
15. Grantham SA, Dick HM, Thompson RC, Jr, Stinchfield FE. Occipito-cervical arthrodesis: indications, technique and results. Clin Orthop 1969;65:118.

16. Chamberlain WE. Basilar impression (platybasia), a bizarre development anomaly of the occipital bone and upper cervical spine with striking and misleading neurlogic manifestations. Yale J Biol Med 1939;11:487.
17. Henderson DRF. Vertical atlantoaxial subluxation and rheumatoid arthritis. J Rheumatol 1975;14:31.
18. McGregor W. The significance of certain measurements of the skull in the diagnosis of basilar impression. Br J Radiol 1948;21:171.
19. Kricum, ME. Imaging Modalities in Spinal Disorders. Philadelphia: Saunders, 1988:154.
20. Fischgold H, David M, Bregeat P. La tomographie de la base du crane en neuro-chirurgie et neuro-ophthalmologie. Paris: Masson & Cie, 1952. [Also cited by Hinck VC, Hopkins CE, Savara BS. Diagnostic criteria of basilar impression. Radiology 1961;76:572.]
21. Wiesel SW, Rothman RH. Occipitoatlantal hypermobility. Spine 1979;4:187.
22. Wiesel SW, Kraus D, Rothman RH. Atlanto-occipital hypermobility. Orthop Clin North Am 1978;9:969.
23. Georgopoulos G, Pizzutillo PD, Lee MS. Occipitoatlantal instability in children. A report of 5 cases and a review of the literature. J Bone Joint Surg 1987;69A:429.
24. Hensinger RN, Lang JE, MacEwen GD. Klippel Feil syndrome: a constellation of associated anomalies. J Bone Joint Surg 1974;56A:1246.
25. Lee CK, Weiss AB. Isolated congenital cervical blocked vertebrae below the axis with neurologic symptoms. Spine 1981;6:118.
26. Winter RB. Congenital Deformities of the Spine. Stuttgart: Thieme-Stratton, 1983:301.
27. Lipson SJ. Dysplasia of the odontoid process in Morquio's syndrome causing quadriparesis. J Bone Joint Surg 1977;59A:340.
28. Holmes JC, Hall JE. Fusion for instability and potential instability of the cervical spine in children and adolescents. Orthop Clin North Am 1978;9:923.
29. Clark CR, Kathol MH, Walsh T, El-Khoury GY. Atlantoaxial rotatory fixation with compensatory counter occipito-atlanto subluxation: a case report. Spine 1986;11:1048.
30. Fielding J, Stillell WT. Chynn K, York S, Efthmios C. Use of computed tomography for the diagnosis of atlantoaxial rotatory fixation: a case report. J Bone Joint Surg 1978;60A:1102.
31. Alker GJ, Jr, Oh YS, Leslie EV. High cervical spine and craniocervical junction injuries in fatal traffic accidents: a radiological study. Orthop Clin North Am 1978;9:1003.
32. Evarts CM. Traumatic occipito-atlantal dislocation. J Bone Joint Surg 1970;52A:1653.
33. Gabrielson TO, Maxwell JA. Traumatic atlanto-occipital dislocation: a case report of a patient who survived. AJR, 1966;97:624.
34. Lipson J, Hammerschlag SP. Atlantoaxial arthrodesis in the presence of posterior spondyloschisis (bifid arch) of the atlas. A report of three cases and an evaluation of alternative wiring techniques by computerized tomography. Spine 1984;9:65.
35. Whitesides TE, Kelley RP. Lateral approach to the upper cervical spine for anterior fusion. South Med J 1966; 59:879.
36. Simmons EH, Dutoit G, Jr. Lateral atlantoaxial arthrodesis. Orthop Clin North Am 1978;9:1101.
37. Bohler J. Anterior stabilization for acute fractures and nonunions of the dens. J Bone Joint Surg 1982;64A:18.
38. Taddonio RF, Jr, King AG. Atlantoaxial rotatory fixation after decompressive laminectomy. A case report. Spine 1982;7:540.
39. Wertheim SB, Bohlman HH. Occipito-cervical fusion: indications, technique, and long-term results in thirteen patients. J Bone Joint Surg 1987;69A:833.
40. Perry J, Nickel VL. Total cervical spine fusion for neck paralysis. J Bone Joint Surg 1959;41A:37.
41. Newman P, Sweetnam R. Occipito-cervical fusion: an operative technique and its indications. J Bone Joint Surg 1969;51B:423.
42. White A, III, Panjabi MM. Clinical Biomechanics of the Spine. Philadelphia: Lippincott, 1978.
43. Robinson RA, Southwick WO. Surgical approaches to the cervical spine. In: Instructional Course Lectures, the American Academy of Orthopaedic Surgeons. St. Louis: Mosby, 1960;17:299.
44. Grantham SA, Dick HM, Thompson RC, Jr, Stinchfield FE. Occipito-cervical arthrodesis: indications, technique and results. Clin Orthop 1969;65:118.
45. Heywood AWB, Learmonth RD, Thomas M. Internal fixation for occipito-cervical fusion. J Bone Joint Surg 1988;70B:708.
46. Wiesel SW, Rothman RH. Occipitoatlantal hypermobility. Spine 1979;4:187–191.
47. Nagashima HC. Surgical treatment of irreducible atlanto-axial dislocation with spinal cord compression. A case report. J Neurosurg 1973;38:374.
48. Eismont FJ, Bohlman HH. Posterior methylmethalcrylate fixation for cervical trauma. Spine 1981;6:347.
49. Kriegen JC. Internal fixation of the unstable rheumatoid cervical spine. Ann Rheum Dis 1966;25:242.
50. Ransford AO, Crockard HA, Pozo JL, Thomas NP, Nelson RW. Craniocervical instability treated by contoured loop fixation. J Bone Joint Surg 1986;68B:173.
51. Roy-Camille R. Rachis cervical superieur. In: Cinquiemes journees d'orthopedie de la pitie masson Paris, 1986.
52. Greenberg AD. Atlantoaxial dislocations. Brain 1968;91:655.
53. Conaty JP, Mongan ES. Cervical fusion in rhematoid arthritis. J Bone Joint Surg 1981;63A:1218.
54. Lipson SJ. Dysplasia of the odontoid process in Morquio's syndrome causing quadriparesis. J Bone Joint Surg 1977;59A:340.
55. McKusick VA. Heritable Disorders of Connective Tissue. 4th Ed. St. Louis: Mosby, 1972.
56. Kopits SF. Orthopaedic complications of dwarfism. Clin Orthop 1976;114:153.
57. Betham D. Os odontoideum in chondrodystrophia calcifans congenita: a case report. J Bone Joint Surg 1982;64A:1385.
58. Spitzer RL, Rabinowitch JY, Wybar KC. A study of the abnormalities of the skull, teeth and lenses in Mongolism. Can Med Assoc J 1961;84:567.
59. Isu T, Myasaka K, Abe H, Ito T, Iwasaki Y, Tsuru M,

Kitaoka K, Tsunoda M. Atlantoaxial dislocation associated with neurofibromatosis. J Neurosurg 1983;58:451.
60. McRae DL. Bony abnormalities in the region of the foramen magnum: correlation of the anatomic and neurlogic findings. Acta Radiol 1953;40:335.
61. List CF. Neurologic syndromes accompanying developmental anomalies of the occipital bone, atlas and axis. Arch Neurol Psychiatr 1941;45:577.
62. Spranger JW, Langer LO, Jr, Wiedermann HR. Bone Dysplasias. An Atlas of Constitutional Disorders of Skeletal Development. Philadelphia: Saunders, 1974.
63. White AA, III, Panjabi MM. Clinical Biomechanics of the Spine. Philadelphia: Lipponcott 1978:71.
64. Hohl M, Baker HR. The atlantoaxial joint. J Bone Joint Surg 1964;46A:1739.
65. Louis R. Surgery of the Spine. Surgical Anatomy and Operative Approaches. Berlin-Heidelberg-New York: Springer-Verlag, 1983:58.
66. Jackson H. The diagnosis of minimal atlantoaxial subluxation. Br J Radiol 1950;23:672.
67. Fielding JW, Hawkins RJ, Ratzan SA. Spine fusion for atlantoaxial instability. J Bone Joint Surg 1976;58A:400.
68. Steel HH. Anatomical and mechanical considerations of the atlantoaxial articulations. J Bone Joint Surg 1968;50A:1481.
69. Hecker P. Appareil ligamenteux occipito-atloidoaxoidien: etude d'anatomie comparee. Arch Anat Hist Embryol 1923.
70. McRae DL. The significance of abnormalities of the cervical spine. AJR 1960;84:3.
71. Greenberg AD. Atlantoaxial dislocations. Brain 1968;91:655.
72. Itoh T. An isolated congenital narrow canal of the atlas. In: Kehr P, Weidner A, eds. Cervical spine I. New York: Springer-Verlag, 1987:317–321.
73. Roach JW, Duncan D, Wenger DR, Maravilla A, Maravilla K. Atlantoaxial instability and spinal cord compression in children diagnosed by computerized tomography. J Bone Joint Surg 1984;66A:708.
74. Arey LB. Developmental Anatomy. 6th Ed. Philadelphia and London: Saunders 1954.
75. Hensinger RN, MacEwen GD. Congenital anomalies of the spine. In: Rothman RH, Simeone FA, eds. The Spine. 2d Ed. Philadephia: Saunders 1982.
76. Fielding JW, Hensinger RN, Hawkins RJ. Os Odontoideum. J Bone Joint Surg April 1980;62A:376.
77. Parke WW. The vascular relations of the upper cervical vertebrae. Orthop Clin North Am 1978;9:879.
78. Guinn JO, Smith JO. Congenital absence of the odontoid process. AJR, 1962;88:424.
79. Kricun M. Imaging Modalities and Spinal Disorders. Philadelphia: Saunders, 1988;158.
80. Sheppard CN. Familial hypoplasia of the odontoid process. J Bone Joint Surg 1966;48A:1224.
81. Hensinger RN. Congenital anomalies of the odontoid. In: The Cervical Spine. The Cervical Spine Research Society. Philadelphia: Lippincott, 1983:164.
82. Nagashima C. Surgical treatment of irreducible atlantoaxial dislocation with spinal cord compression: a case report. J Neurosurg 1973;38:374.
83. Sherk HH, Nicholson JT. Rotatory atlantoaxial dislocation associated with ossiculum terminale in Mongolism: a case report. J Bone Joint Surg 1969;51A:957.
84. Sherk HH, Nicholson JT. Chung SMK. Fractures of the odontoid process in young children. J Bone Joint Surg 1978;60A:921.
85. Herzenberg JE, Hensinger RN, Dedrick DK, Phillips WA. Potential hazards of backboards in transport of children with neck injuries. J Bone Joint Surg 1989;71(A):15.
86. Special Olympics Committee. Special Olympics News Release: Participation by individuals with Down's syndrome who suffer from the atlantoaxial dislocation condition. Washington, DC: Special Olympics Inc., March 31, 1983.
87. Martel W, Tishler J. Observations on the spine in Mongoloidism. AJR 1966;97:630.
88. Pueschel SM, Scola FH, Perry CD, Pezzullo JC. Atlantoaxial instability with Down's syndrome. Pediatr Radiol 1981;10:129.
89. Siegfried M, Pueschel SM, Herndon JH, Gelch MM, Senft KE, Scola FH, Goldberg MJ. Symptomatic atlantoaxial subluxation in persons with Down's syndrome. J Pediatr Orthop 1984;4(6):682.
90. Cope R, Olsen S. Abnormalities of the cervical spine in Down's syndrome: diagnosis, risks, and review of the literature with particular reference to Special Olympics. South Med J 1987;80:33.
91. Miller JDR, Capusten BM, Lampard R. Changes at the base of the skull and cervical spine in Down's syndrome. J Can Assoc Radiol 1986;37:85.
92. French HG, Burke S, Roberts JM, Johnston CE, II, Whitecloud T, Edmunds JO. Cervical ossicles in Down's syndrome. J Pediatr Orthop 1987;7:69.
93. Quintana CF, Rebollo VM, Berciano J. Craniocervical anomalies in Down's syndrome. Dev Med Child Neurol 1983;25:252.
94. Rosenbaum DN, Bloomhargen JD, King HA. Atlanto-occipito instability in Down's syndrome. AJR 1986;146:1269.
95. Andrews LG. Myelopathy due to atlantoaxial dislocation in a patient with Down's syndrome and rheumatoid arthritis. Dev Med Child Neurol 1981;23:356.
96. Sherk HH, Pasquariello PS, Waters WC. Multiple dislocations of the cervical spine in a patient with juvenile rheumatoid arthritis and Down's syndrome. Clin Orthop 1982;162:37.
97. Herring JA. Cervical instability in Down's syndrome and juvenile rheumatoid arthritis. J Pediatr Orthop 1982;2:205.
98. Chaudry V, Sturgeon C, Gates AJ, Meyers G. Symptomatic atlantoaxial dislocation in Down's syndrome. Ann Neurol 1987;21:606.
99. Holmes JC, Hall JE. Fusion for instability and potential instability of the cervical spine in children and adolescents. Orthop Clin North Am 1978;9:923.
100. Williams JP, Summerville GM, Minor ME, Riley D. Atlantoaxial subluxation of trisomy 21: another preoperative complication. Anesthesiology 1987;87:253.
101. Griswold DM, Albright JA, Schiffman E, Johnson R, Southwick WO. Atlantoaxial fusion for instability. J Bone Joint Surg 1978;60A:285.
102. Fielding JW, Hawkins RJ, Ratzan SA. Spine fusion for

atlantoaxial instability. J Bone Joint Surg 1976;58A:400.
103. Lipson SJ, Hammerschlag SB. Atlantoaxial arthrodesis in the presence of posterior spondyloschisis (bifid arch) of the atlas. A report of three cases and evaluation of alternative wiring techniques by computerized tomography. Spine 1984;9:65.
104. El-Khoury GY, Clark CR, Cravett AW. Acute traumatic rotatory atlantoaxial dislocation in children; A report of 3 cases. J Bone Joint Surg 1984;66A:774.
105. Jones RN. Rotatory dislocation of both atlanto-axial joints. J Bone Joint Surg 1984;66B:6.
106. Coutts MB. Atlanto-epistropheal subluxations. Arch Surg 1934;29:297.
107. Wortzman G, Dewar FP. Rotatory fixation of the atlantoaxial joint: rotational atlantoaxial subluxation. Radiology 1968;90:479.
108. Fielding JW, Hawkins RJ. Atlanto-axial rotatory fixation (fixed rotatory subluxation of the atlantoaxial joint). J Bone Joint Surg 1977;59A:37.
109. Johnson DP, Ferguson CM. Early diagnosis of atlanto-axial rotatory fixation. J Bone Joint Surg 1986;68B:698.
110. Mixter SJ, Osgood RB. Traumatic lesions of the atlas and axis. Ann Surg 1910;51:193.
111. Gallie WE. Fractures and dislocations of the cervical spine. AM J Surg 1939;46:495.
112. Fried LC. Atlantoaxial fracture dislocation. Failure of posterior C1–C2 fusion. J Bone Joint Surg 1973;55B:490.
113. McGraw RW, Rusch RM. Atlantoaxial arthrodesis. J Bone Joint Surg 1973;55B:482.
114. Brooks AL, Jenkins EB. Atlantoaxial arthrodesis. A wedge compression method. J Bone Joint Surg 1978;60A:279.
115. Mitsui H. A new operation for atlantoaxial arthrodesis. J Bone Joint Surg 1984;66B:422.
116. Guyotat J, Pelissou I, Daherine T, Bachou R. Use of Cotrel-Dubousset material in C1, C2 instability. Neuro Chirurgie 1987;33(3):236–238.
117. Roosen K, Trauschel A, Growte W. Posterior atlantoaxial fusion. A new compression clamp for laminar osteosynthesis. Arch Orthop Trauma Surg 1982;10:27.
118. Sorenson KH, Hugby J, Hine O. Interlaminar atlantoaxial fusion for instability. Acta Orthop Scand 1978;49:341–349.
119. Anderson LD, D'Alonzo RT. Fractures of the odontoid process of the axis. J Bone Joint Surg 1974;56A:1663.
120. Fang HSY, Ong GB. Direct anterior approach to the upper cervical spine. J Bone Joint Surg 1962;44A:1588.
121. Hall JE, Denis F, Murray J. Exposure of the upper cervical spine for spinal decompression by mandible and tongue splitting approach. Case report. J Bone Joint Surg 1977;59A:121.
122. Bonney G, Williams JPR. Transoral approach to the upper cervical spine. A report of 16 cases. J Bone Joint Surg 1985;67B:691.
123. Sakou T, Morizono Y, Morimoto N. Transoral atlantoaxial anterior decompression and fusion. Clin Orthop 1984;187:134.
124. DeAndrade JR, Macnab I. Anterior occipito-cervical fusion using an extra-pharyngeal exposure. J Bone Joint Surg 1969;51A:1621.
125. Robinson RA. Fusions of the cervical spine. J Bone Joint Surg 1959;41A:1.
126. Johnson RN, Southwick WO. Surgical approaches to the cervical spine. In: Rothman RH, Simeone FA. The Spine. Philadelphia: Saunders, 1982:93–147.
127. McAfee PC, Bohlman HH, Riley LH, Jr, Robinson RA, Southwick WO, Nachlas NE. The anterior retropharyngeal approach to the upper part of the cervical spine. J Bone Joint Surg 1987;69A:1371.
128. Henry AK. Extensile Exposure. 2d Ed. London: Churchill Livingstone, 1973:67–72.
129. Whitesides TE, Kelley RP. Lateral approach to the upper cervical spine for anterior fusion. South Med J 1966;59:879.
130. Whitesides TE. Lateral retropharyngeal approach to the upper cervical spine. In: The Cervical Spine. The Cervical Spine Research Society. Philadelphia: Lippincott, 1983:517–527.
131. Van Shrick FG. Die angeborene kyphose. Orthop Chirurg 1932;56:238–259.
132. Winter RB, Moe JH, Wang JF. Congenital kyphosis: its natural history and treatment as observed in the study of 130 patients. J Bone Joint Surg 1973;55A:223.
133. Tsou PM. The embryology of congenital kyphosis. Clin Orthop 1977;128:18.
134. Schmorl G, Junghanns H. The Human Spine in Health and Disease, Wilkes SP, Goins LS, trans. New York: Grune and Stratton, 1959.
135. Mayfield JK, Winter RB, Bradford DS, Moe JH. Congenital kyphosis due to defects of anterior segmentation. J Bone Joint Surg 1980;62A:1291.
136. Montgomery SP, Hall JE. Congenital kyphosis. Spine 1982;7:360.
137. James JIP. Paraplegia in congenital kyphoscoliosis. J Bone Joint Surg 1975;57B:261.
138. Bingold AC. Congenital kyphosis. J Bone Joint Surg 1953;35B:579.
139. Williams F, McCall W, O'Brien JP, Park WM. Severe kyphosis due to congenital dorsal hemivertebra. Clin Radiol 1982;33:445.
140. Lorenzo RL, Hungerford D, Blumenthal BI, Bradford BF, Sanchez F, Bogolu S. Congenital kyphosis and subluxation of the thoracolumbar spine due to vertebral aplasia. Skeletal Radiol 1983;10:255.
141. Greig DM. Congenital kyphosis. Edinburgh Med J 1916;26:93.
142. Winter RB, Moe JH. The results of spinal arthrodesis for congenital spinal deformity in patients younger than five years old. J Bone Joint Surg 1982;64A:419.
143. Bradford DS. Vascularized rib graft. In: Moe's Textbook of Scoliosis and Other Spinal Deformities. Philadelphia: Saunders, 1987:179.
144. Bradford DS. Anterior vascularized pedicle bone grafting for the treatment of kyphosis. Spine 1980;5:318.
145. Morgan R, Brown JC. The effect of laminectomy on the pediatric spinal cord-injured patient. J Bone Joint Surg 1974;56A:1767.

146. Dorr LD, Harvey JP, Jr, Nickel VL. Clinical review of the early stability of spinal injuries. Spine 1982;7:545.
147. Hodgson AR, Yau ACMC. Anterior surgical approaches to the spinal column. In: Appley AG, ed. Recent Advances in Orthopaedics. Baltimore: Williams & Wilkins, 1964:289–323.
148. Bohlman HH, Eismont FJ. Surgical techniques of anterior decompression and fusion for spinal cord injuries. Clin Orthop 1981;154:57.
149. Heinig CF. Eggshell Procedure. In: Luque E, ed. Segmental Spinal Instrumentation. Slack, 1984:231–234.
150. Herbinaux G. Traite sur divers accouchemens laborieux, et sur les polypes de la matrice. Bruxelles: DeBoubers, 1982.
151. Neugebauer FL. A new contribution to the history and etiology of spondylolisthesis. (Reprinted from 1895.) Clin Orthop 1976;117:4.
152. Wiltse LL, Newman PLT, MacNab I. Classification of spondylolysis and spondylolisthesis. Clin Orthop 1976;117:23.
153. Killian HF. Schilderungen never beckenformen und ihres verhaltens im leben. Mannheim: Verlag von Bassermann und Matheg, 1854.
154. Robert. Monatsschr Geburtsk Frauenkrank 1855;5:81.
155. Rowe GG, Roche MB. The etiology of the separate neural arch. J Bone Joint Surg 1953;35A:102.
156. Borkow SE, Kleiger B. Spondylolisthesis in the newborn. Clin Orthop 1971;81:73.
157. Stewart TD. The age incidence of neural-arch defects in Alaskan natives. J Bone Joint Surg 1953;35A:937.
158. Albanese M, Pizzutillo PD. Family study of spondylolysis and spondylolisthesis. J Pediatr Orthop 1982;2:496.
159. Wynne-Davis R, Scott JHS. Inheritance and spondylolisthesis. J Bone Joint Surg 1979;61B:301.
160. Rosenberg NJ, Bargar WL, Friedman B. The incidence of spondylolysis and spondylolisthesis in non-ambulating patients. Spine 1981;6:35.
161. Jackson DW, Wiltse LL, Civincione RJ. Spondylolysis in the female gymnast. Clin Orthop 1976;117:68.
162. Hutton WC, Stott JRR, Cyron BM. Is spondylolysis a fatigue fracture? Spine 1977;2:202.
163. Letts M, Smallman T, Afanasiev R, Gouw G. Fracture of the pars interarticularis in adolescent athletes: a clinical-biomechanical analysis. J Pediatr Orthop 1986;6:40.
164. Wiltse LL, Widell EH, Jackson DW. Fatigue fracture: the basic lesion in isthmic spondylolisthesis. J Bone Joint Surg 1975;57A:17.
165. Fredrickson BE, Baker D, McHolick WJ, Yuan HA, Lubicky JP. The natural history of spondylolysis and spondylolisthesis. J Bone Joint Surg 1984;66A:699.
166. Harris IE, Weinstein SL. Long-term follow-up of patients with grade III and IV spondylolisthesis. J Bone Joint Surg 1987;69A:960.
167. McPhee IB. Symptomatic spondylolisthesis with scoliosis. J Bone Joint Surg 1979;61B:237.
168. Sherman FC, Rosenthal RK, Hall JE. Spine fusion for spondylolysis and spondylolisthesis in children. Spine 1979;4:59.
169. Dubowitz B, Friedman L, Papert B. The oblique cranial tilt view for spondylolysis. J Bone Joint Surg 1987;69B:421.
170. McAfee PC, Yuan HA. Computed tomography in spondylolisthesis. Clin Orthop 1982;166:62.
171. Sherman FC, Wilkinson RH, Hall JE. Reactive sclerosis of a pedicle and spondylolysis in the lumbar spine. J Bone Joint Surg 1977;59A:49.
172. Meyerding HW. Spondylolisthesis. Surg Gynecol Obstet 1932;54:371.
173. Meyerding HW. Low backache and sciatic pain associated with spondylolisthesis and protruded intervertebral disc. J Bone Joint Surg 1941;23A:461.
174. Saraste LT. Symptoms in relation to the level of spondylolysis. Int Orthop 1986;10:183.
175. Nicol RO, Scott JHS. Lytic spondylolysis. Repair by wiring. Spine 1986;11:1027.
176. Pedersen AK, Hagen R. Spondylolysis and spondylolisthesis. J Bone Joint Surg 1988;70A:15.
177. Saraste AV, Brostrom LA, Aparisi T. Prognostic radiographic aspects of spondylolisthesis. Acta Radiol Diagn 1984;25:427.
178. Saraste LT. Long-term clinical and radiological follow-up of spondylolysis and spondylolisthesis. J Pediatr Orthop 1987;7:631.
179. Hensinger RN, Lang JR, MacEwen GD. Surgical management of spondylolisthesis in children and adolescents. Spine 1976;1:207.
180. Pizzutillo PD, Mirenda W, MacEwen GD. Posterolateral fusion for spondylolisthesis in adolescence. J Pediatr Orthop 1986;6(3):311.
181. Stanton RP, Meehan P, Lovell WW. Surgical fusion in childhood spondylolisthesis. J Pediatr Orthop 1985;5:411.
182. Johnson JR, Kirwan EO'G. The long-term results of fusion in situ for severe spondylolisthesis. J Bone Joint Surg 1983;65B:43.
183. Kiviluoto O, Santavirta S, Pentti S, Pauli M, Pauli P. Postero-lateral spine fusion. Acta Orthop Scand 1985;56:152.
184. Bradford DS. Treatment of severe spondylolisthesis. Spine 1979;4:423.
185. Bradford DS, Gottfried Y. Staged salvage reconstruction of grade IV and V spondylolisthesis. J Bone Joint Surg 1987;69A:191.
186. Dick W. The "fixateur interne" as a versatile implant for spine surgery. Spine 1987;12:882.
187. Matthiass HH, Heine J. The surgical reduction of spondylolisthesis. Clin Orthop 1986;203:34.
188. McPhee IB, O'Brien JP. Reduction of severe spondylolisthesis. Spine 1979;4:430.
189. McQueen MM, Court-Brown C, Scott JHS. Stabilization of spondylolisthesis using Dwyer instrumentation. J Bone Joint Surg 1986;68B:185.
190. Sijbrandij S. Reduction and stabilization of severe spondylolisthesis. J Bone Joint Surg 1983;65B:40.
191. Steffee AD, Sitkowski DJ. Reduction and stabilization of grade IV spondylolisthesis. Clin Orthop 1988;227:82.
192. McPhee IB, O'Brien JP. Scoliosis in symptomatic spondylolisthesis. J Bone Joint Surg 1980;62B:155.

■13■

Fusion Techniques for Scoliosis

William A. Phillips and Robert N. Hensinger

Arthrodesis of the spine by the posterior approach is the most common surgical treatment for many spinal deformities of childhood and adolescence. In this chapter, we discuss our technique for posterior spinal fusion for a variety of conditions, emphasizing surgical management of idiopathic scoliosis. Operative treatment of congenital scoliosis and neuromuscular scoliosis is also briefly discussed. Preoperative planning, intraoperative control of blood loss, and postoperative management are discussed as well as the important role of the anesthesiologist.

History

Posterior spinal fusion for scoliosis was first described by Hibbs in 1911.[1] From his experience with tuberculosis of the spine, he surmised that arthrodesis of the spine would probably prevent progression of idiopathic scoliosis. Hibbs' technique emphasized meticulous dissection, careful hemostasis, and prolonged postoperative immobilization.[2] No autogenous iliac crest bone graft was used nor were the facet joints violated.

Over the next 40 years, arthrodesis of the spine for scoliosis met with limited success.[3] There was an unacceptably high rate of failure of fusion, and the amount of correction that could be obtained was limited. The use of additional bone graft from the iliac crest was helpful. Moe[4a] emphasized careful excision of the facet joints to improve the chance for a successful arthrodesis.

In the early 1960s, Harrington[4b] reported on the use of distraction and compression rods for internal stabilization of spinal deformities and ushered in the modern era of spinal fusion for scoliosis. The past 10 years have seen tremendous growth in the number of devices available for internal fixation of the spine. Today the scoliosis surgeon must not only master the techniques of exposure and arthrodesis of the spine, but must also become familiar with the various types of internal fixation and how to use them.

Preoperative Planning

Patient Selection

The major goals in spinal fusion for scoliosis are to prevent progression of the curve to the point that the patient is disabled by cardiorespiratory compromise, pain, or neurological deficit[5–7] and to correct the deformity. The psychological effects of a large spinal deformity are incompletely understood, but may be very important to the patient. Partial correction of the scoliosis is possible, but patients must be informed that their spine will never be normal, because correction of the curve and arrest of progression are obtained at the cost of reduced spinal motion.

Because the operation is performed to prevent progression, the curve should be at significant risk for progression. Factors used to assess the risk of progression include the age and maturity of the patient, the magnitude of the curve, and the location of the curve.[8] The Risser method of grading the ossification of the iliac apophysis is helpful in assessing the degree of maturity and determining the risk of scoliosis progression.[9] Curves in patients of Risser stage 3 or higher are much less likely to progress than curves in patients of Risser stage 2 or less.[8] In idiopathic scoliosis, curves below 40° Cobb angle are unlikely to progress after skeletal maturity and seldom require fusion. Curves above 50° Cobb are more likely to progress after skeletal maturity, particularly those in the thoracic spine.[10] Curves between 40° and 50° Cobb represent a gray zone where observation may be indicated for skeletally mature patients in good alignment, and arthrodesis should be considered in skeletally immature patients who are at risk for further progression during their remaining growth.

Thoracic and thoracolumbar curves are more likely to progress than lumbar curves.[10]

The deformity that results from scoliosis can vary greatly, even for curves of the same magnitude. Idiopathic scoliosis is a three-dimensional spinal deformity. Alterations in spinal alignment such as decreased thoracic kyphosis and increased vertebral rotation contribute to the unsightly "rib hump," but may not be apparent on the anteroposterior radiograph. The scoliosis may result in the head not being centered over the pelvis. A slender patient's deformity may be more apparent than that of a patient who is obese.

Radiograph Assessment

Although the decision for surgery is based mainly on the spinal deformity in the frontal plane, a lateral radiograph of the spine should be taken before surgery to assess the sagittal alignment of the spine and to rule out concomitant problems such as spondylolisthesis.

To aid in selection of fusion levels, the flexibility of the spine should be evaluated.[11a] Radiographs can be obtained with the patient lying down[11b,12a] while someone attempts to reduce the deformity with manual pressure or traction, or with the patient standing with instructions to lean as far to each side as possible.

Large Curves

In curves of large magnitude (more than 90° Cobb), a two-stage arthrodesis of the spine may be advisable. The first stage consists of an anterior release of the spine, followed possibly by halo traction. Posterior spinal fusion is performed a week or two later. Careful attention has to be paid to the patient's nutritional status between the two operations. Hyperalimentation should be strongly considered to minimize the catabolic effects of the first procedure and to limit complications.[12b]

Selection of Fusion Levels

Before surgery, the levels of fusion and instrumentation sites should be selected. Deciding how much to fuse depends on curve location and flexibility of the compensatory curves. Too short a fusion may result in further progression of the deformity, while too long a fusion requires a larger operation and costs the patient motion segments. There are several ways to determine the extent of a planned spinal fusion. A rule of thumb is to fuse one or two vertebrae above and below any structural curves. A structural curve is defined as one that does not reverse on bending films and in which the spinous processes are rotated toward the midline.

In addition, instrumentation should be placed in such a way to center the head over the pelvis. The lower hook should be seated within Harrington's stable zone, which is defined by vertical lines extending up from the sacroiliac joints.[13] King and his colleagues from Minneapolis emphasized the importance of fusing from neutrally rotated vertebra to neutrally rotated vertebra—that is, a vertebra whose spinous process is equidistant from the two pedicles on the anteroposterior radiograph.[11a] King also pointed out that many compensatory lumbar curves do not require fusion if they are more flexible than the accompanying structural thoracic curve.

Fusion to the last lumbar vertebra (usually the fifth) has been associated with a high incidence of back pain and should be avoided.[14a]

Blood Replacement

Substantial blood loss should be anticipated from the extensive exposure required, making blood replacement almost always necessary. To minimize the risk of transfusion-acquired illnesses,[14b] we prefer to have our patients donate their own blood preoperatively for retransfusion later. Patients are allowed to donate 1 unit per week up to 10 days before their surgery. With new preservatives, this allows them to donate 3 to 4 units in the month before surgery. Our patients are instructed to take ferrous sulfate, and the blood bank will continue to draw blood for autotransfusion as long as the patient's hematocrit remains above 30%.

Intraoperative Management

Patient Monitoring

With the blood loss and fluid shifts that inevitably occur during scoliosis surgery, close monitoring of the patient is essential. A foley catheter should be inserted to monitor urine output. The state of the circulatory system can be measured in several ways. An arterial catheter can measure peripheral blood pressure. A central venous pressure line can be inserted to administer large amounts of fluids rapidly. The reliability of monitoring the central venous pressure in the prone position is questionable.

The most accurate way to assess the circulatory system is with a right atrial (Swan–Ganz) catheter that directly monitors cardiac output. A Swan–Ganz catheter is more difficult to insert than a central venous or arterial catheter. A possible advantage of a Swan–Ganz line is the ability to aspirate air embolism, if it occurs, from the right side of the heart. A Doppler stethoscope taped to the chest can detect this rare but catastrophic complication.[15]

A major concern in scoliosis surgery is protection of neurological function. Earlier recognition of neurological compromise allows a more rapid response, which may increase the chance of neurological recovery. Intraoperative assessment of spinal cord function has become routine for most scoliosis surgeons.

Spinal cord function can be assessed intraoperatively by the wake-up test,[16,17] the clonus test,[18] or somatosensory-evoked potentials (SSEP).[19] The wake-up test is performed by bringing the patient up to a light level of anesthesia. The patient is instructed to squeeze the anesthetist's hand to make certain the patient is awake enough to follow commands. The patient is next told to move the feet. Once this has been observed, the anesthesia is deepened and the procedure continues. The wake-up test requires some comprehension on the patient's part, although most do not recall the episode later. Rehearsal with the patient before surgery enhances its reliability.

Close cooperation with the anesthesiologist is crucial. Gradual lightening of the level of anesthesia can allow rapid performance of the wake-up test when the surgeon wants it. Care must be taken to avoid complete reversal of anesthesia, or the patient's blood pressure may rise excessively and the patient's movements may disengage the fixation and dislodge the endotracheal tube.

The clonus test is performed on a patient at the same level of anesthesia as a wake-up test, but requires no patient cooperation. Instead of commanding the patient to move the feet, an examiner rapidly dorsiflexes the ankles. The production of sustained clonus indicates preservation of spinal cord function.

Many centers perform intraoperative assessment of spinal cord function by SSEPs. Stimulating electrodes are placed over the posterior tibial and popliteal nerves. Electrodes on the skull record the signals transmitted through the spinal cord from the legs. SSEP signals of diminished amplitude or increased latency indicate possible problems with spinal cord function.[19] SSEPs monitor only posterior column (afferent nerve) function, and there have been instances of paralysis without SSEP change.

The use of SSEPs places additional demands on the anesthesiologist. Inhalation agents such as halothane cannot be used in large dosages. Extra care must be taken to maintain the patient's core temperature, because hypothermia can alter the SSEP signals. Wrapping the extremities in blankets before surgery, and heating and humidifying the inspired anesthetic gases, can help reduce intraoperative heat loss.[20]

Intraoperative Positioning

Careful positioning of the patient can also help reduce blood loss. Placing the patient prone on a Relton–Hall frame allows the abdomen to hang free, taking pressure off the vena cava.[21] This reduces the blood flow through Batson's plexus, which surrounds the spinal cord.[22]

A spinal fusion is a relatively long procedure. The patient will be in the prone position on the Relton–Hall frame for 4–6 hours. The legs should be wrapped in elastic bandages to help prevent thrombus formation and to reduce heat loss. Bony prominences, in particular the patellae and iliac crests, should be carefully padded. In females, care must be taken in positioning on the frame to ensure that the breasts are not under too much pressure. The arms should be placed with the shoulders in less than 90° abduction or brachial plexus palsies can result. An x-ray plate should be placed beneath the patient to allow intraoperative radiographic localization of the levels exposed.

Selection of Instrumentation

The use of internal fixation as an adjunct to a well-performed arthrodesis of the spine has greatly improved the results for surgical management of scoliosis. With spinal instrumentation, greater correction can be obtained; the rate of pseudarthrosis is reduced, and patients can be mobilized more quickly.[23]

Today's scoliosis surgeon is faced with a bewildering array of devices for internal fixation of the spine. Each type of instrumentation has its own advantages and disadvantages, and each surgeon needs to be familiar with his own abilities to use the different forms of instrumentation. Use of internal fixation devices facilitates correction of deformity, but may decrease the amount of bone exposed and available for arthrodesis. The benefit of slightly increased correction must be weighed against the difficulty of application of a specific spinal instrumentation system and the risk of complications. If a major problem is encountered intraoperatively, the ultimate fallback is to use no instrumentation and obtain correction with a Risser localizer cast postoperatively.

Unfortunately, the ideal spinal instrumentation system does not exist. The ideal system would have a high degree of safety and reliability with a minimum risk of neurological injury. The rate of complications such as failure of fixation and implant breakage would be low. The system would be strong enough to resist loads and moments from all directions, perhaps without external support. It would be easy to apply, with little increase in operative time over that needed to perform an arthrodesis. The ideal system would restore normal spinal contours and not create new deformities.

Each of the currently available spinal instrumentation systems achieves some of these criteria. None meets them all. No one device is the best choice for every surgeon to use on every patient. Surgeons vary in technical ability and experience, and patients vary in their needs and desires. In interviews with patients, parents, and physicians, lack of postoperative immobilization was not regarded to be as important as the avoidance of neurological complications.[24]

We briefly review here the various devices commonly in use to augment posterior spinal fusion in the management of idiopathic scoliosis. These include the Harrington distraction and compression rod system, the Luque method of sublaminar wire fixation, the Wisconsin method of fixation with spinous process wires, and the newest addition to the armamentarium of the spinal surgeon, the Cotrel–Dubousset system. Recent modifications and improvements made in these systems are also discussed.

Harrington Instrumentation

The spinal implants developed by Dr. Paul R. Harrington of Houston remain the most widely used today. The instrumentation originally consisted of a distraction rod applied to the concave side of the curve and a compression rod applied to the convex side.[4b] After installation of Harrington rods, a generous area of lamina remains accessible for decortication and bone grafting. An average curve correction of 50% can be obtained using Harrington rods in adolescent idiopathic scoliosis.[25] Several factors limit further correction. Excessive distraction may be associated with neurological injury, presumably from stretch-induced spinal cord ischemia. Prompt removal of distraction will sometimes reverse the neurological injury.[26] Intraoperative assessment of spinal cord function by SSEP, the wake-up test, or the clonus test may help lessen the risks of this potentially catastrophic complication.

A second limiting factor to curve correction by Harrington rod is the decreased efficiency of axial distraction as the curve magnitude reduces.[27,28] Axial distraction corrects a spinal curvature by applying a force parallel to the spine acting across a moment arm that runs perpendicularly to the apex of the curve. As the curve is reduced, this moment arm is decreased, so greater applied force results in less correction. With Harrington distraction rods, all the distraction force is applied only at the two laminae where the hooks are seated. If the load exceeds the strength of the lamina, fracture and loss of correction can result.[29] Because the thoracic laminae are thinner, failure is more likely to occur at the upper hook site.

To avoid overdistraction, some surgeons incorporate strain gauges into their distraction devices.[30] Others rely on "feel" for when to stop distracting.[31] Studies of instrumented spines have demonstrated that the load on the distraction rod diminishes in a few minutes because of the viscoelasticity of the spine's soft tissues (creep).[25,29,32] Repeated distraction over time can gradually overcome much of the viscoelasticity and allow further correction. Repeated distraction of the Harrington rod can overcome the creep to some extent, but a problem arises; as the spine is lengthened, the ratcheted portion of the rod below the hook becomes longer. This increases the stress on the junction of the ratcheted (thin) portion of the rod and the smooth (thick) portion of the rod, and increases the risk of rod fracture at the junction.[33,34] Distraction rods with short ratcheted segments are now manufactured to minimize the risk of rod fracture, but these limit the ability to repeatedly distract the spine.

Distraction of the spine can also be done with an outrigger device attached to the hooks. By using the clothespin-like hook clamps devised by Zielke, it is possible to keep the spine closer to the final length while placing a distraction rod that has a short ratcheted portion.

One method of reducing the risk of lamina fracture is to share the load between two adjacent laminae. With regular ratchet end hooks this is difficult, because the sagittal curve of the spine may not allow placement of the hooks in a line straight enough to allow passage of the distraction rod through two hooks. Bobechko[35] devised a hook with a sliding barrel (Fig. 13.1A) that allows placement of two hooks on the ratchet end of the rod. A special spreader is used to load both hooks simultaneously. The sliding barrel hook is taller than a regular hook, and may be prominent or even subcutaneous in thin individuals. This construct uses a straight distraction rod that reduces not only scoliosis but also the normal sagittal plane curves.

The Harrington distraction rod elongates the spine. This elongation results in reduction of spinal curves in both the coronal and sagittal planes. The coronal plane curve, that is, scoliosis, is pathological. The sagittal plane curves, that is, thoracic kyphosis and lumbar lordosis, are physiological. If the spine is instrumented to the lower lumbar region with a straight distraction rod, the normal lumbar lordosis is reduced and a "flatback" syndrome can result.[36,37] To walk upright, affected patients must either hyperextend their hips or walk in a crouched position.[38a] Neither is desirable, and both are uncomfortable and unsightly.

To overcome this problem, Moe modified the Harrington rod by making the inferior end of the rod, and the corresponding hole in the lower hook, square shaped (Fig. 13.1B). This allows the rod to be contoured to preserve lumbar lordosis while preventing unwanted rotation of the rod. While the use of contoured rods diminishes the loss of sagittal plane curves, it has not completely eliminated this problem.[38b] Contoured rods are weakened and more likely to break, and the mechanical efficiency of the rod for distraction is reduced. Square-ended contoured rods are also more difficult to install. A special pusher[39] or clamp is very helpful, because rotation must be controlled to seat the rod in the square-holed Moe hook.

The strength of a Harrington rod construct depends on how well the hooks are attached to the lamina. In axial loading, the limiting factor is the strength of the lamina in which the hooks are seated. The spine fails

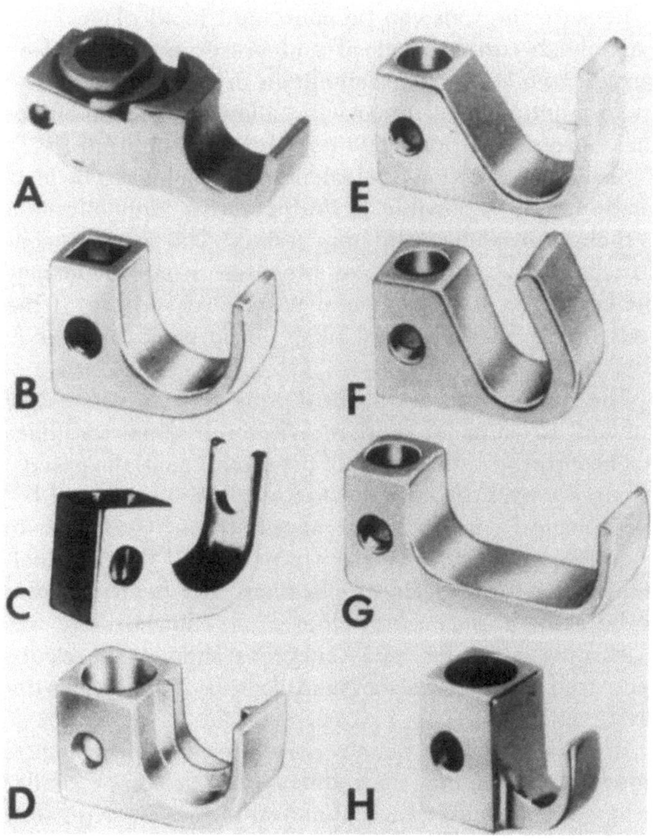

Figure 13.1. Modified hooks for Harrington distraction rods. **A.** Bobechko's sliding barrel hook. **B.** Moe's square-ended hook. **C.** Zielke bifid hook. **D.** Ribbed hook. **E.** Leatherman hook. **F.** Andre hook. **G.** Moe alar hook. **H.** Pediatric hook. (Reprinted with permission from Phillips WA, Hensinger RN. Wisconsin and other instrumentation for posterior spinal fusion. Clin Orthop 1988;229:46. Illustration courtesy of Zimmer, Incorporated, Warsaw, Indiana.)

before the Harrington rod breaks. With bending and particularly twisting of the trunk, hooks can be dislodged fairly easily, resulting in loss of fixation. Because of the risk of dislodgement, most surgeons use some form of external immobilization, such as a cast or brace, after Harrington instrumentation.

Several hook modifications have been developed to help prevent accidental dislodgement. Zielke devised a ratchet-end hook with a bifid shoe (Fig. 13.1C) designed to fit tightly around the pedicle of the thoracic vertebra. A ratchet-end hook with a sharp rib in the shoe (Fig. 13.1D) can also be used. The rib helps prevent lateral displacement of the hook, but can weaken the bone and lead to lamina fracture.

Leatherman designed a series of collar-end hooks with extended shoes (Fig. 13.1E) that help improve seating of the hook in a spine with increased lumbar lordosis. One problem is that if a Leatherman hook shifts or tilts, it can narrow the spinal canal. Andre hooks are angled (Fig. 13.1F) so that the rod insertion site is no longer parallel to the shoe. This hook conforms better to the lamina and is less likely to shift or tilt.

For instrumentation to the pelvis, a variety of hooks have been designed to attach to the sacrum. While the Moe alar hook (Fig. 13.1G) is best known, its mouth is so wide that the risk of accidental dislodgement is increased in smaller patients. Leatherman hooks with a smaller mouth may conform better to the ala in small patients and may fit better in some cases. Another method of instrumenting to the pelvis is placement of a threaded rod through both posterior iliac crests just above the sacrum. The distraction rod can be attached by either an eyelet threaded on the sacral rod or a special collar-end hook with threads on its shoe to interlock with the sacral rod. Zielke developed a hinged rod that is driven into the ilia bilaterally. It is less prominent, an advantage in thin patients.

Prominence of the hardware beneath the skin poses a serious problem in young children or thin patients, particularly when the spine is instrumented into the upper thoracic region (T3 and above). A simple solution is to invert the rod and hooks and place the smaller collar-end hook cephalad. The ratchet-end hook can then be placed caudad where more muscle is available to cover it. Pediatric hooks with smaller shoes and bodies (Fig. 13.1H) are also available. A threaded rod can be used for distraction in smaller patients, although it is thinner than the standard distraction rod and not as strong.

Compression Rods

The Harrington compression rod entails placement of multiple hooks linked on a threaded rod around either the transverse processes or laminae. Nuts adjacent to each hook are moved along the rod by a wrench to apply the compressive force. While the threaded rod is flexible, proper placement of the hooks can be difficult and time consuming.

Keene[40] and his coworkers at Wisconsin modified the compression hooks to make them easier to apply. Instead of threading all the hooks on the rod before installation, special hooks with an upward-opening groove are individually placed. The rod is pushed into the hook and a bushing is slid into the hook around the rod, locking the rod and hook together. The wrench used to tighten the nuts generates a large torque without the sensory feedback of the distraction rod spreader; thus, overtightening the nuts can lead to lamina fracture.

Currently, the compression rod is less frequently used because many surgeons report good results with just the distraction rod. Correction is not increased substantially with use of the compression rod, but the stability of the instrumented spine (the ability to resist external loads) may be increased by transverse loading (linking the compression rod to the distraction rod.[41–43] The compression rod tends to increase lordosis in the instrumented segment because it is applied posteriorly on the spine.[44] Because many patients with thoracic scoliosis are already hypokyphotic, an additional flattening of the thoracic spine is undesirable. The compression rod has been recommended to help preserve lumbar lordosis in fusions of the lumbar spine.[45]

In summary, how closely does Harrington instrumentation approach our ideal? It is reasonably safe, if excessive distraction is avoided. In most forms, external support is advisable postoperatively. It is easy to install. It corrects scoliosis, but care must be taken to prevent unwanted decreases in sagittal plane curves. Now in use for almost a quarter of a century, the Harrington rod continues to enjoy wide acceptance and excellent clinical results.

Luque Instrumentation

In the mid 1970s, Dr. Eduardo Luque of Mexico City developed a different approach to spinal instrumentation to meet the needs of his patients. Faced with a large number of patients with paralytic scoliosis (from polio) and a climate that made prolonged postoperative immobilization impractical, Dr. Luque developed what he called segmental spinal instrumentation (SSI).[46,47a,b] SSI consists of 2 contoured smooth rods fixed to the spine by multiple sublaminar wires. Rods of either 3/16- or 1/4-in.diameter are available.

Passage of sublaminar wires requires laminotomies with excision of the ligamentum flavum at each instrumented level.[47a,b] This increases operative time by at least 45 minutes when compared with Harrington rod instrumentation.[48] Luque recommended bending the rods preoperatively, but many surgeons contour the rods intraoperatively, which can be very time consuming, particularly with the stiff 1/4-in. rod. Use of a malleable aluminum rod as a template is helpful. The placement of hardware at every level limits the amount of exposed bone available for fusion.[35]

The Luque system corrects by transverse loading.[28] Its moment arm extends perpendicularly from the apex to the end of the curve. As the curve is reduced, the spine elongates and the moment arm increases. The increasing corrective force as the curve is reduced means that overcorrection with an increased risk of neurological injury is possible. To reduce the risk of overcorrection, the rods should be contoured to include the residual scoliosis achieved on preoperative bending films. A Luque-instrumented spine resists bending and twisting well, but may settle with axial loading.[49,50]

Because the rods can be contoured in all planes, it is possible to correct scoliosis and preserve sagittal plane curves[48] while the "L" shape helps prevent rotation. The use of multiple sublaminar wires allows correction of thoracic lordosis by pulling the spine to a contoured rod.[51]

Scoliosis correction equivalent to that achieved by Harrington rods is possible.[48] Postoperative immobilization is thought by some to be unnecessary. The resulting construct is so strong that rod breakage from fatigue may not occur for at least several years post surgery. If the rods break, they are most likely to do so at the apex of their contour.[52]

The major drawback of the Luque system is its use of sublaminar wires for fixation. While the spinal cord does not occupy the entire width of the spinal canal, the passage of curved wires can impinge on the dura and spinal cord.[53] Neurological complications ranging from hypesthesia to complete paralysis have been reported.[48,54–57] The incidence of neurological complications has been reported to be as high as 17%.[57] Wilber et al. showed there was a learning curve for many surgeons and, as experience increased, the incidence of neurological complications decreased.

Broken wires have been reported to cause neurological injury by "springing" more deeply into the canal, similar to opening a safety pin.[58] Removal of broken wires may be hazardous as well, because the wire may spring further into the canal as it is extracted.[59] This is perhaps more of a concern in the acute setting. Later the formation of scar tissue around the wire may offer some protection to the dura during wire removal.

Because the spine is viscoelastic, the initial tension in the wires holding the rod diminishes with time. If not properly secured, the rod can migrate or spin. If the rod migrates, it can slip off some wires and become more prominent. If the rod spins, the contour of the rod in the sagittal plane can add to the scoliosis and result in loss of correction. To help prevent rod migration and spin, McCarthy[60] devised a collar that locks to the rod with a bolt. The collar has a hole for passage of a wire to secure it to the spine.

Fixation of Luque rods to the pelvis can be accomplished by putting the transverse portion of the L through a hole in the ilium, not unlike a sacral bar. More secure pelvic fixation can be achieved by the Galveston technique, that is, driving the rod into the pelvis between the inner and outer tables just above the sciatic notch.[61] Contouring the rod to accomplish this is very demanding, but can be done preoperatively.

Moseley has developed a special rod for use in paralytic scoliosis associated with muscular dystrophy.[62] Spin and migration are prevented with his "unit rod" because the entire construct is one long precontoured rod with a hairpin turn at the top. Use of a closed loop, either a commercially available welded ring (Zimmer, Warsaw, Indiana) or a rod bent into a rectangle, can also help prevent rod migration and spin. Contouring these rods to accommodate the residual three-dimensional spine deformity after correction of scoliosis may be difficult.

In summary, the Luque system is strong, although many surgeons still prefer to use some form of brace for postoperative immobilization. It can correct scoliosis and preserve and even improve sagittal plane curves. In most hands there is a greater risk of neurological injury, which is a major drawback. The risk of neurological injury appears to be at least partially related to surgical experience with the technique. The passage of sublaminar wires and the need to contour the rod substantially increases operative time when compared with the time needed to install a Harrington rod. While very useful for paralytic scoliosis, the use of Luque rods for routine adolescent idiopathic scoliosis is difficult to recommend because of the increased risk of neurological injury.

Wisconsin Segmental Instrumentation

After Dr. Luque popularized the use of sublaminar wires, many surgeons began securing Harrington distraction rods to the spine with sublaminar wires (Harri–Luque or "Tex-Mex" technique). This was attractive because both axial and transverse loading were used to correct the scoliosis, and the resulting construct was very strong. The risk of neurological injury remained, not only from the sublaminar wires but also from the possibility of the hooks being pulled horizontally further into the spinal canal as the Harrington rod was loaded transversely and pulled to the spine.[63]

Drummond and his colleagues at the University of Wisconsin developed an alternate technique of segmental fixation.[64,65] With their Wisconsin system, the risks from sublaminar passage of wires are avoided. Wires are passed through a hole made in the base of the spinous process. Each wire is a closed loop that contains a steel button. After the doubled wire is passed, the button is pulled against the spinous process, giving Wisconsin wires a pull-out strength almost equal to that of sublaminar wires.

In Drummond's description of the technique, Wisconsin wires were used to secure a contoured Harrington distraction rod on the concave side of the curve and a contoured Luque rod with L bends at both ends on the convex side (Fig. 13.2). While obviously more time consuming than placing a standard Harrington rod, installation of the Wisconsin system is easier, quicker, and neurologically safer than the Luque system. However, Wisconsin instrumentation of double-curve-pattern scoliosis can be challenging, because the recommended technique is to overlap the supporting Luque rods for the two curves by several levels. Leaving the L bend off the overlapping end of one or both Luque rods makes it easier to place them, but increases the potential for rod migration. As with the Luque technique, the multiple rods used by the Wisconsin system limit the area available for bone graft placement.

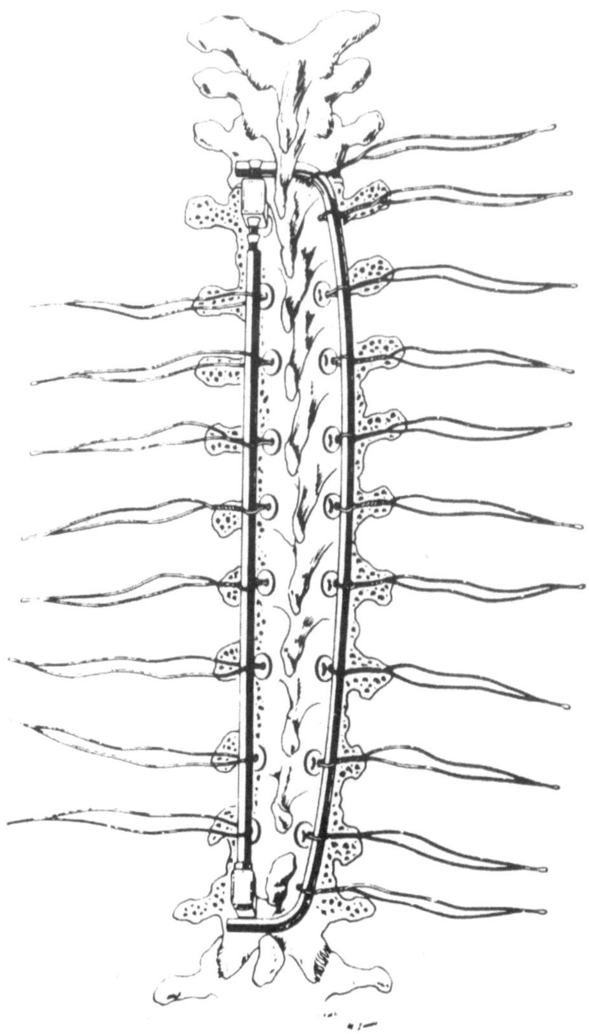

Figure 13.2. Wisconsin segmental spinal instrumentation. (Reprinted with permission from the Spinal Instrumentation Catalog, Section D, 1987, Zimmer Inc., Warsaw, Indiana, p. D–30.)

The Wisconsin system allows for both axial and transverse loading to correct the scoliosis. Theoretically this is the ideal method of correction.[27,28] Because the rods are contoured and segmentally fixed, and sagittal plane curves can be preserved. The resulting construct is claimed to need minimum postoperative immobilization, perhaps just a corset.

In summary, in idiopathic scoliosis, the Wisconsin system is as safe as a Harrington rod and nearly as strong as a Luque construct.[64,66] It can be installed relatively easily. By contouring the rods and fixing them to the

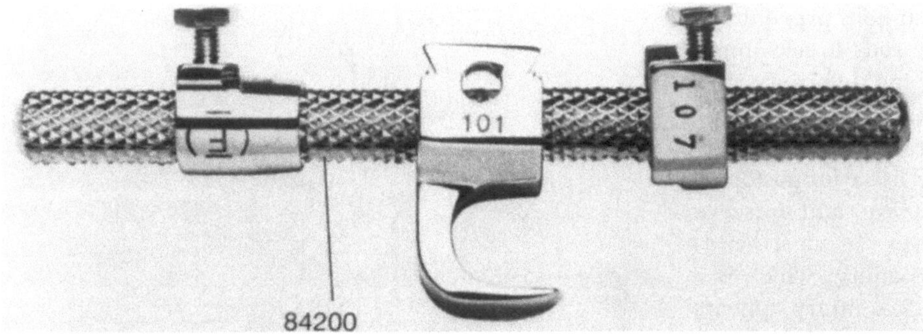

Figure 13.3. Cotrel–Dubousset rod and hook. Rod is knurled; hook blocker (left) slides in to open hook (center) to secure hook to rod. Security bolt (right) is used when large loads are anticipated. (Reprinted with permission from Universal Instrumentation [CD] for Spinal Surgery brochure, Stuart, Inc., Greensberg, Pennsylvania, p. 5.)

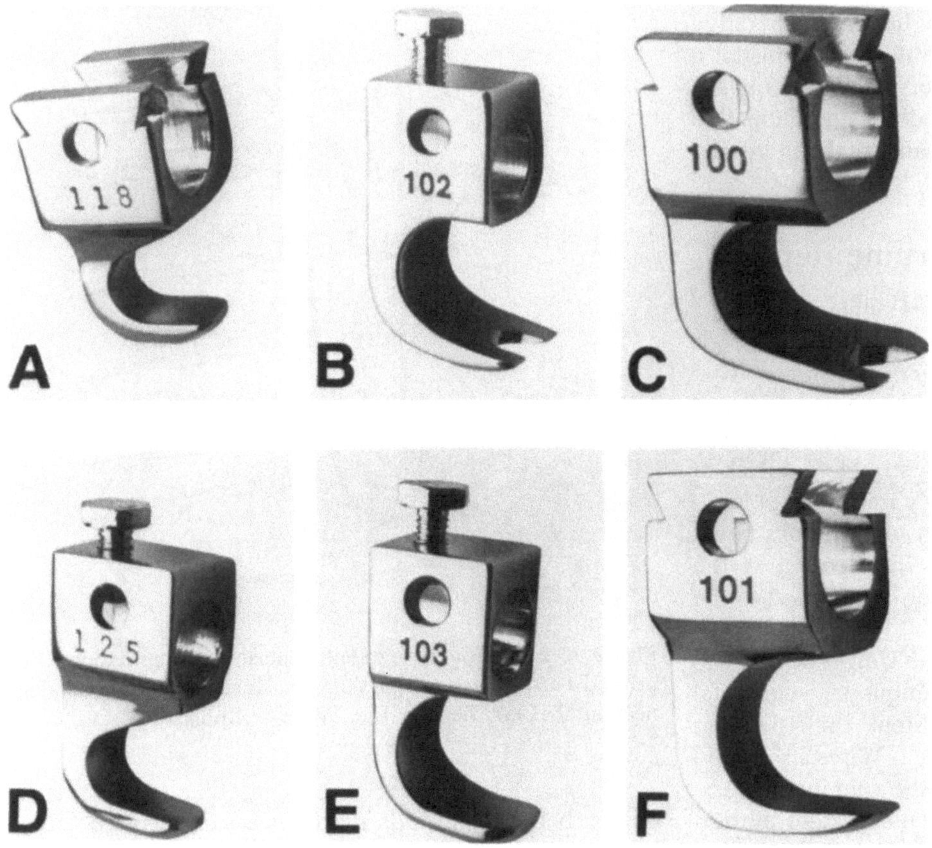

Figure 13.4. Cotrel–Dubousset hooks. **A.** Open thoracic laminar hook. **B.** Closed pedicle hook. **C.** Open pedicle hook. **D.** Closed thoracic laminar hook. **E.** Closed lumbar laminar hook. **F.** Open lumbar laminar hook. Note difference in shoe shape and size between thoracic and lumbar laminar hooks. (Reprinted with permission from Universal Instrumentation [CD] for Spinal Surgery brochure, Stuart, Inc., Greensberg, Pennsylvania, pp. 5–7.)

spine in a segmental fashion, sagittal curves can be preserved while correcting the scoliosis. The Wisconsin system is the instrumentation of choice for routine idiopathic scoliosis at the present time in our institution.

Cotrel-Dubousset (C–D) Instrumentation

A recent addition to the armamentarium of the spinal surgeon is Cotrel–Dubousset (C–D) instrumentation. The rod for the C–D system is knurled (Fig. 13.3), allowing hooks to be placed pointing in either direction (cephalad and caudad) with any degree of rotation. This ability to place hooks in either direction anywhere on the rod allows compression and distraction of different portions of the spine with a single rod. The hooks for the C–D system are available in several shoe shapes, both open and closed (Fig. 13.4). Hooks at the ends of the rod are closed on top and the rod has to be threaded through them. Additional hooks along the rod are open on top and the rod is dropped into them. The open hooks are locked to the rod by hook blockers (Fig. 13.3) that are similar in function to the bushings of the Wisconsin compression system. The C–D rod can be rotated while maintaining its attachment to the spine, theoretically allowing correction of

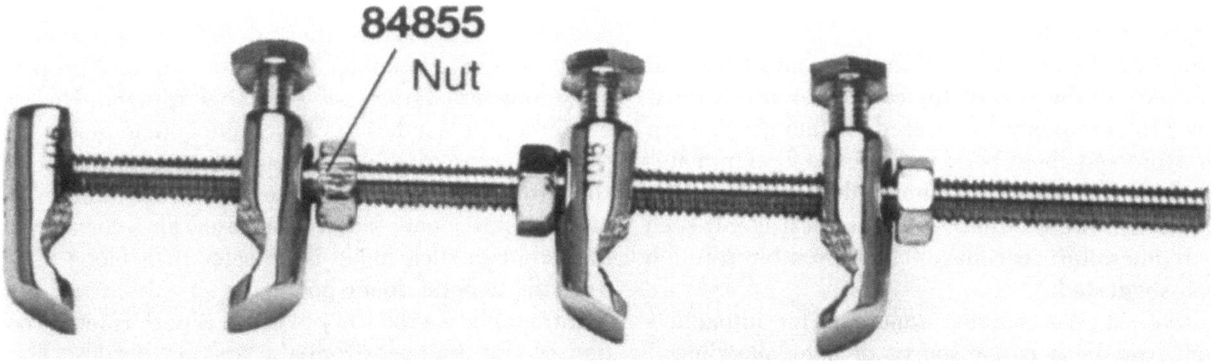

Figure 13.5. Transverse traction rod. Adjustable clamps are knurled to tightly fit rod. (Reprinted with permission from Universal Instrumentation [CD] for Spinal Surgery, Stuart, Inc., Greensberg, Pennsylvania, p. 6.)

rotational deformities and reducing the rib prominence. Two rods are inserted and linked with an adjustable transverse traction rod (Fig. 13.5). Postoperative immobilization is claimed to be unnecessary.

Careful preoperative planning is crucial with the Cotrel–Dubousset (C–D) apparatus. Bending radiographs are needed to plan the multiple hook placement sites. Usually four hooks are placed along the concave side of the curve and four along the convex side. Hook site preparation is similar to that required for Harrington hooks. Fitting the contoured rod to the multiple hooks can be very demanding. Special instruments are available to help place the rod in the hooks. While helpful, these instruments can exert enough force to pull the hook out by fracturing the lamina. Decortication is recommended before instrument insertion because it is difficult after C–D instrumentation is inserted. Given the time it takes to install a C–D rod, this may increase blood loss. C–D instrumentation is much more difficult to install and should be learned from a surgeon experienced in its use. Its theoretical ability to correct the spinal deformity in all planes makes it an exciting new device. Early reports on the C–D system are encouraging.[67–69]

The quest for the ideal spinal instrumentation system will probably never end. Further improvements of the current systems will inevitably appear, new concepts will be developed, and spinal surgeons will continue to be faced with the need to compare the advantages and disadvantages of different systems. Each surgeon should select what will work best in his or her hands for each patient.

Control of Blood Loss

Control of blood loss during scoliosis surgery has always been a primary concern for surgeons. Excessive blood loss slows down the operation and increases the risks for the patient. As Hibbs noted in an early report on spinal fusion for scoliosis, "only in an operative field that is free from hemorrhage can the operator see to exercise the care necessary for thorough work."[2] Excessive blood loss requires replacement, and the risk of diseases transmissible by blood transfusion such as AIDS[70] and hepatitis,[71] makes it important to minimize the need for allogeneic blood transfusions.

By combining surgical and anesthetic techniques that minimize blood loss with the use of autotransfusions, it is now possible to complete a routine posterior spinal fusion without using allogeneic blood transfusions.

The surgeon's role in controlling blood loss begins with selection of the appropriate operation for a given patient. Preoperative bending films should be used to plan the extent of spinal fusion required.[11a] Because blood loss during spinal fusion generally increases as operative time increases,[16] the time necessary to properly install a spinal instrumentation system must be weighed against its advantages.

Operative control of blood loss can begin before the skin incision. When the patient is lying prone the intraabdominal pressure is increased, resulting in vena caval compression which increases the pressure in the venous channels around the spine (Batson's plexus). This can cause increased bleeding during exposure of the spine. Positioning the patient on a device that allows the abdomen to hang free, such as the Relton-Hall frame, avoids the increase in intraabdominal pressure that leads to compression of the vena cava.[21]

Infiltration of the skin and paraspinous muscles with a dilute (1:500,000) solution of epinephrine has been recommended.[72] This is thought to reduce bleeding by producing local vasoconstriction and is claimed to facilitate dissection in the proper plane. There is a transient, although apparently hemodynamically insignificant, rise in serum levels of epinephrine with injection of a 1:500,000 solution.[73,74] Sponges soaked in epinephrine solution can be packed into the wound to control local bleeding.[72] Careful surgical technique can reduce blood loss. Subperiosteal dissection avoids tearing the numerous vessels in the paraspinous muscles.

Bleeding from bone can be difficult to control but can be minimized by the use of topical hemostatic agents. Bone wax has commonly been used. Although concern has been expressed about bone wax being a foreign material, pathological studies have shown that it is resorbed and replaced by fibrous tissue.[75] Other topical agents such as Avitene (microfibrillar collagen) and thrombin solution have been suggested.

The iliac crest, the common donor site for autogeneic bone graft, can be a major source of bone bleeding.[76] Bone wax can be used here as well. Use of cadaver bone graft avoids bleeding from the bone graft donor site entirely. Availability is not a problem, as there are several commercial sources of freeze-dried allogeneic cancellous bone, and many institutions also maintain their own bone banks. Reports suggest that fusion rates are comparable to those with autogenous bone graft.[77]

The primary area of bone bleeding during scoliosis surgery is the spine itself. Excision of the facet joints and thorough decortication of the laminae add to intraoperative blood loss, but increase the likelihood of a successful arthrodesis, the primary goal of the procedure.[4a] Thrombin-soaked gelfoam can be temporarily packed into the excised facet joints to aid in hemostasis and removed when the cancellous plugs are inserted. Decortication should be performed as late in the procedure as possible to minimize the time of uncontrollable bone bleeding and allow visualization in the wound for as long as possible.

From the foregoing discussion, it should be obvious that an operation of the magnitude of a spinal fusion will inevitably result in some loss of blood. In patients who cannot or will not receive blood transfusions, such as Jehovah's Witnesses,[78–80] it may be necessary to stage the procedure by exposing and fusing a limited part of the spine, stopping when the blood loss reaches a level compatible with normal function without transfusion, and returning to surgery when the patient's blood count has increased.

If a patient is going to receive a blood transfusion, the safest blood is the patient's own: autotransfused blood. Two common methods of autotransfusion are preoperative collection and preservation of a patient's blood.[81] and intraoperative salvage of blood lost in the wound.

Preoperative collection of blood for autotransfusion requires that the patient donate blood to be preserved and refrigerated just like allogeneic donated blood. At the authors' institution, patients are allowed to donate one unit per week until 10 days before surgery. Because a new preservative, citrate phosphate dextrose with adenine (CPDA-1), allows a shelf life as long as 35 days, typically three units can be obtained in the month before surgery. Patients are put on supplemental iron to keep the hematocrit above 30% to allow these donations. Children or patients weighing less than 90 pounds can have proportionately smaller aliquots of blood withdrawn. No special equipment is needed to collect autogeneic blood beyond the resources of a blood bank. It is now the policy of the authors' blood bank to allow parents and other family members to donate blood designated for a certain patient even though such blood is no safer than blood obtained from the general donor pool.

Intraoperative recovery of blood is performed by collection of the drainage from the suction bottles. The red cells are filtered, washed, and concentrated, and then reinfused into the patient. The Cell-Saver system is the most widely used of the several commercially available machines designed for this purpose.[82] The cost of the special equipment and of the technician necessary to operate it has perhaps limited its use.

Both autotransfusion methods are limited in the amount of blood loss that can be replaced. Intraoperative blood recovery systems can recover about 50% of the lost red cells.[82] Donations for autotransfusion are limited by the effectiveness of the preservative, although in special circumstances it is possible to freeze blood for as long as 3 years. Blood substitutes such as fluorocarbon compounds or stroma-free hemoglobin are still experimental. If too much blood is lost, allogeneic transfusions are still needed.

Although good surgical technique can minimize blood loss,[83] even the most careful spinal surgeon may find a wide variation in blood loss during what appears to be a standard procedure. To learn more about the mechanisms of blood loss during scoliosis surgery, a study was designed and carried out at our institution. All the patients had the same diagnosis (adolescent idiopathic scoliosis), the same anesthesia (hypotensive), the same operation (posterior spinal fusion), and the same surgeon, who used a consistent technique.

The working hypothesis was that variations in the patient's hemodynamic status, even under hypotensive conditions, could account for variations in blood loss. The patient's hemodynamic status was monitored with Swan–Ganz, central venous, and radial artery catheters. Because the autonomic nervous system and the renin-angiotensin system both play a major role in hemodynamic regulation, their roles were examined by assaying blood samples for levels of epinephrine, norepinephrine, renin, and angiotensin II. All these variables were measured at set intervals during surgery and whenever the surgeon judged the bleeding to be excessive.

Two important findings came from this study:[73] (1) when the surgeon thought there was more bleeding, he was correct; one or more of the hemodynamic parameters had changed; and (2) blood loss correlated most closely with left ventricular stroke work index (LVSWI), a measure of blood flow. Since LVSWI is computed from systemic vascular resistance, cardiac output, and heart rate, an increase in cardiac output at a constant blood pressure, even at hypotensive levels, would increase LVSWI and increase blood loss. With induced hypotension, increases in cardiac output were mediated by increased activity in either the autonomic nervous system, the renin-angiotensin system, or both.

In a broad sense, the surgeon's control of blood loss is related to his skill in controlling the number and size of bleeding points and how long they stay open. Because bleeding from bone is unavoidable, the surgeon's ability to control blood loss is limited. The only thing the surgeon can do is to go faster. The anesthesiologist controls blood flow, or how fast blood is lost through the open vessels. Given the inevitable bone bleeding and a limit to how quickly any surgeon can operate, this means the anesthesiologist becomes the primary determinant of blood loss. The anesthesiologist thus plays an important part in controlling blood loss during spinal surgery. Two major techniques used by anesthesiologists to control blood loss are hemodilution and induced hypotension.

Hemodilution decreases the loss of red cell mass by reducing the hematocrit of the blood lost intraoperatively. The patient is phlebotomized in the operating room and several units of blood are removed and preserved. Circulating volume is maintained by crystalloid replacement. The operation is performed at normal or reduced blood pressure. At the end of the procedure, the patient is diuresed of excess fluid, and the patient's own blood is retransfused. Despite the lower oxygen-carrying capability of the blood, the decreased viscosity of the diluted blood allows better tissue perfusion so tissue oxygenation is maintained. Good results have been reported with hemodilution.[84] It requires no specialized equipment and is simple to perform. However, if one of the goals of minimizing blood loss is to keep the operative field dry as well as to minimize the need for transfusion, intraoperative hemodilution appears less attractive. Blood with a hematocrit of 20 is as difficult to see through as blood with a hematocrit of 40.

Blood loss can also be reduced by decreasing blood flow. Although commonly referred to as hypotensive anesthesia, these techniques are actually directed at reducing the left ventricular stroke work index. Arterial blood pressure is a relatively convenient way of assessing the patient's hemodynamic status, although as previously noted, it is not necessarily the best overall measure of hemodynamic status.

A major concern about hypotensive anesthesia during scoliosis surgery has been the potential for increasing the risk of spinal cord injury.[33] It was feared that hypotensive anesthetic techniques would leave a narrower margin of safety because of reduced spinal cord blood flow.[26] With reduced spinal cord blood flow, an insult to the spinal cord such as distraction or invasion of the spinal canal could be more likely to cause a neurological deficit. However, a growing body of evidence suggests there is little if any increased risk of neurological injury with hypotensive anesthetic techniques. Several investigators have demonstrated experimentally that spinal cord blood flow can be autoregulated independently of systemic blood flow under controlled hypotension.[85–88]

Somatosensory evoked potentials (SSEP), a noninvasive means of intraoperatively assessing spinal cord function, have been shown not to change significantly with moderate hypotension.[89] Experimental[86,87] as well as clinical[89–92] reports have found that distraction of the spine under moderate hypotension appears no more hazardous than distraction of the spine at normal blood pressure.

The anesthesiologist has several alternatives to produce hypotensive anesthesia. High levels of halothane can produce hypotension and reduce blood flow by acting as a vasodilator, by decreasing systemic vascular resistance, and by a direct inhibitory effect on the myocardium, decreasing cardiac output. Like most inhalation agents, halothane anesthesia makes it impossible to monitor SSEPs intraoperatively[19] and to safely and reliably perform a wake-up test. This makes halothane less attractive for routine use in scoliosis surgery. To allow intraoperative spinal cord monitoring and easy reversibility for a wake-up test, balanced anesthesia with nitrous oxide supplemented with narcotics has become popular. Reduction of blood flow can be obtained with intravenously administered hypotensive agents. The two agents most commonly used in this country are sodium nitroprusside and trimethaphan.

Sodium nitroprusside is a peripheral vasodilator that relaxes the smooth muscle in the walls of the arterioles and venules. It is administered by constant infusion. Sodium nitroprusside-induced hypotension is difficult for the anesthesiologist to regulate. The blood pressure varies, and the infusion rate must be constantly altered. The induced hypotension quickly reverses when the infusion is stopped. Sodium nitroprusside does not block the catecholamine release that occurs in response to diminished blood pressure[73] and which can cause rebound hypertension with increased bleeding. Rebound hypertension may be noted intraoperatively, but more typically will be evidenced in the recovery room by excessive drain output and a blood-soaked dressing. While the rebound effect can be partially blocked with beta blockers such a propanalol,[73,93] there is little advantage to the patient in decreasing intraoperative blood loss only to increase blood loss that night or the next day.

Trimethaphan acts as both a peripheral vasodilator and

a ganglionic blocker, so rebound hypertension is not a problem.[73] Trimethaphan is also administered by constant intravenous infusion. Unlike sodium nitroprusside, trimethaphan-induced hypotension does not reverse quickly when the infusion is stopped.

While both sodium nitroprusside and trimethaphan have been used clinically with good results, there are some experimental differences between these hypotensive agents and their effect on spinal cord blood flow. Spinal cord blood flow in dogs was decreased for the first 30 minutes of sodium nitroprusside-induced hypotension. As autoregulatory mechanisms came into play, spinal cord blood flow then returned to normal levels. With sodium nitroprusside-induced hypotension, there were no deleterious effects from spinal distraction once the spinal cord blood flow had returned to normal.[86]

In contrast, spinal cord blood flow during trimethaphan-induced hypotension decreased and paralleled the decrease in mean arterial pressure. There was no autoregulatory compensation observed with trimethaphan. When the trimethaphan infusion was stopped, there was a slow return of spinal cord blood flow to normal. However, distraction of the spine did not cause any problems even with this diminished spinal cord blood flow.[88]

Recent experiments with nitroglycerine-induced hypotension in dogs have shown that spinal cord blood flow was maintained at control levels throughout the period of induced hypotension.[87] This is potentially a great advantage, and clinical trials with this agent are in progress. It is uncertain how much data from the canine spinal cord blood flow model can be extrapolated to clinical cases. However, regulatory mechanisms of blood flow in the spinal cord appear to be similar in most mammals.

Controlling blood loss during scoliosis surgery is a challenge to both the surgeon and the anesthesiologist. Both have other concerns during the procedure. In addition to minimizing blood loss, the surgeon's primary goal is a safe, successful arthrodesis. The anesthesiologist's technique must allow intraoperative assessment of spinal cord function either by SSEP or a wake-up test or both. Successful control of blood loss allows the patient to receive a better operation and significantly reduces the patient's risk of acquiring transfusion-related illnesses.

Surgical Technique

The surgical technique for posterior spinal fusion is divided into two parts. The first part discusses exposure and arthrodesis of the spine, independent of the type of instrumentation. The second part discusses techniques for implanting different instrumentation for correction of scoliosis.

Exposure and Arthrodesis

A straight-line incision gives a better cosmetic result. Skin scratches should be avoided. A heavy suture pulled taut from the spinous process of T1 to the gluteal cleft can be pressed lightly to the spine and the planned incision marked with a skin scribe. The skin and subcutaneous tissues can be infiltrated with a 1:500,000 solution of epinephrine to facilitate hemostasis. The incision is carried down to the fascia overlying the spine. Bleeding can be controlled with electrocautery. Self-retaining retractors should be used to keep the tissues under tension and facilitate dissection in the proper plane. Superficial dissection continues until the tips of the spinous processes are palpable in the slight depression between the paraspinal muscles. It may be necessary to undermine the skin slightly to palpate the spinous processes at the apex of the curve. Using a kelly clamp, each spinous process is straddled while the fascia over it is divided with coagulating cautery. The fascia between the spinous processes is divided by "connecting the dots."

Subsequent dissection takes advantage of the thicker periosteum in children and adolescents. A careful subperiosteal dissection reduces blood loss and can usually be accomplished without difficulty. Dissection should start at the caudal end of the wound and proceed cranially to facilitate stripping muscle fibers from their origins on the spine. Using a Cobb elevator, the surgeon should start on the side of the spinous process, come down onto the lamina, and sweep toward the facet joints. Sponges soaked in 1:500,000 epinephrine solution are packed in the wound to facilitate hemostasis. If there is bleeding from the bone, electrocautery or bone wax is used to control it. The assistant alternates dissecting with the surgeon, stripping and packing on one side of the spine, then on the other. At that point a check radiograph should be obtained to determine the levels exposed. A towel clip is placed on the base of a spinous process. The spinous processes in the thoracic spine point caudally, and a towel clip placed near the tip of the spinous process may be superimposed over the next caudal vertebral body on the radiographs. Placing the towel clip near the thoracolumbar junction is helpful since the ribs are convenient landmarks.

No attempt should be made to expose the tips of the transverse processes on the first pass or excessive bleeding will result. Once the entire extent of the spine has been partially exposed, the epinephrine-soaked sponges are removed, self-retaining retractors are replaced deeper in the wound, and a second pass is made beginning caudally and proceeding cranially. On the second pass, soft tissue should be stripped from the spine to the tips of the transverse processes.

The interspinous ligaments and facet joint capsules in

the lumbar spine are removed with a combination of rongeurs and curettes, taking care to preserve the facet joint capsules and interspinous ligaments between the last vertebra in the fusion and its caudal neighbor. Working up into the thoracic spine, curettes are used to work along the superior and inferior aspect of each lamina to expose the facet joint.

Meticulous hemostasis is essential. Bleeding should not be excessive if the dissection remains subperiosteal. If there is excessive bleeding, the anesthesiologist should be informed because the blood pressure and cardiac output may have increased.

Now that the entire spine over the levels to be fused has been subperiosteally exposed to the tips of the transverse processes, all the facet joints are visible and the soft tissues are held back by self-retaining retractors.

Facet Excision

The next step is ablation of the facet joints. Care should be taken to preserve, for the time being, the facet joints at sites where hooks are to be inserted. There are two popular techniques for ablation of the thoracic facet joints.[72] Moe described directing a gouge onto the facet obliquely from medial to lateral, raising a flap off the inferior aspect of the lamina to expose the superior facet joint of the caudal vertebra. The facet can then be denuded of cartilage with a gouge or curette and a chunk of cancellous bone can be lightly impacted into the joint (Fig. 13.6). Hall described using a Capener gouge directed straight down on the facet joint on the inferolateral aspect of the lamina, exposing the superior facet joint of the vertebra below. The articular cartilage can be curetted or gouged out. Again, a chunk of cancellous bone should be inserted (Fig. 13.7). The lumbar facets can be excised with a carefully directed osteotome and curette (Fig. 13.8). Instead of placing bone graft in each facet joint as it is excised, thrombin soaked gelfoam can be packed in to aid in hemostasis. It should be removed before bone graft insertion.

Bone Graft

The ideal bone to use for posterior spinal fusion is autogenous bone. Most commonly, bone graft is harvested from the posterior iliac crest. If the fusion extends to the lumbar region, the posterior iliac crest can be exposed by caudal extension of the incision and dissection above the lumbar dorsal fascia. A separate incision along the posterior iliac spine can be made if a thoracic level fusion is being performed. The posterior iliac crest is split sharply and the outer table is then exposed subperiosteally. The outer table is removed and strips of cancellous bone taken using a gouge. Care should be taken to avoid penetration of the sacroiliac joint near the posterior inferior spine of the iliac crest. The superior gluteal artery passing through the sciatic notch should be avoided. Once the bone graft is harvested, bone wax can be laid over the raw surfaces to aid hemostasis. A drain is inserted; a large towel can be packed in the wound, and the fascia over the crest can then be towel clipped shut until closure.

Insertion of Instrumentation

To this point, the exposure of the spine has been made in a standard fashion regardless of instrumentation.

Preparation of Hook Sites

Both the Harrington and Cotrel–Dubousset (C–D) systems require distraction hooks be placed on the inferior aspect of upper thoracic lamina and the superior aspect of lower thoracic or lumbar lamina. Both may also require compression hooks to be placed around transverse processes in the upper thoracic spine or on the inferior aspect of the lamina in lower thoracic or lumbar vertebrae.

The C–D system has special instruments to facilitate exposure of the hook sites, but the principles remain the same. To prepare a distraction hook site in the thoracic spine, a narrow osteotome is used to make a cut in the lamina parallel to the long axis of the spinous process. The cut should carefully go through both cortices. A second cut is made perpendicularly removing the inferolateral corner of the lamina. This should expose the underlying superior facet of the next caudal vertebra. The osteotome used to make these cuts should be very sharp and should be controlled carefully to avoid penetration into the spinal canal. Some surgeons direct the second cut slightly cranially toward the midline to reduce the risk of lateral hook dislodgement. The space under the lamina can then be opened with a small Penfield-style elevator, a sharp Harrington hook, or the pedicle finder from the C–D instrumentation set. Care should be taken to get below both cortices of the lamina (Fig. 13.9). The aim is to release any remaining soft tissue and to locate the pedicle if desired for hook placement. The intended hook can be inserted and gently impacted into place.

For placement of compression hooks in the upper thoracic spine, an elevator or a sharpened hook is used to strip the soft tissue from the transverse processes. In the lower thoracic spine the compression hooks must be placed sublaminarly because the transverse processes are usually too small to hold the hook. The laminotomy is started with a Leksell rongeur, biting away the ligamentum flavum in the midline until epidural fat is visible. Part of the downward-pointing spinous process from the superior vertebra usually needs removal as well. Any bone removed

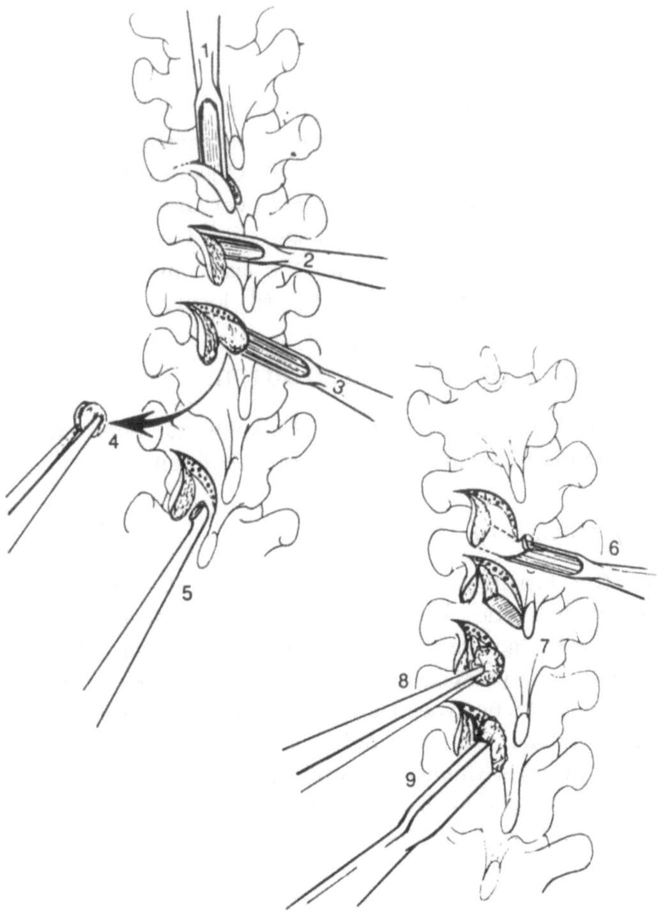

Figure 13.6. Moe's technique of thoracic facet fusion. (Reprinted with permission from Bradford DS, et al. Moe's Textbook of Scoliosis and Other Spinal Deformities. 2d Ed. Philadelphia: Saunders, 1987:140.)

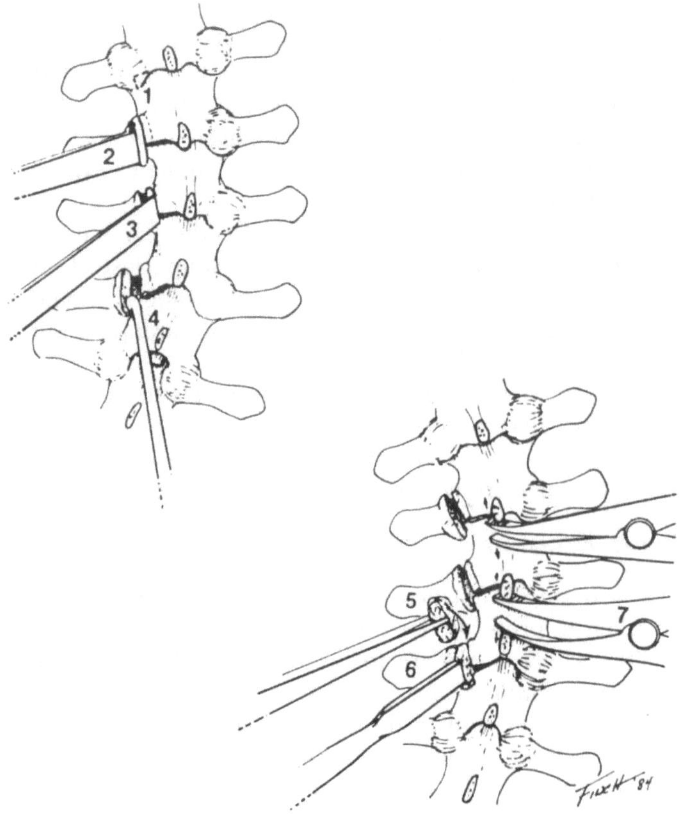

Figure 13.8. Lumbar facet fusion. (Reprinted with permission from Bradford DS, et al. Moe's Textbook of Scoliosis and Other Spinal Deformities. 2d Ed. Philadelphia: Saunders, 1987:141.)

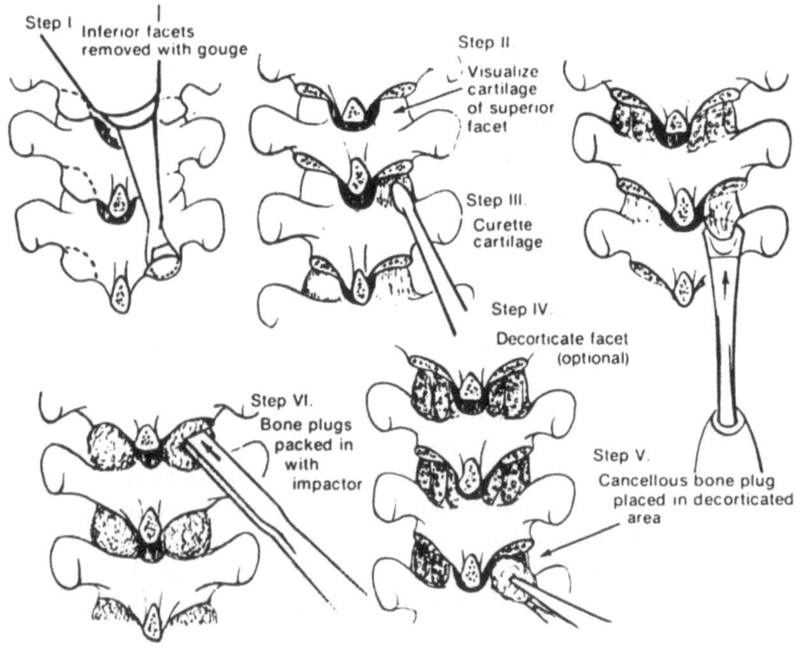

Figure 13.7. Hall's technique of thoracic facet fusion. (Reprinted with permission from Bradford DS, et al. Moe's Textbook of Scoliosis and Other Spinal Deformities. 2d Ed. Philadelphia: Saunders, 1987:140.)

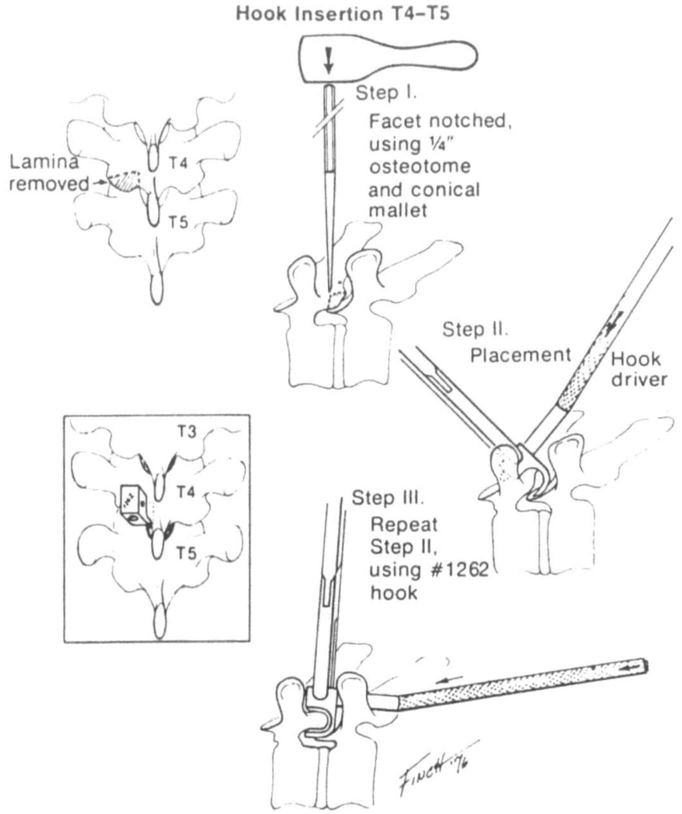

Figure 13.9. Upper hook site preparation. (Reprinted with permission from Bradford DS, et al. Moe's Textbook of Scoliosis and Other Spinal Deformities. 2d Ed. Philadelphia: Saunders, 1987:144.

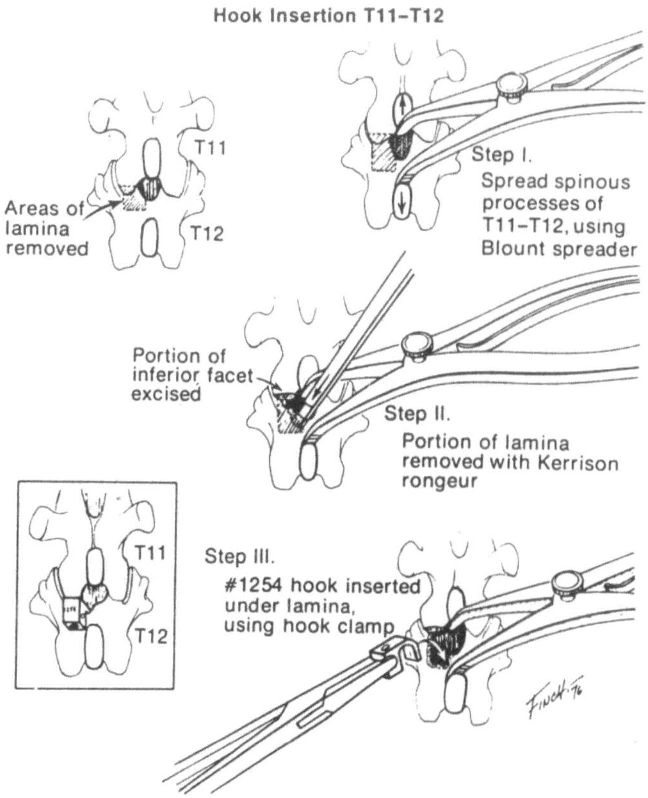

Figure 13.10. Hook insertion in lower thoracic spine. Similar technique is used in lumbar spine. (Reprinted with permission from Bradford DS, et al. Moe's Textbook of Scoliosis and Other Spinal Deformities. 2d Ed. Philadelphia: Saunders, 1987:144.)

can be saved for grafting. A Kerrison rongeur is used to remove the rest of the ligamentum flavum and square off the inferior aspect of the lamina for better seating of the hook.

In the lower thoracic lumbar spine, laminotomies are needed for insertion of compression or distraction hooks. The ligamentum flavum is excised, exposing the edge of the lamina. A laminar spreader may facilitate exposure. A Kerrison rongeur is used to make a square cut in the lamina (Fig. 13.10). If instrumentation is to be carried out in the lower lumbar spine it is often helpful to use a large Leksell rongeur to thin out the lamina immediately above the hook site. This will facilitate pushing the rod low enough to seat the hook completely below the lamina. If a lamina is damaged during the preparation of a hook site, an adjacent lamina, superiorly or inferiorly, can be prepared for hook placement.

Insertion of Harrington Instrumentation

Installation of the two hooks for the ratcheted distraction rod requires laminotomies with minimum invasion of the spinal canal. Some surgeons use the forked hook designed by Zielke to straddle the pedicle, which minimizes penetration into the spinal canal.

Once both hooks have been placed, the clothespin-like Zielke hook clamps can be attached to the hooks. The Harrington distraction outrigger can then be attached to the Zielke hook clamps. Using the outrigger, the spine can be repeatedly distracted to overcome the viscoelasticity of the spine and gradually gain more correction over a period of time. With the outrigger in place, excision of the facet joints can be performed, often resulting in further mobilization of the spine and additional correction.

While the outrigger is under tension, the wound can be packed with sponges and the iliac crest bone graft can be harvested. By the time the bone graft has been harvested, the outrigger can usually be further distracted.

If a square-ended Harrington rod is to be used, it should be contoured appropriately to preserve lumbar lordosis and thoracic kyphosis. With the Zielke hook holders holding the outrigger, it may be possible to insert the Harrington distraction rod with the spine distracted. If the rod is contoured a great deal, rod insertion with the distractor in place may be difficult. Removal of the distractor, expeditious insertion of the rod, and redistraction may be less frustrating and time consuming. Care should be taken using the Harrington rod spreader to apply force gradually to minimize the risk of lamina fracture.

Once the distraction rod has been inserted, the compression apparatus can be inserted if desired. The Keene modification of the compression system allows placement of all needed bushings and nuts on the threaded, flexible compression rod. The hooks are placed under the laminae or transverse processes and the rod dropped into the top opening slot. A bushing is slid along the rod to engage each hook, locking the rod down.

After all the bushings are engaged, the hexagonal nuts are tightened. Care should be taken when tightening the compression apparatus because the wrench does not give the sensory feedback that the distractor gives; the first sign of overtightening may be fracture of the transverse process. In the thoracic spine, overtightening can reduce thoracic kyphosis. After the compression rod is inserted, it can be cross-linked to the distraction rod by the transverse loading device of Cotrel or wire loops for additional stability.

After installation of Harrington rods, a generous area of lamina remains accessible for decortication of bone grafting.

Application of the Wisconsin Wires

After the Harrington distraction hooks and outrigger are placed, angled awls are used to drill a hole in the base of each spinous process. A doubled Wisconsin wire is passed from each side and threaded through the button of the opposite wire. Each wire is pulled taut against the base of the spinous process and the button can be lightly impacted into place with a punch. The wire loops are opened up on the concave side, and a previously contoured Harrington rod is inserted. The spine is distracted and the wires twisted loosely to approximate the rod to the spine. Next, a contoured Luque rod with at least one L-bend is passed through the open loops on the convex side of the curve. The wires are loosely twisted around the Luque rod. The distraction rod is retightened. Each rod is then pushed to the spine and the wires tightened.

Insertion of the Cotrel–Dubousset (C–D) Apparatus

Use of C–D instrumentation is very challenging, and supervised, hands-on training is essential. The components give the spinal surgeon tremendous flexibility and allow use of the C–D for virtually any condition or problem in the spine. However, a discussion of every possible use of the C–D system is beyond the scope of this chapter.

For scoliosis surgeons, the major appeal of the C–D system is its purported ability to correct thoracic scoliosis while maintaining or restoring thoracic kyphosis and improving rotational alignment of the spine. The technique for C–D instrumentation of a thoracic scoliosis is presented here. The spine is exposed in standard fashion. Hook sites on both sides are prepared. The facets are excised and grafted and the laminae decorticated on each side before the rod is inserted.

Routine C–D instrumentation of thoracic scoliosis usually requires placement of eight hooks and two rods. Correct hook placement is essential. Selection of hook sites is based on the preoperative anteroposterior, lateral, and side-bending radiographs of the spine. The neutral vertebrae are at the ends of the curve and they should be in neutral rotation; that is, the spinous process should be halfway between the pedicles. The apical vertebra appears most rotated and has a vertical convex border. The intermediate vertebrae are the end vertebrae of the rigid portion of the curve, which usually extends over four or five levels with the apical vertebra in the center.

The concave side is instrumented first. Hook sites are prepared on the two neutral and two intermediate vertebrae. Hook selection is as follows: for the cephalad neutral vertebra, a closed pedicle hook; for the cephalad intermediate vertebra, an open pedicle hook; for the caudad intermediate vertebra, an open laminar hook; and for the caudad neutral vertebra, a closed laminar hook. Depending on the size of the patient, the laminar hooks can be the larger lumbar or smaller thoracic hook. The cranial two hooks point cranially; the caudal hooks point caudally because this rod is intended to distract the spine. Using a template, if necessary, a rod of appropriate length is contoured to roughly parallel the scoliosis. As the rod is rotated, it will in a sense convert the thoracic scoliosis to thoracic kyphosis. Excessive contour in the rod makes it easier to seat it on the hooks, but makes it more difficult to spin the rod and restore thoracic kyphosis. Insufficient rod contouring will reduce the possible correction of rotation and will leave the rod functioning more like a Harrington distraction rod.

Inserting the rod and sliding the blockers into place is similar in principle to applying the Wisconsin compression apparatus with its open hooks and bushings. However, the C–D rod is not flexible, and the hook blockers must be rotated as well as pushed along the rod to seat in the open hooks. Fortunately the C–D instrument set includes special instruments for facilitating rod placement in the hooks. These include rod and blocker pushers as well as a hook clamp with a lever that can pull the seated hook up to the rod. Note that fracture of the lamina can occur if excessive force is used.

After the rod and the hook blockers are inserted, C-rings are placed behind the blockers at the two intermedi-

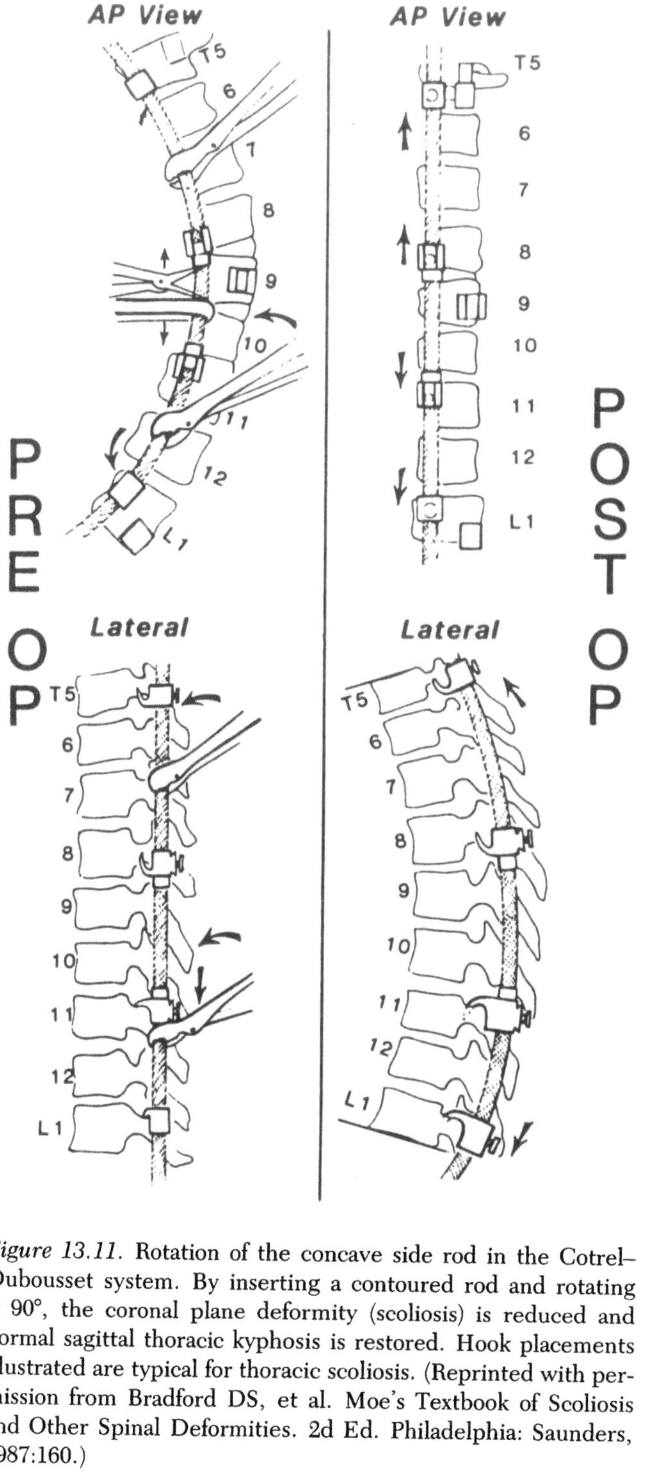

Figure 13.11. Rotation of the concave side rod in the Cotrel–Dubousset system. By inserting a contoured rod and rotating it 90°, the coronal plane deformity (scoliosis) is reduced and normal sagittal thoracic kyphosis is restored. Hook placements illustrated are typical for thoracic scoliosis. (Reprinted with permission from Bradford DS, et al. Moe's Textbook of Scoliosis and Other Spinal Deformities. 2d Ed. Philadelphia: Saunders, 1987:160.)

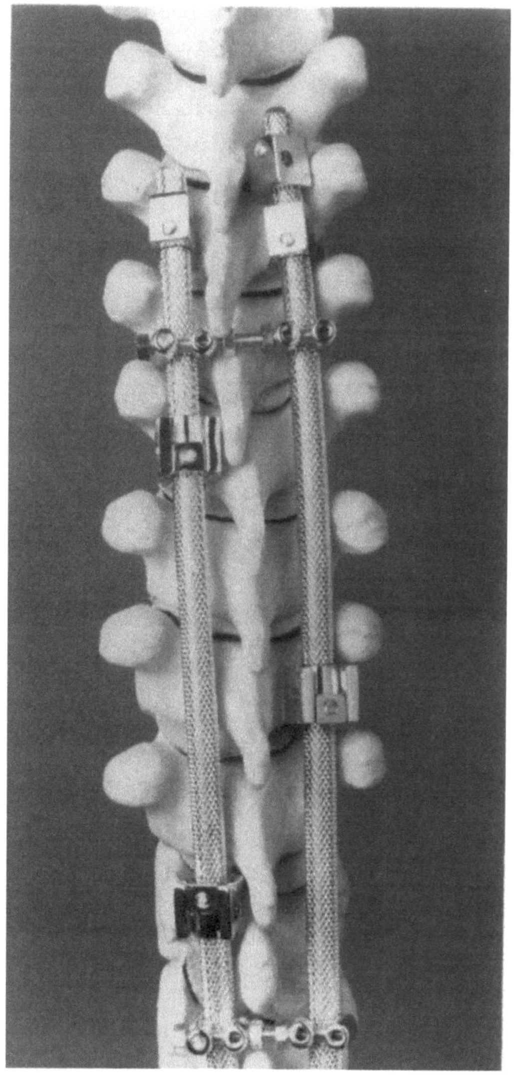

Figure 13.12. Cotrel–Dubousset instrumentation in place. Bolt heads have been broken off hooks locking them into place on rod, and transverse traction rods have been applied. (Reprinted with permission from Universal Instrumentation [CD] for Spinal Surgery brochure, Stuart Inc., Greensberg, Pennsylvania, p. 3.)

ate vertebrae. The C-rings should be placed so that they can easily be removed when they are spun 90°. The lock nut on one C-ring is tightened; then the rigid segment is distracted by pushing against the other C-ring, which is then locked into place. The hooks in the neutral vertebrae at the ends of the curve are left loose to allow the rod to spin inside them.

Using the two large rod clamps, the rod is slowly rotated while the C-rings keep the intermediate hooks in place. As the contoured rod rotates, the spine is straightened in the frontal plane, the thoracic scoliosis is reduced, while the spine is contoured more in the sagittal plane, the thoracic kyphosis is restored (Fig. 13.11).

The flexibility and degree of curvature of the spine and the contour of the rod affect how much correction can be obtained. As with distraction of a Harrington rod, gradual correction to overcome the spine's viscoelasticity is important. Excessive rotation may result in lamina fracture and pulling out of the intermediate hooks.

When the desired rotation has been achieved, the lock nuts on the two hook blockers are tightened and the C-rings removed. Additional distraction is applied to the two neutral vertebrae hooks to further correct the scoliosis. The spine may now look almost straight. The nuts on all the hooks and blockers are now tightened.

Placement of the convex rod is designed to push the lamina at the apex of the curve more anteriorly, further derotating the spine while reducing the height of the rib prominence. Hook placement for the convex rod is as follows: on the cranial neutral vertebra, a "claw" consisting of a closed laminar hook around the transverse process and a closed pedicle hook; on the apical vertebra, an open pedicle hook; and on the caudal neutral vertebra, a closed laminar hook. Again the choice of lumbar (large) on thoracic (small) laminar hooks depends on patient size.

The convex rod is contoured with bends about one-fifth of the way from each end. The upper fifth is bent into kyphosis, the lower fifth into lordosis. These bends result in a rod with a gentle "S" curve when viewed from the side. The rod and blocker for the open pedicle hook is seated. The two hooks of the claw are pulled together and locked to the rod. Compression is applied at the apical and distal hooks, resulting in further correction of the scoliosis.

If desired the wake-up test can now be performed. The nuts on all the hooks and blockers are tightened until they shear off, locking everything in place. The two rods are linked with the device for transverse traction (DTT) proximally and distally to increase the rigidity of the construct (Fig. 13.12). Instrumentation of double curves requires more hooks, using each rod to distract the concave side of a curve and compress the convex side.

To ensure a solid arthrodesis of the spine, decortication precedes rod placement. With all the hooks and blockers, rod placement, rod rotation, and tightening the hooks can be time consuming, possibly resulting in increased blood loss with C–D instrumentation.

Intraoperative Spinal Cord Monitoring

After the spine has been corrected to its maximum extent, a wake-up test, or clonus test, can be performed. The level of anesthesia is lightened while the operative field is flooded with warm saline to minimize risk of air embolism. Once the wake-up test is successfully completed, anesthesia can be reinstituted and wound closure can begin.

Wound Closure

The muscle and fascia are closed with interrupted stitches of absorbable suture. Drains below the fascia, directly against the bleeding bone, will not allow formation of a hematoma that can help tamponade further bleeding. Also, a drain is placed above the fascia and brought out through a stab wound. To leave a better cosmetic result the skin is reapproximated and closed with a running subcuticular stitch.

Intraoperative Complications

Neurological Injury

The most dreaded intraoperative complication of spinal surgery is paralysis. MacEwen[26] reported a 1:400 incidence of spinal cord injury with scoliosis surgery. The risk of neurological injury may be increased with excessive distraction and with certain devices, such as sublaminar wires.

Injury to the spinal cord from overdistraction is thought to be on the basis of compromise of spinal cord blood flow. Injuries from invasion of the spinal canal are probably from direct trauma.

Increased latency and reduced amplitude of the SSEP signal may indicate neurological compromise, but may also be the result of excessive spinal cord cooling or inappropriate levels of inhaled anesthetic agents; irrigating with warm saline or altering the anesthesia may return the signal to normal. Alteration of the SSEP signal or failure of a wake-up or clonus test require immediate action. Reduction of distraction by loosening or removal of the rod should be quickly performed. It may be advisable to discontinue hypotensive anesthesia to allow maximum blood flow to the spinal cord. The role of steroids in possible injuries to the spinal cord remains controversial.

Intraoperative Hardware Problems

When too large a force is applied, the lamina or transverse process may fracture, requiring an adjacent vertebra to be instrumented. Lamina fracture is probably more common in the thoracic spine where smaller laminae and smaller hooks result in a larger concentration of forces.

If a wire is overly tightened, breakage can result. Breakage of Wisconsin wire is usually not a problem. The wire can often be replaced, and if not, one less wire does not decrease stability much. If a sublaminar wire breaks, acute removal is controversial. Leaving a broken sublaminar wire in place may allow the wire to spring back into the canal somewhat like opening up a safety pin. But the wire may also spring more deeply into the canal as it is removed. We recommend removal of the wire if possible.

Improper contouring of a rod may not become apparent until after insertion. Special instruments are available to help recontour the rod in situ. Alternately, the rod can be removed and a new properly contoured rod inserted.

Other Intraoperative Problems

Excessive bleeding can be the result of poor surgical technique but may be a consequence of poor anesthetic control of blood flow. Any sudden increase in blood loss without obvious cause should be brought to the attention of the anesthesiologist. If excessive bleeding continues, it may be judicious to terminate the procedure, inserting any available bone graft.

Intraoperative cardiac arrest, which has been rarely reported, may result from hypovolemia, air embolism, or transfusion reaction. Air embolism is thought to result from an increased negative intrathoracic pressure that can pull air in through the exposed sinusoids of the laminae and result in a large bolus of air going to the heart. The wake-up test is a period of increased risk because the patient's ventilation is less controlled and the patient may breathe spontaneously. Flooding the field with saline before the wake-up test helps prevent this catastrophic complication.

A dural tear can result in cerebrospinal fluid (CSF) leak. If possible, the tear should be immediately repaired. If the tear is inaccessible it is often sealed off by the hematoma from the wound. If a dural tear occurs the patient should be kept flat in bed for 5 days postoperatively. This prevents the rise in CSF pressure that accompanies the upright position, which could reopen the tear.

Postoperative Management

While still intubated, the patient is carefully rolled onto a bed or stretcher. The patient is extubated in the operating room or recovery room. The instruments should be kept sterile, and the operating team should be prepared to reopen the wound and remove the instrumentation in the event the patient demonstrates loss of neurological function on awakening. If the fusion included the thoracic spine, a portable radiograph is taken in the recovery room to rule out a pneumothorax.

Postoperative use of the Stryker frame has decreased as the stability of internal fixation of the spine has increased. Our patients are log rolled and positioned with pillows on a regular bed. Patients are kept on their backs for about 6 hours after surgery in an effort to reduce bleeding by maintaining pressure on the wound.

Serial neurological examinations should be performed in the first 24 hours postoperatively because not all neurological complications become apparent immediately postoperatively. Epidural hematoma may result in spinal cord compression and delayed paraplegia. Postoperative facial edema is common from the dependent position and will resolve as the patient mobilizes his/her third-space fluid.

Improper positioning of the patient can result in postoperative nerve compression syndromes. The lateral femoral cutaneous nerve of the thigh can be compressed from the Relton–Hall frame, resulting in lateral thigh numbness. The brachial plexus may be stretched if the arms are abducted or extended excessively during surgery.

Syndrome of Inappropriate Diuretic Hormone

Many patients who undergo posterior spinal fusion for idiopathic scoliosis develop the syndrome of inappropriate antidiuretic hormone (SIADH)[94] in the immediate postoperative period. The exact etiology is poorly understood, but the increase in antidiuretic hormone results in a decrease in urine output despite decreasing serum sodium levels.[94] The danger is that SIADH may be mistaken for a hypovolemia and excessive intravenous fluid may thus be administered, resulting in fluid overload and pulmonary edema.

SIADH tends to present in the middle of the night when the operating surgeon may not be readily available and the patient may be under the care of a junior house officer. SIADH usually resolves without any treatment and fluid restoration is seldom necessary. If urine output is unsatisfactory, a small amount (5 mg) of furosemide (Lasix ®) will restore good urine flow.

Superior Mesenteric Artery Syndrome

Superior mesenteric artery (SMA) syndrome is occlusion of the third part of the duodenum by the superior mesenteric artery at its oblique takeoff from the aorta. The lengthening of the trunk seen with distraction instrumentation is thought to be a contributory factor. Thin patients seem more susceptible, perhaps because they have less retroperitoneal fat to cushion the duodenum. Affected patients present with symptoms of an upper gastrointestinal tract obstruction such as vomiting. Treatment consists of nasogastric suction until the obstruction resolves, usually in a few days. Occasionally hyperalimentation is needed if the obstruction persists.[95]

Wound Infection

Postoperative wound infections are uncommon in scoliosis surgery. The preferred treatment for a deep wound infection is thorough debridement and closure over drains.[96] Removal of the hardware is not always necessary and may be contraindicated. Fusion can proceed in spite of infection, and is probably more likely to occur if motion in the spine is kept to a minimum.

Postoperative Care

The need for postoperative immobilization depends on the type of internal fixation, how well it is inserted, and the preference of the surgeon. Some forms of internal fixation are claimed to be stable enough that no external immobilization is necessary (this is discussed more fully in Chapter 16). We prefer our patients to be fitted with a plastic bivalved thoracolumbosacral orthosis (TLSO). After the TLSO is fitted, the patient is mobilized, usually by about the fourth or fifth day postoperatively, and discharged from the hospital about 7 days postoperatively. By this time the patient is able to walk and climb stairs.

The patient is instructed to wear the brace at all times except when taking a shower and is restricted to lifting not more than 10 pounds. Most patients are able to return to school or work by 3 to 4 weeks after surgery. The brace is worn for 6 months postoperatively. Activity is restricted for 1 year, at which time resumption of normal activities is permitted with the exception of gymnastics and contact sports such as football, hockey, and wrestling.

Follow-up radiographs are taken at 1, 3, 6, and 12 months, and then yearly for 5 years.

Long-Term Follow-Up

Relaxation in the tension in the soft tissues of the spine results in a gradual loosening of the instrumentation. Typically this results in only a minimum (less than 5°) loss of correction, and usually occurs in the first few months after surgery.

Loosening or dislodgement of an internal fixation device can result in a substantial loss of correction. Breakage of an internal fixation device is usually a fatigue failure, and strongly suggests the presence of pseudarthrosis. The pseudarthrosis may not be readily visible on routine radiographs, and tomograms may be necessary to locate the exact site. The need for reoperation depends on the patient's symptoms, the degree of deformity, and any progression in deformity. Revision of the fusion with additional bone grafting is usually successful.

The use of an insufficiently contoured rod into the lower lumbar spine can result in loss of lumbar lordosis and the so-called flat back syndrome. Affected patients walk with an awkward, crouched gait. In fusions extending into the lower lumbar spine, great care should be taken to preserve lumbar lordosis by contouring the rod.

Posterior translation (retrolisthesis) of the vertebra at the caudal end of a distraction rod has been reported to be associated with an increased incidence of pain in one long-term follow-up study.[14a] To minimize the occurrence of retrolisthesis, Bradford[72] described passing a wire loop around the two most caudad spinous processes before distraction.

A spinal fusion puts an increased load on the disc and at the end of the fusion. This increased load can lead to premature disc degeneration, degenerative facet hypertrophy, and spinal stenosis. At present these problems are mostly associated with fusion to the lower lumbar spine. However, the modern era of spinal fusion dates back only 25 years. The adolescent girls who underwent fusions then are now only entering their forties. It is possible that with more time there will be more problems.

Posterior Fusion in Other Forms of Scoliosis

The operative management of idiopathic scoliosis has been discussed in detail. Other forms of scoliosis may require different techniques.

Congenital Scoliosis

Operative management of congenital scoliosis is in many ways similar to management of idiopathic scoliosis. Instrumentation to correct the deformity is used less frequently, because there appears to be an increased association with incidence of neurological complications. If the use of corrective instrumentation is contemplated, a preoperative myelogram is advisable to rule out problems such as diastematomyelia. If the goal of surgery is prevention of further progression, an in situ fusion may be sufficient.

Special care is needed to determine intraoperatively the levels to be fused because the anatomy is distorted. Usually less of the spine is fused in cases of congenital scoliosis; often the abnormal vertebra(e) is fused to the two adjacent normal vertebrae. Compensatory curves should not progress once the congenital curve is fused.[97] After the segments to be fused have been exposed and decorticated and the facet joints excised, metallic clips are placed on the spinous processes of the cranial and most caudal vertebrae to mark the extent of fusion and to serve as references for measuring growth and possible curve progression. Autogenous bone graft should be used whenever possible. Postoperative immobilization with either a cast or brace is maintained for 6 to 12 months.

Neuromuscular Scoliosis

Scoliosis in neurologically impaired patients presents special challenges to the spinal surgeon. Patient cooperation is often unobtainable. The bone in the spine may be of poor quality because of disuse osteoporosis, the use of antiseizure medication, poor nutrition, or a combination of all these. Postoperative immobilization is often difficult to maintain. Patients with neuromuscular diseases often have poor temperature-regulating mechanisms. The use of heated, humidified anesthetic gases can help prevent excessive heat loss during surgery. The need for secure fixation of the spine with minimum postoperative immobilization is often best served by the use of segmental spinal instrumentation, that is, an instrumentation system with multiple attachments to the spine. The three major forms of segmental spinal instrumentation are (1) the sublaminar wires and L-rods popularized by Luque; (2) the intraspinous process wires of the Wisconsin system; and (3) the use of multiple hooks of the Cotrel–Dubousset (C–D) system. (Use of the C–D system and Wisconsin wires has already been discussed in the section on idiopathic scoliosis.)

Luque (SSI) Instrumentation

Luque or L-rod instrumentation consists of two smooth, contoured, L-shaped rods attached to the spine with multiple sublaminar wires. Rods of ³⁄₈-in. and ¹⁄₄-in. diameter are available. The smaller rods are easier to bend and cut, but the larger rods are twice as strong. Luque recommended contouring the rods preoperatively based on bending films, but contouring can also be done intraoperatively. It is important to realize that rarely can perfectly straight rods be inserted without increasing the risk of neurological injury from overcorrection of the deformity. An exception to this is the collapsing curve seen in muscular dystrophy, which can be well managed with Moseley's unit rod or two straight L-rods. In addition, the rods should be contoured in the sagittal plane to preserve thoracic kyphosis and lumbar lordosis.

Operative Technique

The exposure of the spine has been described. The spine is exposed subperiosteally to the tips of the transverse processes; the facet joints are excised and bone grafted. Good hemostasis is essential to minimize the risks of sublaminar wire passage. Passage of the sublaminar wires requires removal of the ligamentum flavum at each level and usually a small laminotomy as well. In the thoracic spine the downward-pointing spinous processes often need to be removed. A transversely directed large rongeur can be used to carefully bite down in the interspace between two laminae and remove the superficial layers of ligamentum flavum just until the epidural fat shows through. Then a smaller Leksell or Kerrison rongeur can remove the remainder of the ligamentum flavum. Bleeding epidural vessels can be coagulated with bipolar cautery or packed off with thrombin-soaked gelfoam.

A doubled 16- or 18-gauge wire is contoured into an arc just long enough to span the lamina with a rounded, slightly upwardly bent tip. Wires are passed most easily in a caudal-to-cranial direction with a continuous gently upward pull to avoid too deep an incursion into the spinal canal. The tip of the wire should always be in contact with the undersurface of the lamina (Fig. 13.13). If there is resistance, the wire should be withdrawn and a new attempt made. When the tip appears in the next interspace, it should be firmly grasped with a large needle holder or similar instrument. While maintaining a constant upward pull, the wire is carefully advanced until half the length is on each side of the lamina.

The tip is cut off (taking care to ensure it does not fall in the wound) and the two loops of wire are pulled apart, one to each side of the spine. From this point on, care must be taken to avoid jostling the wires and pushing the loops further into the spinal canal.

To help keep the wires from unintended penetration into the spinal canal, the loop can be crimped over the lamina, then bent back out of the wound and secured with a clamp. Yngve[98] described looping the wire on itself to accomplish the same thing, prevention of spinal cord injury by accidental jostling of the wires.

To insert the contoured L-rod, the two ends of each wire can be pulled to opposite sides of the wound and the rod laid along the laminae. Alternately, the clamped loops of wires can be pulled open and the rod threaded up. While rod pushers push the rod to the spine, the wires are tightened, starting at the apex of the curve. Pulling the rod to the spine by tightening the wires is likely to result in wires cutting through the lamina. A distraction rod can be substituted for the contoured Luque rod. This so-called Tex/Mex or Harri–Luque system allows for axial distraction as well as transverse correction. Once both rods are inserted, the wires are retightened and the two rods are tied together at 7 levels by wire loops.

In neuromuscular scoliosis, the fusion may need to be extended to the pelvis. Luque rods can be fixed to the pelvis in several ways. The "L" of the rod can be pushed through a hole drilled transversely across the posterior ilium, just above the sacrum, similar to implanting a Harrington sacral bar.

More secure pelvic fixation results from the "Galveston technique."[61] The end of the rod is driven into a hole predrilled in the ilium just above the sciatic notch. A series of bends over the sacrum direct the remainder of the rod up the spine. This technique is quite demanding, and preoperative bending of the lower portion of the rod is recommended. Less bone graft is available after installation of L-rods with the Galveston technique, so excision

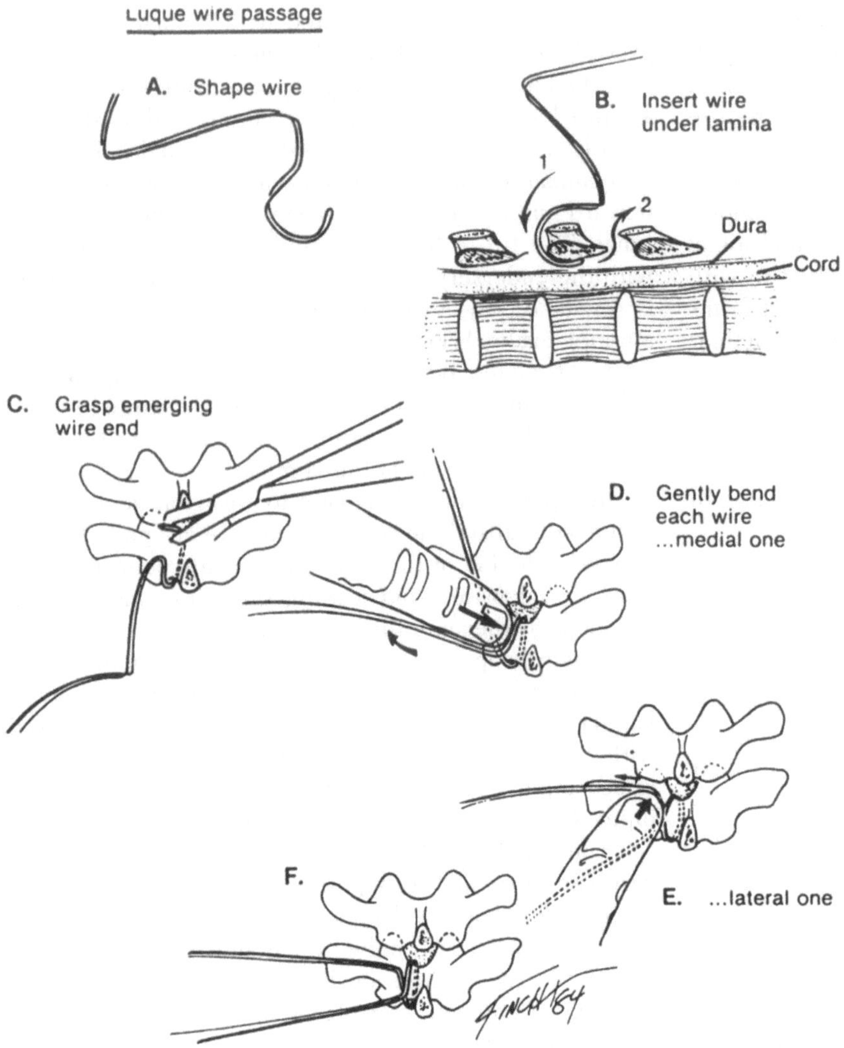

Figure 13.13. Passage of sublaminar Luque wires. (Reprinted with permission from Bradford DS, et al. Moe's Textbook of Scoliosis and Other Spinal Deformities. 2d Ed. Philadelphia: Saunders, 1987:151.)

and grafting of the facet joints is important to secure a solid arthrodesis.

Scoliosis in Myelomeningocele

The lack of bony elements posteriorly in this condition may require an anterior approach with discectomy and interbody fusion as an initial procedure. Dissection through the scar tissue posteriorly may be difficult, and the assistance of a neurosurgeon is often helpful, particularly in cases where tethering of the spinal cord is present.

Instrumentation in Myelomeningocele

The paucity of posterior elements in the lower part of the spine in the myelomeningocele patient presents special challenges. Segmental instrumentation is often possible, either by passing Luque wires around the everted laminae or by carefully mobilizing the dura and passing Wisconsin wires through the upturned laminae. Luque rods can be extended into the pelvis by the Galveston technique, or a contoured Harrington rod with a sacral hook can be inserted onto the sacral ala. Many children have a pelvis too small for a Moe-style sacral hook, and a Leatherman hook can be used instead. Above the dysraphic levels of the spine, sublaminar or spinous process wires are used. Lumbar lordosis must be maintained to allow the child to sit forward on his thighs.

Special postoperative complications in myelomeningocele include acute hydrocephalus, particularly if the cord is transected and oversewn. Surgery of this magnitude can result in shunt malfunction for reasons poorly understood, and excessive lethargy postoperatively should be investigated. The rate of infection and pseudarthrosis are higher in this group of patients; if postoperative immobilization is needed, a removable body jacket allows for inspection of the skin.

Conclusion

Posterior spinal fusion for childhood spinal deformity requires careful preoperative planning, familiarity with the anatomy of the spine, and familiarity with the planned instrumentation. Close cooperation with the anesthesiologists intraoperatively is essential to minimize the need for blood replacement. If these steps are taken, a variety of childhood spinal deformities can be safely managed.

References

1. Hibbs RA. An operation for progressive spinal deformities. NY Med J 1911;93:1013.
2. Hibbs RA. A report of fifty-nine cases of scoliosis treated by the fusion operation. J Bone Joint Surg 1924;6:3.
3. American Orthopaedic Association Research Committee: End result study of the treatment of idiopathic scoliosis. J Bone Joint Surg 1941;23:963.

4a. Moe JH. A critical analysis of methods of fusion for scoliosis. J Bone Joint Surg 1958;40A:529.

4b. Harrington PR. Treatment of scoliosis. Correction and internal fixation by spine instrumentation. J Bone Joint Surg 1962;44A:491.

5. Nachemson A. A long-term followup study of non-treated scoliosis. Acta Orthop Scand 1968;3A:466.
6. Nilsonne U, Lundgren, KD. Long-term prognosis in idiopathic scoliosis. Acta Orthop Scand 1968;39:456.
7. Weinstein SL, Zaval DC, Ponseti IV. Idiopathic scoliosis: long-term followup and prognosis in untreated patients. J Bone Joint Surg 1981;63A:702.
8. Lonstein JG, Carlson JM. Prognostication in idiopathic scoliosis. J Bone Joint Surg 1984;66A:1061.
9. Risser JC. The iliac apophysis: an invaluable sign in the management of scoliosis. Clin Orthop 1958;11:111.
10. Weinstein SL, Ponseti IV. Curve progression in idiopathic scoliosis: long-term followup. J Bone Joint Surg 1983;65A:447.

11a. King HA, Moe JH, Bradford DS, Winter RB. Selection of fusion levels in thoracic idiopathic scoliosis. J Bone Joint Surg 1983;65A:1302.

11b. Bjerkreim I, Carlsen B, Korsell G. Preoperative Cotrel traction in idiopathic scoliosis. Acta Orthop Scand 1982;53:901.

12a. Nachemson A, Nordwall A. Effectiveness of preoperative Cotrel traction for correction of idiopathic scoliosis. J Bone Joint Surg 1977;59A:504.

12b. Mandelbaum B, Tolo VT, McAfee P, Buresh P. Nutritional deficiencies after staged anterior and posterior spinal surgery. Orthop Trans 1986;10:32.

13. Harrington PR. Technical details in relation to the successful use of instrumentation in scoliosis. Orthop Clin North Am 1972;3:49.

14a. Cochran R, Irstam L, Nachemson A. Long-term anatomic and functional changes in patients with adolescent idiopathic scoliosis treated by Harrington rod fusion. Spine 1983;8:576.

14b. Kruskall MS, Umlas J. Acquired immunodeficiency syndrome and directed blood transfusions. Arch Surg 1988;123:23.

15. McCarthy RE, Mertz JD, Lonstein JE, Kuslich SD. Air embolism in spinal surgery. Orthop Trans 1985;9:484.
16. Hall JE, Levin CF, Sudhir KH. Intraoperative awakening to monitor spinal cord function during Harrington instrumentation and spine fusion. J Bone Joint Surg 1978;60A:533.
17. Vauzelle L, Stagnara P, Jouvinroux P. Functional monitoring of spinal cord activity during spinal surgery. Clin Orthop 1973;93:173.
18. Hoppenfield S, Gross AM, Andres C. The ankle clonus test. Orthop Trans 1985;9:118.
19. Bunch WH, Scarff TB, Trimble J. Current concepts review. Spinal cord monitoring. J Bone Joint Surg 1983;65A:707.
20. Kling TF, Pandit U, Hensinger RN, Phillips WA. Efficacy of heated/humidified inspired anesthetic gas in maintaining body temperature during scoliosis surgery. Orthop Trans 1986;10:29.
21. Relton JGS, Hall JE. An operation frame for spinal fusion. A new apparatus designed to reduce haemorrhage during operation. J Bone Joint Surg 1967;49B:327.
22. Batson OV. The function of the vertebral veins and their role in the spread of metastases. Ann Surg 1940;112:138.
23. Goldstein LA. Treatment of idiopathic scoliosis by Harrington instrumentation and fusion with fresh autogenous iliac bone grafts. J Bone Joint Surg 1969;51A:209.
24. Bunch WH, Chapman RG. Patient preferences in surgery for scoliosis. J Bone Joint Surg 1985;67A:794.
25. Dunn HK, Daniels AU, McBride GG. Intraoperative force measurements during correction of scoliosis. Spine 1982;7:448.
26. MacEwen GO, Bunnell WP, Sriram K. Acute neurological complications in the treatment of scoliosis. J Bone Joint Surg 1975;57A:404.
27. Schultz A, Hirsch C. Mechanical analysis of Harrington rod correction of idiopathic scoliosis. J Bone Joint Surg 1973;55A:983.
28. Wenger DR, Carollo JJ, Wilkerson JA, Jr. Biomechanics of scoliosis correction by segmental spinal instrumentations. Spine 1982;7:260.
29. Waugh TR. Intravital measurements during instrumental correction of idiopathic scoliosis. Acta Orthop Scand (Suppl) 1966;93:1.
30. Nachemson A, Elfstrom G. A force-indicating distractor for the Harrington rod procedure. J Bone Joint Surg 1969;51A:166.
31. Ashworth MA, Lowe PJ, Bryant JT. A force indicating spreader. A tool for teaching the Harrington technique. Spine 1982;7:80.
32. Nachemson A, Elfstrom G. Intravital wireless telemetry of axial forces in Harrington distraction rods in patients with idiopathic scoliosis. J Bone Joint Surg 1971;53A:445.
33. Cook SD, Barrack RL, Georgette FS, Whitecloud TS, II, Burke SW, Skinner HB, Renz EA. An analysis of failed Harrington rods. Spine 1985;10:313.
34. Erwin WD, Dickson JH, Harrington PR. Clinical review of patients with broken Harrington rods. J Bone Joint Surg 1980;62A:1302.

35. Akeson J, Bobechko WP. Treatment of scoliosis by instrumentation with double upper hooks and posterior fusion. Orthop Trans 1986;10:35.
36. Grobler LJ, Moe JH, Winter RB, Bradford DS, Lonstein JE. Loss of lumbar lordosis following surgical correction of thoracolumbar deformity. Orthop Trans 1978;2:239.
37. Moe JH, Denis F. The iatrogenic loss of lumbar lordosis. Orthop Trans 1977;1:131.
38a. Wasylenko M, Skinner SR, Perry J, Antonelli DJ. An analysis of posture and gait following spinal fusion with Harrington instrumentation. Spine 1983;8:840.
38b. Casey M, Asher M, Jacobs RR, Orrick J. The effect of Harrington rod contouring on lumbar lordosis. Orthop Trans 1985;9:125.
39. Nordwall A. Briefly noted: a new instrument: the Harrington rod director. Spine 1986;11:498.
40. Keene JS, Drummond DS, Narechania RG. The Wisconsin compression system. Spine 1982;7:83–85.
41. Armstrong GW, Connock SH. A transverse loading system applied to a modified Harrington instrumentation. Clin Orthop 1975;108:70.
42. Gaines RW, McKinley LM, Leatherman KD. Effect of the Harrington compression system on the correction of the rib hump in spinal instrumentation for idiopathic scoliosis. Spine 1981;6:489.
43. Herndon WA, Ellis RD, Hall JA, Millis MG. Correction with a transverse loading system in the operative management of scoliosis. Clin Orthop 1982;165:168.
44. Ogilvie JW, Millar EA. Comparison of segmental spinal instrumentation devices in the correction of scoliosis. Spine 1983;8:416.
45. Gaines RW, Leatherman KD. Benefits of the Harrington compression system in lumbar and thoracolumbar idiopathic scoliosis in adolescents and adults. Spine 1981;6:483.
46. Luque ER. Segmental spinal instrumentation for the correction of scoliosis. Clin Orthop 1982;163:192.
47a. Luque ER, Cardoso A. Segmental correction of scoliosis with rigid internal fixation. Preliminary report. Orthop Trans 1977;1:136.
47b. Allen BL, Jr, Ferguson RL. The Galveston technique for L-rod instrumentation of the scoliotic spine. Spine 1982;7:276.
48. Phillips WA, DeWald RL. A comparison of Luque segmental spinal instrumentation with Harrington rod instrumentation in the management of idiopathic scoliosis. Orthop Trans 1985;9:437.
49. Nasca RJ, Hollis JM, Lemons JE, Cool TA. Cyclic axial loading of spinal implants. Spine 1985;10:792.
50. Wenger DR, Carollo JJ, Wilkerson JA, Jr. Laboratory testing of segmental spinal instrumentation versus traditional Harrington instrumentation for scoliosis treatment. Spine 1982;7:265.
51. Winter RB. Thoracic lordoscoliosis in neurofibromatosis: treatment by a Harrington rod with sublaminar wiring. J Bone Joint Surg 1984;66A:1102.
52. Johnston CE, II, Ashman R, Sherman M. Mechanical consequences of rod contouring and residual scoliosis in sublaminar pelvis SSI. Orthop Trans 1986;10:5.
53. Zindrick M, Knight G, Bunch W, Miller M, Butler D, Azarkia, B. The depth of wire penetration of intrasegmental wire in the neural canal at insertion. Orthop Trans 1986;10:6.
54. Herring JA, Wenger DR. Segmental spinal instrumentation: a preliminary report of 40 consecutive cases. Spine 1982;7:285.
55. Johnston CE, II, Happel LT, Norris R, Burke SW, King AG, Roberts, JM. Delayed paraplegia complicating sublaminar segmental spinal instrumentation. J Bone Joint Surg 1986;68A:556.
56. Thompson GH, Wilber RG, Shaffer JW, Scoles PV, Nash CJ, Jr. Segmental spinal instrumentation in idiopathic scoliosis. A preliminary report. Spine 1985;10:623.
57. Wilber RG, Thompson GH, Shaffer JW, Brown RM, Nash CL, Jr. Postoperative neurologic deficits in segmental spinal instrumentation: a study utilizing spinal cord monitoring. J Bone Joint Surg 1984;66A:1178.
58. Bernard TN, Jr, Johnson CE, II, Roberts JM, Burke SW. Late complications due to wire breakage in segmental spinal instrumentation. Report of two cases. J Bone Joint Surg 1983;65A:1339.
59. Nicastro JF, Traina J, Lancaster M, Hartjen C. Sublaminar segmental wire fixation anatomic pathways during their removal. Orthop Trans 1984;8:172.
60. McCarthy RE. Experience with a locking collar for Luque rods. Orthop Trans 1986;10:7.
61. Allen BL, Jr, Ferguson RL. The Galveston technique of pelvic fixation with L-rod instrumentation of the spine. Spine 1984;9:388.
62. Moseley C, Mosca V, Lawton L, Koreska J. Improved stability in segmental instrumentation of neuromuscular scoliosis. Orthop Trans 1986;10:5.
63. Rossier AB, Cochran TP. The treatment of spinal fractures with Harrington compression rods and segmental sublaminar wiring. A dangerous combination. Spine 1984;9:796.
64. Drummond D, Guadagni J, Keene JS, Breed A, Narechania R. Interspinous process segmental spinal instrumental. J Pediatr Orthop 1984;4:397.
65. Guadagni J, Drummond D, Breed A. Improved postoperative course following modified segmental spinal instrumentation and posterior spinal fusion for idiopathic scoliosis. J Pediatr Orthop 1984;4:405.
66. Mino DE, Stauffer ES, Davis PK, Hester J. Torsional loading of Harrington distraction rod instrumentation compared to segmental sublaminar and spinous process supplementation. Orthop Trans 1985;9:119.
67. Bridwill KH, Pruitt D, Capelli A, Schoenecker PL. Experience with 100 Cotrel-Dubousset instrumentations. Orthop Trans 1987;11:183.
68. Millis MB, Hall JE. Early experience with CD instrumentation in an American orthopaedic center. Orthop Trans 1987;11:50.
69. Shufflebarger HL, Clark RN. Cotrel–Dubousset instrumentation in adolescent idiopathic scoliosis. Orthop Trans 1987;11:48.
70. Curran JW, Lawrence DN, Jaffe H, Kaplan JE, Zyla LD, Chamberlan M, Weinstein R, Lui K, Schonberger LB, Spira TJ, Alexander WJ, Swinger G, Ammann A, Solomon S, Auerbach D, Mildvan D, Stoneburner R, Jason JM, Haverkos MW, Evatt BL. Acquired immunodeficiency syndrome

(AIDS) associated with transfusions. N Engl J Med 1984;310:69.
71. Widmann FK. Untoward effects of blood transfusion. Postgrad Med 1981;69:40.
72. Bradford DS. Techniques of surgery. In: Bradford DS, Lonstein JE, Moe JM, Ogilvie JW, Winter RB, eds. Moe's Textbook of Scoliosis and Other Spinal Deformities. 2d Ed. Philadelphia: Saunders, 1980.
73. Knight PR, Lane GA, Hensinger RN, Bolles RS, Bjoraker DG. Catecholamine and renin-angiotensin response during hypotensive anesthesia induced by sodium nitroprusside or trimethaphan camsylate. Anesthesiology 1983;59:248.
74. Low JM, Harvey JT, Cooper GM, Prendiville WJ. Plasma concentrations of catecholamines following adrenaline infiltration during gynaecological surgery. Br J Anaesth 1984;56:849.
75. Sorrenti SJ, Cumming WJ, Miller D. Reaction of the human tibia to bone wax. Clin Orthop 1984;182:293.
76. Moleno R, Dommisse GF. Spinal surgery: minimizing blood loss. J Bone Joint Surg 1975;57B:259.
77. McCarthy RE, Peek RD, Morrissy RT, Hough AJ. Allograft bone in spinal fusion for paralytic scoliosis. J Bone Joint Surg 1986;68A:370.
78. Bowen JR, Angus PD, Huxster RR, Mace Wan, DC. Posterior spinal fusion without blood in Jehovah's Witness. Clin Orthop 1985;198:284.
79. Winter RB, Swayze C. Severe neurofibromatosis kyphoscoliosis in a Jehovah's Witness. Spine 1983;8:39.
80. Wong KC, Webster LR, Coleman SS, Dunn HKL. Hemodilution and induced hypotension for insertion of a Harrington rod in a Jehovah's Witness patient. 'Clin Orthop 1980;152:237.
81. Cowell HR, Swickard JW. Autotransfusion in children's orthopaedics. J Bone Joint Surg 1974;56A:908.
82. Flynn JC, Metzger CR, Csencsitz TA. Intraoperative autotransfusion in spinal surgery. Spine 1982;7:432.
83. Ernst T, Cook DR. Surgical technique is a major determinant of blood loss during Harrington rod instrumentation. Read at American Academy of Pediatrics, Anesthesiology Section, Las Vegas, Nevada, April 19, 1980.
84. DuToit Q, Relton J, Gillespie R. Acute hemodilution autotransfusion in the surgical management of scoliosis. J Bone Joint Surg 1978;6.B:178.
85. Jacobs HK, Lieponis JV, Bunch WH, Barber MNB, Salem MR. The influence of halothane and nitroprusside on canine spinal cord hemodynamics. Spine 1982;7:35.
86. Kling TF, Fergusson NV, Leach AB, Hensinger RN, Lane GA, Knight PR. The influence of induced hypotension and spine distraction on canine spinal cord blood flow. Spine 1985;10:878.
87. Kling TF, Spargo PM, Hensinger RN, Knight PR. The effect of nitroglycerin-induced hypotension with and without spine distraction on canine spinal cord blood flow. Orthop Trans 1986;10(1):19.
88. Kling TF, Wilton N, Hensinger RN, Knight PR. The influence of trimethaphan (Arfonad) induced hypotension with and without spine distraction on canine spinal cord blood flow. Spine 1986;11:219.
89. Grundy BL, Nash CL, Brown RH. Deliberate hypotension for spinal fusion: prospective randomized study with evoked potential monitoring. Can Anaesth Sco J 1982;29:452.
90. Malcolm-Smith NA, McMaster MJ. The use of induced hypotension to control bleeding during posterior fusion for scoliosis. J Bone Joint Surg 1983;65B:255.
91. McNeill TW, DeWald RL, Juo KN, Bennett EJ, Salem MR. Controlled hypotensive anesthesia in scoliosis surgery. J Bone Joint Surg 1974;56A:1167.
92. Patel NJ, Patel BS, Paskin S, Laufer S. Induced moderate hypotensive anesthesia for spinal fusion and Harrington rod instrumentation. J Bone Joint Surg 1985;67A:1384.
93. Knight PR, II, Lane GA, Nicholls MG, Tait AR, Nahrwold ML, Hensinger RN, Cohen PJ. Hormonal and hemodynamic changes induced by pentolinium and propranolol during surgical correction of scoliosis. Anesthesiology 1980;53:127.
94. Bell GR, Gurd AR, Orlowski JP, Andrish JT. The syndrome of inappropriate antidiuretic-hormone secretion following spinal fusion. J Bone Joint Surg 1986;68A:720.
95. Munns SW, Morrissy RT, Colladay ES, McKenzie CH. Hyperalimentation for superior mesenteric artery (CAST) syndrome following correction of spinal deformity. J Bone Joint Surg 1984;66A:1175.
96. Transfeldt EE, Lonstein JE, Winter RB, Bradford D, Moe J, Mayfield J. Wound infections in reconstructive spinal surgery. Orthop Trans 1985;9:128.
97. Hoffinger SA, Renshaw TS, Murphy J. The compensatory curve in congenital scoliosis. Presented at 22nd Annual Meeting, Scoliosis Research Society, September 18, 1987.
98. Yngve DA, Burke SW, Price CT, Riddick MF. Sublaminar wiring. J Pediatr Orthop 1986;6:605.

14

Fusion Techniques for Adult Spinal Deformity

David S. Bradford and William C. Lauerman

Introduction

The adult patient with spinal deformity represents one of the most challenging problems for the spinal surgeon. The scope of this problem appears to be increasing as the result of prolonged life expectancy and increased reader awareness in the lay and medical press. A recent survey of members of the Scoliosis Research Society revealed that more than one in three operations for scoliosis are performed on adults.[1]

Adult spinal deformities fall into one of several categories. Scoliosis, idiopathic, is the deformity requiring surgical treatment in the adult. Kyphotic deformities of various etiologies and spinal deformities secondary to previous surgery are also frequently seen.

Treatment of these patients is complicated by a lack of clear-cut surgical indications in the adult, a higher complication rate, and coexisting medical problems such as diabetes, heart disease, and lung disease, secondary to a long history of cigarette smoking. It is imperative to adequately assess these patients from a medical viewpoint before undertaking major spinal reconstructive surgery in this population. An internist or pulmonary medicine expert may prove invaluable.

Scoliosis

Principles

The adolescent with scoliosis is usually a passive participant in the referral process, while the adult is a more active one. It is important to determine whether the presenting complaint is pain, cosmesis, pulmonary problems, or progression of the curve. Curve progression may be interpreted by the patient as a sensation that the body and chest is becoming more "unbalanced"; or a feeling of losing height. On the other hand the patient may have been told, on the basis of serial radiographs, that the curve is indeed progressing.

The etiology of scoliosis seen in the adult population is similar to that in the adolescent. Idiopathic scoliosis is by far the most common, with paralytic, congenital, and other known causes presenting with a frequency similar to that seen in the adolescent.

In attempting to achieve longlasting patient satisfaction, determining the patient for whom surgical treatment is appropriate is as important as choosing the surgical technique. The most common indication for treating the adult patient is pain. Although the relationship of scoliosis in the adult to back pain is controversial,[2–6] most authors agree that pain is more common in lumbar curves and curves of larger magnitude. Documented recent curve progression is also believed by most to represent a clearcut indication for surgery. Progressive pulmonary insufficiency, the patient's concern over cosmesis, or functional decompensation may also be indications for surgery.

Nonoperative treatment is the mainstay or certainly should be considered the initial mode of therapy in adult patients with scoliosis and back pain. After ruling out other more common causes of back pain, treatment, for the most part, consists of the standard care for back pain; heat, analgesics, nonsteroidal antiinflammatory medications, instructions in proper back care and mechanics, exercises supervised by a competent therapist, and occasionally external neuroaugmentive devices. Other treatment modalities include local facet injections and a semirigid, well-lined underarm body brace.[7]

The surgical treatment of an adult with spine deformity may prove a complex undertaking. The approach to the adult differs from the adolescent in several specific areas. While curve correction is of major importance in the surgical treatment of the adolescent, pain relief with curve correction and stabilization are the primary goals of surgery

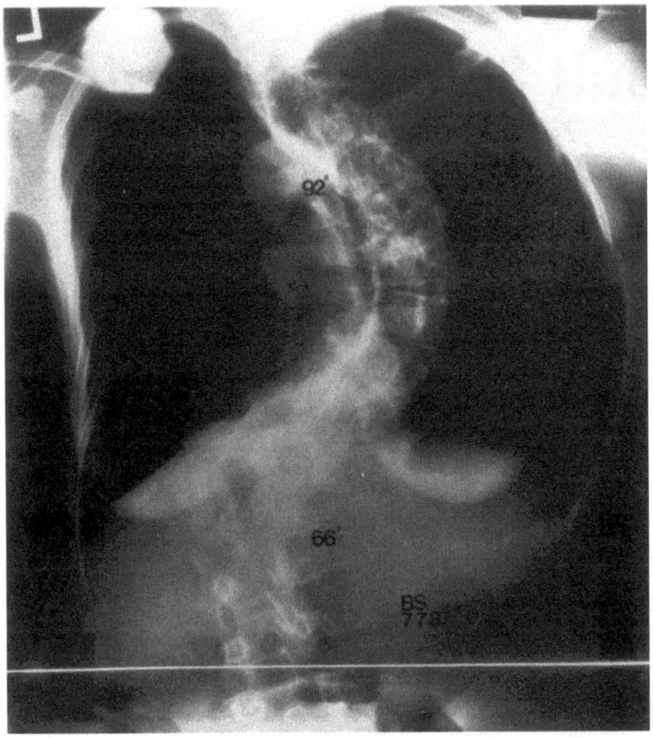

A

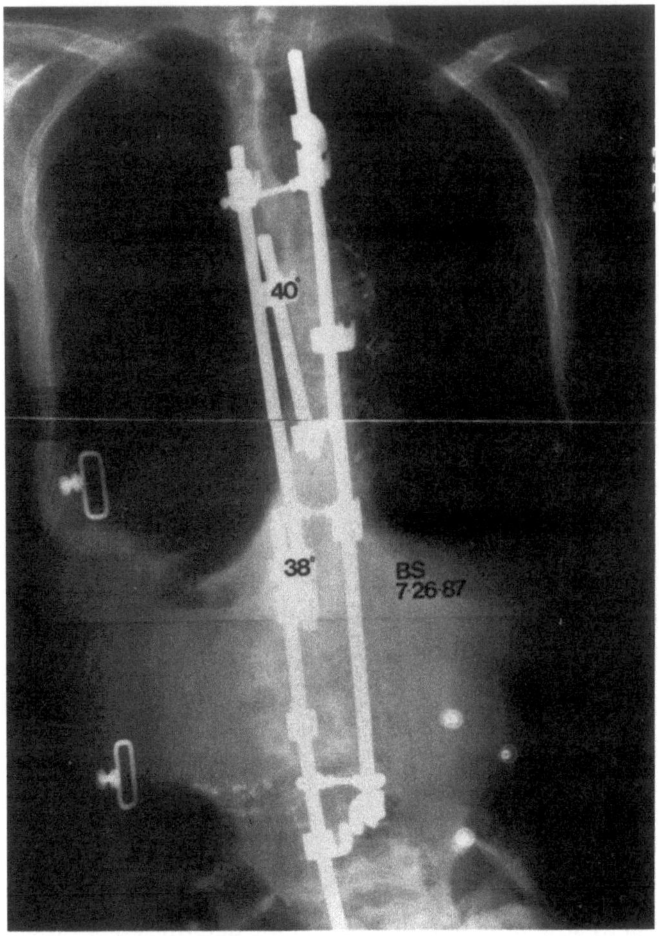

B

Figure 14.1. 53-year-old woman with osteopenia and severe, painful scoliosis. **A.** Severe, rigid double major curve. Marked decrease in bone density seen. **B.** Treatment consisted of staged anterior and posterior fusion with the use of multiple hooks and rods in the Cotrel–Dubousset system to distribute the corrective force. Symptomatic cutout of the upper hook occurred in first postoperative week.

in the adult. Osteopenia is a common finding in the adult population with spinal deformity and may jeopardize attempts at rigid spinal fixation. A greater distribution of corrective forces must be considered. This can be achieved with the use of compression rods, multiple distraction rods, the use of sublaminar or spinous process wiring, or the use of the Cotrel–Dubousset implant (Fig. 14.1). The lack of satisfactory or sufficient bone for grafting, the possible need to supplement fusion with allograft bone, and the importance of sagittal plane alignment are additional areas that add complexity to any surgical management scheme.

Surgical Treatment

Single Thoracic Curve

Patients requiring treatment who present with thoracic curvatures may be managed by one of several different techniques, which vary depending on the severity of the curve and its flexibility. Curvatures of approximately 70° or less and which are more flexible, with correction on side-bending of 40% to 50%, may be managed quite satisfactorily with a single-stage posterior spinal fusion and instrumentation by any one of several constructs. Instrumentation options include Harrington, Luque, or the use of the Cotrel–Dubousset instrumentation. Stability of the Harrington implant may be augmented by using two or three distraction rods in the concavity of the curve, two proximal hooks with the distraction rod, a Harrington distraction rod with sublaminar wires, or a distraction rod in the concavity of the curve with a compression rod on the convexity.

Recently, the Cotrel–Dubousset (C–D) system has been used extensively in adults at the Twin Cities Scoliosis Center. While the fixation furnished by this implant appears superior to other available constructs, it also has several disadvantages. The use of C–D in correcting rigid three-plane deformities of the thoracic or lumbar spine is less effective in adults than in adolescents and children. Derotation by rotating the rod 90° is often not feasible and may result in dislodgement or hook pullout of the concave intermediate hooks. On the other hand, the fixation furnished by this implant appears superior to other available constructs.[8]

Thoracic curves greater than 70°, particularly the more rigid curves, represent a more difficult problem. Single-stage posterior surgery in these curves has led to less than optimal results with a high rate of pseudarthrosis, inadequate curve correction, and/or loss of curve correction postoperatively.[9–11] A recent review from the Twin Cities Scoliosis Center reported superior results in these larger, more rigid curves with the use of a staged anterior fusion without instrumentation followed by a posterior spinal fusion with instrumentation.[12]

The first stage consists of a transthoracic anterior discectomy and osteotomy as necessary at each level; all the intervertebral disc material and osteophytes are removed back to the posterior longitudinal ligament. After removal of the bony endplates with an osteotome, a periosteal or osteoperiosteal flap is reflected off the anterolateral aspect of each vertebral body and a trough is cut into each vertebra. Harvesting cancellous bone graft from each vertebral centrum provides grafting material to be used in addition to the morselized rib. An interbody trough-type fusion is then done at each level using cancellous and cortical bone chips (Fig. 14.2).

One week later, a second-stage procedure is carried out that consists of total facetectomies and posterior osteotomies as necessary, along with instrumentation as previously described. Facet fusion, consisting of excision of the inferior articular facet and removal of all cartilage on the underlying superior facet, followed by cancellous bone grafting, is essential in achieving a solid fusion in the adult. Decortication is performed out to the tips of the transverse processes in both the thoracic and lumbar spine (Fig. 14.3). In the lumbar spine, decortication and bone grafting are not performed in the midline or over the lamina to avoid the development of post fusion stenosis. The use of more complex implants subtracts noticeably from the area available posteriorly for bone grafting; this underscores the importance of performing a thorough facet fusion. The ideal material for bone grafting is autogenous corticocancellous and cancellous bone from the iliac crest. Other autogenous sources such as local bone from the spinous processes, and, when available, rib graft, are also used. Unfortunately adult patients, particularly women, frequently have a significant degree of osteopenia limiting the amount of autogenous bone available. In this situation, allograft is mixed with the harvested autograft. Fresh or frozen bone, such as femoral head or tibial plateau, would appear to be the optimal source of allograft.

In the instrumentation of these more rigid curves, the use of stacked C–D rods in the concavity has proven helpful. In this technique a short distraction rod is placed between the intermediate vertebrae, frequently from T7 to T10, and a longer distraction rod placed between the end vertebrae. The apex of the curve is then pulled toward the midline with the use of two DTT (Device for Transverse Traction) devices between the two rods, tightened in compression (Fig. 14.4). The convex rod is applied in the usual fashion, and standard upper and lower DTTs are used. The use of this two-stage technique on larger, more rigid curves has resulted in a decrease in the pseudarthrosis rate as well as an increase in correction with less loss of correction postoperatively.[12]

In curves exceeding 90° and demonstrating rigid ankylosis, a greater degree of correction can be obtained by vertebrectomy or a technique of vertebral column resection.[13] If a total vertebrectomy is performed, a posterior

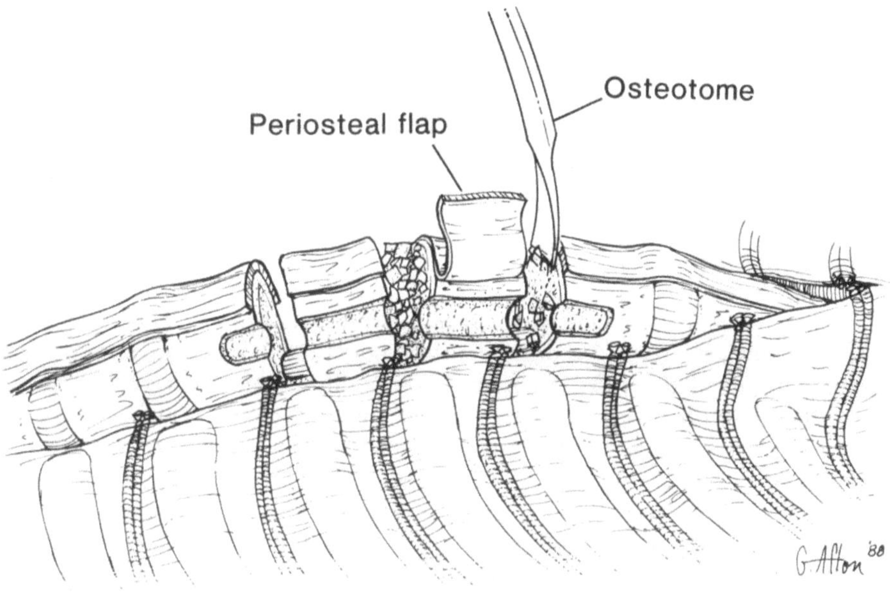

Figure 14.2. Anterior trough-type interbody fusion. After complete disc excision, bony endplate is removed with osteotome and periosteal flap is elevated off body. Trough is then cut into body; from this, bone can be directly harvested. This bone, with morselized rib, is packed into interspace.

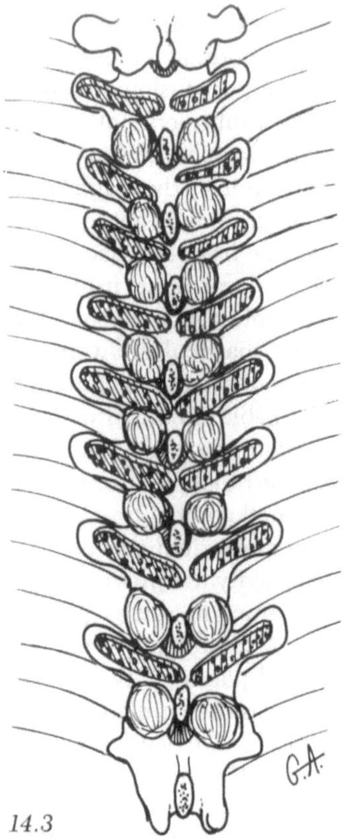

14.3

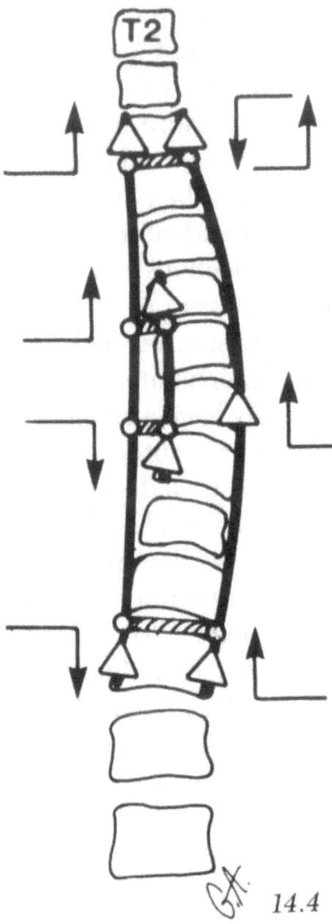

14.4

Figure 14.3. Posterior fusion technique before placement of instrumentation. Facet fusion with excision of inferior articular facet and removal of all cartilage on superior facet is performed with decortication out to tips of transverse processes. Decortication and bone grafting are not performed in midline and over laminae in lumbar spine.

Figure 14.4. Stacked C–D distraction rods in concavity for severe thoracic curves.

distraction implant is ill advised. In this situation, L-rods with sublaminar wires or the C–D system is used to realign the spine by correcting at least two of the three plane deformities (Fig. 14.5).

Thoracoplasty

For many patients, the most cosmetically displeasing aspect of their scoliosis is the prominent rotational rib deformity, referred to as the rib hump. When this is the case, usually with rib prominences greater than 3.5 cm, a thoracoplasty through the same incision should be considered. If derotation with the C–D implant is possible, the need for a thoracoplasty is usually obviated, but in the adult a full 90° of derotation is frequently not possible.

Rib resection is performed through the same midline incision used to expose the spine, and may precede or follow the spinal fusion with instrumentation. The trapezius muscle is detached from the midline fascia, and dissection proceeds dorsal to the paraspinal musculature to the rib prominence. The number of ribs resected depends on the appearance of the deformity. A common mistake is to remove too few ribs or to leave residual rib prominences proximally or distally; usually, six to eight ribs are removed. A wide exposure is achieved allowing visualization of the ribs to the posterior axillary line, and the periosteum overlying the prominent ribs to be excised is incised in a longitudinal fashion. The rib is subperiosteally exposed and detached, first at the posterior axillary line and then, using a Cobb elevator, from the transverse process and the vertebral body disc junction. The ribs should be removed intact, and prominent transverse processes on the convex side should also be removed to maximize the cosmetic result. A chest tube is inserted if any air leaks are apparent on wound irrigation; if not, a hemovac drain is placed and brought up to the skin laterally. The trapezius muscle is reattached to the midline. The bone obtained serves as a valuable source of bone graft.

Postoperatively, the patients may have some transient decreased pulmonary function, which should resolve within 3 months after surgery. Long-term diminution in pulmonary function after thoracoplasty is unusual. The major complication of the procedure is a development of a pleural leak, which is treated intraoperatively or postoperatively with placement of a chest tube.[14]

Thoracolumbar or Lumbar Curve

Patients with thoracolumbar or lumbar curvatures can be treated surgically with either a single-stage anterior fusion with Zielke instrumentation or a posterior fusion with instrumentation. For flexible curves less than 80° and without significant lumbosacral pathology or a significant thoracic curve, the authors' preferred technique is the anterior approach with Zielke instrumentation. The advantages of this technique are the shorter fusion that is required, optimal correction, and low incidences of pseudarthrosis. Some flattening or partial loss of lumbar lordosis is common with this implant system. Therefore, attention to detail is of paramount importance.[15]

The fusion levels are selected by instrumenting all vertebrae adjacent to the intervertebral discs that are wedged open to the convexity of the curve or that are significantly translated (greater than 0.5 cm) from the subjacent vertebrae. A portion of the concave outer annulus is left in place to act as a tether to prevent overcorrection. Loss of lumbar lordosis can be minimized by the placement of a screw posteriorly, in a posterior-to-anterior direction, into the apical vertebral body. Placement of anterior inter-

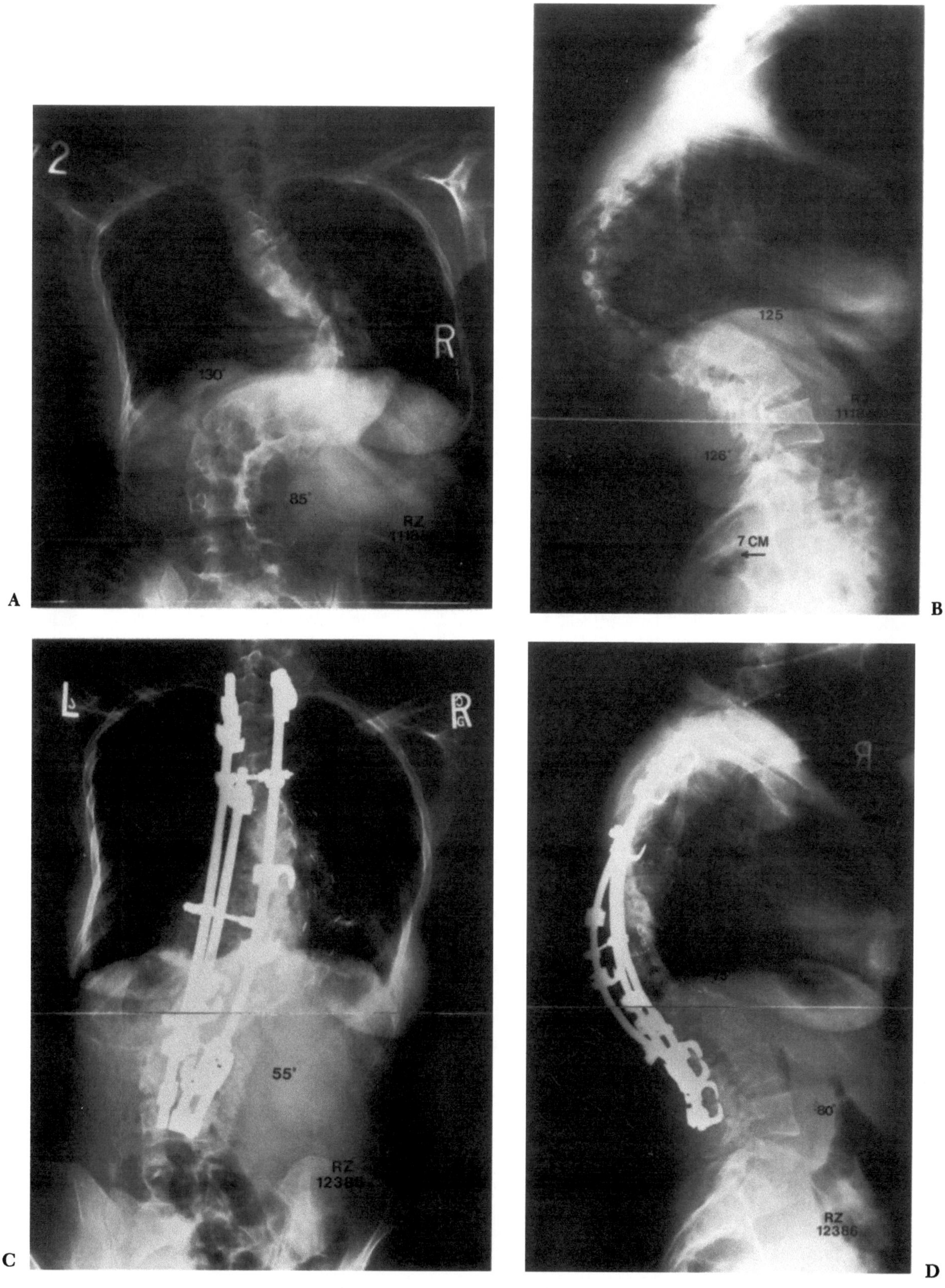

Figure 14.5. 38-year-old woman with severe kyphosing scoliosis and pain. **A** and **B.** Preoperative radiographs show magnitude of deformity. **C** and **D.** Treatment consisted of staged anterior and posterior osteotomies with T10 vertebrectomy, fusion, and stabilization with C–D implant. Use of distraction implant after vertebrectomy may lead to neurological compromise.

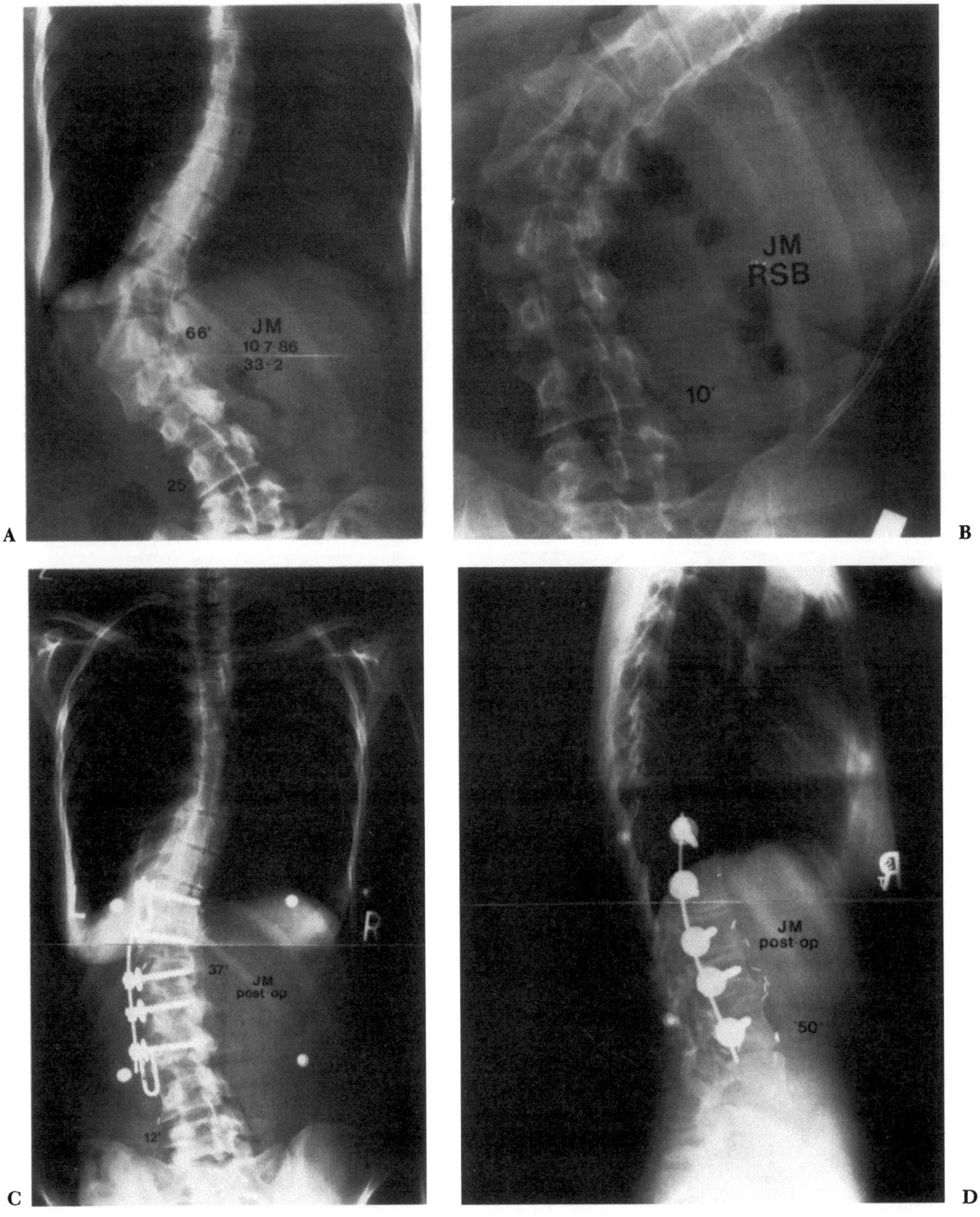

Figure 14.6. 33-year-old woman with painful thoracolumbar scoliosis. **A.** Preoperative radiograph demonstrates 66° T–L curve with 25° lumbosacral fractional curve. **B.** L3 corrects to 10° over sacrum on side-bending. **C.** Use of Zielke implant allows maintenance of one motion segment more than with posterior implant. **D.** Correct screw placement and use of anterior bone blocks to maintain total lumbar lordosis.

body bone blocks has also been beneficial in preventing the development of implant kyphosis.[15] (Fig. 14.6).

Although a single-stage posterior approach with instrumentation is a viable option, use of a distraction implant across the lumbar spine can lead to significant loss of lordosis. Square-ended Harrington rods prebent into lordosis, Luque instrumentation, or the C–D system may be used with this approach.

The C–D system provides greater stability and improved fixation in the area of the spine, which is at significant risk of pseudarthrosis. Lumbar lordosis can be maintained with the C–D implant, using the technique described by Cotrel.[8] Generous facetectomies are performed to improve mobility of the curve and to allow posterior approximation into lordosis. Typically, there are two apical vertebrae into which are placed open hooks on the convexity. Hooks are only placed into the end vertebrae on the concavity of the curve. A mild distraction force may be provisionally applied across the concavity, although this is not always necessary, and the convex rod applied. Compression is then applied across all four hooks and held with C-rings, and the convex rod is rotated within the four rings toward the convexity. This rotation produces lumbar lordosis and corrects the scoliosis at the same time. The convex rod is then locked into the hooks in the usual fashion; further distraction, athough not excessive, is applied across the concave rod and this too is locked. (Fig. 14.7).

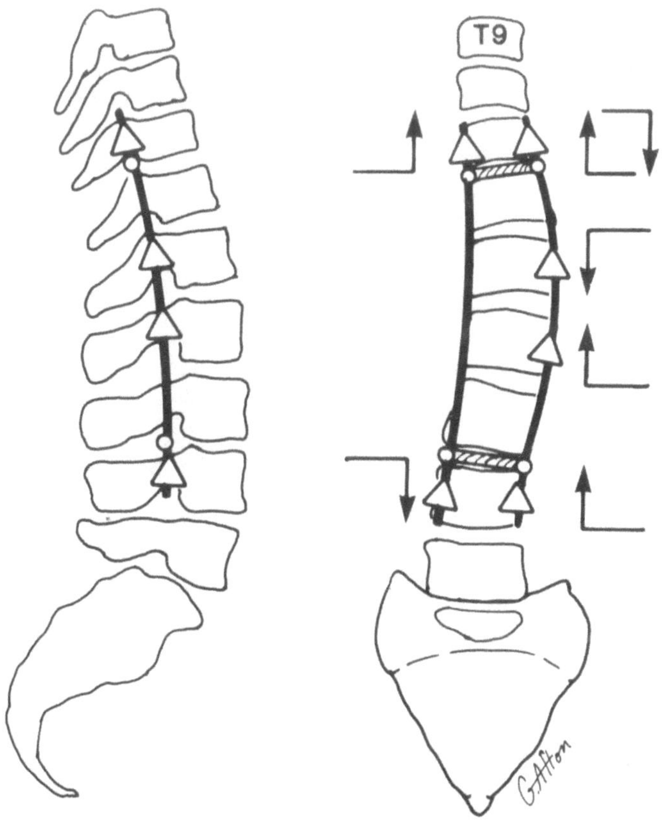

Figure 14.7. Convex first technique for use of C–D system in lumbar scoliosis to preserve lordosis.

It is essential, with the use of posterior instrumentation and fusion in the lumbar spine, to address the sagittal contour. The upper end of the instrumentation cannot end at the apex of a significant thoracolumbar or thoracic kyphosis. It is occasionally necessary to instrument well up into the thoracic spine to prevent the development of a junctional kyphosis.

A history of neurogenic claudication with radiculopathy is uncommon but may be seen with lumbar scoliosis. Nerve root compression is seen at the apex of the lumbar curve in the concavity or in the concavity of a lumbosacral fractional curve and may be caused by hypertrophic facets, a descended pedicle, or uncinate spurs.[16] When surgery is necessary, treatment options include instrumentation and fusion, decompression, or a combination of the two. In milder cases, correction of the curve with instrumentation will usually afford adequate decompression.[17] More severe nerve root compression may need formal decompression, and it is the authors' experience that this should be combined with spinal fusion. Decompression alone requires significant bony resection and commonly leads to progression of the curve, increased back pain, and recurrence of radicular pain from pedicular kinking and nerve root entrapment.

If there is a significant lumbar curvature associated with radicular stenotic pain (more than 30°–40°), anterior interbody fusion followed by posterior decompression with instrumentation has been used (Fig. 14.8). Flexible lumbar curvatures of less than 40° may be seen, which arise de novo in the elderly population, associated with osteoporosis or degenerative disc disease.[18–20] In this situation, and in the presence of reasonable bone stock, a posterior approach alone with decompression and instrumentation with a transpedicular implant may be sufficient. At 6 months after surgery, any evidence of delayed healing may be managed by either posterior augmentation of the bone graft or anterior interbody fusion.

Double Thoracic and Lumbar Curves

A thoracic and lumbar double-curve pattern in which the lumbar curve is smaller in magnitude and more flexible than the upper curve may be managed by a selective thoracic fusion.[21] While these guidelines have proven quite useful in adolescents, their applicability to adults is not as clear cut. Adult lumbar curves tend to be more rigid, and will not spontaneously correct as reliably as those in the adolescent. Furthermore, the presence of a junctional kyphosis between the two curves, which is commonly seen in the adult, eliminates the possibility of instru-

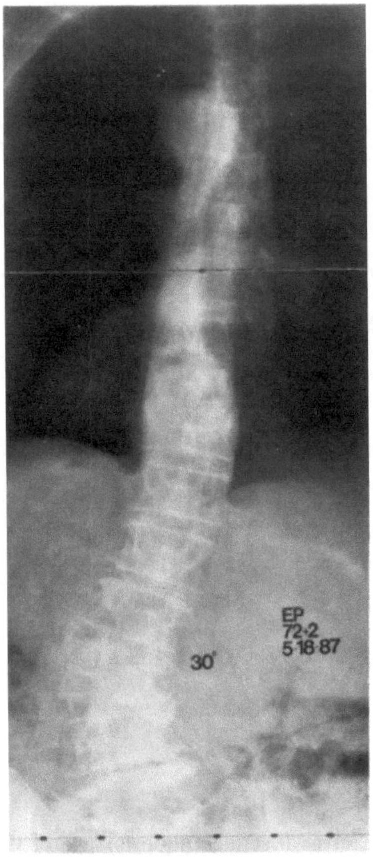

A

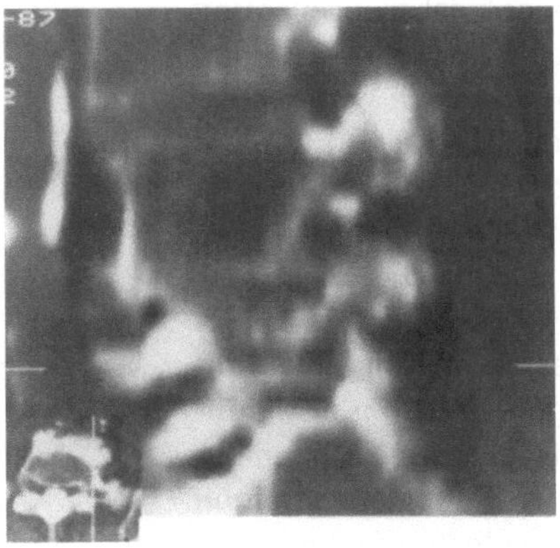

B

Figure 14.8. 72-year-old man with degenerative scoliosis and back and leg pain. **A.** Preoperative radiograph shows marked degenerative changes throughout lumbar spine. **B.** CT scan demonstrates foraminal compromise from uncinate spurring and descended concave pedicle. Facet hypertrophy also contributes to spinal stenosis in these patients. **C** and **D.** Treatment consisted of staged anterior and posterior approach with use of C–D implant for fusion down to sacrum. Frontal plane correction is of minimal concern in such a case; maintenance of lumbar lordosis is essential.

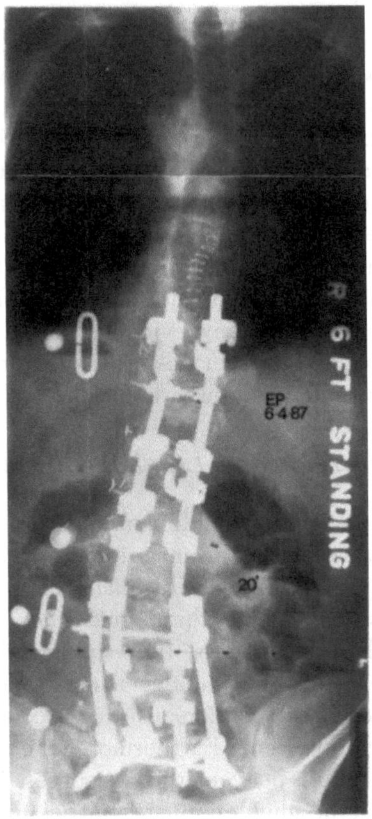

C

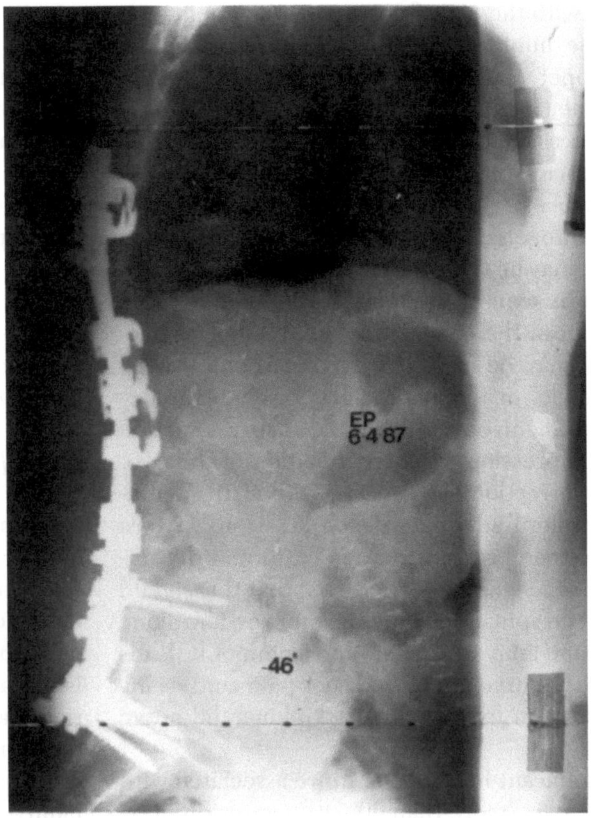

D

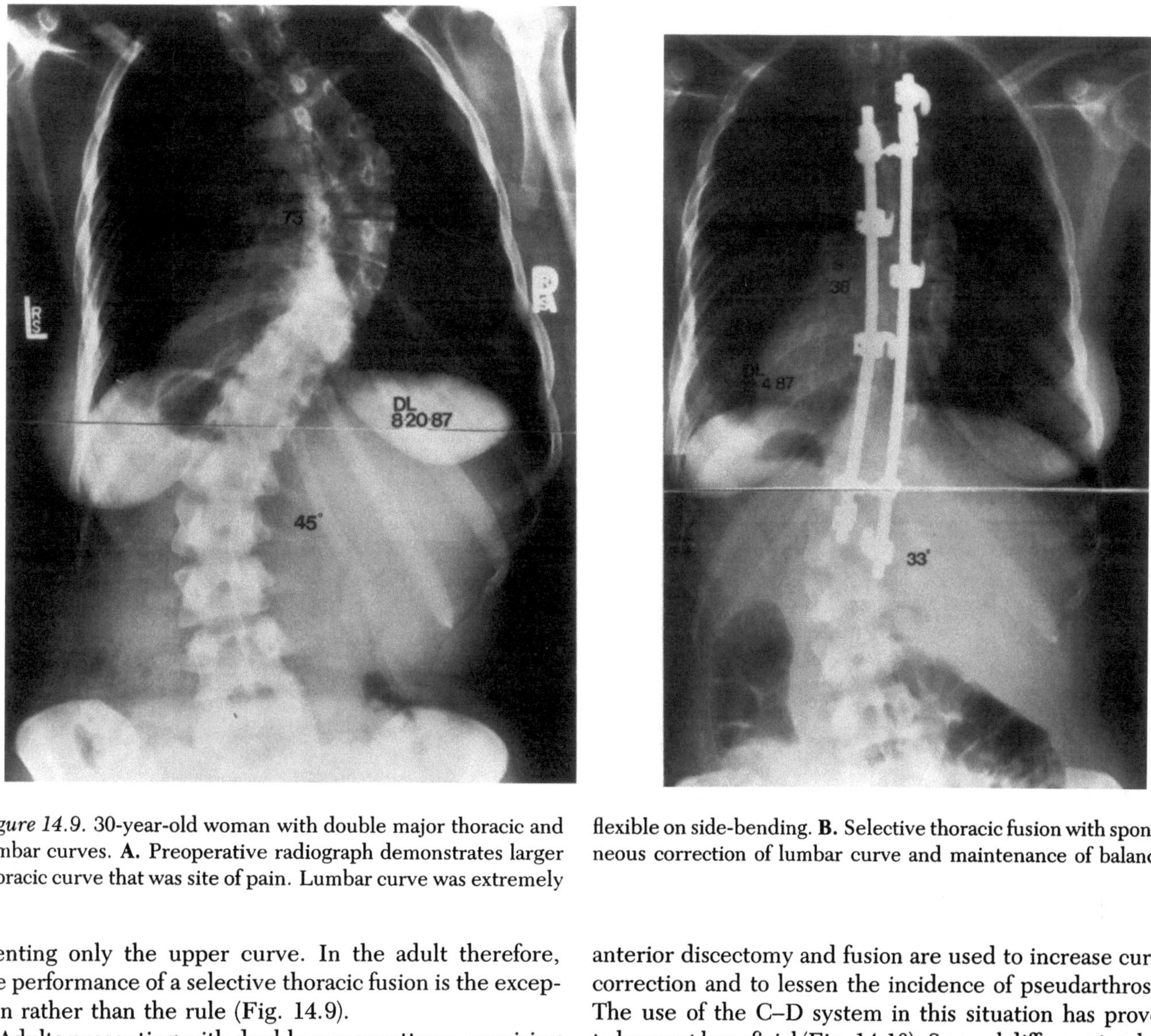

A B

Figure 14.9. 30-year-old woman with double major thoracic and lumbar curves. **A.** Preoperative radiograph demonstrates larger thoracic curve that was site of pain. Lumbar curve was extremely flexible on side-bending. **B.** Selective thoracic fusion with spontaneous correction of lumbar curve and maintenance of balance.

menting only the upper curve. In the adult therefore, the performance of a selective thoracic fusion is the exception rather than the rule (Fig. 14.9).

Adults presenting with double-curve patterns requiring fusion of both curves pose a difficult problem. Balanced curves of lesser magnitude (less than 50°) and with good flexibility may be managed satisfactorily with single-stage posterior spinal fusion and instrumentation. Choices of instrumentation include a single Harrington distraction rod, distraction and compression rod, a double distraction dollar sign rod, distraction rods plus sublaminar wires, the L-rod system, or the C–D system. Balanced correction with maintenance of sagittal plane contours must be achieved.

In larger, more rigid curves, or in patients with imbalanced deformity where the lumbar curvature is greater and more rigid, combined procedures should be considered. A first-stage procedure consisting of an anterior thoracoabdominal approach with fusion of the thoracolumbar and lumbar spine without instrumentation is followed after 1 week by a posterior fusion with instrumentation. The anterior discectomy and fusion are used to increase curve correction and to lessen the incidence of pseudarthrosis. The use of the C–D system in this situation has proved to be most beneficial (Fig. 14.10). Several different implant configurations may be used for instrumenting double curves. In less severe curves, a single rod on either side of the spine may be used with the placement of apical hooks into the convex apical vertebrae but without the use of intermediate hooks on the concave side of either curve (Fig. 14.11). Rotation of these prebent rods permits simultaneous correction of the scoliosis with maintenance of sagittal plane curvature, although in the adult this rotation is technically difficult. More severe curves can be instrumented with a three- or four-rod construct[8] with the use of double-barreled hooks above and below the junctional vertebrae. The corresponding concave rod goes into the enclosed inner channel while the lateral opening of the double hook accepts the convex rod (Fig. 14.12). Insertion of the lumbar convex rod may be facilitated by a moderate amount of provisional distraction across the curve with the concave rod, but the convex rod across

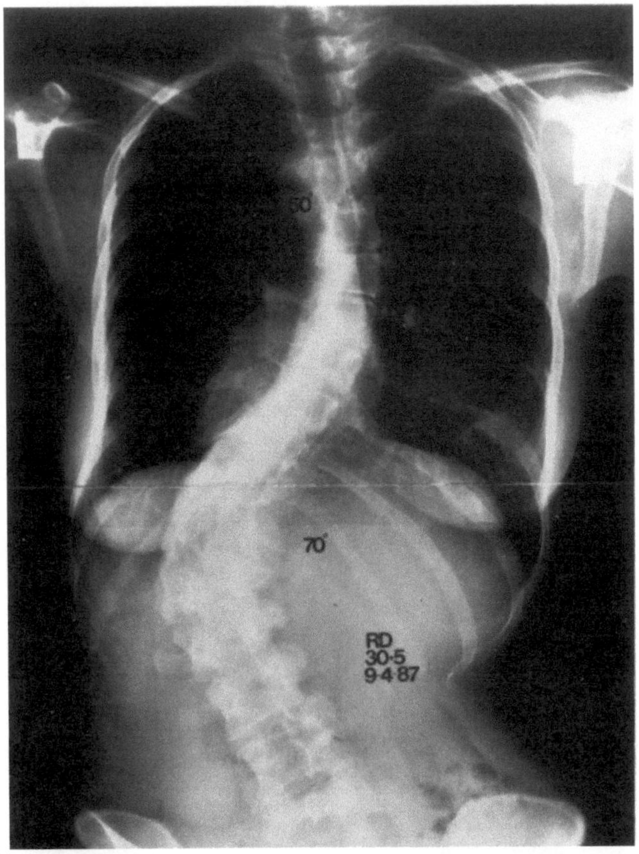

A

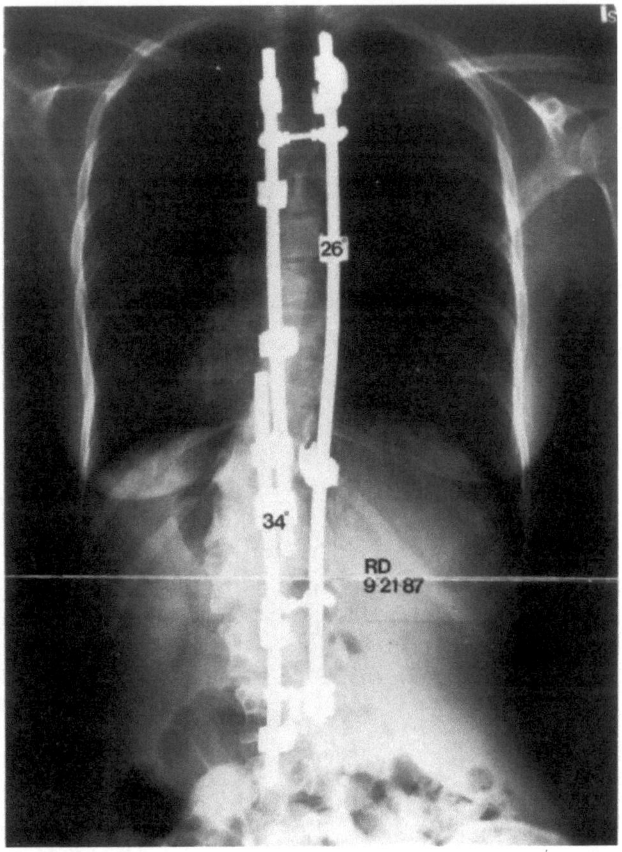

B

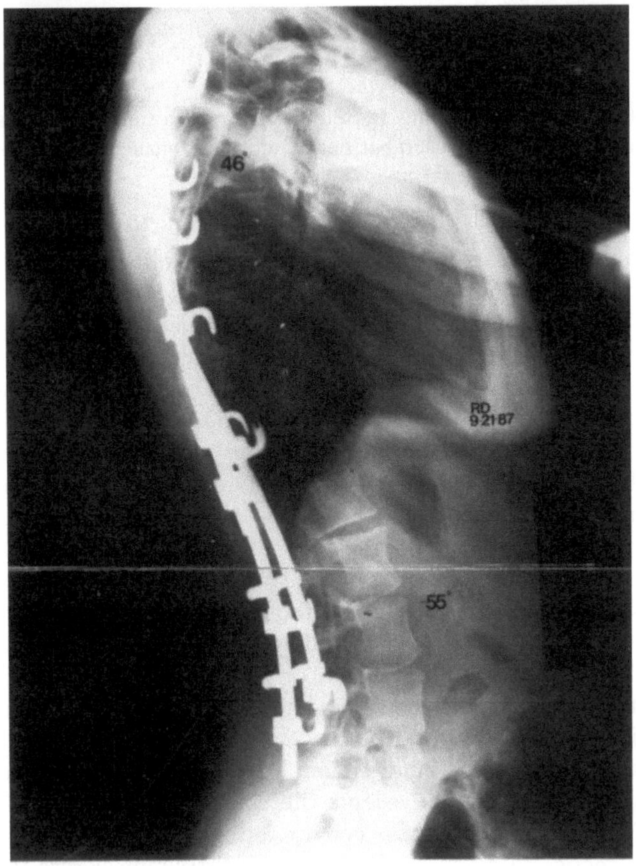

C

Figure 14.10. 30-year-old woman with double major curve with larger, more rigid lumbar curve. **A.** Preoperative appearance. **B.** Staged anterior discectomies and fusion and posterior fusion with instrumentation allowed excellent correction. Loss of correction and pseudarthrosis rates are decreased with this approach. **C.** Good maintenance of sagittal contours.

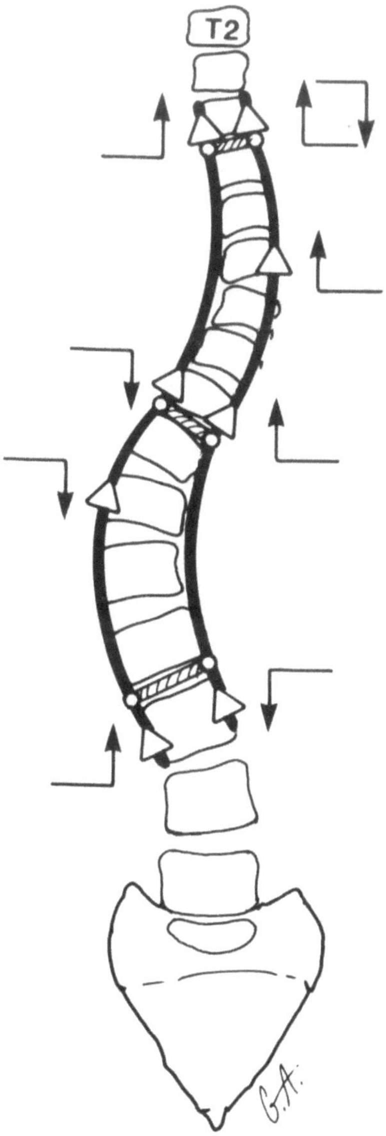

Figure 14.11. Double major curve instrumented with two long rods.

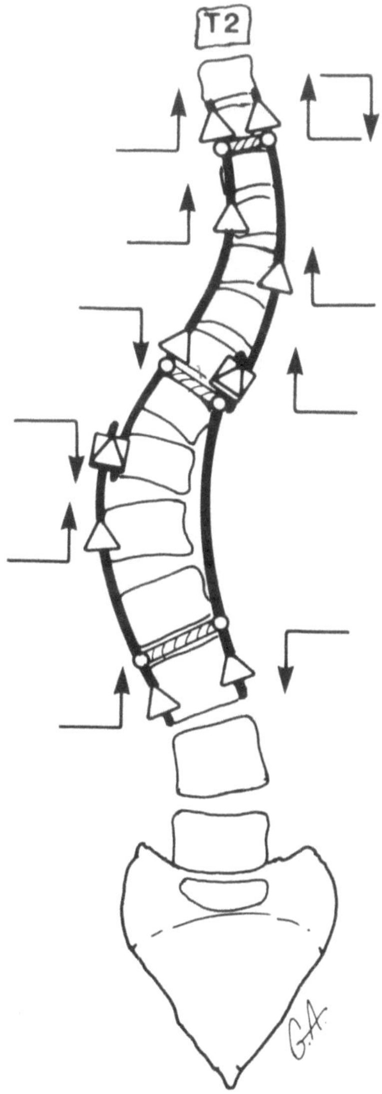

Figure 14.12. Four-rod technique for severe double major curve. Double-barreled hooks are placed above and below neutral vertebrae.

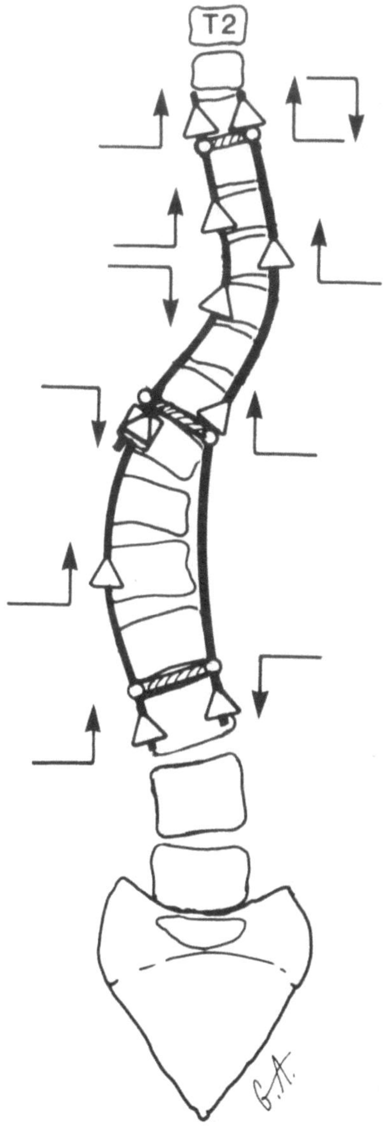

Figure 14.13. Three-rod technique. Provisional distraction rod across lumbar curve is removed after convex lumbar rod is applied and compressed, and single long rod is applied.

the lumbar spine should be compressed before final distraction of the opposite rod to prevent the development of an implant kyphosis at this level.

In the authors' experience, a three-rod construct has proven useful in this situation. In this technique a distraction rod across the concavity of the thoracic curve, using standard intermediate hooks and ending in a double-barreled supralaminar hook, is placed first; tension is then applied with C-rings, which are rotated if possible. A provisional distraction rod is then placed across the concavity of the lumbar curve to facilitate correction of this curve, followed by a placement of a convex rod across the lumbar curve, utilizing the double-barreled hook, which is tightened into compression to maintain lumbar lordosis. The initial lumbar rod is then removed and a single long rod is placed in compression over the thoracic curve and in a moderate degree of distraction across the lumbar curve (Fig. 14.13). Three DTTs are used in this construct. It is of utmost importance that any implant used not produce a thoracolumbar or lumbar kyphosis.

Fusion to the Sacrum

Rarely is fusion to the sacrum necessary in the adult with idiopathic scoliosis. Indications for this most difficult spinal fusion include severe lumbar curves with continuation into the sacrum producing an "oblique take-off," severe degenerative disc disease below a lumbar curve, or a rigid lumbosacral fractional curve that does not correct on side-bending. Evaluation of lumbosacral pathology before attempting arthrodesis to the sacrum may include discography to assess disc status and the production of symptomatic pain and/or the use of facet blocks.

The use of a single-stage posterior spinal fusion of a long curve to the sacrum has produced uniformly poor results.[22] The incidence of pseudarthrosis, loss of lumbar lordosis, and implant failure continues to be high with any form of treatment, but has been seen at the Twin Cities Scoliosis Center to be diminished with the use of a staged anterior and posterior approach.[23] The first stage consists of an anterior thoracoabdominal approach with fusion of the lumbar curvature to the sacrum without instrumentation. The second stage consists of instrumentation with a posterior spinal fusion. The use of L-rods with segmental instrumentation and transiliac fixation with the Galveston technique,[24] or the use of the C–D system with transpedicular fixation, has led to improved results when attempting to instrument down to the sacrum. Any rods used must be contoured to maintain lumbar lordosis and must be extended up into the thoracic spine if there is significant thoracic deformity.

Complications of transpedicular fixation include the possibility of nerve root injury, dural laceration, and loss of fixation in osteopenic bone.[25,26] The use of two or three screws on either side optimizes fixation. To facilitate this procedure technically, the surgeon may place a short rod through the transpedicular sacral screws with linkage between this rod and a rod through the rest of the curvature with the use of a domino (see Fig. 14.8). It should be noted however that the use of two rods and a domino results in a somewhat less rigid construct than is achieved with the use of a single rod. Also, L-rod fixation across the pelvis occasionally results in sacroiliac pain which may necessitate rod removal.

Results and Complications

A high percentage of satisfactory long-term results can be obtained in the surgical stabilization of adult scoliosis,[27] but the variable results obtained in terms of pain relief, curve correction, and reversal of pulmonary dysfunction have discouraged some authors.[28] Pain relief is often incomplete after surgical correction of adult scoliosis, a point meriting serious consideration when undertaking such surgery with pain as the primary indication. Despite the lack of complete pain relief after surgery, the experience of most authors has been that an acceptable reduction in pain with a high level of patient satisfaction is obtained.[9,10,27] Curve correction is less in the adult than in the adolescent with idiopathic scoliosis. While curve correction of more than 60%–70% is obtained with the use of newer implants in the flexible adolescent spine, the average correction in most adult series has ranged from 30%–40%. In addition, all authors report a significant loss of correction postoperatively.[10,11] Improvement in pulmonary function after surgical correction of adult scoliosis has been unpredictable, with most patients returning to their baseline pulmonary status.

Surgical complications in the adult are similar to those in the adolescent patient treated for scoliosis, but appear to occur with much greater frequency. Pseudarthrosis is the most common major complication in adults, occurring in 7%–17% of patients. In a recent review of patients with adult idiopathic scoliosis treated at the Twin Cities Scoliosis Center, a 15% rate of pseudarthrosis was seen with single-stage posterior fusion with Harrington instrumentation.[11] By comparison, a review of patients treated by staged anterior and posterior approaches revealed no failures of fusion in 26 patients after an average of 4 years.[12] Wound and urinary tract infections, cardiopulmonary problems, neurological damage, thrombophlebitis, and loss of lumbar lordosis are all complications of scoliosis surgery in the adult.

Finally, in the evaluation of the adult treated surgically for adult scoliosis, it is evident that the age of the patient plays a significant part in the expected outcome of surgery. The approach to spinal deformities in the elderly represents a major undertaking. The results are significantly less satisfactory than in the young adult. Kostuik recently reported his results in patients over the age of 50, and related an extremely high complication rate including a 27% pseudarthrosis rate, a loss of lumbar lordosis in 13 of 73 patients, kyphosis above the fusion secondary to osteoporosis in 9 cases, and in general a 25% chance of poor results.[29] This underscores the importance of approaching these elderly patients with extreme caution.

Salvage Surgery

Repeat surgery on an adult who has undergone previous spinal fusion for spinal deformity is one of the most difficult undertakings facing the spinal surgeon. The patient's most common presenting complaint is pain. Increasing deformity, commonly in the sagittal plane, respiratory failure, and occasionally neurologic dysfunction are also seen.[30] One or more pseudarthroses are frequently present in this situation, but loss of curve correction either through bending of a solid fusion mass or adding on above or below previously fused segments may occur in the case of a solid fusion.

Pseudarthrosis

In all series failure of fusion is highest in the thoracolumbar and lumbar spine, particularly when single-stage posterior fusion is performed. The etiology of the deformity includes idiopathic, paralytic, and congenital scoliosis, as well as kyphotic and post traumatic deformities.

Successful repair of a pseudarthrosis requires even more rigid adherence to technique than primary spinal fusion. Meticulous resection of any fibrous tissue at the pseudarthrosis site is essential. While no statistics exist documenting the superiority of rigid internal fixation in this setting, it is certainly the preferred technique at this time. The C–D implant, used in compression, affords stabilization and the capability for correction where indicated. Decortication of the preexisting fusion mass down to bleeding bone and the addition of autologous iliac crest graft enhance the chances of achieving successful fusion. Even under these ideal circumstances the successful repair of pseudarthrosis in adults, particularly in the lumbar spine, is by no means assured, and consideration should be given to an anterior spinal fusion to enhance the results.

The experience at the Twin Cities Scoliosis Center has been that, more often than not, more than one pseudarthrosis is found when any single pseudarthrosis exists.[31] It is therefore essential to explore the entire fusion mass carefully. A lamellated outer cortical shell of bone may be suspended from one level to the next appearing to signify a solid fusion, but when this thin shell of bone is removed, gross motion is frequently found. It is not uncommon to surgically document a pseudarthrosis at a level that has been believed, on the basis of a previous exploration, to be solidly fused.

Loss of curve correction may occur secondary to a pseudarthrosis or in the face of a solid fusion. When the magnitude of the deformity and its rigidity are such that adequate correction cannot be obtained with standard instrumentation techniques, an osteotomy may be performed. The osteotomy technique is useful in the presence of ankylosed facets; it may be performed at the level of the pseudarthrosis or through a solid fusion.[30,32]

The fusion mass is exposed to its most lateral extent or to the tips of the transverse processes bilaterally. The transverse processes are usually identifiable even under the most solid of fusions. The osteotomy will proceed from the midline across the facet joint midway between the pedicles above and below, and out between, the corresponding transverse processes. A gouge or osteotome is used to remove the outer cortical shell of the fusion mass and then a gouge, osteotome, or high-speed air drill is used to carefully thin out the cancellous bone down to the level of the inner cortex. The inner cortex is carefully broached using either an air drill or curette. This may be easiest in the midline where the inner cortex is the thinnest. Once the dura is adequately visualized the osteotomy can be extended to either side using a Kerrison rongeur, passing between the pedicles and the transverse processes.[30] Adequate bone should be resected to ensure that with compression no bony impingement on the neural elements occurs. It is most important to generously undercut the osteotomy site to ensure that no damage to the neural elements occurs.

Depending on the number and levels of osteotomies, correction may be achieved in two planes. The nature of the deformity will dictate the instrumentation chosen. Bilateral compression implants are used with kyphotic deformities, and distraction coupled with compression implants are used for a frontal plane curvature (Fig. 14.14).

More severe deformities, which cannot be corrected with simple posterior osteotomy and instrumentation, can be addressed in one of two ways. Staged posterior exploration and osteotomy with interval halo femoral traction to obtain correction followed by posterior instrumentation, as described by Cummine and coworkers,[30] is a viable treatment option. Another approach in these severe problems is the use of vertebral resection. This may consist of either a posterior, transpedicular decancellation or open vertebral decancellation performed through an anterior approach.

Flat Back Syndrome

Symptomatic loss of lumbar lordosis has been noted to occur, most commonly after the use of distraction instrumentation across the lumbar spine, although this symptom complex may be seen occasionally in patients who have had lumbar spine fusion without instrumentation.[33,34] The patients present most commonly with the inability to stand erect and with back pain. Loss of lumbar lordosis or the presence of thoracolumbar kyphosis is seen on standing lateral radiographs, and the patient's forward list is noted by dropping a vertical line from the body of C7 that falls anterior to the sacral promontory.

The treatment of this syndrome is extremely difficult. One or more posterior closing wedge osteotomies, as described previously, and fixed with compression instrumentation using either the C–D system or heavy Harrington compression rods, are performed. An average of 20° of correction can be obtained per osteotomy level.

The ability to maintain correction obtained at surgery relates to the initial ability to center the body of C7 over the sacrum on standing. Postoperative loss of correction, particularly when such sagittal plane imbalance is present, is a significant problem but it occurs less commonly when an anterior interbody fusion is performed[33] (Fig. 14.15). In the series reported by Lagrone and coworkers, most patients stated they benefited from their corrective osteotomies. However, more than 50% of patients continued

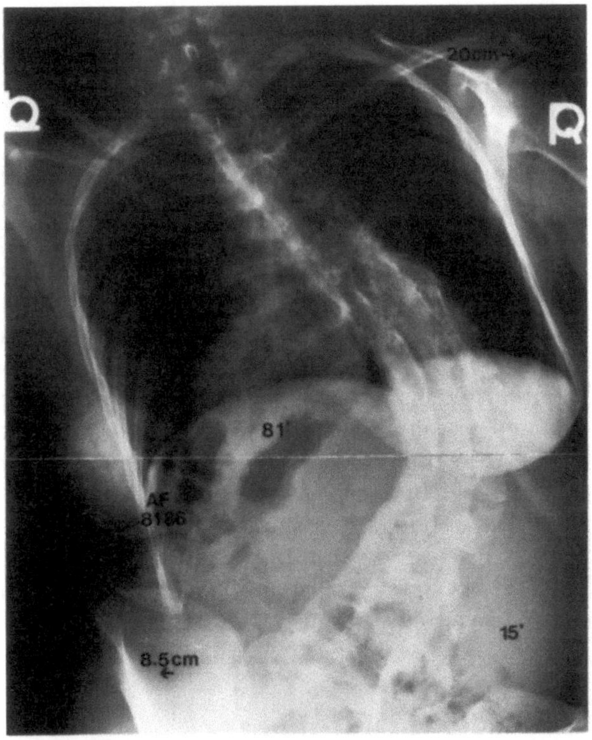
20cm
81°
AF
8186
8.5cm
15°

A

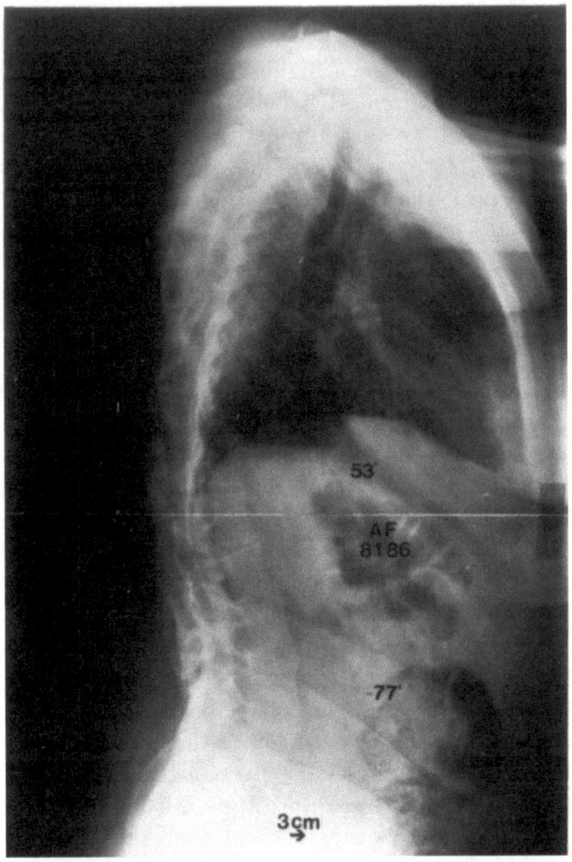
53°
AF
8186
-77°
3cm

B

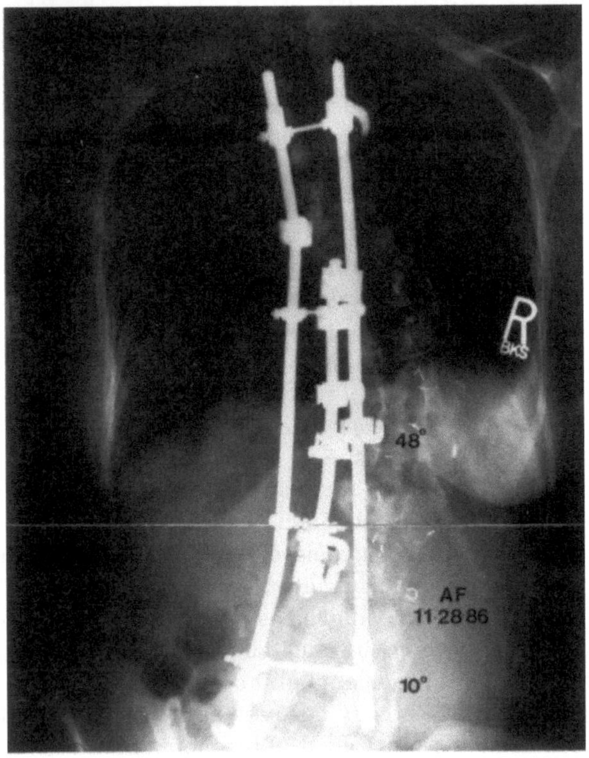
R
BKS
48°
AF
11 28 86
10°

C

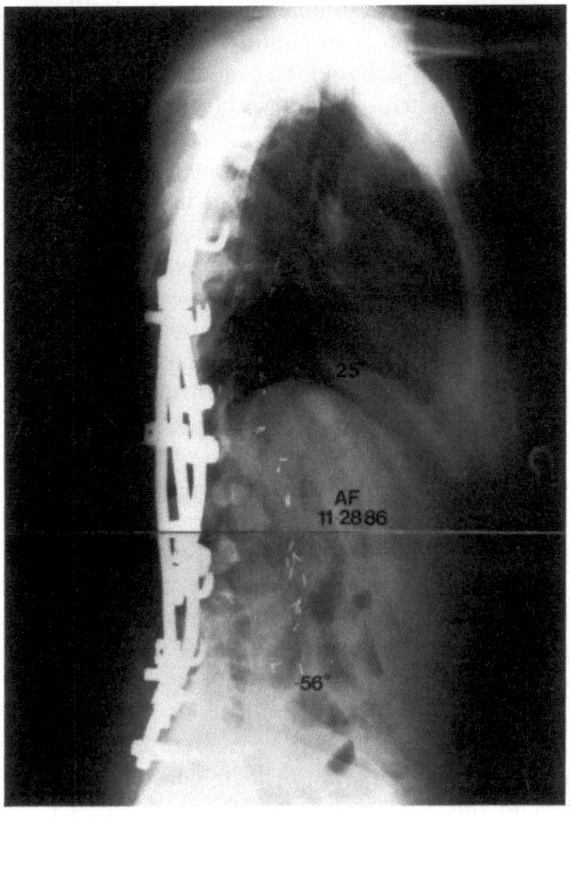
25°
AF
11 28 86
-56°

D

Figure 14.15. Flat back syndrome. **A.** Despite previous attempts at correction with use of Harrington compression implant, inability to center body of C7 over sacrum with knees straight has recurred. **B.** Anterior and posterior osteotomies and correction with C–D implant in compression bilaterally allowed restoration of sagittal balance. Achievement of sagittal balance is essential for maintenance of correction.

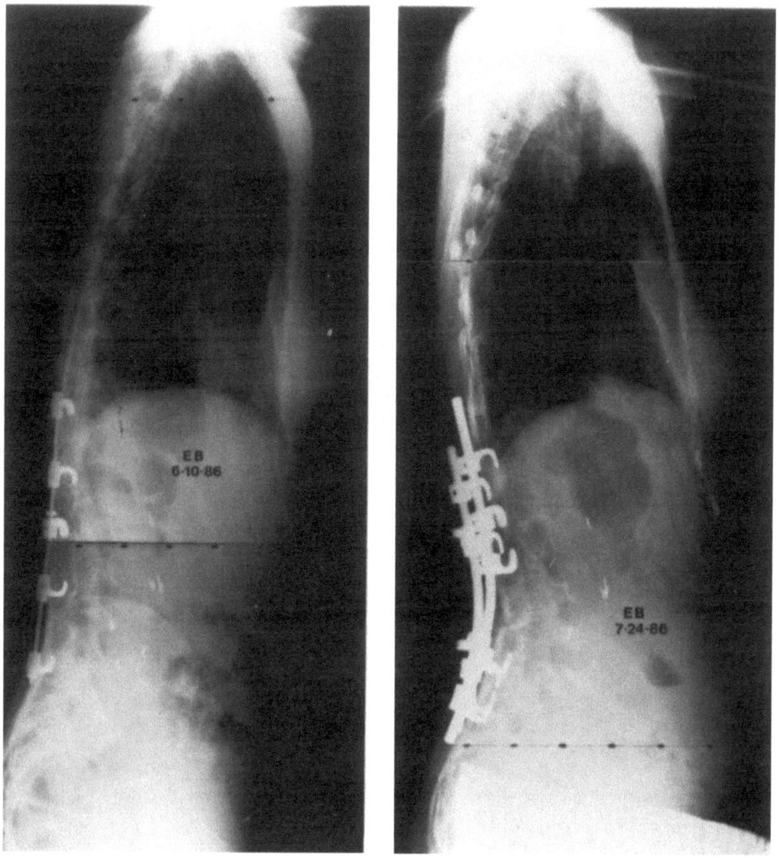

A B

to lean forward, and many patients continued to have moderate to severe back pain. As in any of the foregoing salvage techniques, pseudarthrosis, dural tears, failure of fixation devices and neuropraxia are associated complications.[33]

Kyphosis

Kyphosis in the adult may arise from a number of causes including untreated Scheuermann's kyphosis, congenital deformity, neuromuscular disease, osteopenia, and spondylitis (see following). A variety of surgical approaches may be considered. Preoperative medical evaluation and treatment of the patient are imperative, particularly in the older patient with progressive kyphotic collapse secondary to osteopenia.

The curve should be evaluated to determine the relative rigidity, measuring maximal correction on supine lateral extension radiographs. The possibility of neurological involvement, which has been reported in all these entities, should be appreciated;[35,36] the use of magnetic resonance imaging (MRI) to assess cord compression of the thoracic spine has been extremely helpful. Finally, the adequacy of bone stock should be assessed.

Supple curves correcting to less than 55°, without anterior cord compression, or curves of less than 55° in which correction is not necessary, may be treated by a single-stage posterior fusion with instrumentation. Dual heavy Harrington compression rods, L-rods, and the C–D implant used in compression bilaterally are implant options (Fig. 14.16). Use of the L-rod technique in these kyphotic deformities has been associated with a high incidence of progressive kyphosis above or below the fusion with less than an optimal result,[37] and is therefore not favored in the treatment of most kyphotic deformities.

If significant cord compression exists anteriorly, decompression is necessary before any attempt at correction.

Figure 14.14. 26-year-old woman with pseudarthrosis and increasing deformity and displacement in two planes. **A** and **B.** Preoperative radiographs show magnitude of deformity; loss of frontal plane balance is particularly marked. **C** and **D.** Postoperative radiographs. Anterior and posterior approaches with multiple osteotomies and L1 vertebrectomy allowed correction of curvature as well as centering occiput over sacrum in both planes.

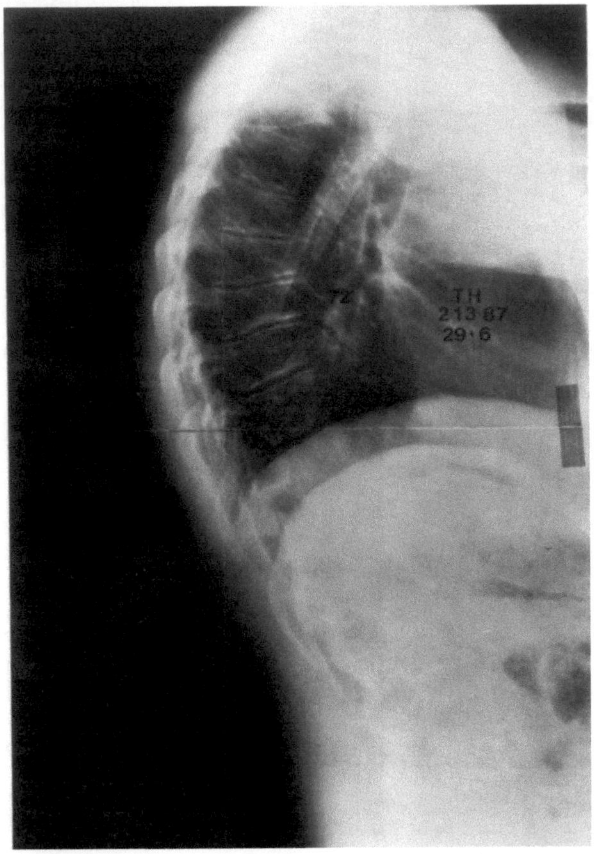

A

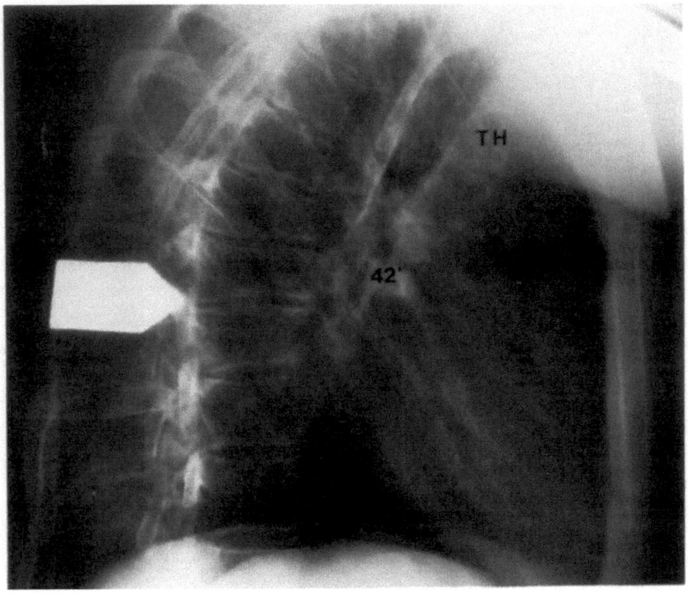

B

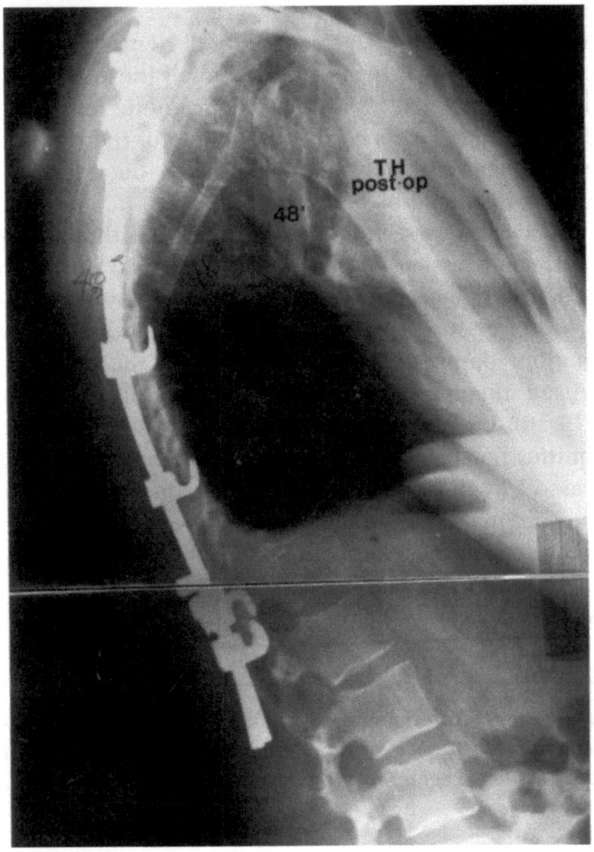

C

Figure 14.16. 29-year-old man with pain and idiopathic round-back deformity. **A.** Preoperative radiograph. **B.** Correction on hyperextension to 42°. **C.** In this patient, in whom appearance was not a major concern, adequate correction is obtained with single-stage posterior instrumentation and fusion.

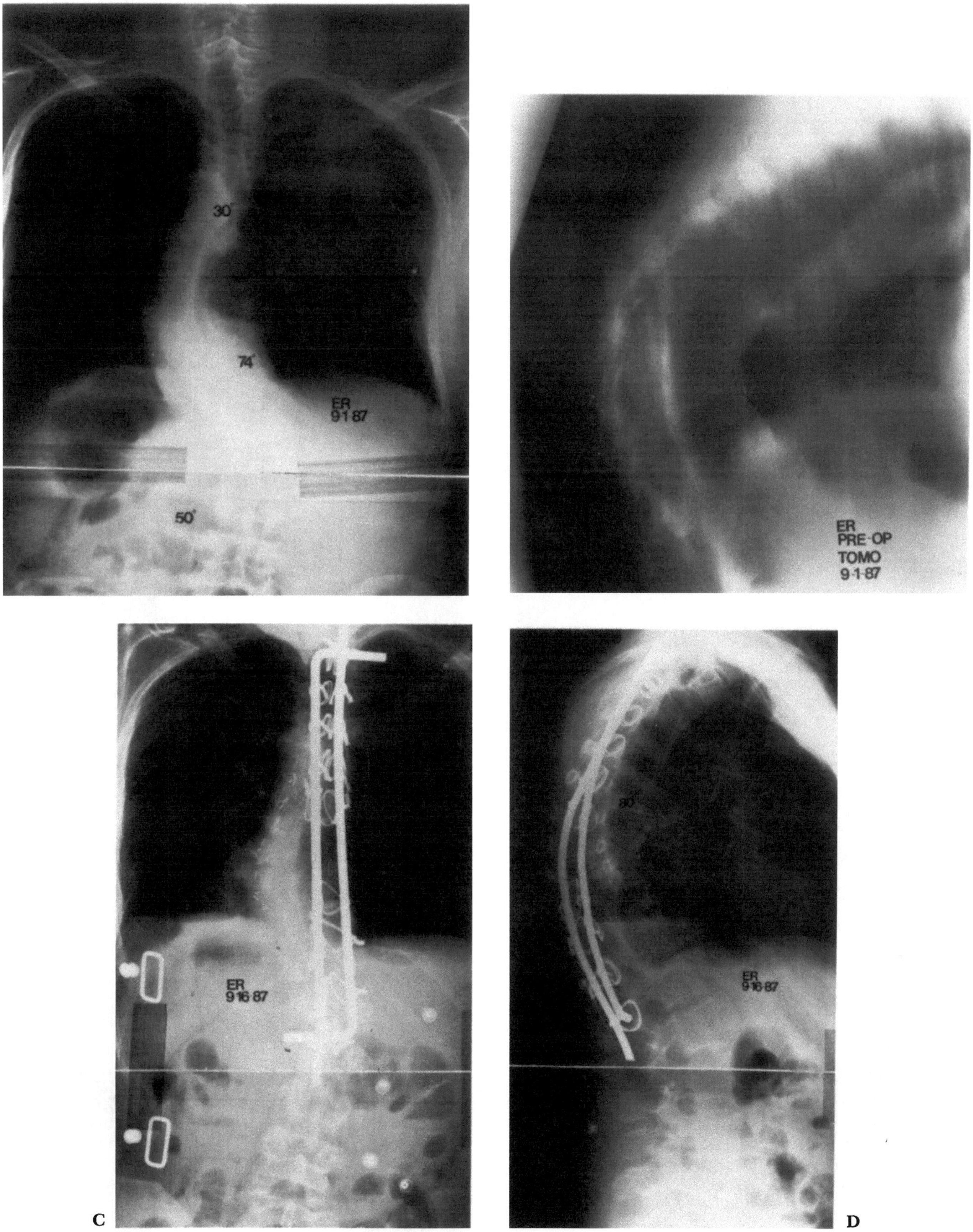

Figure 14.17. 40-year-old man with severe kyphoscoliosis. **A** and **B.** Preoperative plain PA radiograph and lateral tomogram demonstrate magnitude of deformity. **C** and **D.** Treatment consisted of anterior and posterior osteotomies and vertebrectomy at T9 with Luque instrumentation.

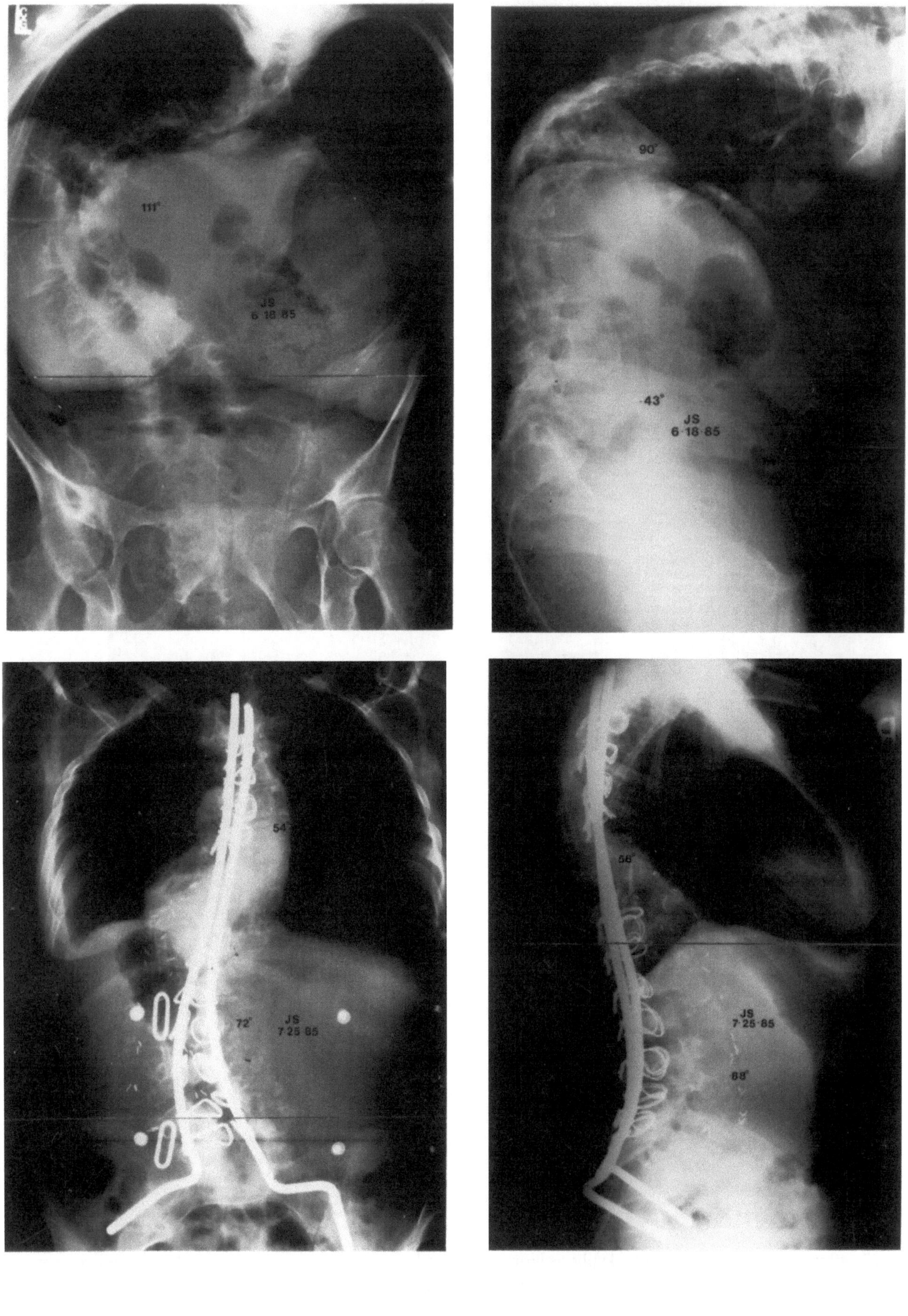

A B C D

E

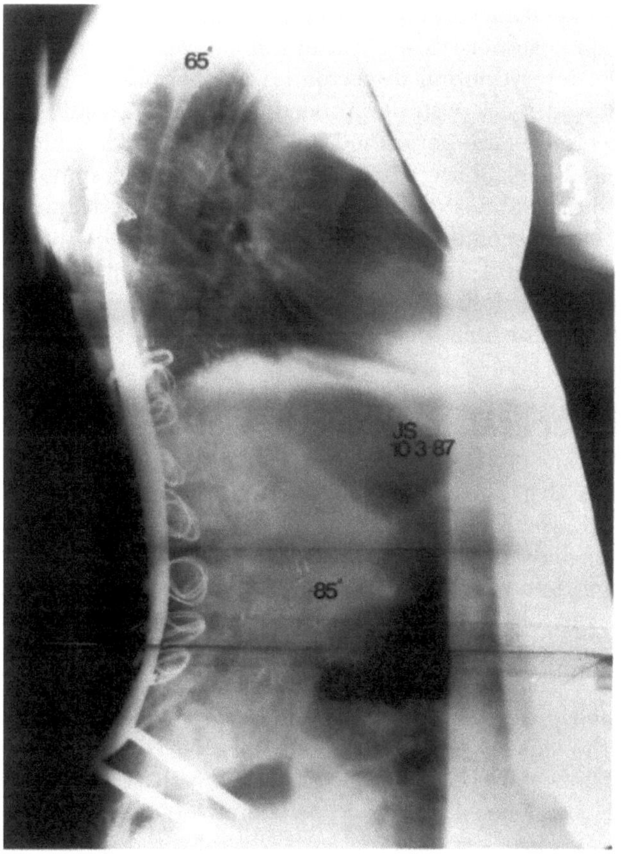

Figure 14.18. 42-year-old woman with ankylosing spondylitis. **A** and **B.** Preoperative radiographs demonstrate severity of deformity. Simple kyphosis is more common in spondyloarthropathies than two-plane deformity such as this. Note sagittal imbalance. **C** and **D.** Anterior and posterior osteotomies and L1 vertebrectomy with stabilization utilizing Luque–Galveston technique. **E.** With restoration of sagittal balance, long-term correction is maintained.

Preoperative traction is contraindicated in the treatment of kyphotic deformities with cord compression. Decompression may be performed through an anterior transthoracic or thoracoabdominal approach, a posterolateral costotransversectomy approach, or a Michelle–Krueger approach involving the resection of the transverse process and pedicle, affording visualization of the vertebral body and anterior cord. The anterior approach is preferred as it appears to be safer, affords better visualization for decompression, and certainly enhances one's ability to perform an anterior approach.

Rigid or more severe curves require an anterior approach. In cases in which correction is not desired, discectomy and anterior spinal fusion in situ utilizing a strut graft technique is performed. Correction can be achieved with the use of a two-stage approach; the first stage is an anterior release, which may require a discectomy and osteotomy in the case of a type II congenital kyphosis, or release of the anterior longitudinal ligament in Scheuermann's kyphosis (Fig. 14.17); the second stage consists of a posterior fusion with instrumentation as previously described.

Spondyloarthropathy

Ankylosing spondylitis is the most common of the rheumatic disorders, including psoriatic arthropathy, Reiter's syndrome, arthropathy associated with inflammatory bowel disorders, and rheumatoid arthritis, which can lead to fixed spinal deformity. These patients present with progressive kyphotic deformity of the cervical or thoracic spine or loss of lumbar lordosis. This is initially associated with pain, but eventually results in a painless ankylosis.[38] In more severe cases, the patient is unable to stand upright even with knee flexion, producing a severe functional disability.

Beginning with Smith-Petersen, Larson, and Aufranc in 1945,[39] several authors have described spinal osteotomy for correction of this deformity. Concern over reports of death and neurological complications following this procedure, particularly in the series presented by Law,[40] limited the acceptance of this technique.

Evaluation of the patient is essential because the source of the deformity may occur at any one of several sites.[41] The flexed posture may be related to hip flexion contractures, which, if present, should be addressed before attempting spinal surgery. Spinal deformity may occur in the lumbar spine, the thoracic spine, or at the cervicothoracic junction. The most common site of pathology in the spine is in the lumbar region, with loss of lumbar lordosis and pelvic tilting. The lumbar spine is the safest site to perform an extension osteotomy, which is generally performed between L2 and L3, or between L3 and L4.

The technique of the osteotomy is similar to that previously described. As much as 2 cm of bone and a portion of each pedicle may be resected to achieve maximum correction. It is essential that the apex of the osteotomy lie anterior to the dural tube so that the neural elements are not stretched when the osteotomy is closed down. The ideal apex is at the junction of the posterior longitudinal ligament with the intervertebral disc. As described by McMaster,[42] correction occurs by virtue of fracturing through the ossified anterior longitudinal ligament and disc space in tension. As in other deformities of sagittal imbalance, the key to maintaining correction has proven to be the ability to center the plumb line from C7 over the sacrum (Fig. 14.18).

Occasionally the primary deformity from ankylosing spondylitis is in the thoracic spine. When possible it is preferable to perform a compensatory extension osteotomy through the lumbar region, because this is safer. If correction and stabilization through the thoracic spine is necessary, a two-stage procedure consisting of a first-stage anterior osteotomy and interbody fusion followed by posterior osteotomies with compression instrumentation is the preferred approach.

Kyphotic deformity of the cervical spine at the cervicothoracic junction is sometimes seen in the spondyloarthropathies. Most authors recommend performing surgery at this level under local anesthesia with the patient immobilized in a halo and in a sitting position. Osteotomy at the C7–T1 level is considered safest because the vertebral artery is anterior to the transverse processes at this level, and injury to the nerve root at risk, C8, is likely to cause less disability than at other cervical roots. Wide laminectomies from C6 to T2 with decompression and visualization of the C8 nerve root bilaterally and slow, controlled correction has proven safe and efficacious, as described by Simmons.[43]

With the evolution of newer techniques, whereby a spinal shortening procedure is performed, the correction of these crippling deformities has proven a viable undertaking. The complications of any spinal osteotomy, such as pseudarthrosis, neurological damage, dural laceration, and implant failure, also exist for this procedure; further particular attention should be paid to postoperative ileus, which is common in these patients and should be treated prophylactically with the institution of nasogastric drainage.

Thoracic Lordosis

Thoracic lordosis or hypokyphosis is most commonly seen in primary scoliotic deformities, and the surgical management of this condition consists of that described for scoliosis. The occasional patient is seen in whom primary thoracic lordosis leading to a decrease in chest volume necessitates treatment. Scoliotic deformities also exist in which the thoracic lordosis is a significant treatment consideration and is not addressed by the use of standard instrumentation techniques.

Treatment of thoracic lordosis can be through either a single-stage or two-stage technique. Single-stage posterior instrumentation and fusion with the L-rod system and sublaminar wires afford some correction of thoracic lordosis, but it is generally inadequate in the rigid adult spine when significant sagittal plane correction is necessary. Similarly, while adolescent patients with thoracic lordoscoliosis can be instrumented with the C–D system and, through rod rotation can achieve correction into thoracic kyphosis, the more rigid deformity with inadequate bone stock found in the adult makes this technique less reliable.

A combined technique has been described,[44] consisting of a first-stage anterior approach in which rib osteotomies at the posterior rib angle at multiple levels and multiple-level intervertebral discectomies are performed. This is followed by a posterior procedure in which similar rib osteotomies are performed on the opposite side and segmental sublaminar wires are used to pull the spine and the attached posterior rib cage to the prebent distraction by L-rods, creating thoracic kyphosis. This technique has proven useful in the treatment of patients having rigid thoracic lordosis greater than −30° and presenting with incipient or frank pulmonary dysfunction.

Postoperative Management

Other than in cases in which vertebrectomy is performed or in which spinal stability is believed to be severely compromised, the patients are allowed out of bed between stages to a bedside chair or with a walker. Most patients are out of bed within 2 to 3 days postoperatively and are allowed to begin walking. A standing mold is taken for a removable thoracolumbosacral orthosis (TLSO) which the patient wears fulltime except when in bed or in the shower. Adult patients with good bone stock who are believed to have been rigidly fixed with a C–D implant are occasionally managed postoperatively without an orthosis. However, most patients treated with the C–D system, and all patients treated with Luque or Harrington instrumentation, are advised to wear a brace after surgery.

Traction is rarely used between stages as it has not been found to lead to increased curve correction. The occasional patient with paralytic scoliosis and significantly diminished pulmonary function may be managed by preoperative halo-wheelchair traction to optimize respiratory capacity, which is then continued between stages. Patients are usually discharged 7 to 10 days after surgery. Walking 1 to 2 miles is encouraged in the early postoperative period. If roentgenograms show the implant to be in satisfactory condition with no loss of correction, patients are allowed to return to work 2 to 4 months after surgery, as well as to resume sexual activities.

Conclusions

The spectrum of adult spinal deformities is varied, but several common threads may be seen in these difficult problems. In an increasingly older patient population, it is imperative to adequately evaluate the patient's preoperative medical condition as well as to exhaust all possibilities for conservative management. The indications for surgery in any given case need to be carefully evaluated and compared to the sometimes disappointing results and complications seen in these conditions. Reliance on newer implants to compensate for inadequate preoperative planning, lack of attention to the complex three-plane deformities seen, or failure to carry out meticulous fusion techniques are factors contributing to certain failure. On the other hand, many adults with complex spinal deformities may be helped with the new techniques available to the spinal surgeon.

References

1. Lowe TG. Report of the Morbidity and Mortality Committee, Scoliosis Research Society, 1987.
2. Collis DK, Ponseti IV. Long-term follow-up of patients with idiopathic scoliosis not treated surgically. J Bone Joint Surg 1969;51A:425.
3. Fowles JV, Drummond DS, l'Ecuyers S, Roy L, Kassab MT. Untreated scoliosis in the adult. Clin Orthop 1978;134:212.
4. Nachemson A. Adult scoliosis and back pain. Spine 1979;4:513.
5. Kostuik JP, Bentivoglio J. The incidence of low-back pain in adult scoliosis. Spine 1981;6:268.
6. Jackson RP, Simmons EH, Stripinis D. Incidence and severity of back pain in adult idiopathic scoliosis. Spine 1983;8:749.
7. Bradford DS. Adult scoliosis: current concepts of treatment. Clin Orthop 1988;229:70.
8. Cotrel Y. New Instrumentation for Surgery of the Spine. London: Freund, 1986.
9. Kostuik JP, Israel J, Hall JE. Scoliosis surgery in adults. Clin Orthop 1973;93:225.
10. Swank S, Lonstein JE, Moe JH, Winter RB, Bradford DS. Surgical treatment of adult scoliosis. A review of two-hundred and twenty-two cases. J Bone Joint Surg 1981;63A:268.
11. Van Dam BE, Bradford DS, Lonstein JE, Moe JH, Ogilvie JW, Winter RB. Adult idiopathic scoliosis treated by posterior spinal fusion and Harrington instrumentation. Spine 1987;12:32.
12. Byrd JA, Scoles PV, Winter RB, Bradford DS, Lonstein JE, Moe JH. Adult idiopathic scoliosis treated by anterior and posterior spinal fusion. J Bone Joint Surg 1987;69A:843.
13. Bradford DS. Vertebral column resection. Presented at the Annual Meeting of the American Orthopaedic Association, Hot Springs, Virginia, 1986.
14. Steel HH. Rib resection and spine fusion in the correction of convex deformity in scoliosis. J Bone Joint Surg 1983;65A:920.
15. Moe JH, Purcell GA, Bradford DS. Zielke instrumentation (VDS) for the correction of spinal curvature. Clin Orthop 1983;180:133.
16. Epstein JA, Epstein BS, Jones MD. Symptomatic lumbar scoliosis with degenerative changes in the elderly. Spine 1979;4:542.
17. Simmons EH, Jackson RP. The management of nerve root entrapment syndromes associated with the collapsing scoliosis of idiopathic lumbar and thoracolumbar curves. Spine 1979;4:533.
18. Vanderpool DW, James JIP, Wynne-Davies R. Scoliosis in the elderly. J Bone Joint Surg 1969;51A:446.
19. Robin GC, Span Y, Steinberg R, Makin M, Menczel J. Scoliosis in the elderly. A follow-up study. Spine 1982;7:355.
20. Grubb SA, Lipscomb HJ, Coonrad RW. Collapsing degenerative scoliosis. Presented at the Annual Meeting of the Scoliosis Research Society, Vancouver, British Columbia, 1987.
21. King HA, Moe JH, Bradford DS, Winter RB. The selection of fusion levels in thoracic idiopathic scoliosis. J Bone Joint Surg 1983;65A:1302.
22. Steenaert BA. Posterior spinal fusion including the sacrum in scoliosis. J Bone Joint Surg 1981;63B:289.
23. Balderston RA, Winter RB, Moe JH, Bradford DS, Lonstein JE. Fusion to the sacrum for nonparalytic scoliosis in the adult. Spine 1986;11:824.
24. Allen BL, Ferguson RL. The Galveston technique for L-rod instrumentation of the scoliotic spine. Spine 1982;7:119.
25. Roy-Camille R, Saillant G, Mazel C. Internal fixation of the lumbar spine with pedicle screw plating. Clin Orthop 1986;203:7.
26. Steffee AD, Biscup RS, Sitkowski DJ. Segmental spine plates with pedicle screw fixation. A new internal fixation device for disorders of the lumbar and thoracolumbar spine. Clin Orthop 1986;203:45.
27. Ponder RC, Dickson JH, Harrington PR, Erwin WD. Results of Harrington instrumentation and fusion in the adult idiopathic scoliosis patient. J Bone Joint Surg 1975;57A:797.
28. Sponseller PD, Cohen MS, Nachemson Al, Hall JF, Wohl MEB. Results of surgical treatment of adults with idiopathic scoliosis. J Bone Joint Surg 1987;69A:667.
29. Kostuik JP, Sano S, Okada A. Surgical treatment of spinal deformities in persons over the age of fifty. Presented at the Annual Meeting of the Scoliosis Research Society, Vancouver, British Columbia, 1987.
30. Cummine JL, Lonstein JE, Moe JH, Winter RB, Bradford DS. Reconstructive surgery in the adult for failed scoliosis fusion. J Bone Joint Surg 1979;61A:1151.
31. Lauerman WC, Bradford DS, Transfeldt ET, Moe JH, Ogilvie JW. Results of treatment of pseudarthrosis after scoliosis fusion. Unpublished data, 1987.
32. Floman Y, Penny JN, Micheli LF, Riseborough EJ, Hall JE. Osteotomy of the fusion mass in scoliosis. J Bone Joint Surg 1982;64A:1307–1316.
33. Lagrone MO, Bradford DS, Moe JH, Lonstein JE, Winter RB, Ogilvie JW. Treatment of symptomatic flatback following spine fusion. J Bone Joint Surg 1988;70A(4):569.
34. Moe JH, Denis F. The iatrogenic loss of lumbar lordosis. Orthop Trans 1977;1(2):131.
35. Bradford DS, Garcia A. Neurologic complications in Scheuermann's disease. J Bone Joint Surg 1969;51A:567.
36. Winter RB, Moe JH, Wang JF. Congenital kyphosis. J Bone Joint Surg 1973;55A:223.
37. Coscia MF, Bradford DS, Ogilvie JW. Scheuermann's kyphosis: results in 19 cases treated by spinal arthrodesis and L-rod instrumentation. Presented at the Annual Meeting of the Scoliosis Research Society, Vancouver, British Columbia, 1987.

38. Bradford DS. Ankylosing spondylitis. In: Bradford DS, Lonstein JE, Moe JH, Ogilvie JW, Winter RB, eds. Moe's Textbook of Scoliosis and Other Spinal Deformities. Philadelphia: Saunders, 1987:628.
39. Smith-Petersen MN, Larson CB, Aufranc OE. Osteotomy of the spine for correction of flexion deformity in rheumatoid arthritis. J Bone Joint Surg 1945;27A:1.
40. Law WA. Osteotomy of the spine. Clin Orthop 1969;66:70.
41. Bradford DS, Schumacher WL, Lonstein JE, Winter RB. Ankylosing spondylitis: experience in surgical management of 21 patients. Spine 1987;12:238.
42. McMaster MJ. A technique for lumbar spinal osteotomy in ankylosing spondylitis. J Bone Joint Surg 1985;67B:204.
43. Simmons EH. Kyphotic deformity of the spine in ankylosing spondylitis. Clin Orthop 1977;128:65.
44. Bradford DS, Blatt JM, Rosp FL. Surgical management of severe thoracic lordosis: a new technique to restore normal kyphosis. Spine 1983;8:420.

V
Postoperative Management

15

Imaging of Spinal Fusions

Joel W. Yeakley and John H. Harris, Jr.

Spinal fusions are used as a stabilization method in various types of spinal pathology including trauma, discogenic disease, congenital disorders, infection, and neoplasia.[1,2,3] Imaging of spinal fusions presents a challenging problem in view of the multiple types of fusion that use the different approaches and fusion materials discussed elsewhere in this volume.

The current concern over cost-effectiveness in modern medicine emphasizes that a choice must be made regarding the type of imaging procedure or procedures that will demonstrate the effectiveness of the fusion. Choosing the "best" method of evaluating any particular fusion requires close collaboration between the orthopaedic surgeon and radiologist.

Commonly used imaging methods for evaluation of spinal fusions include the following:

1. Plain radiographs, including lateral flexion/extension or bending views
2. Fluoroscopy with videotape monitoring
3. Polytomography
4. Myelography
5. Computed tomography (CT), including three-dimensional reformation (3DCT)
6. Magnetic resonance imaging (MRI)
7. Single photon emission computed tomography (SPECT) and other radionuclide techniques.[4]

Postfusion sequelae that may be related to the "failed" fusion syndrome include the following:[5–12]

1. Extrusion of a bony plug posteriorly or posterolaterally from the disc space into the spinal canal or neural foramen, respectively
2. Failure of fusion with pseudarthrosis and/or acquired spondylolysis
3. Spinal stenosis
4. Infection with osteomyelitis
5. Arachnoidal adhesion and/or epidural fibrosis[13]
6. Displacement of orthopaedic implants.

The choice of the imaging modality used in the evaluation of a fusion may depend on the type of abnormality suspected clinically.

Plain Film Studies

All imaging examinations of spinal fusions, regardless of the age of the fusions, should begin with plain-film studies in the frontal and lateral projections. "Cone-down" views in the specific area of the fusion provide better skeletal definition. Oblique views may be necessary, especially in the lumbar area. A "baseline" plain film examination should be obtained as soon postoperatively as the patient's condition permits. This becomes the comparison film for all follow-up examinations. Plain film studies are suited to evaluation of spinal fusion because they are the easiest to obtain and can be used in the presence of any type of orthopaedic implant. They are also best suited for comparison purposes because of the ease of reproducibility of patient position. In addition, the cost of the examination is minimal when compared to many of the other methods used to evaluate fusion. Plain radiographs will often demonstrate abnormal gas within soft tissues or focal osseous resorption indicative of infection, as well as displacement of graft material or orthopaedic implants. At the same time, plain films provide an indication of bony union of the fusion mass to underlying vertebral elements.

Flexion/Extension or Bending Views

Routine plain film radiographs provide only static information regarding the status of the fusion. Instability at the fusion site can only be confirmed by demonstration of

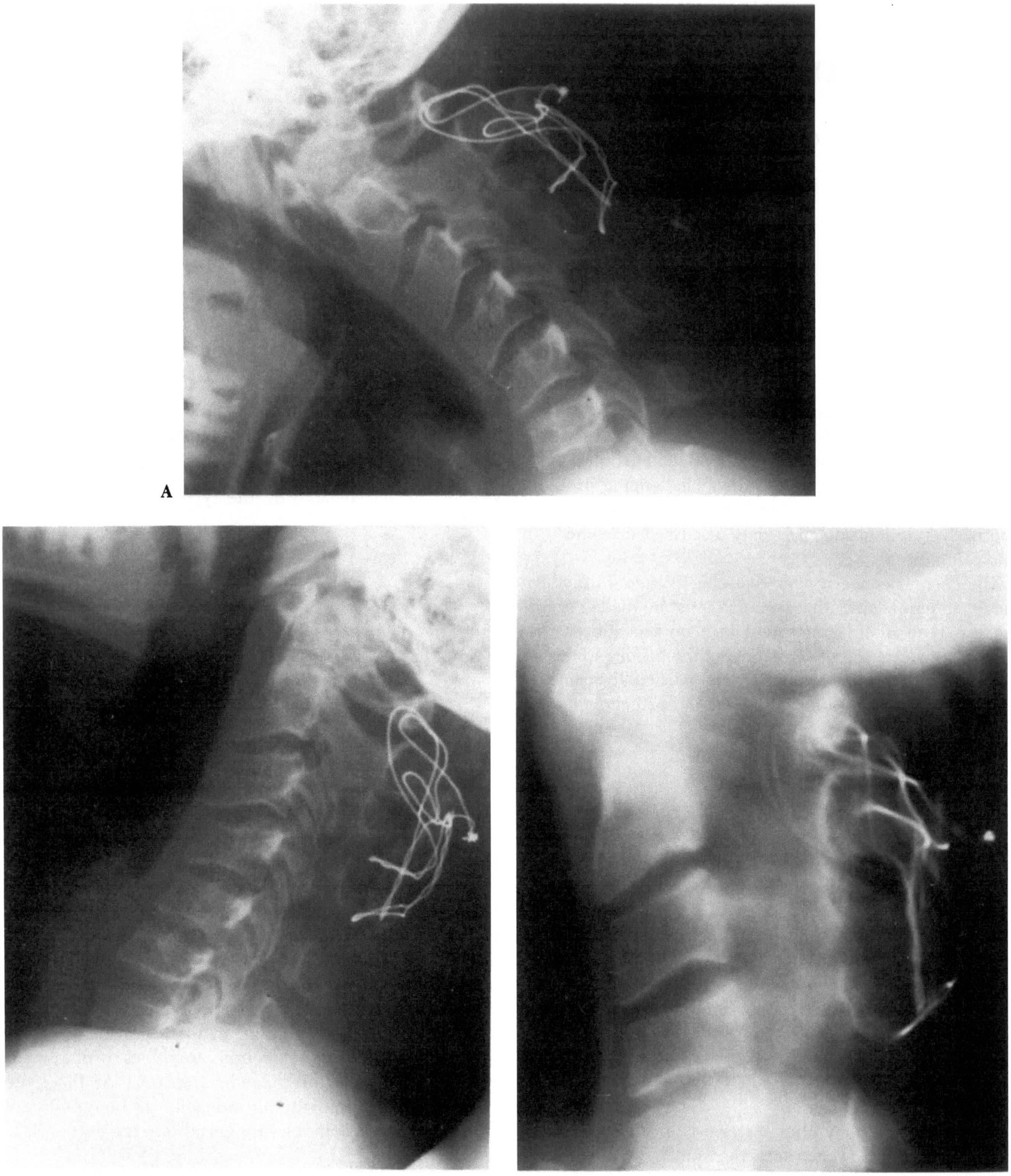

A B C

Figure 15.1. Type II odontoid fracture. After posterior wire fusion of C1–C4, stability is demonstrated on lateral flexion (**A**) and extension (**B**) views. Lateral polytomography (**C**) performed soon after fusion procedure reveals wire fusion posteriorly is well seen despite "ghost" artifacts. Odontoid fracture itself is not yet fused.

change in position of the involved vertebrae or a change in the relative position of the components of the fusion mass during flexion/extension lateral projections or lateral bending views. Flexion/extension or bending views performed with voluntary self-positioning of the patient evaluate both stability and the voluntary range of motion through the fusion area (Fig. 15.1). If, for whatever reason, the patient voluntarily splints the area of the spine being examined during the motion studies, a false-negative examination may be obtained in the presence of a "failed fusion." It is particularly important the radiologist and/or surgeon personally instruct the patient in the necessary maneuvers to "stress" the area of the spine during the examination and personally supervise the examination so that patient motion does not exceed pain threshold.

Fluoroscopy with Videotape Monitoring

Flexion/extension or bending examination may be obtained during fluoroscopic examination, with "spot" filming obtained in any desired position. This technique affords optimum patient positioning to demonstrate the fusion graft and its relation to the vertebral elements. Any motion at the fusion site can be observed and recorded on videotape for subsequent review, analysis, and treatment planning. These dynamic sequences may be replayed as necessary without further radiation to the patient.

Polytomography

Polytomography has been traditionally used in the evaluation of fusion procedures[14,15] with sections of 1.5-, 3-, or 5.0-mm thickness obtained in an anteroposterior (coronal), lateral (sagittal), or oblique projections. Polydirectional tomography may also be performed with the patient in lateral flexed and/or extended position. The high resolution at the level of the tomographic "slice" plane affords exquisite detail of the bony components of the fusion and the relation of the fusion mass to the posterior vertebral elements. The extent and degree of bony fusion, bony overgrowth, and the presence and extent of fractures or fusion failure within the fusion mass are all clearly delineated by polytomography. In areas where bony bridging may appear incomplete, it is generally not possible to distinguish between nonunion and fibrous union with polytomography. However, polytomography has the advantage of producing useful images in the presence of metallic plates, screws, wires, Harrington rods, or other metallic fixation devices or prostheses. Although "ghost" images may be formed by these structures, they can usually be sorted out from the desired bony detail (Fig. 15.2). Remember that some degree of magnification is inherent in polydirectional tomography. Although inclusion of the entire length of the fusion in each tomographic plane is possible, three-dimensional relationships require mental integration of the coronal and sagittal images.

Myelography

Although myelography is not routinely used in the evaluation of spinal fusions, it has unique applications in the evaluation of the spinal canal and cerebrospinal fluid (CSF) spaces. Spinal fluid leaks or pseudomeningocele formation may be accurately defined by myelography. Impingement on the spinal thecal sac by metallic fixation devices, fusion mass, fusion overgrowth, or postoperative hematoma is clearly defined by myelography. Arachnoidal adhesion can also be defined as distortion of the thecal sac and matting or adherence of nerve roots. Myelography can be used in patients in whom metallic fixation devices may cause excessive artifact with other modalities such as CT, and may be performed in association with polytomography if necessary.

Computed Tomography

Computed tomography (CT) has become popular in recent years for the evaluation of spinal fusions.[6,9,14,16,18–20] Axial sections with reformatting in multiple planes selected to optionally demonstrate the fusion mass have resulted in increased accuracy in predicting fusion. The thinner the axial sections, the better the reformatted images. In other words, 5-mm or 10-mm axial sections will not provide nearly as accurate reformatted images as 3-mm axial sections. However, the thinner sections limit the length of spine that can be evaluated by CT because of increased imaging time, tube overheating with excessive number of sections, and greater patient radiation exposure. The area to be examined must therefore be specifically delineated by the attending physician or radiologist based on plain radiographic findings to shorten the time of examination and minimize patient radiation dose.

CT examinations are generally more expensive than polytomographic studies. However, CT allows the patient to remain in only one position (usually supine) during the examination whereas polytomography requires different positioning for each plane of examination. CT also requires a much shorter examination time than polytomography, which is important for patients who become uncomfortable after long periods of time in one position.

Although metallic fixation devices degrade CT images because of "streak" artifacts, detail sufficient to evaluate anatomical alignment and to assess impingement on the

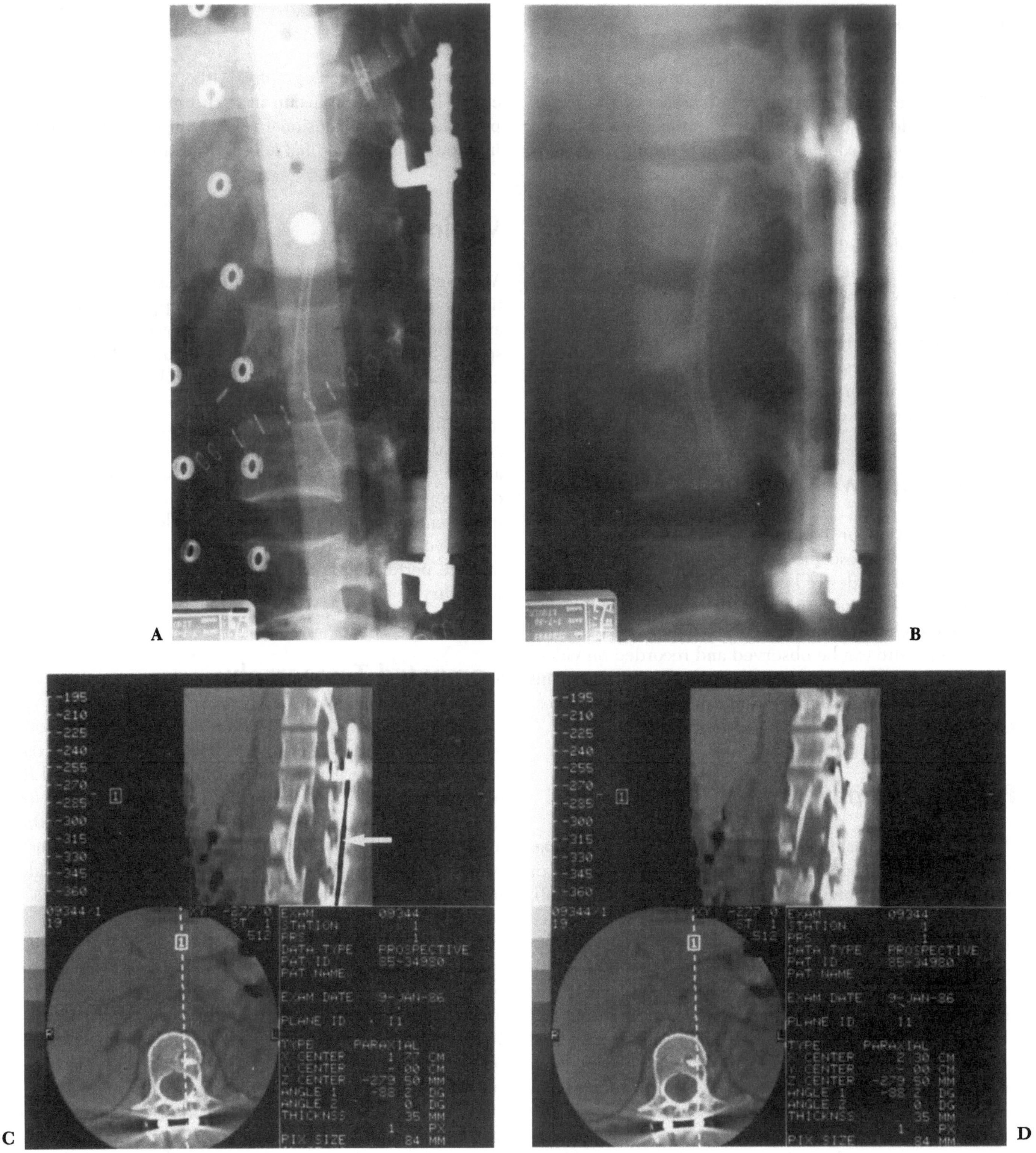

Figure 15.2. Harrington rod T12–L4 with rib graft L1–L3. **A.** Lateral plain radiograph shows Harrington rod and rib graft in place in this patient after L2 burst fracture. **B.** Lateral polytomograph demonstrates position of rib graft from L1–L3 despite ghost images from rods. Note partial resection of L2. **C.** Sagittal reformatted CT shows rib graft well despite black image void artifact from Harrington rod (*arrow*). **D.** Sagittal reformatted CT shows position of Harrington rod and its relation to bony elements despite artifact. **E.** Coronal reformatted CT shows rib graft spanning L1–L3 and partial resection of L2. Distortion of rib graft is from partial section phenomenon. **F.** Final result after removal of Harrington rod shows interbody fusion between L1–L3 despite fractures in rib graft (*arrows*) and some angulation at L1–L2 level.

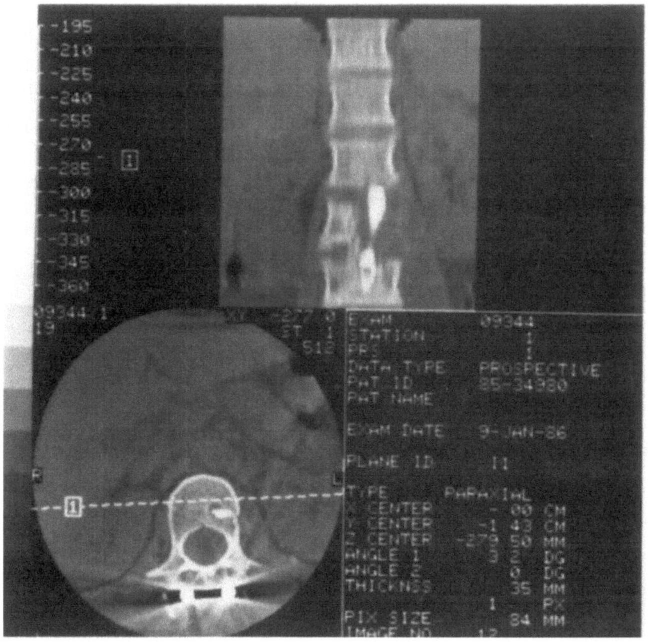

E

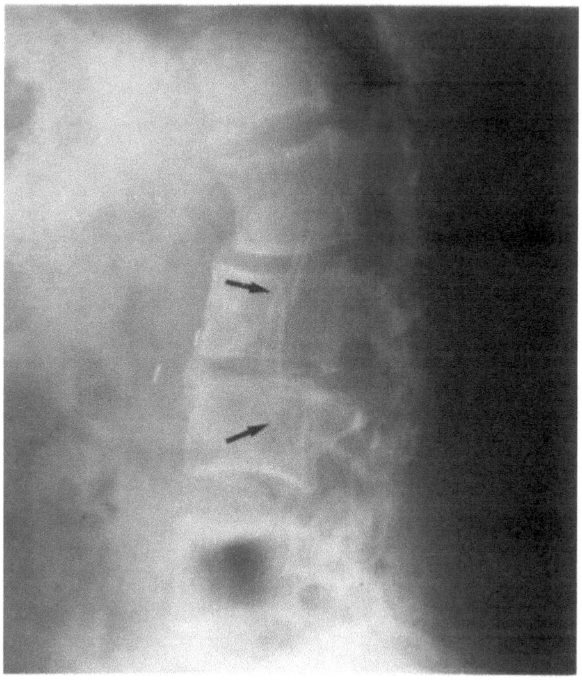
F

Figure 15.2

spinal canal can usually be obtained (Figs. 15.2 and 15.3). Estimation of intrathecal contrast within the spinal canal may be limited by streak artifacts in the presence of metallic fixation devices, however. Harrington rods, Luque devices, and other posterior metallic fixation devices usually produce artifacts that extend lateral to the fixation device while still allowing evaluation of the spinal canal anteriorly (Figs. 15.2 and 15.3). It should be remembered that reformatted images are only as good as the axial images from which they are derived. Thus if artifacts degrade the area of interest in axial views, the reformatted images will also show degraded detail in that area. Fortunately, the worst streak artifacts may lie outside the desired reformatted plane.

In the absence of metallic artifact, axial images give excellent information regarding the bony spinal canal. Although not routinely obtained, axial CT views in flexion and extension may provide additional information regarding the stability of fusions in certain areas such as the craniocervical junction. A few axial sections in flexion and extension may be compared for atlantoaxial subluxation with position changes and thus evaluate posterior fusion procedures aimed at stabilizing this area. As previously mentioned, metallic objects such as wires commonly employed in posterior cervical fusions may result in artifactually degraded images.

Areas of discontinuity between the fusion mass and the underlying vertebrae or within the fusion mass itself are, by themselves, not evidence of a "failed" fusion (Fig. 15.4). Fibrous union produces a similar lucent defect. Incomplete fusion or fusion failure should be established by demonstration of change in position of vertebrae or mass components with changes in patient position. Lucent areas in the fusion caused by infection or pseudarthroses may be better defined by SPECT or MRI, as is discussed subsequently.

CT is particularly valuable in the assessment of postoperative spinal stenosis caused by impingement of the postoperative fusion mass on the bony spinal canal or fusion overgrowth.[14] Axial CT sections uniquely and accurately define the bony spinal canal and also neural foramina in the absence of scoliosis. The status of the thecal sac can be simultaneously defined following administration of intrathecal water-soluble contrast medium. The fusion mass may necessitate the administration of intrathecal contrast medium at a site remote from the area of interest, however. As an example, a large bony fusion in the lumbar area might prohibit lumbar puncture and would therefore require lateral C1–2 puncture as a route for intrathecal contrast medium administration.[21] The contrast material must then be maneuvered to the lumbar area by proper patient positioning.

Arachnoidal adhesion is well defined by CT following intrathecal water-soluble contrast medium administration. Epidural fibrosis and scarring may also be identified by CT, but intravenous (IV) contrast may be required to differentiate this from recurrent or residual disc herniation when a fusion procedure has been associated with discectomy.

In certain cases, three-dimensional CT reformation

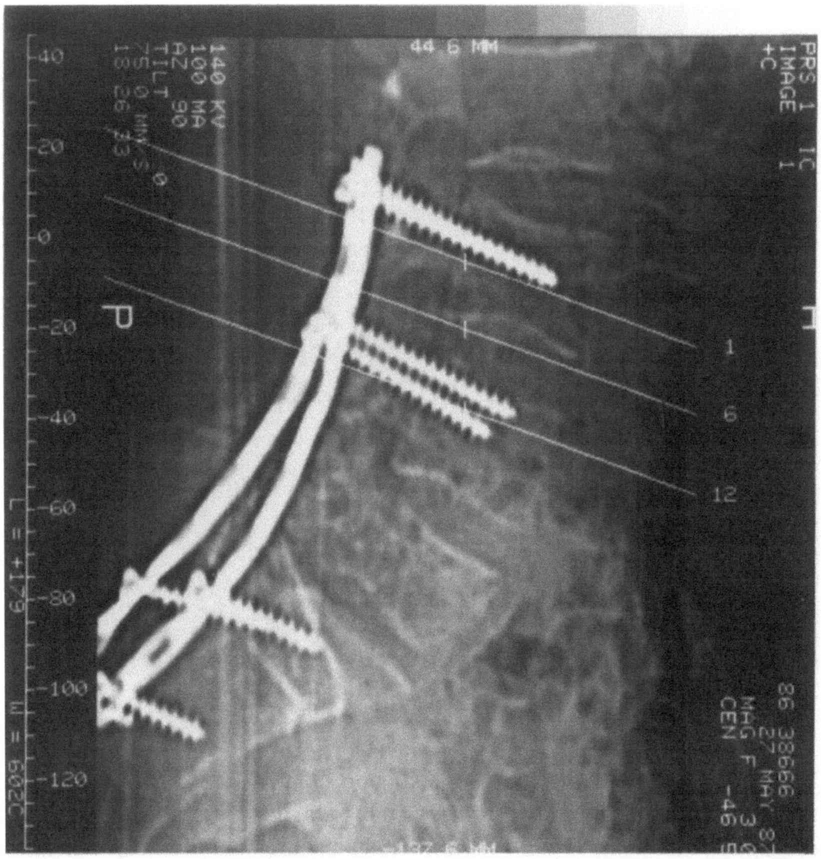

A

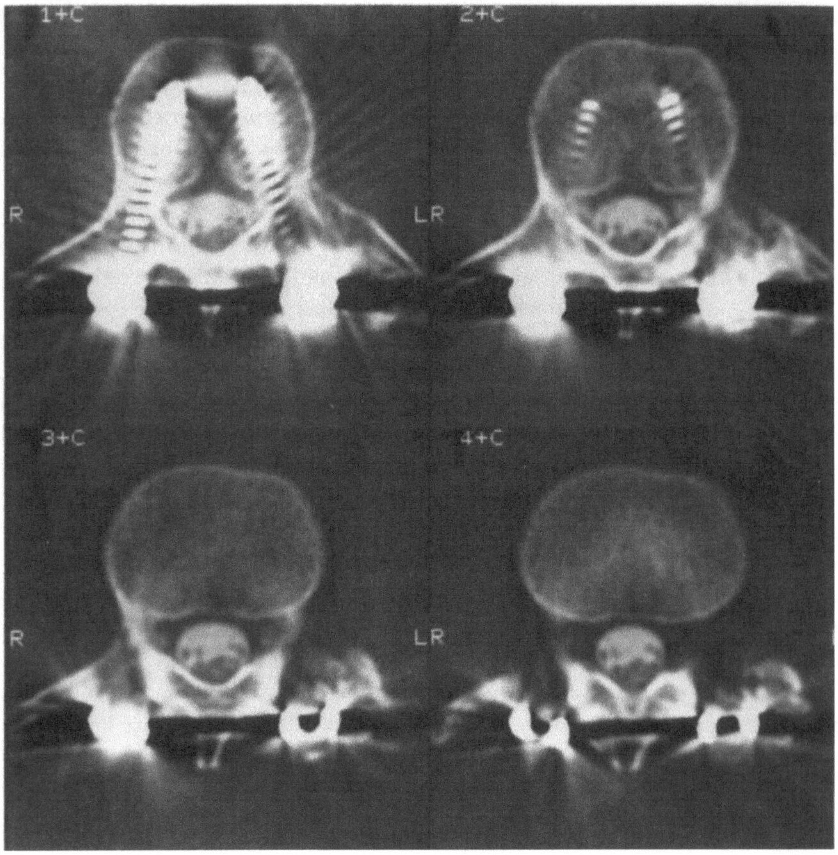

B

Figure 15.3. L3 through S2 fusion using orthopaedic plates with screws. **A.** Lateral digital image shows position of plate and screws. **B.** CT scan following water-soluble contrast material medium shows proper positioning of pedicular screws, and reveals detail of thecal sac and nerve roots despite streak artifact.

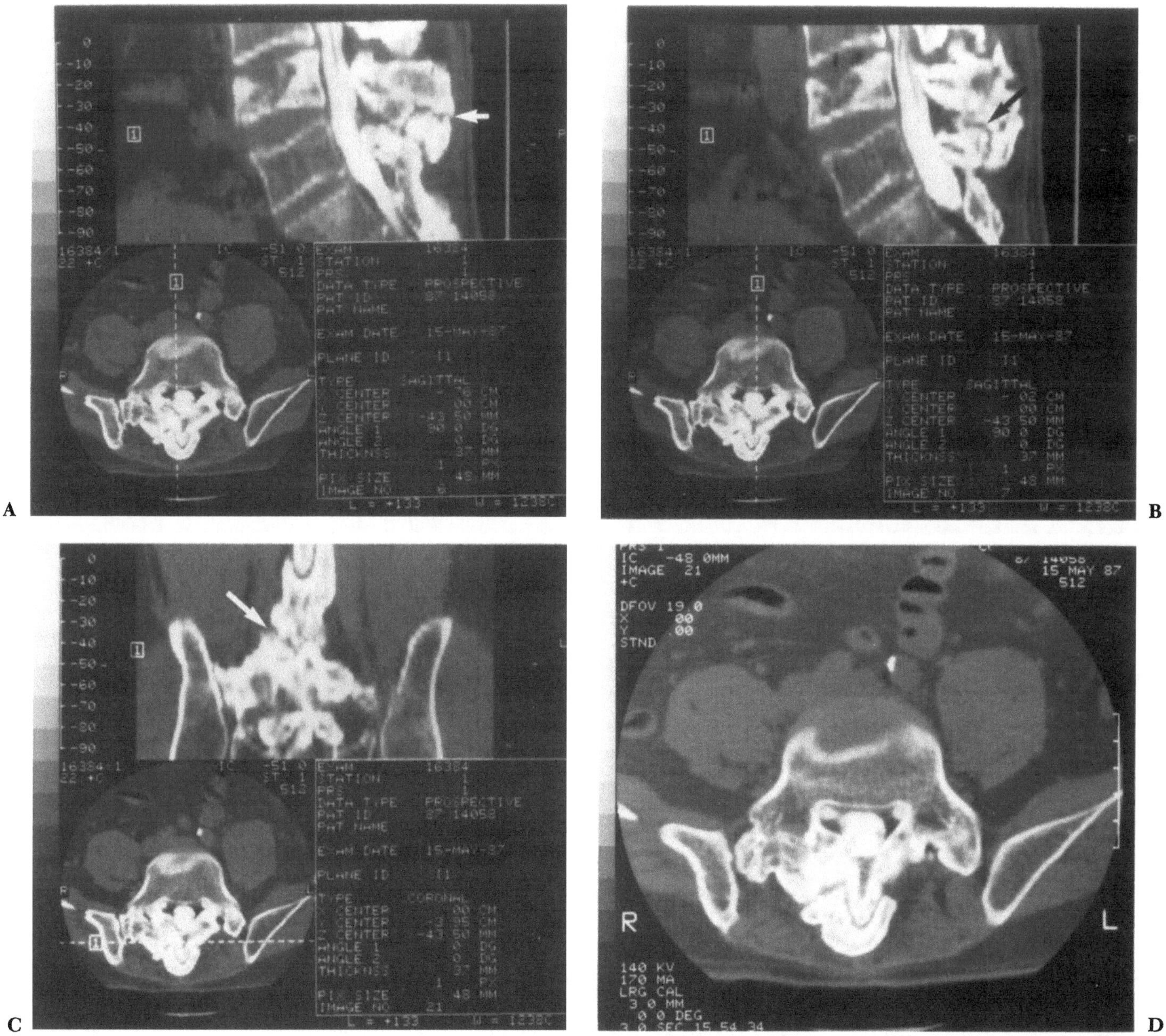

Figure 15.4. Possible fibrous union L4–L5. **A.** Sagittal reformatted CT slightly to right of midline confirms gaps in bony fusion mass at L4–L5 (*arrow*). There appears to be bony bridging across L5–S1. Note distortion of previously fractured L4. **B.** Sagittal reformatted CT slightly to left of midline shows additional gaps in fusion mass at L4–L5. **C.** Coronal reformatted CT shows gaps in fusion mass (*arrow*) at L4–L5, but apparent solid bony fusion at L5–S1 on right. **D.** Axial CT demonstrates gaps in fusion mass near L4–L5 interspace. Although this could represent fibrous union, stability on motion views and lack of abnormal uptake through this area on SPECT scans would be necessary to demonstrate fusion and lack of pseudojoint formation respectively (see text).

(3DCT)[16,22] may be superior to axial CT with sagittal and coronal reformations because of the vastly superior spatial relationships provided by three-dimensional display of the numerically integrated axial CT data (Fig. 15.5). In 3D images, spatial relationships are all clearly discernible by all observers. Further, the 3D images may be rotated in any plane or to any degree, or tilted in any angle along the X, Y, and Z axes. The images can be numerically bisected along any plane so that the interior of the spinal canal can be viewed "from within." Portions of the spinal canal or fusion mass that might obscure other areas may be electronically deleted to provide unobstructed views

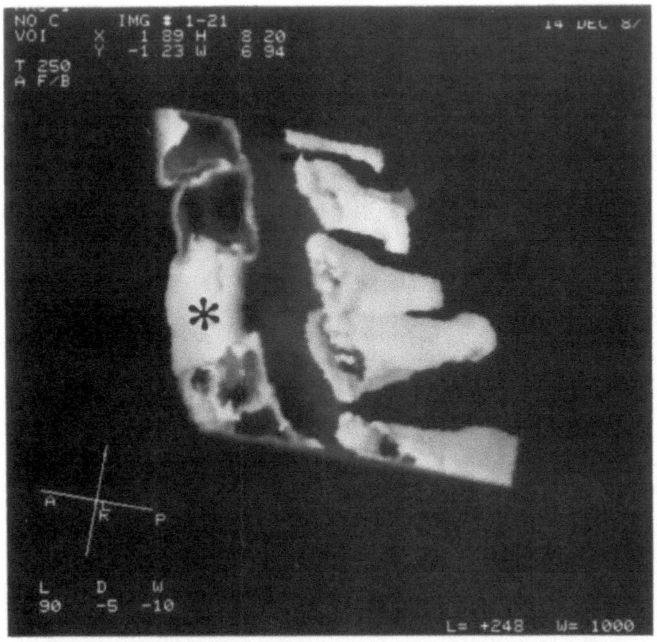

A

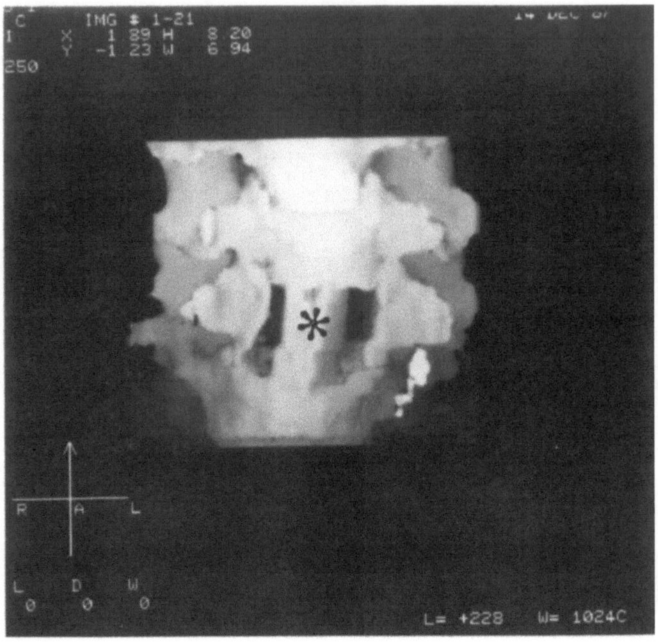

B

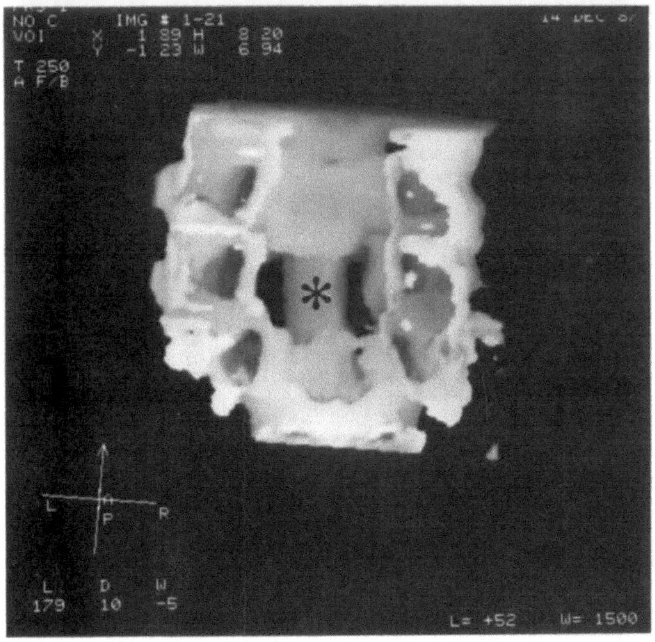

C

Figure 15.5. 3DCT of cervical spine interbody fusion. 3DCT shows proper positioning of interbody bone graft of C5–C7. Lateral (**A**), anterior (**B**), and posterior views (**C**) demonstrate relationship of graft (asterisk) to vertebral elements and spinal canal.

of the fusion components and their relationship to the underlying vertebral segments (Fig. 15.5). As with conventional reformatted images in CT, the three-dimensional reformation is obtained from the axial CT data and requires no additional patient radiation once the axial images have been performed. In the evaluation of posterior and anterior fusions of the spine, 3DCT is able to identify small areas of nonunion when the results of axial and reformatted CT imaging are equivocal.[22]

Magnetic Resonance Imaging

The applications of magnetic resonance imaging (MRI) in the spine have grown enormously during the last few years, especially after the introduction of high-field strength (1.5-T) superconducting magnets and surface coils. While MRI offers the advantage of multiplanar imaging without changing the position of the patient, it has the disadvantage of poor definition of compact cortical bone because of a relative lack of proton content. The cortical bony structures therefore show up as areas of relative absence of signal intensity and appear very black on MR images. The configuration of the compact bone must be inferred from these areas of relative lack of signal. Marrow containing cancellous bone is better defined because of the fatty marrow it contains rather than the actual bony components.

Preliminary experience suggests that these facts may be useful in the imaging fusions. Fragment-onlay-graft or bone-chip types of fusions tend to reorganize into cortical and cancellous elements over a period of time, and if continuity of the marrow signal through a mature graft can be defined, then fusion is present (Fig. 15.6). Ankylosis of the apophyseal joints or relative lack thereof can be defined. MRI should be sensitive to the formation of fractures, pseudojoints, or areas of infection in a fusion mass if there is sufficient edema or fluid in these areas to be

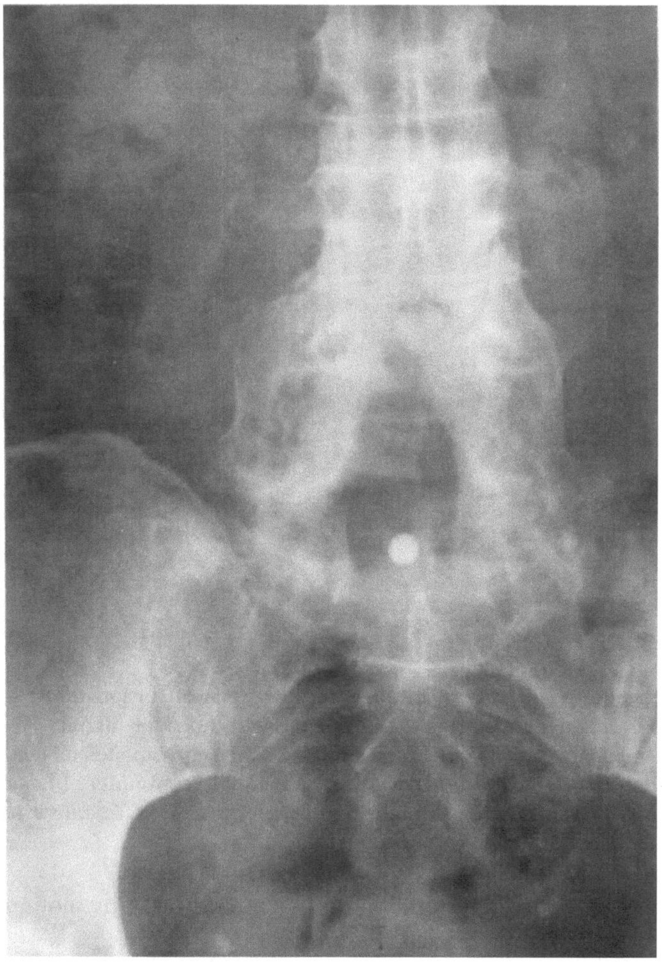

A

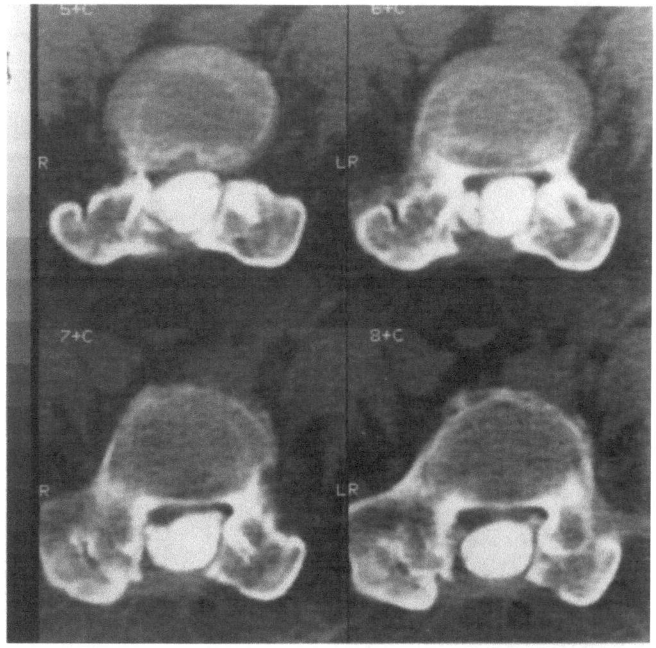

B

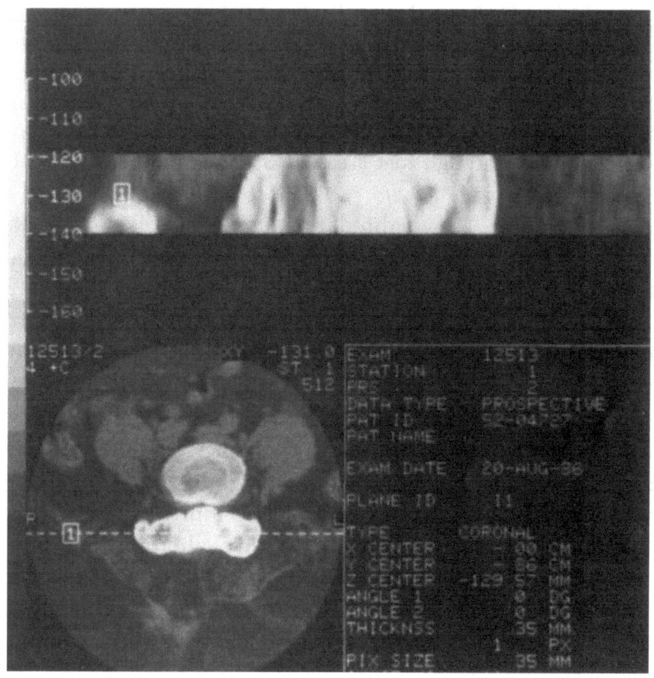

C

Figure 15.6. Lumbar fusion. **A.** Plain radiograph shows fusion spanning L4–L5–S1. **B.** Axial CT shows solid fusion across the L4–L5 area. Note continuity of bone marrow through fused area and ankylosis of facet joints. **C.** Coronal reformatted CT shows solid fusion across L4–L5 area. (Continued)

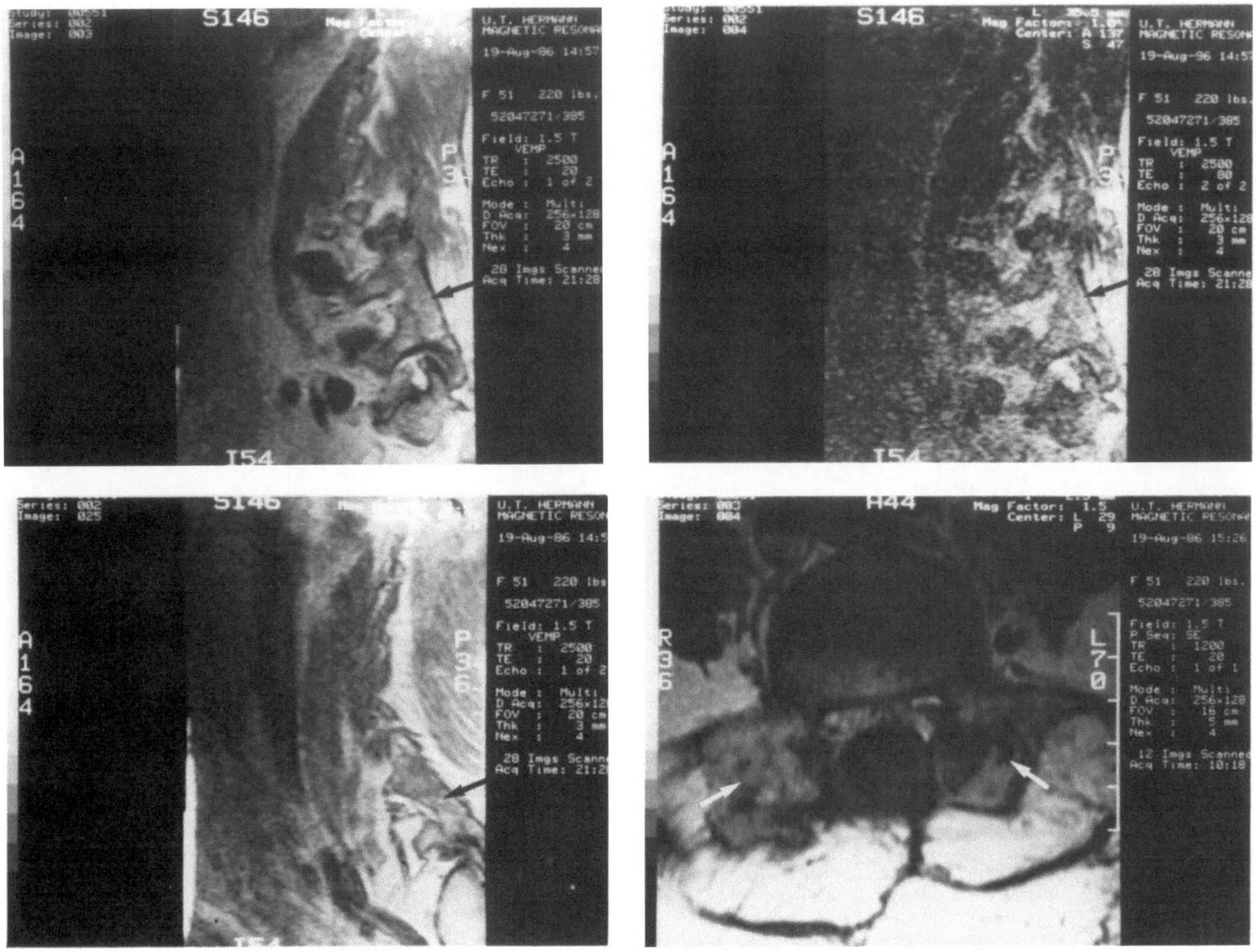

D E F G

Figure 15.6. **D.** Sagittal spin density MRI shows continuity of bone marrow and cortex (*arrow*) across left side of L4–L5 indicating solid fusion. Note lack of ankylosis of left L5–S1 facet joint. **E.** T2-weighted sagittal MR across L4–L5 shows no abnormal high signal intensity through area of fusion mass (*arrow*), confirming continuity through that area. **F.** Sagittal spin-density MRI through right side of fusion indicates apparent fusion through L5–S1 on right as well as through L4–L5 on right (*arrow*). **G.** Axial spin-density MRI through L4–L5 area corresponds in location to axial CT scan shown in **B.** Again note continuity of bone marrow and cortex through fused area, as well as ankylosis of the facet joints (*arrows*).

recognized on T2-weighted images. Lack of continuity of the marrow signal or cortical component through a fusion might also be helpful in that regard.

With special techniques, dynamic MRI motion studies in certain areas such as the cervical spine have become possible. This not only allows evaluation of the fusion stability, but shows the effect of motion on neural structures such as the spinal cord. Recently, a thin flexible surface coil, which permits flexion and extension MRI views, has been used in "whiplash" injuries,[23] and this technique should be applicable to the evaluation of certain types of fusions in the cervical spine as well. Because fibrous tissue has low signal intensity (dark) on virtually all types of currently obtained MR images, fibrous union can be inferred if stability can be demonstrated by motion views (see Fig. 15.7).

While preliminary experience regarding the use of MR in the imaging of spinal fusions is encouraging, its exact role is not yet established, as present experience is somewhat limited. MRI has been determined to be helpful in the definition of arachnoidal adhesion and epidural fibrosis, which may contribute to "failed" back surgery syndrome.[17,24] Arachnoidal adhesions may be identified without intrathecal contrast. Epidural fibrosis may be recognized without contrast, but is perhaps better seen after intravenous gadolinium diethylenetriaminepentaacetic acid (DPTA) administration, which causes "enhancement" of scar tissue much like IV contrast on CT.

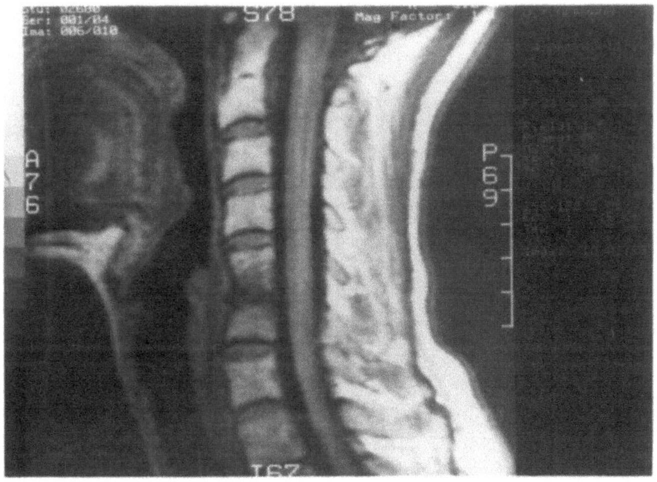
A

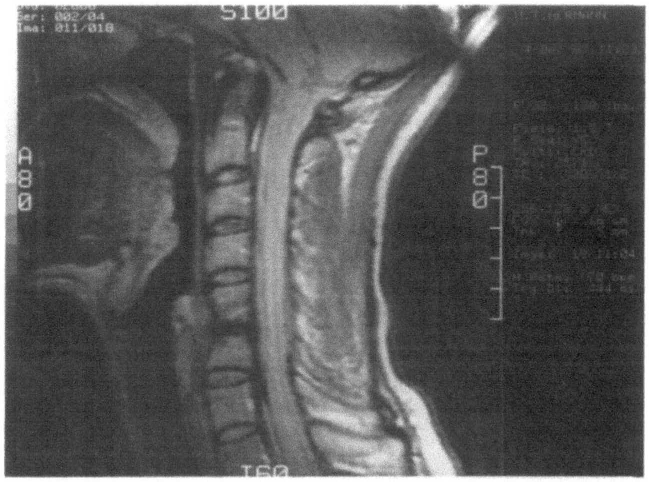
B

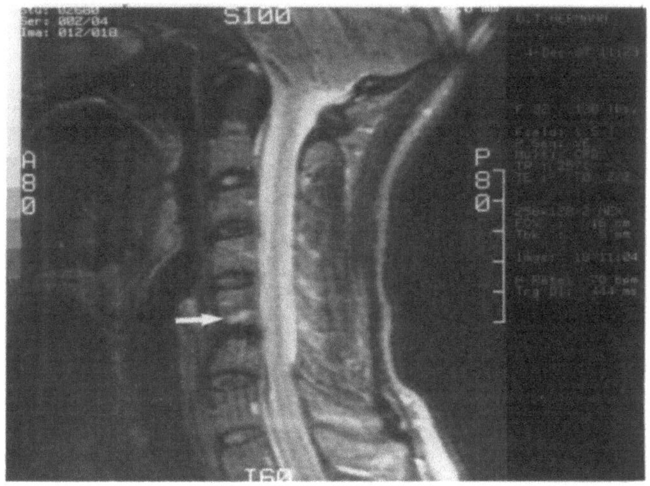
C

Figure 15.7. Fibrous union C5–C6. **A.** T1-weighted sagittal MRI shows fibrous union across C5–C6 stable on motion views. **B.** Spin-density MRI of same area. Low signal intensity is seen through area of the obliterated disc. **C.** T2-weighted sagittal MRI confirms low signal intensity through fibrous union at disc space level. Small area of high signal intensity (*arrow*) in C5 vertebral body may represent small area of edema.

MRI is sensitive in the definition of vertebral discitis/osteomylitis, which may occur when fusion procedures are associated with discectomy. On T1-weighted images there is confluent decreased signal intensity from the vertebral bodies and intervertebral disc space, with an inability to discern a margin between the disc and adjacent vertebral body. On T2-weighted images, there is increased signal intensity from the vertebral bodies adjacent to the involved disc, and an increased signal intensity from within the region of the disc itself. The increased signal from the disc area has an abnormal configuration and is of greater intensity than the usual signal of the normal disc.[25]

MRI has the disadvantage of large field distortion and signal void artifacts in the presence of metallic fixation devices, making its usefulness limited or doubtful in the presence of these objects. One also has to be concerned with possible heat generation in the presence of large metallic objects such as prostheses.

SPECT

SPECT[26] stands for single-photon emission-computed tomography and is a radionuclide technique requiring a special tomographic gamma camera. Pseudojoints are visualized as areas of increased radionuclide uptake in suspicious areas that may not be recognized on plain (nontomographic) radionuclide techniques[27] (Fig. 15.8). Other radionuclide techniques such as gallium-67 or indium-111 leukocyte studies may be helpful in pinpointing areas of suspected infection spinal fusions.

In summary, there are many useful techniques for the evaluation of spinal fusions. The "best" technique or techniques for any individual post-fusion condition will be best determined through close communication between the surgeon and radiologist, and may depend on the type of fusion performed as well as the type of the sequelae expected.

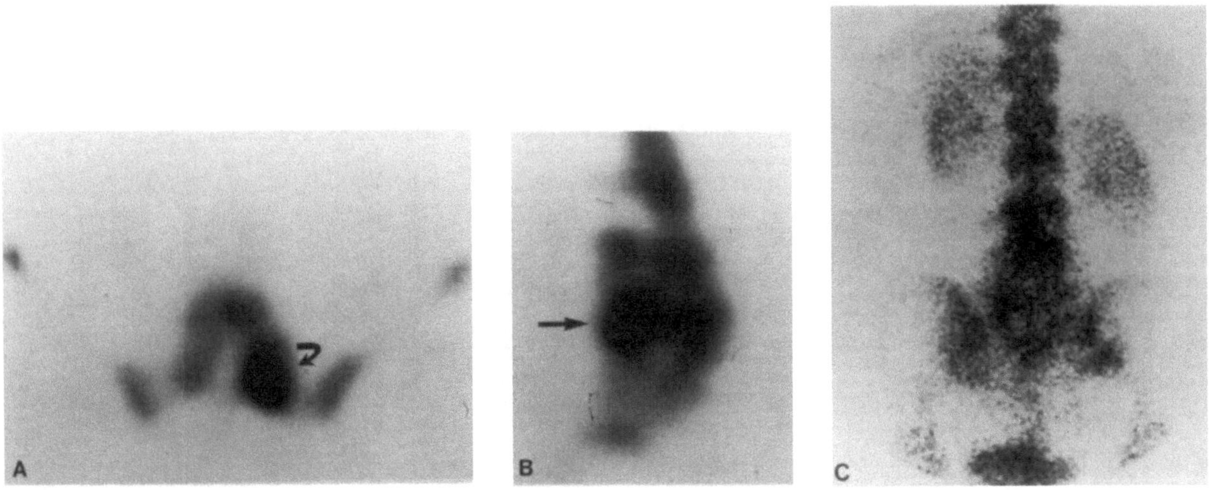

Figure 15.8. Pseudarthrosis of L3 to S1 spinal fusion. Sixty-six-year-old female with continued severe back pain 20 months after spinal fusion. Abnormal focal increased activity is seen on transaxial SPECT image (**A**) at L5 and on a sagittal SPECT image (**B**) through left side of fusion mass (*arrows*). No focal abnormality to suggest pseudarthrosis is seen on planar image (**C**). Pseudarthrosis was confirmed surgically with symptomatic relief following repeat L3–S1 fusion. (Reprinted with permission from D. B. Collier et al.[26])

Acknowledgments. We thank Margaret Pirtle for secretarial support and Jay Johnson for photographic assistance.

References

1. Burton C. Symposium: the role of spine fusion. Spine 1981;6:291.
2. Frymoyer JW. Symposium: the role of spine fusion. Spine 1981;6:284.
3. Wright A. Symposium: the role of spine fusion. Spine 1981;6:292.
4. Harcke HT, Larkin M, Clancy M. Evaluation of spinal fusions by bone scintigraphy. J Nuc Med 1980;21:9.
5. Littleton JT. Conventional pluridirectional tomography. In: Kricun, ME, ed. Imaging Modalities in Spinal Disorders. Philadelphia: Saunders, 1988:289–324.
6. Mall JC, Kaiser JA, Heithoff KB. Postoperative spine. Newton TH, Potts DG (Eds.) Modern Neuroradiology. Computed Tomography of the Spine and Spinal Cord. Clavadel Press, San Anselmo, CA, 1983.
7. Quencer RM, Murtagh FR, Post MJD, Rosomoff HL, Stokes NA. Postoperative bony stenosis of the lumbar spinal canal, evaluation of 264 symptomatic patients with axial radiography. AJR 1978;131:1059.
8. Rothman RH, Booth R. Failures of spinal fusion. Symposium on lumbar spine. Orthop Clin North Am 1975;6:299.
9. Coughlin JD. Extrusion of bone graft after lumbar fusion: CT appearance. J Comput Assist Tomogr 1986;10:399–400.
10. Frymoyer JW, Hanley EN, Howe J, Kuhlmann D, Matteri RE. A comparison of radiographic findings in fusion and nonfusion patients ten or more years following lumbar disk surgery. Spine 1979;4:435.
11. Teplick JG, Teplick SK, Haskin ME. Postoperative lumbar spine. In: Donovan Post, MJ, ed. Computed Tomography of the Spine. Baltimore: Williams & Wilkins, 1984:406–431.
12. Brodsky AE. Post-laminectomy and post fusion stenosis of the lumbar spine. Clin Orthop 1976;115:130.
13. Quencer RM, Tenner M, Ruthman L. The postoperative myelogram: radiographic evaluation of arachnoiditis and dural/arachnoidal tears. Radiology 1977;123:667.
14. Heithoff KB. Computed tomographic assessment of the postoperative spine. In: Geant, HK, ed. Spine Update. San Francisco: Radiology Research & Education Foundation, 1984:243–269.
15. Dawson EG, Clader TJ, Bassett LW. A comparison of different methods used to diagnose pseudarthrosis following posterior spinal fusion for scoliosis. J of Bone and Joint Surg 1985;67:1153.
16. Harris JH Jr., Edeiken-Monroe B. Three-dimensional computed tomography (3D-CT). The Radiology of Acute Cervical Spine Trauma. Baltimore: Williams & Wilkins, 1987:59–60.
17. Ross JS, Masark TJ, Modic MT, Delamater R, Bohlman H, Wilbur G, Kaufman B. MR imaging of lumbar arachnoiditis. AJNR 1987;8:885.
18. Rothman SLG, Glen WV, Jr. CT evaluation of interbody fusion. Clin Orthop 1985;193:47–56.
19. Sachs S. Present status of anterior interbody fusion in the lower lumbar spine. Symposium on the lumbar spine. Orthop Clin North Am 1975;6:275.
20. Stauffer RN, Coventry MB. Anterior interbody lumbar fusion: analysis of Mayo Clinic Series. J Bone Joint Surg 1972;54:756.
21. Murphy MJ, Southwick WO, Riley LH, Jr, Whitesides TE, Sherk HH, Pratt L. Surgical approaches and techniques.

In: The Cervical Spine Research Society, ed. The Cervical Spine. Philadelphia: Lippincott, 1983:496–528.
22. Pate D, Resnick D, Andre M, Sartoris DJ. Three-dimensional computed tomography. In: Kricun, ME, ed. Imaging Modalities in Spinal Disorders. Philadelphia: Saunders, 1988:468–477.
23. Carothers A, Orbach E. Fonar develops surface coil for whiplash injuries. Magn Reson News 1987–1988;3:1.
24. Bundschuh CV, Modic MT, Ross JS, Masaryk TJ, Bohlman H. Epidural fibrosis and recurrent disk herniation in the lumbar spine: MR imaging assessment. Am J Neuroradiology 1988;9:169.
25. Modic MT, Feiglin DH, Pirano DW, Boumphrey F, Weinstein MA, Duchesneau PM, Rehm S. Vertebral osteomyelitis: assessment using MR. Radiology 1985;157:157.
26. Collier DB, Hellman R, Krasnow AZ. Bone SPECT. Semin Nucl Med 1987;17(3):247.
27. McMaster MJ, Merrick MV. The scintigraphic assessment of the scoliotic spine after fusion. J Bone Joint Surg 1980;62B:65.

■16■

Bracing of Spinal Fusions

Victoria M. Dvonch and Wilton H. Bunch

Introduction

The choice of the postoperative orthosis has always reflected the surgeon's perceptions of the strengths and limitations of the surgical construct. Before the development of instrumentation systems, early spinal surgeons focused on creating a surgical procedure that would consistently result in a fusion. They worked out surgical techniques that modified the biology of the surgical site to achieve their desired ends. These surgeons required an orthosis that would not only obtain the desired spinal alignment but would maintain it while fusion took place.

These carefully molded plaster of Paris orthoses were designed with two expectations. First, they were to exert a corrective force on the spine through transverse loading and, in some cases, through distraction. Second, they were fabricated to neutralize the bending and torsional forces that would interfere with bony union. The biomechanical insight of these surgeons, as well as their acceptable success rate, are clearly documented in the literature.[1,2,3]

Spinal surgeons, however, were not satisfied. In an attempt to increase correction and to decrease the rate of pseudarthrosis, instrumentation systems were developed as adjuncts to the fusion procedure. Plaster of Paris postoperative orthoses continued to be used in conjunction with these first implant systems. Gradually, confidence in the implant systems led some to question the role of postoperative orthosis and the biology of the fusion site was displaced, and greater attention was given to the relationship between the orthosis and the internal fixation. Biology was taking a backseat.

This more recent emphasis on the relationship between postoperative immobilization and the perceived biomechanics of the surgical construct can be illustrated in the history of postoperative bracing with Luque instrumentation. When the Luque system of segmental spinal instrumentation (SSI) was introduced, it was believed by many to be significantly more rigid than the Harrington system. This perception was graphically demonstrated when some surgeons decided to forego postoperative immobilization after SSI.[4–17] The supporters of this approach implicitly assumed that SSI could resist all forces on the spine that would disrupt the instrumentation or interfere with the fusion until union could occur. They believed that the advances in internal fixation had eliminated the need for external fixation.

Gradually, papers appeared that questioned the validity of this assumption.[18,19] Groups of patients were identified who required postoperative support, and once again the postoperative orthosis became integral to the treatment plan. The orthosis in large part determined the success or failure of the surgical effort. This gave new life to an orthopedic appliance that a few years earlier seemed doomed to the fate of the Whitman plate.

In the wake of the reports of failure of the Luque device, the role of postoperative spinal orthoses in maintaining biomechanical stability has become clearer. A properly selected orthosis complements the internal fixation by counteracting those forces that would lead to instrumentation failure. It protects the instrumentation in situations in which fusion is delayed and thus allows union to occur prior to metal fatigue.

Thinking About Spinal Orthoses

The decision regarding postoperative immobilization requires a careful evaluation of the biological response of the fusion site and of the biomechanical needs of the instrumentation. These factors must be assessed in light of the underlying physiological and psychological makeup of each patient. Choosing the appropriate orthosis requires careful attention to each patient's problem and the specific surgical solution used. No one instrumentation system exists to meet the range and variety of spinal problems that surgeons must treat. For this reason, postoperative bracing fills an important role in the effective management of spinal fusions.

How does one select an orthosis from among the wide array of designs and materials available? Is there a systematic way to make a selection? Can the spectrum of options be narrowed on the basis of what is available, familiar, or easily fabricated? Can a choice be based on the primary diagnosis, the age, or the functional status of the patient?

At one time in the history of spinal surgery, any one of these methods of selection might have proved adequate. But the variety and complexity of problems presenting today rules out any simple principle of selection. Even the choice of instrumentation can no longer dictate the postoperative regimen. The crossover of instrumentation systems among scoliosis, spinal trauma, degenerative lesions, tumors, and osteoporosis clearly precludes an instrument-oriented approach to orthotic selection.

The surgeon may approach these questions in three different ways. First, the surgeon might establish an absolute rule for all cases, as follows, "I WANT all my patients to receive an "XYZ" orthosis postoperatively." Thus, the orthotic choice need only be made once. This approach assumes that all patients fit into a certain pattern with one style of orthosis addressing all their needs. The method is easy to teach and saves a lot of time. Unfortunately, patients who deviate from the standard pattern are neither appreciated nor well served. Clearly, this approach can lead to poor and unanticipated operative outcomes.

Alternatively, the surgeon might use an intuitive approach, invoking statements such as, "I BELIEVE that this patient needs a body jacket." This course suits those who believe that data cannot be marshalled or predictions made. It denies the role of active problem solving to enhance the odds of a successful outcome. This system, which relies on "luck" or "chance," is deceptively easy to teach. The residents' jargon labels this method "guessing," which highlights its weakness. Lacking reason, principle, or method, it leaves everyone guessing as to the approach to decision making employed by the expert.

Employing the third approach, the surgeon THINKS about the need for postoperative immobilization and sorts out the choices based on the anticipated biological response of the surgical site and the biomechanical needs of the instrumentation. Using this method, the surgeon confronts each patient's problem, as well as its surgical solution, and determines how the postoperative management will influence the final outcome. The patient's problem, as well as the solution, is compulsively evaluated and the potential sources of failure carefully identified. The surgeon who implements this model realizes that no matter how clever the orthotic design or how innovative the modifications, the orthosis must address the biomechanical needs of the patient or else it is merely a rigid postoperative dressing.

A review of the literature on postoperative immobilization for spinal fusion yields an embarrassingly small number of articles, especially in comparison with articles written about other aspects of spinal fusion. A significant proportion describes the replacement of the Risser cast with the plastic body jacket in the management of adolescent idiopathic scoliosis.[20–27] Despite the rather paltry showing in the literature, however, many spine surgeons mull over these issues regularly. The fruits of these ruminations become part of an oral tradition similar to the oral tradition that occurs in trauma and joint arthroplasty.

One limitation of oral tradition, however, is that it relies on the spoken word for the transfer of information. For the students of a laconic spine surgeon, this can present a problem. The residents and fellows watch as the surgeon sizes up the postoperative radiograph, and after a contemplative moment, they receive their instructions. What is going through their boss's head (and supposedly through their own) is a mystery. And because Divine Inspiration is so unreliable, on the day these residents are themselves carriers of the word, they tend to pick a familiar orthosis, even if the underlying situation is different.

This chapter proposes the third mode, the thinking surgeon's approach, for choosing orthoses. The authors will attempt to synthesize the oral tradition and to distill some practical guidelines for decision making.

Choosing the Orthosis: Step One

In assessing an orthosis, four variables need to be examined: (1) the ability of the orthosis to be removed; (2) the weight of the orthosis; (3) the cost of the orthosis; and (4) the counterforces applied by the orthosis. Using these four variables, an ideal orthosis can be described and a reasonable facsimile can be fabricated.

1. The ability to be removed. An orthosis that can be removed for bathing and personal hygiene is clearly a boon to the patient. On the other hand, an orthosis that is constantly being removed in an unsupervised setting is clearly a threat to the success of the surgery. And while the patient is often at fault, there are times when the patient is innocent. Patients who are in institutions or convalescent centers can be victims rather than perpetrators. How many times have patients returned for follow-up with their orthoses on too high, too loose, or even with the front and back reversed? The question that needs to be answered is: Will the orthosis be worn as prescribed? If the answer is unclear, an orthosis that is difficult to remove should be considered.

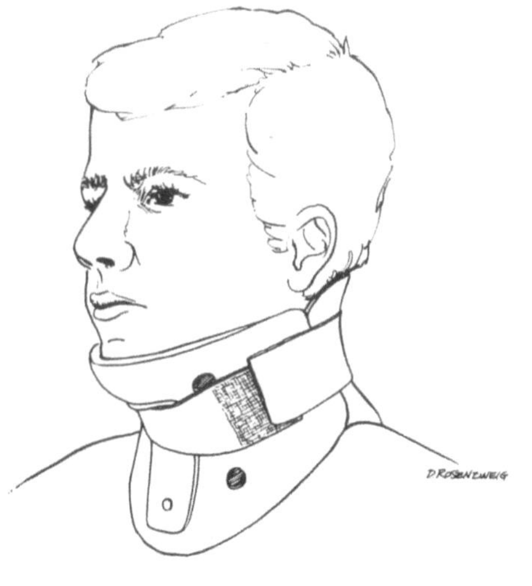

Figure 16.1. Philadelphia collar.

2. Weight: A postoperative orthosis of plaster of Paris weighs 10 to 12 pounds. A fiberglass orthosis weighs several pounds less. A polypropylene orthosis weighs about 4 pounds. For a debilitated patient, a paralyzed patient, or a patient with compromised cardiopulmonary reserve, the extra energy required to move about in a heavier orthosis must be considered.
3. Cost. A plaster of Paris orthosis costs $250. A polypropylene orthosis fabricated by an orthotist can cost from $1000 to $3000. The cast can be applied postoperatively in about 2 hours. The orthotic measurements cannot usually be taken until after surgery, and fabrication time is then necessary. While some skilled orthotists have a very rapid turnover time, most require at least several days. During this time the patient must remain in bed or be placed in a cast. As we move into an era of increasing needs for cost containment, these factors may become increasingly relevant.
4. Counterforces applied. In assessing this factor, one must consider the body region concerned. Various orthoses are addressed accordingly.

Cervical and Cervicothoracic Orthoses

The work of Johnson et al.[28,29] has contributed significantly to the understanding of the biomechanics of cervical orthoses. Those orthoses that encircle the cervical spine with minimal extension onto the thorax provide the least counterforce against cervical spine motion. This group includes orthoses such as the Philadelphia collar (Fig. 16.1). On the whole, these rigid collars are more effective in "controlling" motion than soft cervical collars, which function merely to remind the patient that he has had surgery. Soft collars should not be expected to provide even moderate counterforces, especially to rotation.

The next level of control is provided by cervical orthoses such as the four-poster brace (Fig. 16.2). It does a satisfactory job of controlling flexion over the middle segments but does not control motion in the upper or lower cervical spine significantly. When the orthosis extends onto the thorax, it serves better to control flexion and extension in the mid- and lower cervical spine. This group includes modifications of cervical orthoses such as the four poster

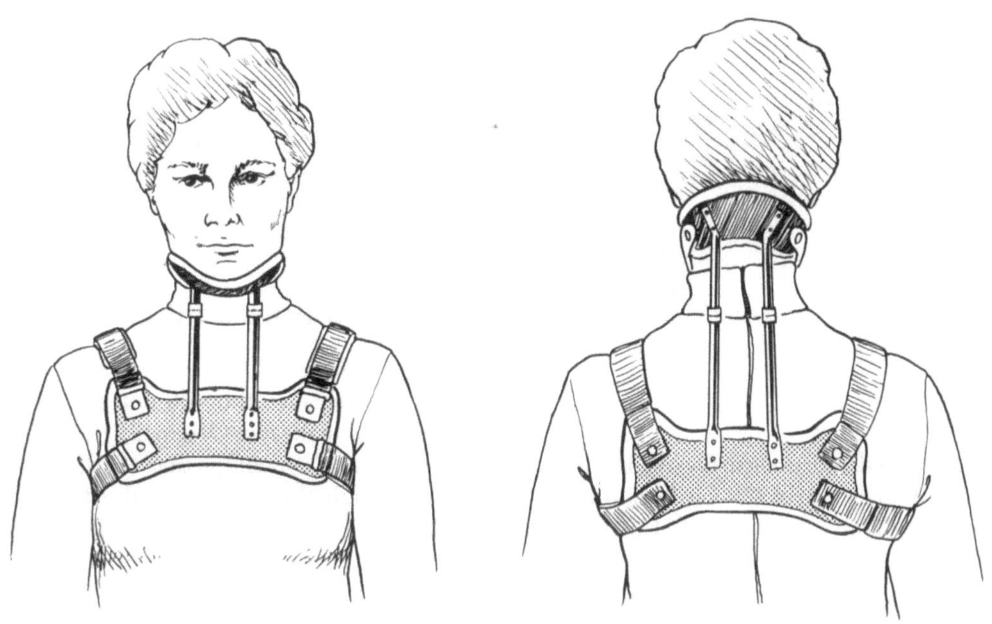

Figure 16.2. Four-poster brace. This model has straps to anchor it more firmly to the trunk.

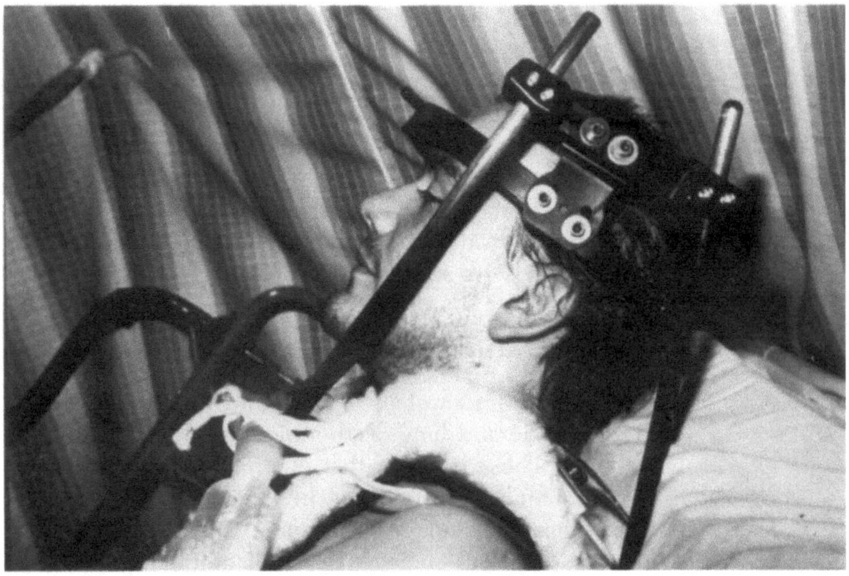

A

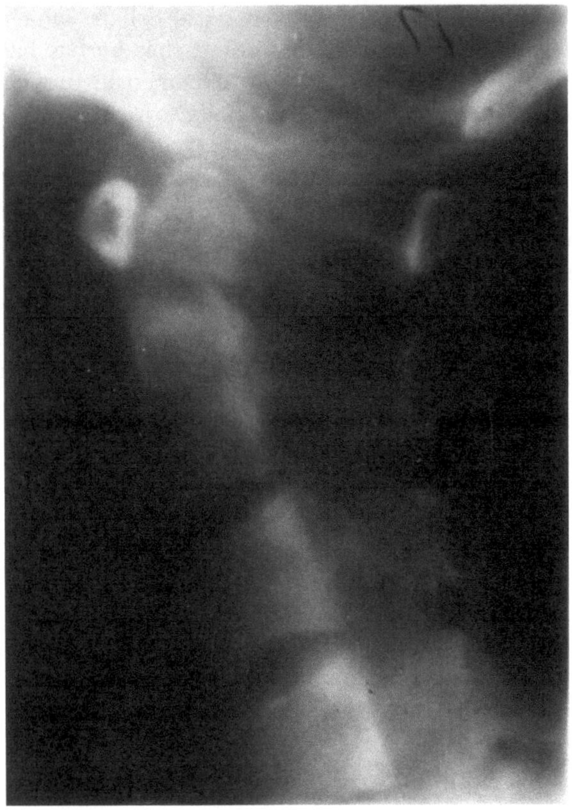

B

Figure 16.3. **A.** Halo vest. **B.** Odontoid fracture treated with halo vest.

so that they are anchored more securely on the trunk. As a group, these orthoses control C1–C2 flexion poorly. The exception to this is the sternal occipital mandibular immobilizer (SOMI) brace, which Johnson found to be uniquely effective in controlling flexion at the atlantoaxial and C2–C3 level. It controlled extension poorly, however.

In general, two additional conclusions can be drawn. First, all conventional removable orthoses do a poor job of controlling rotation and lateral bending over the whole cervical spine. Second, the more controlling a cervicothoracic orthosis is, the more uncomfortable it is; over the long term, patient compliance may become an issue.

Anchoring the orthosis onto the trunk and securing it to the cranium markedly increases the orthotic control of the whole cervical spine. In the Johnson study, the halo/cast provided the maximum stabilization of the cervical spine in flexion/extension/rotation/lateral bending. The halo/vest (Fig. 16.3), with its advantage of less weight, was only slightly less effective. Care should be taken with the halo/vest, however, to be sure that the vest fits properly. Displacement of the fracture in the halo/vest has been reported, and was presumed to be secondary to poor fitting of the vest in nonstandard body types.[30]

It should be remembered that in choosing a postoperative orthosis for the cervical spine, the instability of flexion injuries can be compensated for with posterior instrumentation, thus allowing the use of less rigid supports. Extension injuries are rarely compensated for with internal fixation devices and therefore require a halo/cast/vest orthosis.

Thoracolumbosacral Orthoses

Thoracolumbosacral orthoses (TLSO) are more difficult to discuss, because they do not come in familiar designs like cervical orthoses. Originally designed like postoperative casts, they encompassed the thoracolumbosacral region although the amount of the thoracic spine encased in the orthosis varied (Fig. 16.4). Lantz and Schultz[31] examined the restriction of gross motion in the upper body in a low-profile TLSO. They concluded that a TLSO restricted twisting 21%, lateral bending 48%, flexion 20%, and extension 48%.

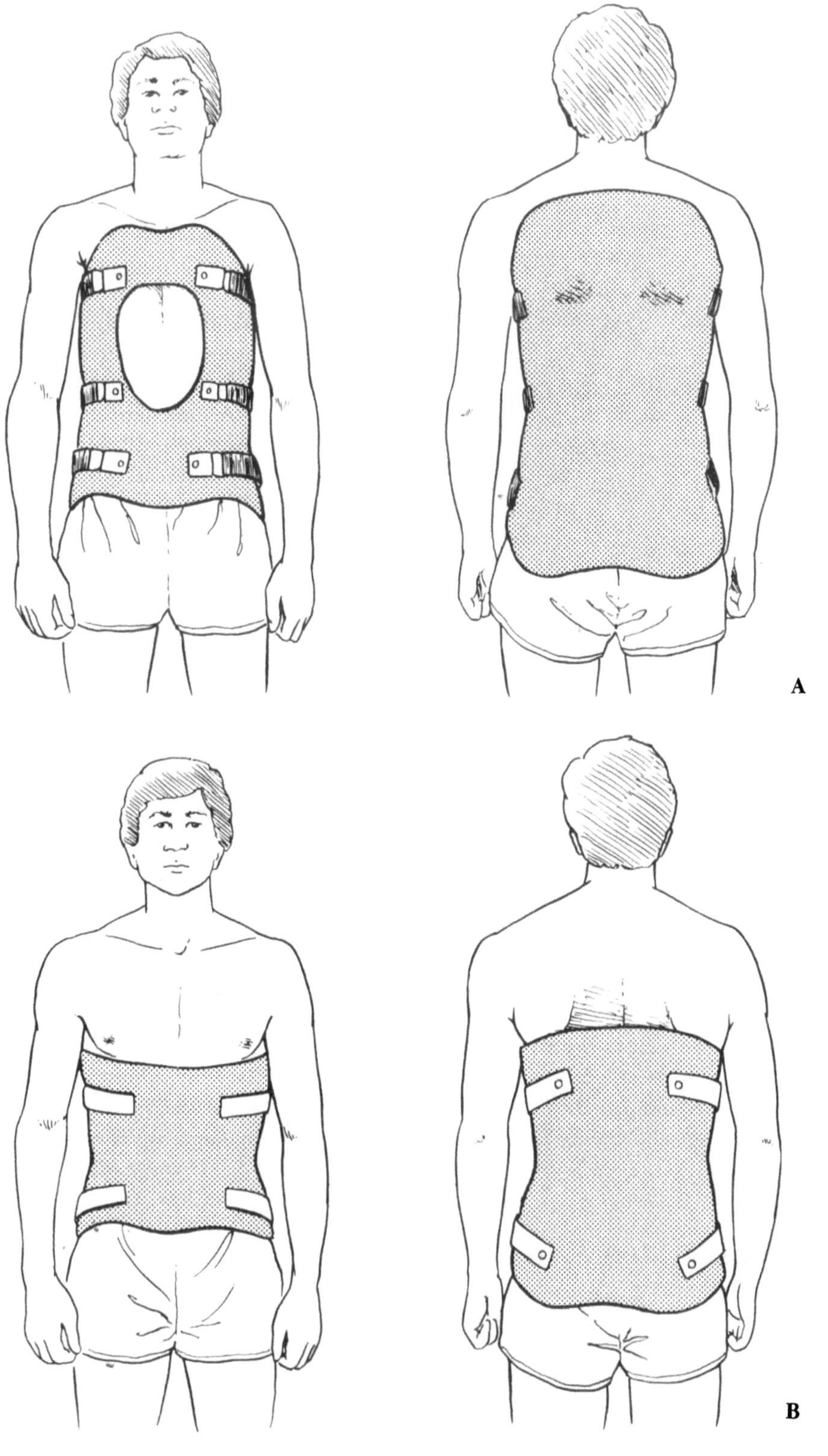

Figure 16.4. **A.** High-profile thoracolumbosacral orthosis (TLSO). **B.** Low-profile TLSO (*continued*).

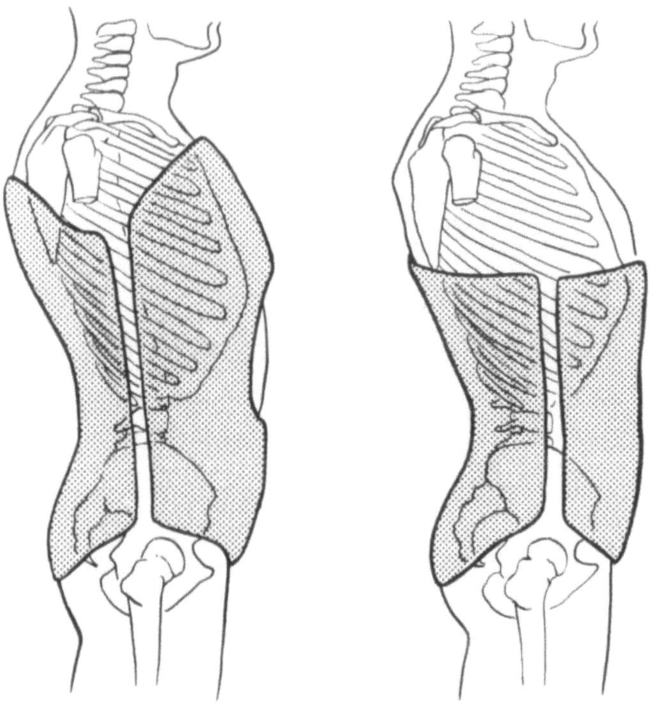

C

Figure 16.4. **C.** Comparison of extent of thoracic spine enclosed by brace.

Most of adult spinal surgery is concerned with the motion of the lumbar vertebrae and the lumbosacral joint. Fidler and Plasmans[32] studied the motion of the lumbosacral spine with no support, with a TLSO, and with single spica in five volunteers; the TLSO extended from the lower ribs to 3 cm below the anterior superior iliac spine in front and to the midpart of the sacrum posteriorly. They found that while the jacket and the spica inhibited motion at L1–L2 and L2–L3 essentially to the same extent, about 51% and 36%, respectively, the spica did a markedly superior job in limiting L4–L5 and L5–S1 motion, 2% and 8%, respectively. The jacket allowed 70% of normal L5–S1 motion.

Choosing the Orthosis: Step Two

Orthotic selection requires a close examination of the factors that influence the success of the operation: the biology of the surgical site, the biomechanics of the instrumentation, and the interplay of the total patient in the treatment plan. Orthotic options should always be evaluated in the light of these considerations.

The Biology of the Fusion Site

The surgeon does not perform a spinal fusion. Rather, he alters the environment of the surgical site to encourage a fusion to take place.[33] The selection of a postoperative regimen is greatly influenced by the success of this alteration. For example, the surgeon's prediction of the time for revascularization and incorporation of the graft into the healing spine figures significantly in decisions about postoperative management. Consider the multiple aspects of the surgical technique that must be reviewed to determine whether a break in technique, an intraoperative complication, or an unexpected finding could have comprised the rate of fusion. Was the stripping of the soft tissue meticulous? Was the blocking of the facets complete? Is the amount of graft sufficient? Is vascular ingrowth impaired by absence of spinal musculature or massive scar tissue? Was the strut graft properly keyed? Was the vascular pedicle patent? Was the fracture really caused by inadequate bone material and not the magnitude of the trauma? These and hundreds of other questions must be answered in assessing the biology of the fusion site and, therefore, the rate of fusion.

The Biomechanics of the Instrumentation

Surgeons cannot afford blind faith in instrumentation systems. An attitude of healthy skepticism is far more appropriate. The complex nature of spinal motion coupled with the infinite variety (and activity) of the human animal have resulted in failure, at some time, of every biomechanical construct. The surgeon must examine his creation for its weaknesses even as he admires it for its strengths.

Although there is a distinct subset of patients who undergo fusion without instrumentation, most patients have fusion in conjunction with a spinal implant. It will be assumed that the system chosen is appropriate and has achieved the desired therapeutic goal and that the postoperative radiograph is judged to be perfect. The surgeon's task is then to think about the particular implant system as it bears on the choice of postoperative immobilization. One question sums up the issues: "What are the forces which, if applied to this construct, will result in instrumentation failure and lead to failure of the fusion?"

Answering this question first involves looking at the failure pattern inherent in the instrumentation itself. For example, a single Harrington distraction rod is vulnerable to hook cutout in forward flexion and rotation. A postoperative orthosis should block this motion.

Second, the surgeon must consider what normal anatomical restraining forces are absent in this patient that are not compensated for by the instrumentation. This is particularly significant in the management of spinal fractures. Consider, for example, the situation in which the anterior longitudinal spinal ligament is disrupted and is not compensated for by two Harrington distraction rods.

Finally, the surgeon must assess how the system will respond to the forces applied as the patient lies in bed, sits, or moves. If anatomical alignment is not achieved, the effect of gravity alone on the upright spine will stress the instrumentation. Bending the instrumentation to accommodate residual deformity induces plastic deformation on the implant system and thus decreases its ability to withstand loading.[34,35] The effect of any additional stresses, such as in a patient who has muscle paralysis or spasticity, must also be estimated.

The Psychosocial Considerations of the Patient

The problem of postoperative immobilization could be solved more easily if the fact that the fusion occurs in a person could be ignored. Not only must one deal with the total physiology of the patient, but one must also contend with the psychology and personality of the person harboring the fusion. As much as we might wish it to be, the patient is more than the vehicle by which our surgical site is transported. The assessment of the total patient contributes significantly to the decision about postoperative bracing.

In assessing the general physiology of the fusion site, one must evaluate the patient's nutrition. Considerable data exist on the role of nutrition in postsurgical healing. A debilitated patient will heal more slowly and could have poorer bone stock at the outset of treatment, thus influencing both the biology and biomechanics of the fusion site. Slower healing results in greater dependence on the instrumentation over time. It also changes the odds in the race between fusion and failure. Other patients for whom problematic physiology plays a critical role would include paralytic and spastic patients, patients with chronic disease, tumor patients, and patients who are immunocompromised.

The patient's attitude toward the fusion and his or her social environment is also a relevant consideration. Through surveys of patient attitudes, Bunch and Chapman[36] found that the presence or absence of a postoperative orthosis after a scoliosis fusion had the least relative importance when compared with such outcomes as nerve injury or reoperation. Idiopathic scoliosis patients are often well prepared for their fusions and are highly invested in the anticipated cosmetic improvement. This is in marked contrast to the patient who requires fusion for a spine fracture accompanied by a neural deficit. This patient goes through well described stages of anger and depression. Even when the indications of the surgery are earefully explained, the patient may harbor the hope that not only will the fracture be stabilized but he will not be paralyzed after the surgery. The profound disappointment associated with the persistent paralysis can make the patient uncooperative.

Certain questions need to be answered for each individual. Will the patient wear the orthosis? Is he reliable enough or is a cast necessary? Is the orthosis so cumbersome that it is impractical and actually impeding the patient's rehabilitation? Is the patient able to understand the instructions provided? Does he need help to get it on and off? Is that help available? Can he use the toilet? Sit in a chair? Ride in a car? Sleep comfortably? A successful fusion in a patient whose rehabilitation is compromised by the inappropriate choice of postoperative orthosis is in many respects a treatment failure.

Applying the Thinking Surgeon's Approach: Case Studies

Case 1: R.T. is a 13-year-old female with idiopathic scoliosis who has a 63° thoracic curve initially treated by electrical stimulation followed by treatment in a Milwaukee brace. An elective spinal fusion is planned using a single Harrington distraction rod (Fig. 16.5).

Biology: In this healthy, previously unoperated young female, the biological factors would be optimal for fusion

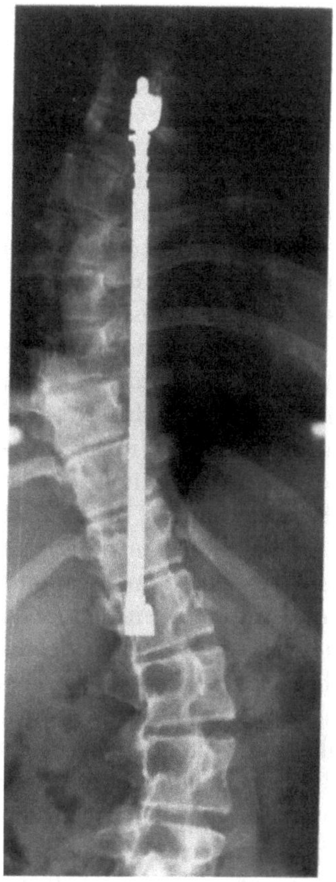

Figure 16.5. Postoperative radiograph shows instrumentation with single Harrington distraction rod.

in the thoracic spine. This does not preclude the need for technically meticulous surgery, however.

Biomechanics: A single Harrington distraction rod fails in rotation and forward flexion. Cyclic rotation in the clockwise direction is a particular problem because in that motion the lamina rotates away from the hook.[37] This system is weakest of the commonly used systems when axial loads are applied, but the load-bearing capacity is not exceeded in the routine patient.

Total Patient: This patient is nutritionally sound and has a good mental attitude toward the surgery. Her family is supportive and the patient is compliant.

Orthotic Choice: Revising her Milwaukee brace, which she is used to, will provide all the motion constraints necessary. The cervicothoracolumbosacral orthosis (CTLSO) limits truncal rotation and forward flexion. Because the patient will not exceed the axial load-bearing capacity of the instrumentation, additional axial support (such as used to be provided by casts or braces molded beneath the mandible) is not necessary. Substituting a TLSO would depend on where the fusion ended. If the instrumentation ended in the upper thoracic spine (T1,T2), the TLSO would need to come far enough cephalad on the chest to block forward flexion over the top of the brace.

Case 2: T.R. is a 19-year-old obese male with a T12–L1 level spina bifida. He has had two prior procedures for his scoliosis. The first attempt resulted in a pseudarthrosis with a broken rod. The attempt to repair the pseudarthrosis resulted in a deep wound infection that was treated by packing. The wound was allowed to heal by secondary intent. He presents with a history of onset of acute back pain while riding his snowmobile.

Biology: This situation is an osteoblast's nightmare. The surgical site is located in previously infected tissue that has a compromised blood supply from massive scarring. The vascular supply is also reduced because the patient lacks the back musculature that normally covers the fusion area. Because of the two previous procedures, the iliac crests are inadequate sources of graft, and bank bone must be used. A delay in fusion time is anticipated.

Biomechanics: This obese male applies considerable stress to a system simply by sitting. Because of his lack of trunk muscles, when he sits he leans forward. This increases his thoracic kyphosis and reverses his lumbar lordosis. When he moves, he uses his arms to move his body and he walks with crutches. These movements generate forces which have a significant distraction component. He was instrumented with dual Harrington compression rods across the pseudarthrosis site and Harrington distraction rods across the area of previous fusion (Fig. 16.6A).

Total Patient: Despite his high-level spina bifida, this patient is extremely active. Living in a rural area, he spends his time either on a snowmobile or an all-terrain vehicle. His general health is good, but his compliance is suspect and he admits to removing his body jackets in the past.

Orthotic Choice: Because of the mode of instrument failure, an orthosis was needed that blocked flexion (Fig. 16.6B). A Milwaukee brace was deemed inadequate, because in this neuromuscular patient a significant extension moment was needed to resist the patient's forward flexions. A broad area of contact was required to dissipate this force on the patient's skin. Because of the patient's size and active lifestyle, a durable, rigid orthosis was needed. Because of the patient's tendency to shed his TLSO, the proper orthosis would have to be difficult to remove. A plaster of Paris orthosis similar in design to a Risser cast was employed and reinforced with fiberglass. It extended up to the sternal notch and over the patient's shoulders. The increased weight slowed the patient down, but this was not detrimental in this young strong male. Thoughtful orthotic management resulted in a successful fusion in a difficult surgical site with an implant construct that many readers would consider primitive.

Case 3: A 39-year-old male was involved in a motor vehicle accident resulting in a fracture with complete paraplegia, at the L1 level (Fig. 16.7A).

Biology: This otherwise healthy young male was profoundly depressed and was refusing to eat. Nutritional support was provided as well as psychiatric counseling.

Biomechanics: Harrington compression rods were placed to resist distraction forces in this very unstable spine. Harrington distraction rods were segmentally fixed using the Wisconsin–Drummond technique to provide greater resistance to forward flexion and rotational stresses than the unwired Harrington distraction rod (Fig. 16.7B).

Total Patient: The treatment plan consisted of transfer of the patient to a spinal cord rehabilitation center after the acute postoperative period. The patient was angry, hostile, and minimally compliant. The nursing staff had difficulty in moving the patient because of his lack of cooperation.

Orthotic Design: Despite the increased stability provided by the segmentally wired instrumentation,[38,39] the combination of paralysis with the lack of patient participation in moving led to a decision for a postoperative orthosis. A removable lightweight TLSO was fabricated to be worn when the patient was moved from bed to chair. The presence of the jacket allowed the nursing staff to move the patient with increased confidence. Three months into the rehabilitation program, the jacket was discontinued as the patient learned to deal with his disability.

Case 4: This 54-year-old man was thrown from a fast-moving car and suffered a fracture of L4 although he remained neurologically intact (Fig. 16.8A). The patient had

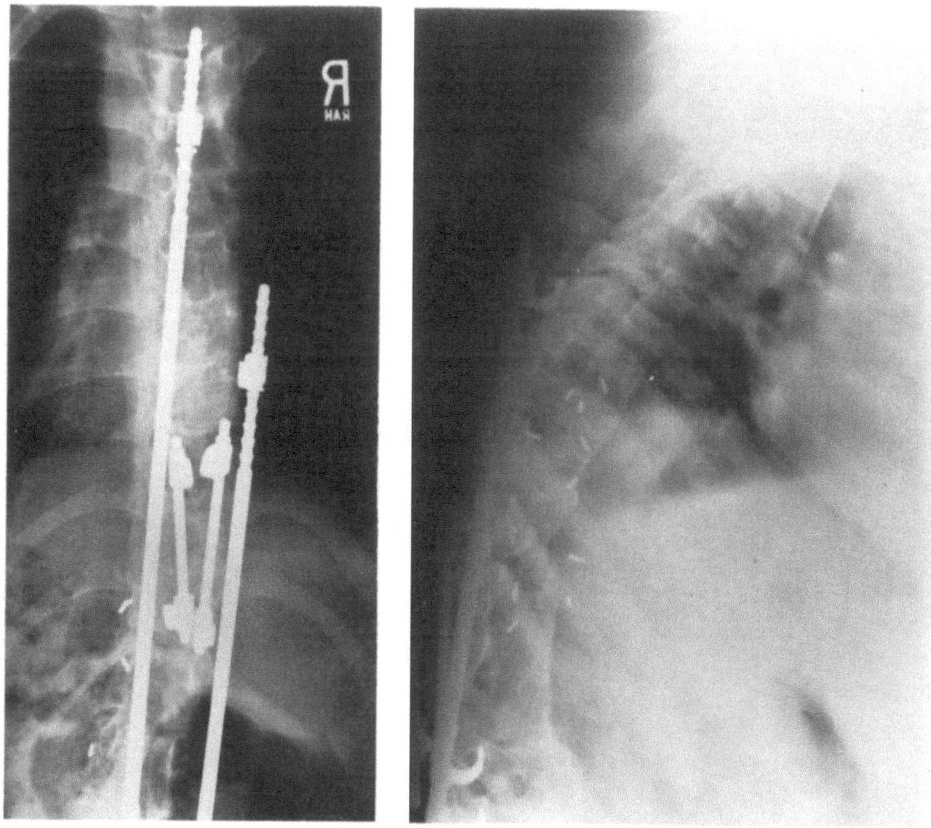

A B

Figure 16.6. **A.** Postoperative radiograph of surgical construct. **B.** Lateral radiograph reveals effect of unrestricted forward flexion on proximal hook of Harrington distraction rod.

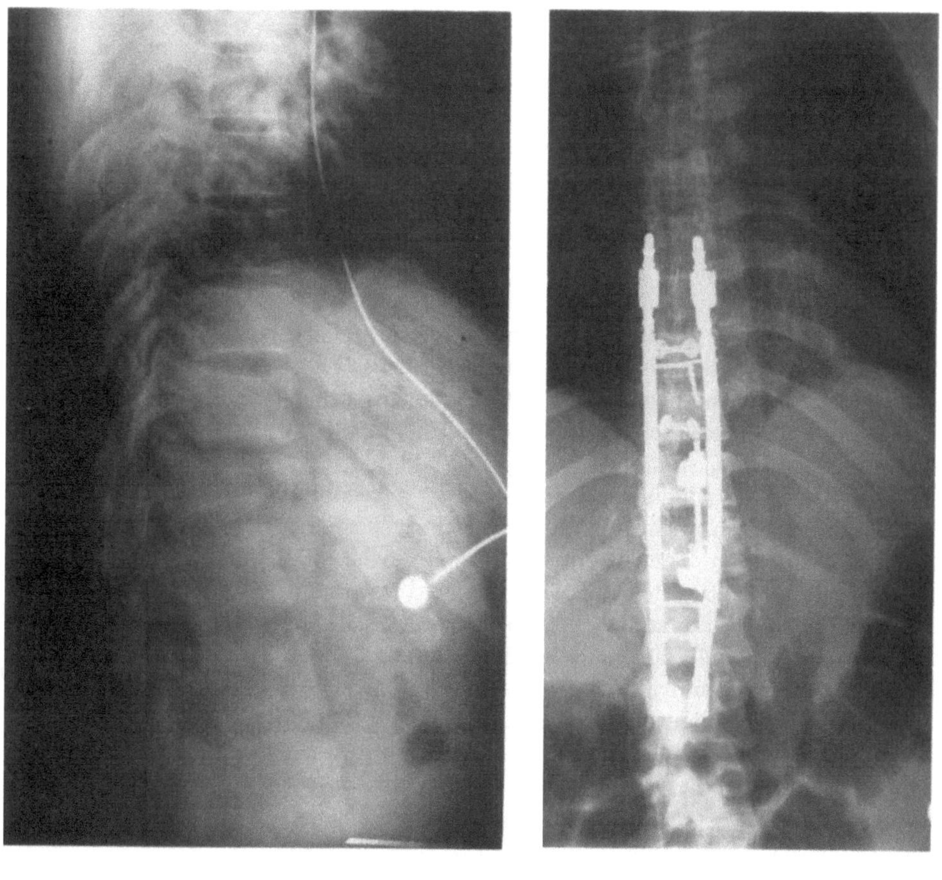

A B

Figure 16.7. **A.** Preoperative lateral radiograph of spinal fracture. **B.** Postoperative radiograph of surgical construct.

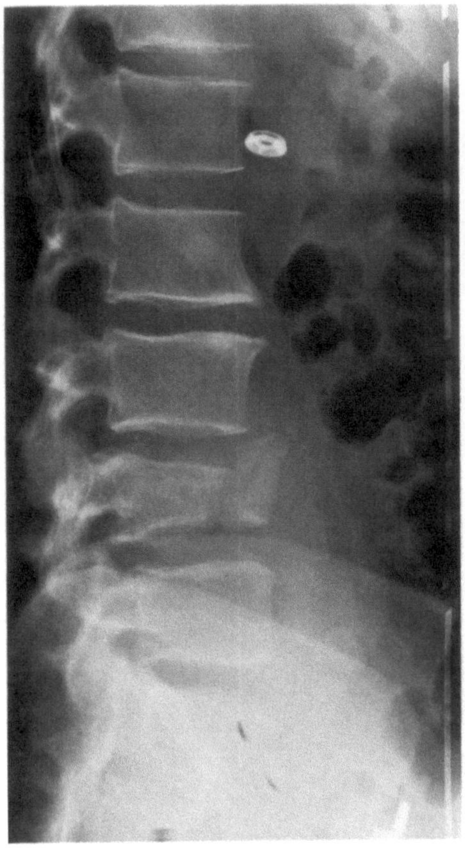
A

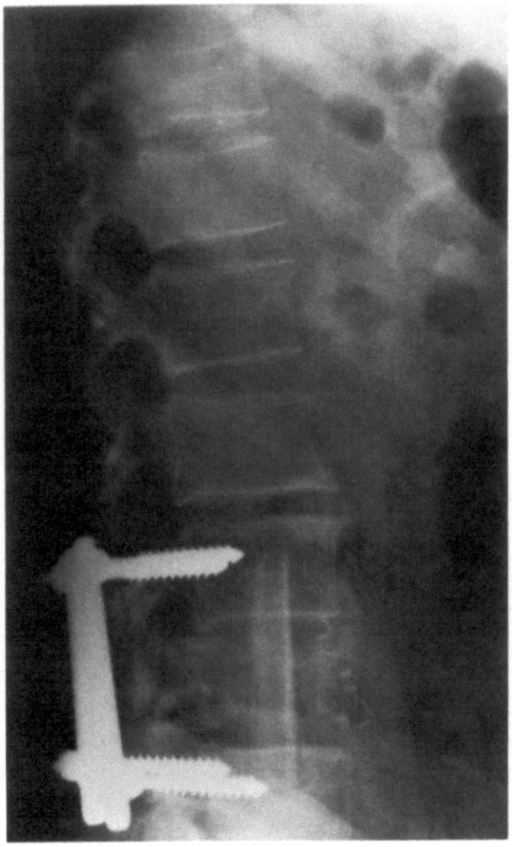
B

Figure 16.8. **A.** Preoperative radiograph shows fracture of L4. **B.** Postoperative lateral view of Steffee plate with anterior strut graft.

a history of significant alcohol intake over many years, and was at bed rest in a small rural community hospital for several weeks undergoing alcohol withdrawal before transfer.

Biology: After years of alcoholism this patient was in poor general condition. No nutritional support was instituted at the time of the injury. At the time of surgery, the quality of bone stock was poor and required supplementation by banked bone.

Biomechanics: The fracture was stabilized by a Steffee plate posteriorly and with a strut graft anteriorly (Fig. 16.8B). Because of the poor quality of the bone, the pull-out strength was presumed to be reduced. Uncontrolled flexion of the lumbar spine had to be prevented.

Total Patient: Although the patient was an agreeable and affable man, his ability to cooperate with the treatment plan was in question. The patient was not employed and the temptation to return to alcohol abuse would be great. Due to financial considerations, no placement option other than returning home was available. The patient had a dedicated wife and family.

Orthotic Choice: Because of the patient's poor bone stock and the presence of the anterior strut, both flexion and extension needed to be blocked in this lumbar spine. Fidler and Plasmans[32] showed that placing a patient in a spica decreased the motion of L3–L4 to 27% of normal and the motion at L4–L5 to 12% of normal. Therefore, the patient was placed in a unilateral spica and discharged to his home. He tolerated the orthosis well, and presented with a solid fusion at the 1-year follow-up. In a more reliable patient, a TLSO with a thigh extension would have provided good stability.

Case 5: A.D. is a 14-year-old female with a T12 spina bifida who underwent a posterior spinal fusion of the thoracic spine for a rapidly progressing scoliosis at age 10. She now presents with a collapsing lumbar spine. She sits with marked lumbar kyphosis (Fig. 16.9A).

Biology: The surgical site has poor overlying soft tissue, and the patient has little muscle mass on her trunk. Because of her lack of ambulation, her bone stock is only fair. Her skin is asensate. She is not obese, and her health is otherwise good. At the fusion site, more than 90% of the bone graft employed was autologous.

Biomechanics: In situations such as this where the problem requires a customized solution, the surgeon needs to be particularly attentive to the biomechanics of the surgical construct. The spine was instrumented with a Dwyer instrumentation system posteriorly, which functions as a tension band in resisting flexion. Because the anterior spinal structures are intact, spinal extension is not a problem. Forward flexion is a concern as the pull-out strength of the Dwyer screws is lessened in the poor

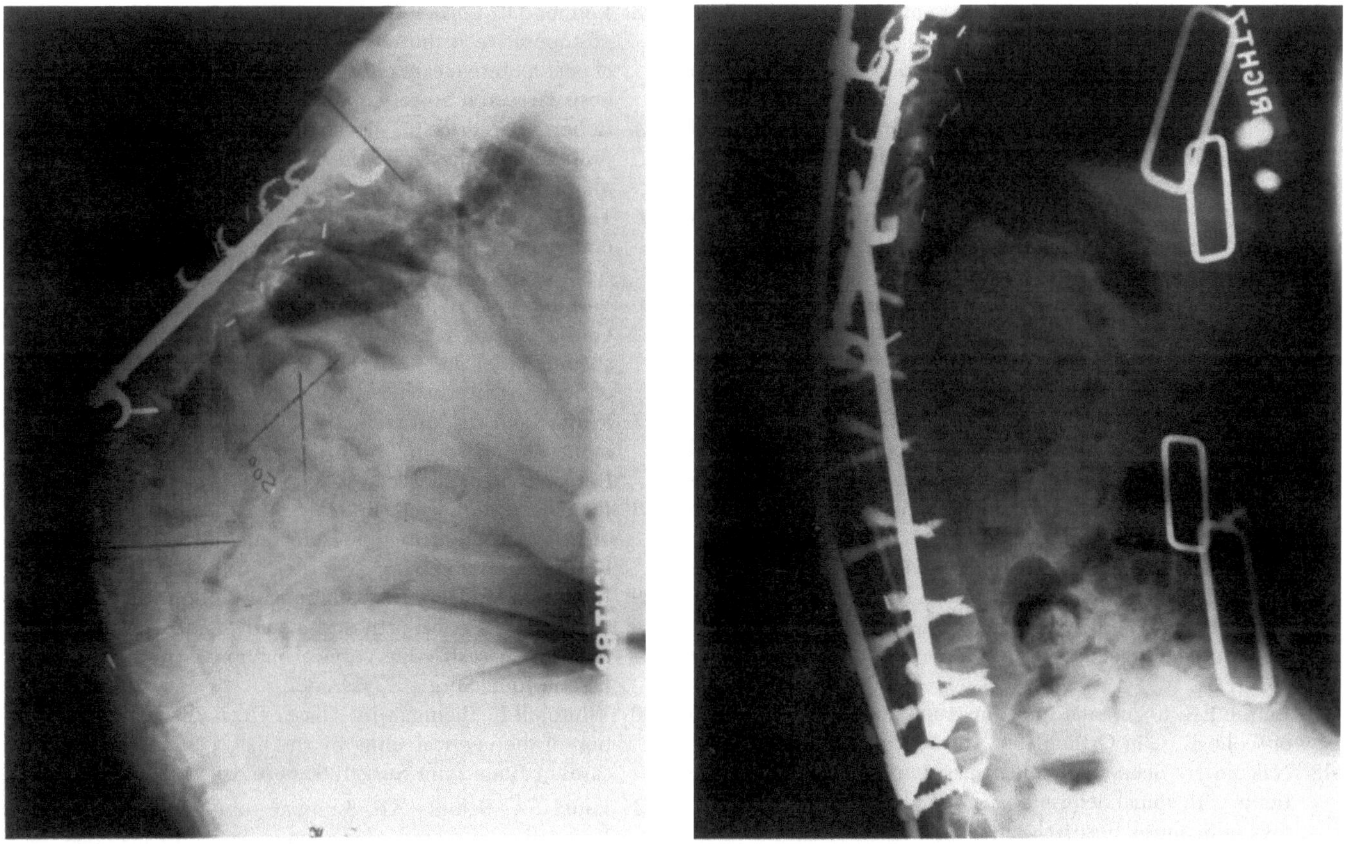

A B

Figure 16.9. **A.** Sitting lateral radiograph of spine. Note reversal of lumbar lordosis. **B.** Postoperative lateral radiograph of surgical construct.

bone stock. The lumbar spine was then spanned with Harrington distraction rods. These rods extend into the region of the previously fused thoracic spine reinforcing the junctional stress point. Because the rods are sensitive to distraction loads, some counterforce to distraction across the lumbar spine is provided by the Dwyer instrumentation (Fig. 16.9B).

Total Patient: The child's family is very supportive and cooperative. The child is very interested in improved trunk height and therefore very motivated. The child is nonambulatory and does not place a significant distraction moment on her spine in her activities of daily living. The mother was instructed on how to care for the child without placing marked distraction or rotational forces on the spine.

Orthotic Choice: Even though the Dwyer screws were well seated in the vertebral bodies, the bodies were small and the bone stock only fair. A significant counterforce to forward flexion was necessary to prevent failure of fixation. A high-profile TLSO was employed to resist the forward flexion of the trunk. The orthosis did not go over the shoulders because a significant distraction force was not anticipated.

Summary

In the absence of an ideal instrumentation system to contend with all the complexities of spinal problems, postoperative bracing will continue to fill an important role in the effective management of spinal fusions. In choosing the appropriate postoperative immobilization, the surgeon must carefully evaluate the biological response of the fusion site and of the biomechanical needs of the instrumentation. These factors must be assessed in light of the underlying physiological and psychological makeup of each patient. This chapter has advocated an active problem-solving approach which takes into account each patient's problem and the unique surgical solution as integral factors in choosing a postoperative orthosis.

References

1. Moe JH. A critical analysis of method of fusion for scoliosis: an evaluation in two hundred and sixty-six patients. J Bone Joint Surg 1958;40A:529.
2. Risser JC, Norquist DM. A followup study of the treatment of scoliosis. J Bone Joint Surg 1958;40A:555.

3. Risser JC. Scoliosis past and present. J Bone Joint Surg 1964;46A:167.
4. Allen BL, Jr. Segmental instrumentation for difficult spine deformities. Orthop Trans 1979;3:4.
5. Allen BL, Jr, Ferguson RL. The operative treatment of myelomeningocele spinal deformity. Orthop Clin North Am 1979;10:845.
6. Allen BL, Jr, Ferguson RL. Segmental instrumentation. A useful adjunct in the treatment of difficult spine deformities. Orthop Trans 1981;5:191.
7. Allen BL, Jr, Ferguson RL. L-rod instrumentation for scoliosis in cerebral palsy. J Pediatr Orthop 1982;2:87.
8. Allen BL, Jr, Ferguson RL. The Galveston technique of pelvic fixation for use with L-rod instrumentation. Proceedings of Scoliosis Research Society, 1983.
9. Ferguson RL, Allen BL, Jr. The evolution of segmental spinal instrumentation in the treatment of unstable thoracolumbar spine fractures. Proceedings of Scoliosis Research Society, 1982.
10. Luque ER. Paralytic scoliosis in growing children. Clin Orthop 1982;163:202.
11. Luque ER, Cardoso A. Treatment of scoliosis without arthrodesis or external support. Preliminary report. Orthop Trans 1977;1:37.
12. Luque ER. Segmental spinal instrumentation for correction of scoliosis. Clin Orthop 1982;163:192.
13. Nakano N. Segmental spinal instrumentation in adult patients with spinal deformity and spondylolisthesis. Proceedings of Scoliosis Research Society, 1982.
14. Renshaw TS. Spinal fusion with segmental instrumentation. Contemporary Orthop 1982;4:413.
15. Taddonio RF. Segmental spinal instrumentation in the management of neuromuscular spinal deformity. Spine 1982;7:305.
16. Taddonio RF, Weller K, Appel M. A comparison of patients with idiopathic scoliosis managed with and without postoperative immobilization following segmental spinal instrumentation with Luque rods: a preliminary report. Orthop Trans 1984;8:172.
17. Guadagni J, Drummond D, Breed A. Improved postoperative course following modified segmental instrumentation and posterior spinal fusion for idiopathic scoliosis. J Pediatr Orthop 1984;4:405.
18. Broadstone P, Leatherman KB. Consider postoperative immobilization of double L-rod. Segmental spinal instrumentation. Orthop Trans 1984;8:171.
19. Herndon WA, Sullivan A, Yngve DA, Gross RH, Dreher G. Segmental spinal instrumentation with sublaminar wires: a critical appraisal. J Bone Joint Surg 1987;69A:851.
20. Bonnet CA, Brown JC, Dietrich T. Post-operative immobilization with the Milwaukee brace after spinal fusion with Harrington rod instrumentation. Orthop Rev 1976;5:39.
21. Erwin WD, Dickson JH, Harrington PR. The postoperative management of scoliosis patients treated with Harrington rod instrumentation and fusion. J Bone Joint Surg 1976;58A:479.
22. Kahn A, III, Snyder MA. Cast versus brace immobilization in spinal fusion. Proceedings of Scoliosis Research Society, 1982.
23. Lehner JT, Lorber C, Haines W, Horwitz M. Immediate postoperative orthotic measurements of co-polymer brace of postoperative care after spinal fusion. Proceedings of Scoliosis Research Society, 1982.
24. Roberts RS, Price CT, Riddick MF. Use of a bivalved polypropylene orthosis in the postoperative management of idiopathic scoliosis. Clin Orthop Rel Res 1984;185:25.
25. Tolo V, Gillespie R. The use of shortened periods of postoperative immobilization in the surgical treatment of idiopathic scoliosis. J Bone Joint Surg 1981;63A:1137.
26. Vasquez-Vela SG, Vasquez-Vela SA. A comparison of postoperative casting versus bracing following Harrington rod instrumentation and fusion for idiopathic scoliosis. Proceedings of Scoliosis Research Society, 1983.
27. Whitecloud TS, Mitchell O, Taylor J. Postoperative management of scoliosis in TLS orthosis. Proceedings of Scoliosis Research Society, 1982.
28. Johnson RM, Owen JR, Hart DL, Callahan RA. Cervical orthoses: a guide to their selection and use. Clin Orthop Rel Res 1981;154:34.
29. Johnson RM, Hart DL, Simmons EF, Romsby GR, Southwick WO. Cervical orthoses, a study comparing their effectiveness in restricting cervical motion in normal subjects. J Bone Joint Surg 1977;59A:332.
30. Whitehill R, Richman JA, Glaser JA. Failure of immobilization of the cervical spine by the halo vest. A report of five cases. J Bone Joint Surg 1986;68A:326.
31. Lantz SA, Schultz AB. Lumbar spine orthosis gearing I. Restriction of gross body motions. Spine 1986;11:834.
32. Fidler MW, Plasmans CMT. The effect of four types of support in the segmental mobility of the lumbosacral spine. J Bone Joint Surg 1983;65A:943.
33. Samuelson WO, Simmons EH. Biological factors affecting success in adult spinal fusion. Proceedings of Scoliosis Research Society, 1987.
34. Johnston CE, II, Ashmon RB, Sjerman MC. Mechanical consequences of rod contouring and residual scoliosis in sublaminar pelvis segmental spinal instrumentation. Orthop Trans 1986;10:5.
35. Johnston CE, II. Mechanical consequences of rod contouring and residual scoliosis in sublaminar segmental instrumentation. J Orthop Res 1987;5:206.
36. Bunch WH, Chapman RG. Patient preferences in scoliosis surgery. J Bone Joint Surg 1985;67A:794.
37. Cool TA. Cyclic torsional testing with force motion analysis of segmental spinal instrumentation and Harrington rod instrumentation. Proceedings of Scoliosis Research Society, 1985.
38. McAfee P, Werner FW, Glisson RR. A biomechanical analysis of spinal instrumentation systems in thoracolumbar fractures: comparison of traditional Harrington distraction instrumentation with segmental spinal instrumentation. Spine 1985;10:214.
39. Mino VE. Torsional loading of Harrington distraction rod instrumentation compared to segmental sublaminar and spine process wiring. Proceedings of Scoliosis Research Society, 1984.

■17■

Complications of Spinal Fusions

Jerome M. Cotler and Andrew M. Star

Introduction

Spinal fusion has associated complications that are similar to those resulting from any other surgical intervention. Thus, whenever a fusion is recommended as part of the care program for a patient these factors must be included in the equation. Are the positive anticipated responses of the procedure sufficient to justify subjecting the patient to the risks? In order to answer this question, the surgeon must be familiar with the complications and have a sense of their prevalence. Much of this data is not really available today, but when possible an attempt for perspective will be offered. A text such as this prepared for orthopaedists, neurosurgeons, fellows and residents will not include complications frequently managed by alternative medical personnel. However, we would expect the reader to be aware of the following complications: hepatitis, renal failure, AIDS, antibiotic toxicity, diffuse intravascular coagulopathy, urinary tract infection, inappropriate antidiuretic hormone release, transfusion reactions, cardiac failure, malignant hyperthermia, drug dependency, atelectasis, pulmonary edema, and pulmonary embolus.

One must not lose sight of the state of the patient's general health which can add to the risk of complications. Included at greater risk here is the obese, nutritionally deprived, or diabetic patient. In addition, patients with gout, rheumatoid arthritis, osteopenia, steroid dependency and multiple prior operations demonstrate added risk factors. The result of this increased risk is often manifested as poor healing of soft and hard tissues as well as high rates of infection.

Complications Common to All Types of Fusions

It is beyond the scope of this review to consider in detail the problem of pain in the postoperative spinal fusion patient. Patients undergoing spinal fusions represent a very diverse group in which the indications for surgery may vary from fusion for scoliosis in an adolescent to fusion for iatrogenic lumbar instability in the multiply operated patient. Clearly, there can be a great deal of psychological overlay in the latter patient, particularly if associated with long-term narcotic use. Even in the most cooperative patient there is no way to objectively measure pain. Moreover, fusion may only represent a peripheral part of the surgical endeavor, such as in the patient with a herniated nucleus pulposis when for individual reasons fusion is elected after disc removal. In this latter case, it is questionable whether to attribute postoperative pain to the disc excision or the fusion. Therefore, although pain is an important sequelae of spinal fusions, it will be omitted from all subsequent discussions of complications unless, like tenderness at a bone graft donor site, it can be directly attributed to the fusion surgery.

Wound Infections

Febrile responses during the first 3 days postoperatively are usually of pulmonary or urinary tract origin. After the third postoperative day, however, fever should direct the surgeon's attention to the possibility of wound infection. Wound erythema, induration, increased pain, and drainage are obvious corroborating evidence, as are systemic responses such as increased white blood cell count. These principles could apply to any surgical patient, but there are certain pieces of information that apply specifically to spine fusion patients.

The incidence of wound infections in the spine fusion literature correlates with several factors such as type of surgery, use of antibiotics, length of operation, and patient factors.[1] For some reason, anterior cervical fusions rarely become infected regardless of whether antibiotics are used. In a review of the literature on complications of anterior spine fusions, Barber[2] found the majority of reported series to demonstrate rates of less than 1% wound infection. Similarly, Tew and Mayfield[3] had only 1 infection in 500 consecutive anterior cervical fusions of the

Smith Robinson type. Anterior spine fusions in a series by Kostuik and Hall[4] were found to have a low infection rate. In fact, all the infections in that series could be attributed to the graft donor site.

Posterior and posterolateral lumbar and lumbosacral fusions have been shown to have a somewhat higher rate of infection. Watkins[5] reported that both posterior Hibbs fusions and intertransverse process fusions had an infection rate of 2.4%. Prothero et al.[6] noted wound infection rates in posterior thoracolumbar fusions with Harrington rods of 3.8% without antibiotics and 2.8% with antibiotics. This difference was not statistically significant. However, higher infection rates occurred in operations of more than 5 hours in length and multiply operated patients. Lonstein et al.[7] reviewed the literature and found a rate of infection of approximately 2% in posterior thoracolumbar fusions without instrumentation. Their study found a 2.8% rate of infection with antibiotics compared with a 9.3% rate without antibiotics.

In summary, the reported infection rates vary with type of operation, but there seems to be a relatively low infection rate in anterior procedures and a somewhat higher incidence in posterior thoracic and lumbar procedures. The influence of antibiotics on posterior fusions appears to be favorable, and there appears to be some tendency for larger and longer procedures, especially when associated with implantation of metallic devices, to cause increased infection rates.

Although the authors certainly support the use of prophylactic antibiotics in anterior spine procedures, the infection rate is already very low, and there is currently no proof that these antibiotics are helpful. We also believe that host factors such as nutritional depletion in major spine trauma patients and the immunocompromising diseases alluded to earlier lead to higher wound infection rates, but there is currently no direct proof of this specific to spine fusion patients.

When wound infection is diagnosed, early intervention is essential. Systemic cultures should be obtained as well as local cultures, and are best obtained under sterile conditions in the operating room. Early wound debridement and thorough pulsed irrigation appear to prevent progressive wound deterioration. If the infection does not appear to progress below the deep fascia, it may be appropriate to leave the fascial sutures intact on the first debridement. However, if the patient does not rapidly show systemic improvement including defervescence and decrease in white blood count, repeat debridement, including the area beneath the fascia, should be performed.

A great dilemma faces the surgeon who is treating a patient with purulent material beneath the fascia. It is a matter of judgment whether bone graft material can be retained. We usually favor leaving the bone graft material in place and packing the wound open, followed by frequent wound debridements with pulsed irrigation in the operating room. Retention sutures may be used to prevent wound spreading. In almost all cases, the instrumentation can be left in place. Other authors disagree and would debride and close the wound primarily, leaving an irrigation-suction system in place.[7]

Spinal Abscesses

Vertebral abscesses may be the result of hematological dissemination or secondary to local surgical intervention. Fortunately, spinal abscesses secondary to open surgical procedures are rare, particularly with the use of perioperative antibiotics.

Infections of the spine often drain into the retrofascial space as defined by Altemeier and Alexander.[8] This potential space lies immediately adjacent to the spinal column and is bordered by the transversalis fascia anteriorly, psoas fascia posteriorly, vertebral column medially, and diaphragm superiorly.[9,10] These abscesses can extend distally along tissue planes and present as masses within the thigh, buttocks, or perineum. Dissection into the psoas sheath can produce symptoms of hip pain. For a complete review of retrofascial and retroperitoneal spaces, the reader is referred to the excellent article by Simons et al.[10] (Fig. 17.1).

Diagnosis of vertebral abscesses is very difficult at an early stage. Symptoms of a nondescriptive origin include abdominal distention, abdominal pain, and generalized fatigue or weakness. The distention is not associated with obstruction, and frequently demonstrates temporary relief with stool passage. Abdominal pain is difficult to localize and the fatigue or weakness is similarly difficult to correlate. Flank or paravertebral tenderness may be very acute with marked muscle spasm, and the patient is usually febrile. Laboratory findings usually include an elevated white blood count with a shift to the left, increased sedimentation rate, and sometimes low hemoglobin.

Routine radiographs often will not demonstrate bony destruction until 2 to 6 weeks have passed. The earliest clinical findings include spinal rigidity and severe pain that is exacerbated with any movement. Suggestion of an active process with high rates of bone destruction and formation can be demonstrated with a three-phase bone scan. The initial vascular phase and the delayed bone image should both demonstrate increased uptake. Bone destruction is well defined via planar tomography or computed tomography (CT). CT scans, in particular, will usually clearly show soft-tissue extension or abscesses whether or not bony destruction is evident. Magnetic resonance imaging (MRI) is also a promising technique for defining these abscesses.

Diagnostic needle aspiration of these vertebral abscesses is performed using plain films, CT, or ultrasound control.

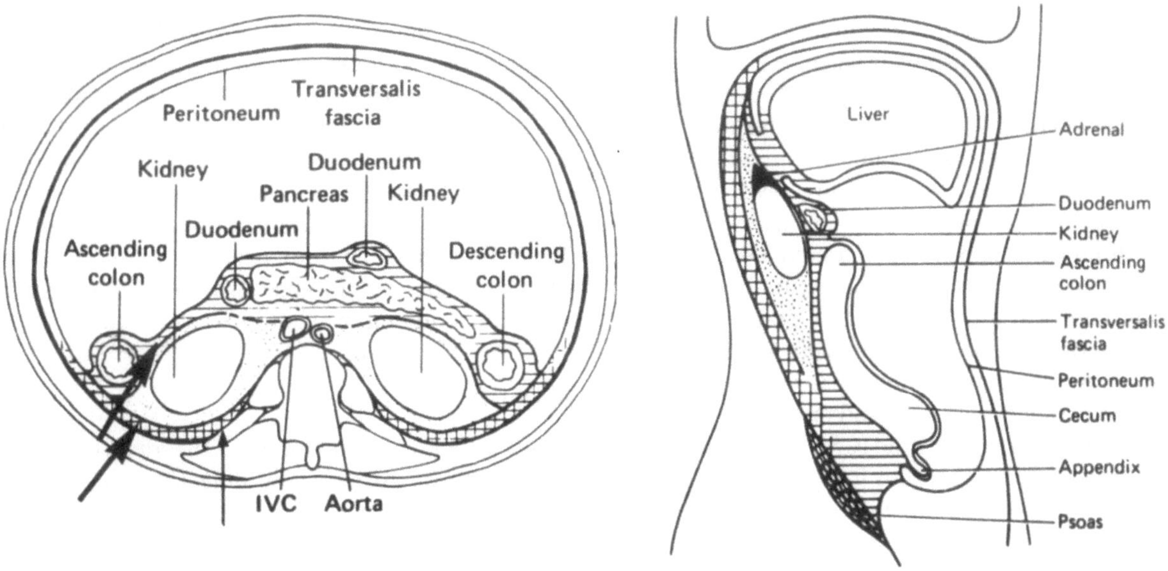

Figure 17.1. Retrofascial (*small arrow*) and retroperitoneal (*large arrows*) spaces. (Reprinted with permission from Meyers MA. Dynamic Radiology of the Abdomen. New York: Springer-Verlag, 1982:110, Fig 4-5.)

Treatment then depends on several factors including the organism cultured, location and size of the abscess, and neurological status. Options for treatment include antibiotics alone, needle/catheter drainage, or open debridement. If open debridement is chosen, a transabdominal approach is contraindicated for fear of introducing an abscess intraperitoneally.

Dural Laceration

In contrast to decompression procedures, fusion of the spine rarely results in dural laceration. The authors' recommendation for treating dural disruption depends on time of diagnosis and location of the laceration.

Dural lacerations that are diagnosed at the time of surgery should be repaired if possible. This may require expanding the surgical exposure to clearly define the edges of the dura. Appropriate magnification and small-diameter suture such as 6–0 nonabsorbable material should be used to provide a complete seal with a minimum of scarring (Fig. 17.2). This can be supplemented, if necessary, with autogenous fascia, fat, or a variety of processed collagen products to produce a watertight seal.[11] Special attention

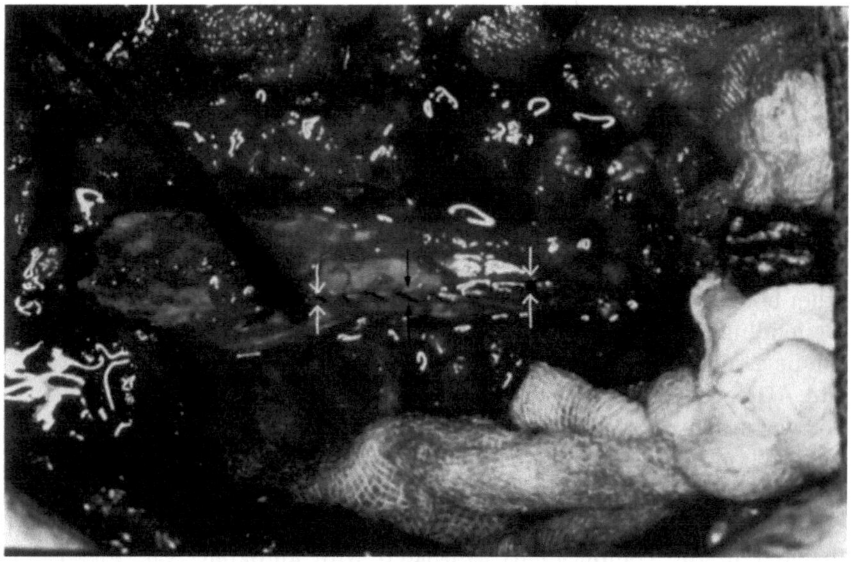

Figure 17.2. Longitudinal dural laceration in lumbar region repaired with running #6-0 silk suture produces watertight seal.

to closure of fascia and skin is required to p oduce a seal that will contain any persistent leakage.

If a dural laceration is diagnosed postoperatively, management is more complicated. Patients with subcutaneous or subfascial collections that are not draining cutaneously should be treated initially with activity restriction to try to reduce the internal pressure and to preserve wound integrity. Often this can be supplemented later with compressive dressings such as an abdominal binder with ultimate resolution of the collection. If a drain is in place, activity restriction should allow the drainage to decrease enough to allow subsequent drain removal.

If a patient presents with a wound or a drain site fistula that is draining cerebrospinal fluid (CSF), the management is more controversial. Sometimes it is possible to perform an open repair if the dural disruption is in an accessible location. This is much easier after posterior approaches where exposure of the large areas of the dura is readily achieved. In contrast, after anterior spine surgery it is often difficult to obtain enough exposure to perform an adequate repair. Sometimes, drainage of CSF using catheters inserted in a remote part of the spine is adequate to reduce the pressure and allow the fistula to close. Obviously, the risk of intradural infection is always present, particularly in an open, draining fistula.

Complications of Bone Grafting

There are currently many possible sources of bone or bonelike materials including cortical or cancellous autografts, cortical or cancellous allografts, and demineralized bone products.[12] A review of these alternatives is presented in Chapter 2. Grafts from the iliac crest have traditionally been the most commonly used source of additional bone material for spine fusions. Some authors would suggest that iliac crest grafts are most desirable because they seem to produce the highest fusion rates.[13–19] This issue is certainly not settled.[20,21a] However, there is no argument that autografts, compared with other sources of bone, are associated with a completely different set of complications related to the bone graft donor site. Complications include vascular, neurological, urinary tract, and abdominal wall injuries. This is not to say that allografts and other bone sources are free of additional complications.[21b] Depending on the method of preparation, donor materials can be associated with transfer of disease such as hepatitis and AIDS for which 100% accurate screening tests are not yet available. Certainly in the patient who is likely to need bone supplementation other than autografts, these risks need to be discussed before surgery.

The remainder of this review of bone grafts will be devoted to the complications associated with autograft acquisition, and will emphasize grafts from the iliac crest because this is the most commonly used donor site.

When harvested with the aid of power equipment, donor bone should be cooled to prevent heat-induced necrosis.[22,23] When harvested, the graft should be maintained in a sponge soaked in autogenous blood. In addition, the graft material should be out of its natural environment for the least possible time, preferably less than 30 minutes. While the graft is dislodged from nutritional support, the ambient temperature should remain below 42°C.[24]

Cosmetic

Most individuals do not find the deformity after bone grafting to be cosmetically objectionable; however, in a very slim individual, particularly a young woman who is very image conscious, harvesting this bone may be very traumatic. Particular areas of concern include the direction and width of the scar, loss of symmetrical contours, and unwillingness to wear swimming attire. Our society is so image conscious and plastic reconstruction oriented that we must be very sensitive to this attitude, which was not prevalent three or four decades ago. The superficial scar may be minimized with the use of subcuticular closures. Loss of contours depends on the volume of bone autograft necessary. If only a relatively small amount of bone is needed, it is possible to develop windows of various sizes between the cortices for access. Desirable sites particularly abundant in cancellous bone anteriorly are under the iliac tubercle and posteriorly under the posterior iliac spine (Fig. 17.3). Alternatives include either splitting the crest, harvesting cancellous material, and partial closure, or obtaining the bone from the inner table (Fig. 17.4). A reported alternative with which the authors have no

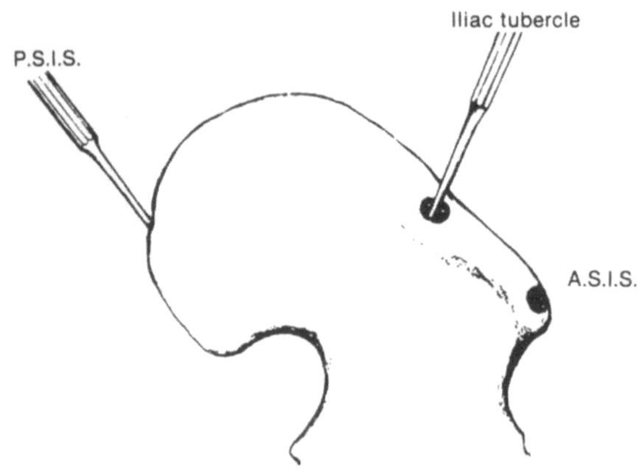

Figure 17.3. Illustration of iliac crest shows removal of cancellous bone through cortical windows. (Reproduced by permission from White AH, Rothman RH, Ray CD. Lumbar Spine Surgery: Techniques and Complications, St. Louis, 1987, The C. V. Mosby Co., Fig. 39-8.)

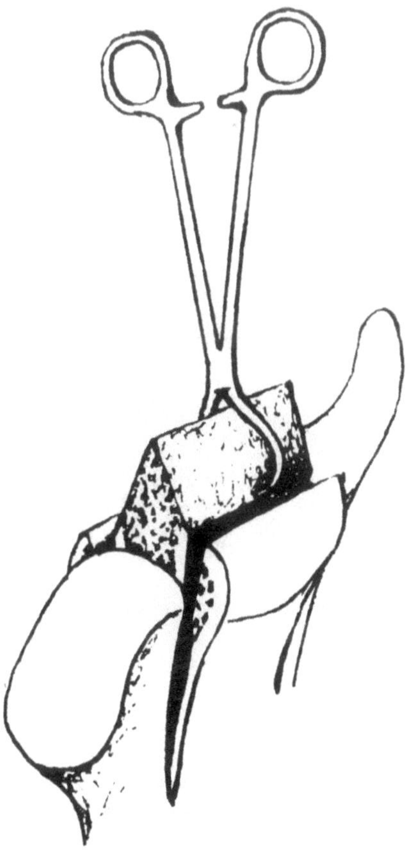

Figure 17.4. Removal of cancellous bone graft by splitting iliac crest. Cortex is reapproximated without leaving cortical defect. (Reproduced by permission from: White AH, Rothman RH, Ray CD. Lumbar Spine Surgery: Techniques and Complications, St. Louis, 1987, The C. V. Mosby Co.)

experience is reconstruction of the contoured pelvis with methylmethacrylate or ceramic (Fig. 17.5). Of necessity, anchor points should be developed to help maintain position of the foreign body.

Pelvic/Hip Fractures and Instability

Fracture of the pelvis or pelvic instability is a rare complication after harvesting bone graft, although there have been several case reports, probably because of the significant consequences. The incidence is not readily available but appears to be less than 1%[25,26] (Fig. 17.6). The most common pattern of instability appears to be sacroiliac joint instability after posterior iliac crest removal with associated pubic ramus stress fracture or symphysis subluxation.[27] Instability appears to be associated with large or multiple grafting procedures[27,28] (Fig. 17.7). The diagnosis requires a high index of suspicion because often the patient will complain only of lumbosacral pain that is similar to the pain of spinal origin for which the patient originally sought treatment. Tenderness is usually localized over the sacroiliac joint but can be difficult to palpate in obese patients. If there is symphysial pain and tenderness associated with radiographic changes showing either anterior ring fracture or subluxation, then the diagnosis should be obvious. However, these may not present until sacroiliac joint instability has been present for a long time. Provocative testing by either applying downward pressure on the lateral aspect of the pelvis with the patient in the lateral position or applying a hip abduction stress with the opposite side of the pelvis firmly fixed (FABER test—flexion-abduction-external rotation) can be very helpful. Radiographic views with the patient standing on first one foot then the other may be diagnostic.[27] Treatment usually involves fusion of the involved sacroiliac joint with either fusion or resection of the symphysis pubis.

Propagation of fractures into the acetabulum is very rare and carries all the risks of any acetabular fracture. The treatment of these complications is really prevention by careful attention to the anatomy of the pelvis and the location of any osteotomies that are performed. When these fractures occur, they should be treated accordingly to location and amount of displacement.

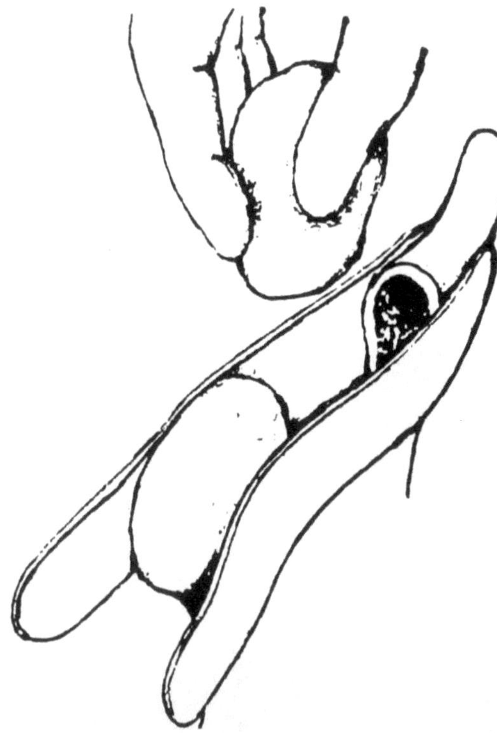

Figure 17.5. Method of application of methylmethacrylate to eliminate cortical defect produced after removing bone for grafting. (Reproduced by permission from: White AH, Rothman RH, Ray CD. Lumbar Spine Surgery: Techniques and Complications, St. Louis, 1987, The C. V. Mosby Co., Fig. 39-20.)

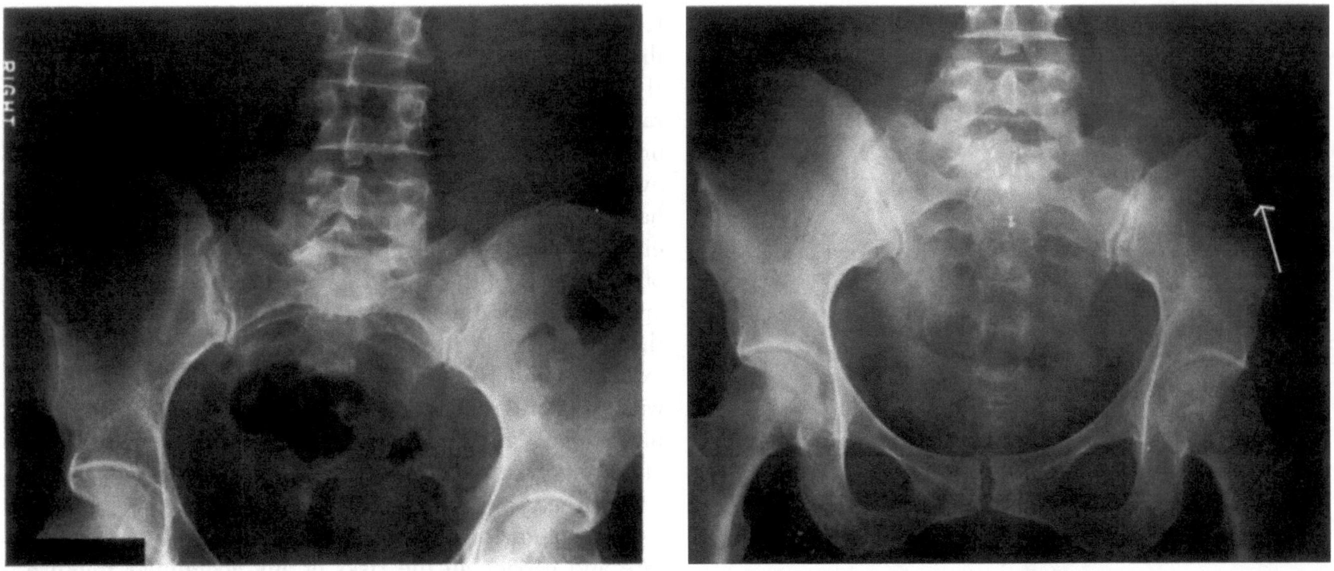

A B

Figure 17.6. Preoperative view (**A**) and postoperative view (**B**) show iliac wing fracture (*arrow*) that occurred after removal of large iliac tricortical graft.

Hip subluxation is an extremely rare complication that is usually associated only with extensive iliac resection.[25] Once again, knowledge of anatomy and a careful operative technique should prevent this complication.

Gait Disturbance

Observation of altered gait is usually a very transient finding, transient in this instance meaning days or weeks (usually not more than 3 to 6 weeks). Its usual etiology is difficult to distinguish, be it pain or freeing of muscles from their normal attachments. Nothing more than symptomatic treatment and time is necessary in these instances. Of necessity one should consider whether any element of nerve damage is an etiological factor. Unless the nerve is a major one (sciatic or femoral), only observation and supportive care is necessary.

Hematoma

The occurrence of large hematomas after harvesting pelvic bone was more prevalent in the past. Factors that predis-

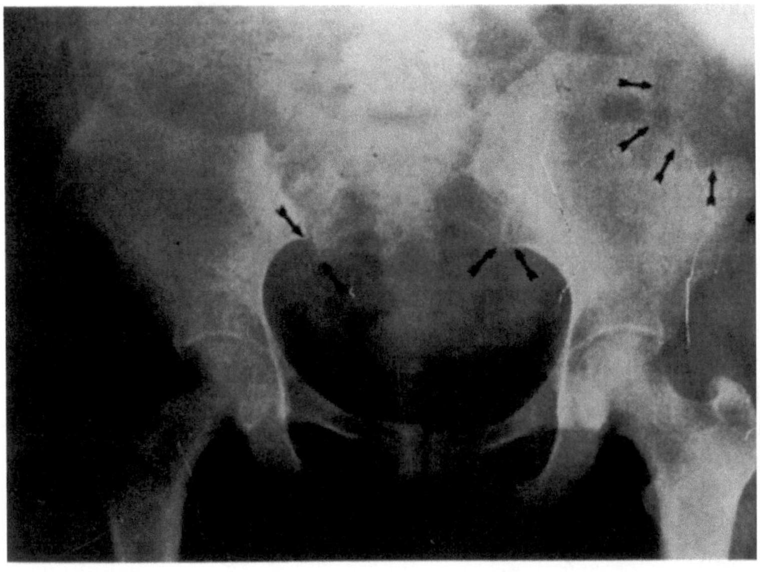

Figure 17.7. Dislocation of left sacroiliac joint and stress fracture of pubic rami associated with obtaining multiple iliac crest grafts. (Reprinted with permission from Lichtblau S. Dislocation of the sacroiliac joint. J Bone Joint Surg 1962;44A:195, Fig. 3.)

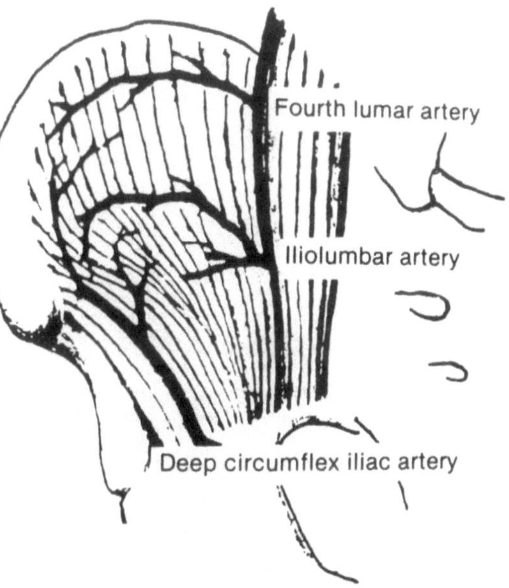

Figure 17.8. Illustration of position of fourth lumbar artery, iliolumbar artery, and deep circumflex iliac artery along medial surface of the ilium. (Reproduced by permission from: White AH, Rothman RH, Ray CD. Lumbar Spine Surgery: Techniques and Complications, St. Louis, 1987, The C. V. Mosby Co., Fig. 39-16.)

pose graft donor sites to postoperative bleeding are the large exposed cancellous surfaces and extensive vasculature of the pelvic musculature. Current practices to prevent this complication include electrocoagulation, electrodissection, careful contiguous subperiosteal dissection, application of local substances [thrombin, gelfoam (Upjohn), avitene (Alcon PR)] to augment blood coagulation, and bone wax application. The advent of closed suction drainage, which allows a portal for egress of accumulated blood over a period of a few days, has probably done the most to prevent large hematomas.

When a hematoma is diagnosed, the authors have not routinely performed open drainage unless the hematoma is very large and the patient becomes hypotensive. In the latter case, major vessel disruption should be suspected and an attempt should be made to control bleeding. This is discussed further in the section on vascular injuries. If a hematoma begins to drain, it is probably wise to reexplore and decompress the wound in the operating room and then perform a primary closure alone or over a drain.

Hemorrhage

There are many vessels around the pelvis that are potential sources of hemorrhage. These vessels lie medial to the area of bone removal. From an anterior to posterior direction, they are (1) the deep circumflex iliac artery, (2) the superior gluteal artery (in the greater sciatic notch, a branch from the internal iliac), (3) the iliolumbar artery, and (4) the fourth lumbar artery (Fig. 17.8).

Damage to these vessels can be minimized by following a few simple rules. (1) Remain subperiosteal during the dissection. This is simple in the young patient who presents for scoliosis fusion because he/she usually will have a thick periosteum. Subperiosteal dissection is somewhat more difficult in older patients where the periosteum is usually thin. (2) Careful muscle retraction including placement of retractors. In a report by Escalas and DeWald in 1977, a Taylor retractor placed in the sciatic notch produced an A-V fistula involving the superior gluteal artery as well as causing a ureteral laceration.[29] (3) Careful appraisal of the relationship between the region of bone removal and the sciatic notch. Although it is not a very common occurrence, laceration of the superior gluteal artery near the sciatic notch is the most frequent arterial injury (Fig. 17.9). It is worthwhile to dissect this vessel in the anatomy laboratory to appreciate its diameter of 6 to 8 mm. This vessel is most vulnerable as it exits the sciatic notch and turns cephalad to supply the gluteus medius and minimus muscles.

A landmark to prevent its injury is to remain above an imaginary line drawn from the posterior superior iliac spine to the anterior iliac spine. Bleeding from this vessel can commonly produce several liters of blood loss in a short time. With adequate assistance and lighting, these bleeding points can usually be controlled with vascular clips.[30] If the end of the artery has retracted behind the

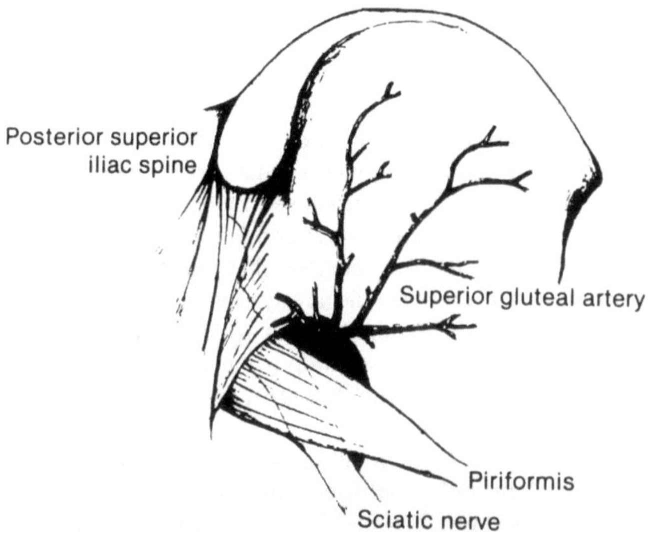

Figure 17.9. Position of superior gluteal artery exiting greater sciatic notch along external surface of ilium above piriformis. (Reproduced by permission from: White AH, Rothman RH, Ray CD. Lumbar Spine Surgery: Techniques and Complications, St. Louis, The C. V. Mosby Co., Fig. 39-14.)

sciatic notch, digital pressure can often control the bleeding to allow slow advancement to the bleeding site and subsequent ligation. Exposure may be augmented by rongeuring away part of the sciatic notch[30] or if all else fails, then boldly splitting the pelvis longitudinally with a Gigli saw.[31] Additional alternatives include catheter embolization or turning the patient supine to enter the pelvis anteriorly. This latter alternative, although often mentioned, is logistically difficult to perform successfully.

Occasionally a patient exhibits postoperative hypotension, and the diagnosis of delayed arterial rupture is entertained.[2,30] Whether this represents delayed rupture or delayed diagnosis is not often clear, but these problems may be amenable to a trial of arterial embolization before operative exploration.

Hernia

Full-thickness harvesting of iliac bone may predispose to hernia formation. As with hernias in any location of the body, predisposition is also associated with tissues demonstrating weaker collagen. Usually the iliopsoas muscle and its inner periosteal base are strong enough to resist this complication, but any factors associated with weakening this barrier may result in a hernia. Clinically the hernia is observed as painful or painless swelling. Pain may result from local tissue tension or intestinal obstruction.[32–37] Intestinal obstruction in this area may be reversible but may also proceed to strangulation.

Prevention of hernia may be aided by several factors. Being careful not to violate the periosteum of the inner pelvic wall, when combined with secure fascial suture, should provide a strong resistance to herniation of abdominal contents. Particularly in the very obese patient, the tissues are often poorly defined and difficult to identify. Moreover, Bosworth[38] reviewed iliac crest defect herniations and found they were caused by extensive resection of the midportion of the crest leaving an opening in this region (Fig. 17.10). He reported that removal of the midportion of the crest should always include the complete crest in a relatively straight line to avoid leaving a midportion iliac opening. These midportion hernias can be repaired by leveling off the iliac crest and then transferring fascia into the defect.

Treatment is the same as for any hernia. If local tissues are prevalent and of sufficient quality, they may be garnered for local reinforcement of the reduction. Bosworth[38] described such a technique in 1955. Without the luxury of local tissue, alternative foreign material such as methylmethacrylate, Marlex®, tantalum, and Dacron® have been suggested.

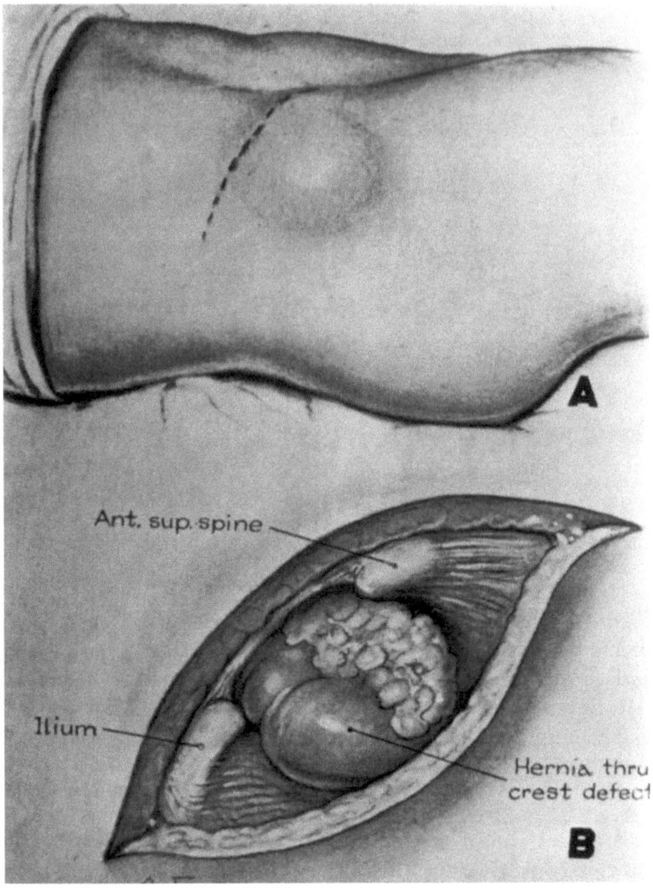

Figure 17.10. **A.** Appearance of herniation through defect in midportion of iliac crest. **B.** Dissection shows herniation. (Reprinted with permission from Bosworth DM. Repair of hernia through iliac-crest defects. J Bone Joint Surg 1955;37A:1071, Fig. 3.)

Heterotopic Bone Formation

Heterotopic bone formation is a rare complication of bone graft harvesting from the iliac crest. When present, it is usually at a distance from the hip joint and rarely causes any functional disability.[26] One might consider prophylaxis in patients such as ankylosing spondylitics who are known to form large amounts of heterotopic ossification; however, any plans for prophylaxis must be considered in light of the minimal morbidity that usually occurs from the heterotopic bone. The current treatments include Indomethacin 25 mg twice a day (bid), radiotherapy in various dosages, and diphosphonates. In the authors' experience, none of these prophylactic treatments should be necessary, but the literature on treatment of heterotopic ossification is still evolving.

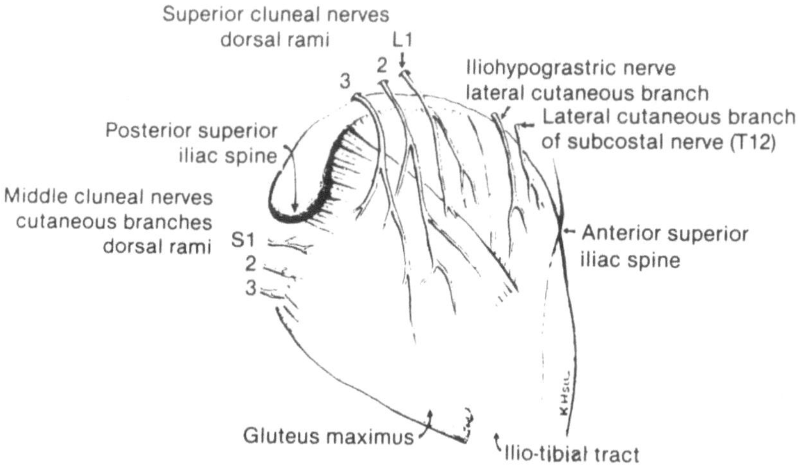

Figure 17.11. Position of cutaneous nerves along posterolateral surface of ilium. (Reproduced by permission from White AH, Rothman RH, Ray CD. Lumbar Spine Surgery: Techniques and Complications, St. Louis, 1987, The C. V. Mosby Co., Fig. 39-13.)

Nerve Injury

Nerve injury, particularly of sensory nerves, is common during harvesting of large iliac crest grafts.[39] Fortunately it is rare for these sensory nerve injuries to be associated with significant morbidity. The significant nerves are (Fig. 17.11) the lateral femoral cutaneous, iliohypogastric, superior cluneal, middle cluneal, ilioinguinal, and genitofemoral nerves.

Lateral Femoral Cutaneous Nerve

This is the most anterior nerve that is encountered. It is a branch of L1, L2, L3 and emerges from the lateral border of the psoas muscle. It then runs downward on the surface of the iliacus muscle, passes under the inguinal ligament, and appears 1 cm from the anterior superior iliac spine medial to the sartorius muscle. It then passes laterally over the surface of the sartorious muscle[40] (Fig. 17.12).

Injury to this nerve is reported in as many as 14% to less than 1% of anterior iliac crest approaches.[25,41,42] The syndrome associated with this injury is known as meralgia paresthetica.[43] This is associated with paresthesia and numbness along the anterolateral surface of the thigh in an area corresponding to the distribution of the lateral femoral cutaneous nerve. The nerve can either be directly injured or can be trapped by scar tissue that forms later. Most of these symptoms will subside with nonoperative treatment, but occasionally release or division is necessary. To prevent this injury, it is recommended that 2 cm of the anterior iliac crest contiguous with the anterior superior iliac spine be left undisturbed if possible.

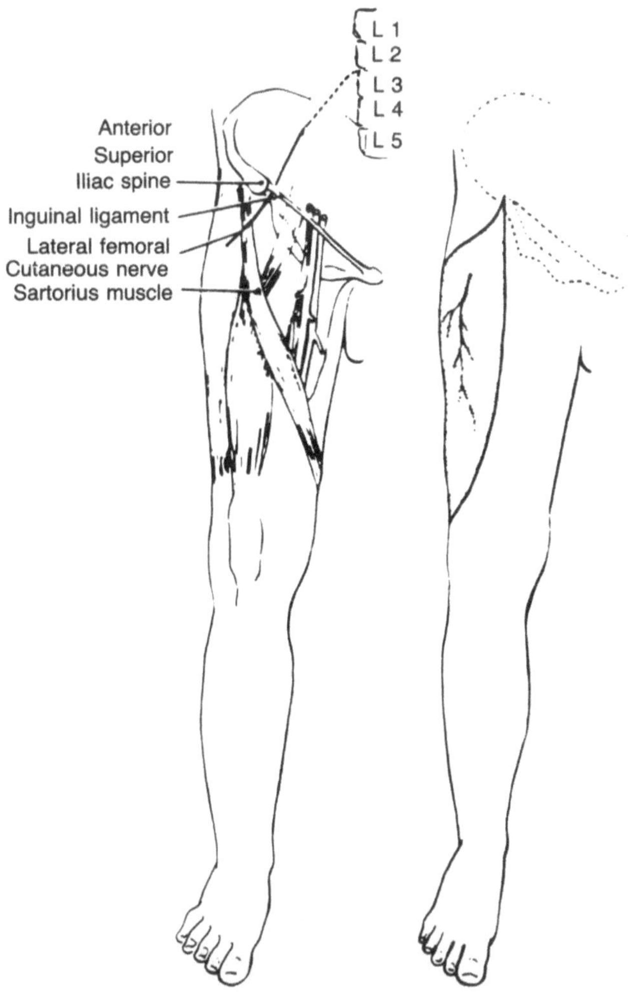

Figure 17.12. Position of lateral femoral cutaneous nerves with respect to anterior superior iliac spine, inguinal ligament, and sartorius muscle. (Reprinted with permission from Weikel AM, Habal MB. Meralgia paresthetica: a complication of iliac bone procurement. Plast Reconstruct Surg 1977;60:573, Fig. 1.)

Ilioinguinal Nerve

This is a branch of L1 that runs along with the iliohypogastric nerve obliquely downward across the quadratus lumborum along the posterior abdominal wall (Fig. 17.13). It enters the transversus abdominus above the iliac crest. It emerges through the superficial inguinal ring and supplies part of the penis and scrotum in the male, and the mons pubis and labia majora in the female.[44]

The mechanism of injury is believed to be compression from a retractor when the abdominal wall is retracted medially away from the iliac crest. Patients with injury to this nerve complain of pain radiating medially toward the inguinal and genital regions and have increased pain with extension and internal rotation of the hip. Ilioinguinal nerve block has been successful in relieving the pain in two persistent cases.[45]

Genitofemoral Nerve

This nerve is formed from L1, L2, and after exiting the psoas muscle divides into genital and femoral branches. The genital branch supplies the skin of the scrotum or labium major, and the femoral branch passes under the inguinal ligament to supply the middle of the anterior thigh.

Injury to this nerve is very rare; the authors could only find one reported case.[41]

Cluneal Nerves

These nerves cross the iliac crest in a longitudinal fashion, and supply sensation to the middle portion of the buttock. They are branches of the first three lumbar and sacral nerve roots. Injury to these nerves is very common during approaches to the posterior iliac crest, particularly when using a transverse incision. Longitudinal skin incisions seem to avoid most of these branches. Review of eight cases of cluneal nerve injury with persistent symptoms indicated that the cause of disability can be proven by infiltration with local anesthetic. Resection then permanently relieved the symptoms in all cases.[46]

General Treatment of Cutaneous Nerve Injuries

Symptoms for all these nerve injuries usually include burning, numbness, paresthesia, or stabbing pain along the appropriate nerve distribution. Usually symptoms can be controlled with various nonoperative techniques such as analgesics, local heat, local nerve blocks, reassurance, transcutaneous electrical stimulation, and time. Only in the occasional patient who has persistent substantial symptoms should operative exploration and neuroma resection be considered.

Noncutaneous Nerve Injuries

The femoral nerve may be injured with extensive medial retraction of soft tissues and usually produces self-limiting disability that spontaneously corrects. Deficit includes quadriceps deficiency which, when severe, can result in the need to manually support the thigh for knee stabilization.

The sciatic nerve takes exit from the pelvis inferior to or through the piriformis muscle. It is mandatory for dissection in this region to remain subperiosteal and apply

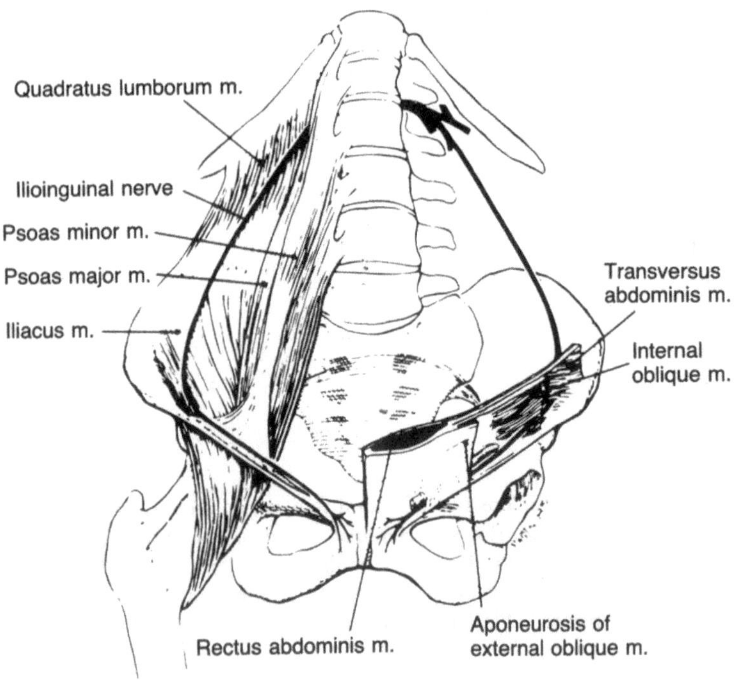

Figure 17.13. Course of ilioinguinal nerve through inguinal ring to become subcutaneous. (Reprinted with permission from Smith SE, De Lee JC, Ramamurthy S. Ilioguinal neuralgia following iliac bone-grafting. J Bone Joint Surg 1984;66A:1306–1308, Fig. 1.)

as little tension as possible to the nerve, thus preventing a traction neurapraxia and foot drop. Fortunately this nerve is only rarely injured.

The superior gluteal nerve provides motor supply to the gluteus medius and minimus. Without its function the patient will walk with a positive Trendelenberg gait. Usually the deficit is a neurapraxia and will correct with time.

Peritoneal Injury

The relevance of this injury is unknown. In a patient with good musculature (iliopsoas muscles) and careful subperiosteal dissection, this structure should not be seen. However, if injury is observed, then careful assessment should be made to be certain that no viscera has been violated. If any of these structures, including the peritoneum, are injured they should be repaired. Repair could be carried out by the orthopaedist or, if necessary, by a general surgeon.

Ureteral Injury

This is an extremely rare injury. To the best knowledge of the authors, only one instance has been reported[29] (Fig. 17.14).

Pain at the Donor Site

As previously noted, pain evaluation in a group of patients who are presenting for operative therapy to relieve pain from a wide variety of sources is impossible to measure objectively. As a means to summarize this section on bone graft complications, it should be realized that between 0.6% and 37% of patients will complain of pain well localized to the donor site.[2,3,47,48] In most patients examined, these symptoms will be mild and transient, but 6% of patients in one series still required narcotics for bone graft donor site pain 10 years postoperatively, although many of these patients also had back pain. Variables such as length of incision, size of graft, surgical skill, and quality of the patients' tissues all seem to have an impact on the overall rate.

Tibia

This bone has modest cancellous reserves available in the proximal metaphysis. In the older adult much of the hematopoietic function has passed from this area, resulting in an atrophied osteopenic source. Premier material available from the tibia remains its cortical stores. This is most accessible from the anteromedial surface with the crest representing its most lateral border. The price for harvesting this cortical material is prolonged weakness in torsion and bending requiring external tibial support for varying periods extending to a year.[49] Total incorporation of cortical graft is difficult to determine, but the construct is usually weakest at 6 months when most cancellous grafts are strongest.[50]

Fibula

This bone has even less cancellous reserves than are found in the tibia. Even for grafts where structural stability is necessary, the authors prefer to use corticocancellous grafts from the iliac crest. Iliac grafts have sufficient cortical bone to provide strength, and much more cancellous bone to provide rapid incorporation.

Nonunion or Graft Collapse

The significance of nonunion or graft collapse obviously varies with the type of graft and location (Figs. 17.15A–17.15C and Fig. 17.16). Graft collapse can be quite serious

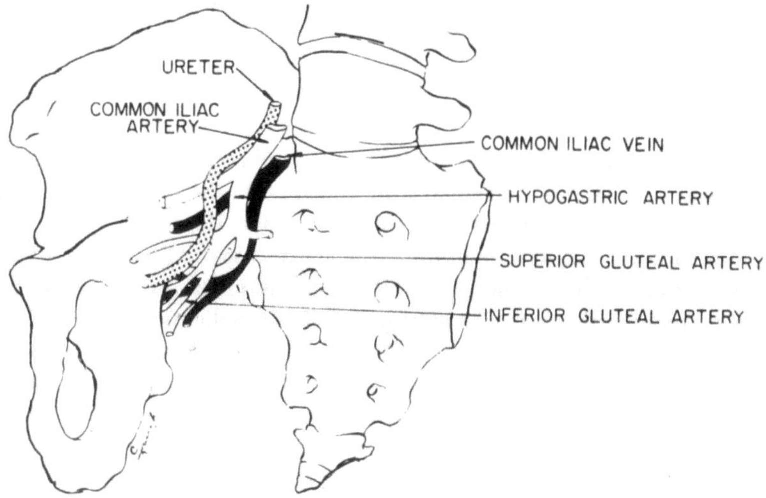

Figure 17.14. Position of ureter along inner surface of the ilium. (Reprinted with permission from Escalas F, DeWald RL. Combined traumatic arteriovenous fistula and ureteral injury: a complication of iliac bone-grafting. J Bone Joint Surg 1977;59A:270, Fig. 1.)

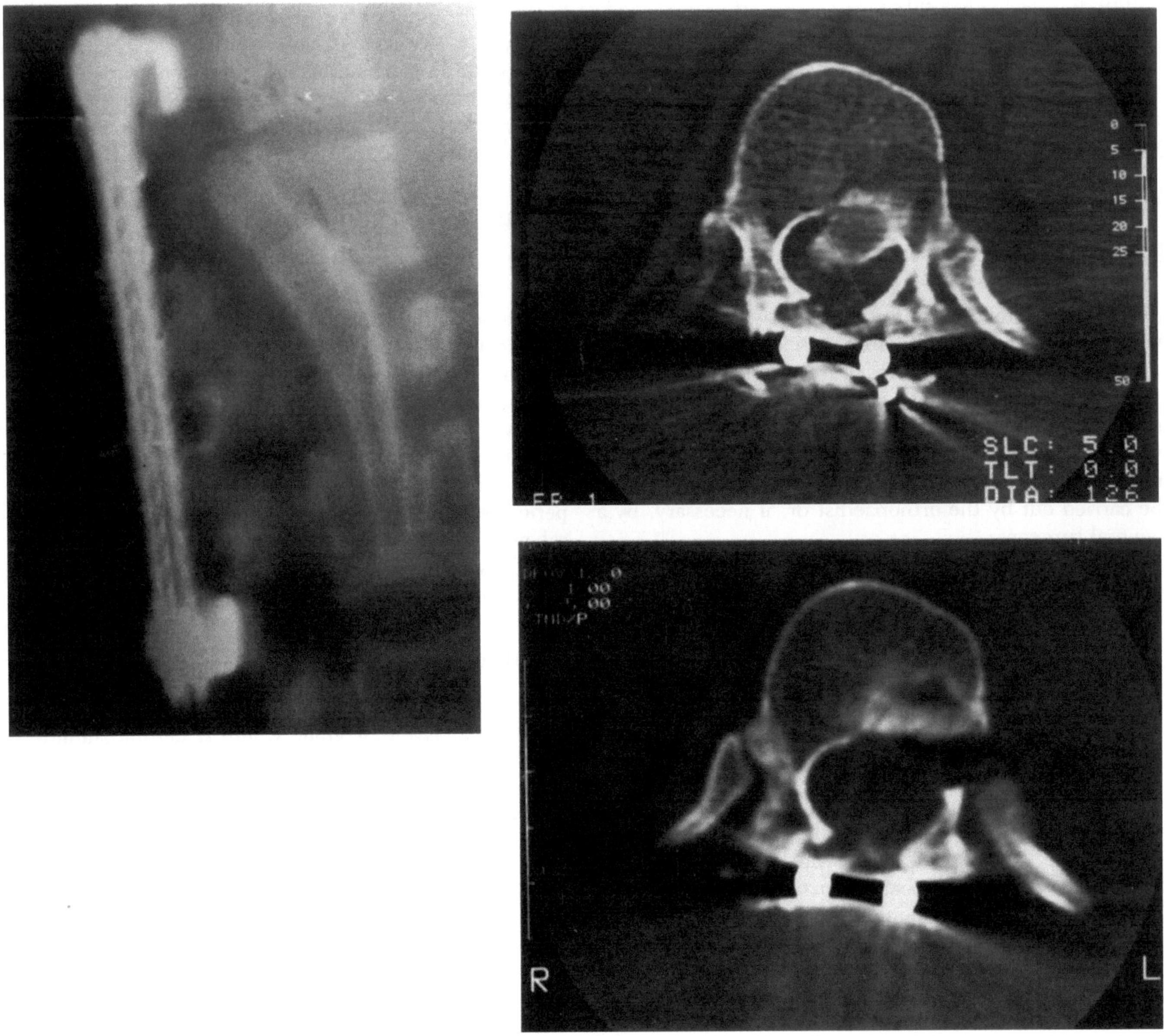

Figure 17.15. Lateral tomogram (**A**) and computerized axial tomography scan (**B**) show tricortical iliac crest strut graft that has migrated into spinal canal. **C.** CAT scan after revision of graft.

if it occurs in a graft used for anterior vertebral reconstruction and results in neural canal compromise. On the other hand, nonunion of a posterior lumbar fusion does not seem to correlate with symptoms in many cases. Moreover, although the diagnosis of graft collapse is quite apparent on plain radiographs, nonunion is difficult to diagnose.

Several authors have shown that the radiologic diagnosis of nonunion did not correlate with the diagnosis based on reexploration and the radiographs tended to underestimate the incidence. However, this must be interpreted in light of poor correlation with symptoms and the apparent acceptability of fibrous union in certain locations.

The authors' approach to graft nonunion or collapse involves determining the following information:

1. Is the patient symptomatic from the nonunion, for example, does graft collapse cause compromise of adjacent structures such as spinal cord or esophagus?
2. Is the patient at risk for sudden collapse or progressive displacement that could compromise adjacent structures?

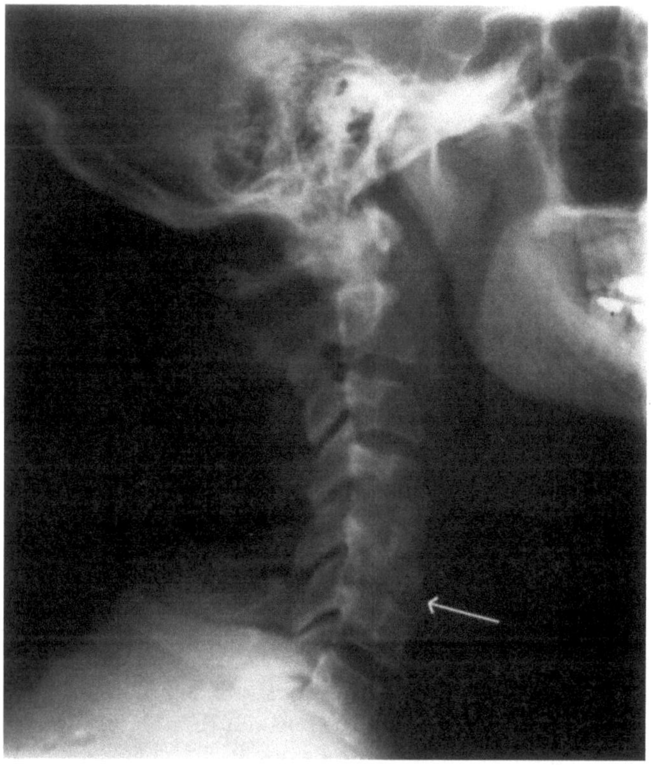

Figure 17.16. Nonunion of anterior cervical fusion after interbody tricortical iliac crest graft.

If either of these questions is answered in the affirmative, then the authors recommend further intervention to stabilize the graft. In early cases, this may only involve bracing to allow the area to stabilize over time. Otherwise, graft replacement, augmentation of fusion mass, addition or alteration of instrumentation, or fusion at another location to provide additional stability (such as posterior fusion after a previous anterior fusion) may be necessary.

Local and systemic factors can significantly affect the healing of bone grafts of all types. Incorporation of grafts requires the presence of blood vessels and osteoprogenitor cells within the grafted area. Local factors such as previous irradiation will injure osteoprogenitor cells and cause significant scarring that can impair the ability of the local blood supply to deliver cells to the region.[51] Systemic factors such as chemotherapeutic agents have been shown to adversely affect bone metabolism.[52]

Anterior Cervical Fusion

This discussion is limited to complications associated with anterior fusion of the middle and lower cervical vertebrae. Anterior fusions of the upper cervical spine are relatively uncommon because of their difficulty and ensuing high complication rate. Fortunately, most fusions of the upper cervical spine can be performed posteriorly.

To understand the complications associated with anterior cervical fusions, it is important to review the anatomy of several key anterior neck structures: the laryngeal nerves, vertebral artery, thoracic duct, thyroid arteries, carotid sheath, and sympathetic chain.

Laryngeal Nerves

The innervation of the muscles of the larynx is through bilateral superior and inferior laryngeal nerves. The superior laryngeal nerve is a branch of the inferior ganglion of the vagus nerve that descends anterior to the vagus nerve in the neck. It travels along with the superior thyroid artery to innervate the cricothyroid muscle. The function of this muscle is to tense the vocal cord during speech. Damage to this nerve often results in hoarseness.[53]

The inferior laryngeal nerve is a branch of the vagus nerve that innervates all of the muscles of the larynx except the cricothyroid. Therefore, interruption of this nerve results in paralysis of the vocal cord on the affected side, which can produce hoarseness and, in some cases, aspiration of liquid because of loss of sensation in the larynx.[53] In most people, a branch of the left vagus nerve leaves the carotid sheath at the level of the aortic arch and turns around the aorta from anterior to posterior to travel upward toward the laryngeal muscle within the groove between the trachea and esophagus to become the inferior laryngeal nerve. The pathway on the right side is similar except the recurrent nerve travels around the subclavian artery. Because it is more common for the right inferior laryngeal nerve to be nonrecurrent (travel directly from the vagus nerve and carotid sheath to the larynx), some surgeons always approach the cervical spine from the left side where the nerve location is more consistent (Fig. 17.17). The incidence of nonrecurrent laryngeal nerve on the right side is reported as 1%.[54a]

Damage to these laryngeal nerves usually results in hoarseness, but hoarseness in the postoperative anterior cervical spine fusion patient is certainly not always from laryngeal nerve laceration. Barber[2] reviewed the literature on anterior cervical fusions in 1978 as well as presenting his own series of 100 Cloward fusions. He found that hoarseness was present in 5% of his own patients and in 4% to 10% of other series reviewed, but only in 1% did it persist beyond 5 weeks after surgery. Bulger et al.[53] reported on vocal cord paralysis associated with anterior cervical fusions and emphasized the difficulties in assessing the incidence. These authors stated that many patients have impaired vocal cord mobility preoperatively. They also believed that vocal cord paralysis can result from

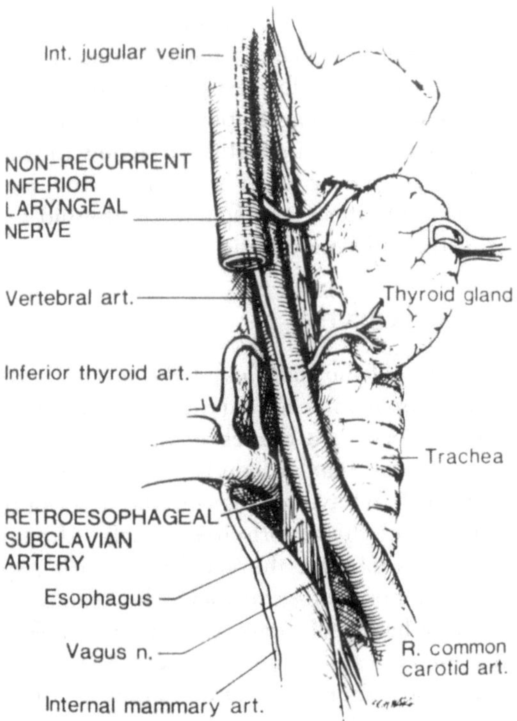

Figure 17.17. Path of nonrecurrent inferior laryngeal nerve passing directly from carotid sheath to larynx. In this position, nerve is directly in surgical field and at high risk for injury. (Reprinted with permission from Bulger RF, Rejowski JE, Beatty RA. Vocal cord paralysis associated with anterior cervical fusion: considerations for prevention and treatment. J Neurosurg 1985;62:659, Fig. 1.)

endotracheal intubation with compression of the recurrent nerve by the endotracheal cuff. Further, as a result of edema from surgery, patients may have hoarseness with normal vocal cord mobility. They performed laryngeal examinations on 102 patients after surgery, and found an incidence of 1% recurrent nerve palsy that resolved within 6 months, despite performing all these operations on the right side where the anatomy of the nerve is known to be less consistent. They also found one patient with a superior laryngeal nerve palsy.

In another series, Heeneman[54b] reported on 85 cases of anterior cervical fusion; 11% of his cases had significant vocal cord paralysis. Six of these had altered vocal cord mobility that resolved within 3 months, and three others had more permanent hoarseness which in one case had to be surgically reconstructed by transplant of rib cartilage to support the paralyzed abducted cord.[55] The author stressed that postoperative hoarseness may result from nerve laceration, edema, or nerve contusion by overly zealous retraction.

Evaluation of hoarseness following anterior cervical spine surgery should include laryngoscopy at about 6 weeks if symptoms persist. Inferior laryngeal nerve injury results in paralysis of all the laryngeal muscles except the cricothyroid, which is innervated by the superior laryngeal nerve. When examined, patients with an inferior laryngeal nerve palsy will demonstrate complete paralysis of the cord in a paramedian position (Fig. 17.18). If this latter injury is bilateral, the patient may have difficulty maintaining an airway; however, this is a very rare occurrence because procedures are not usually performed bilaterally, so usually one side is spared.[56] Paralysis of the cricothyroid muscle alone, which is caused by isolated superior laryngeal nerve palsy, will result in loss of the ability to effectively tense the cord. Patients with this injury will have a mobile cord that is not as straight as the opposite side (Fig. 17.19). Superior nerve paralysis alone often produces only minor symptoms such as easy fatiguing of the voice.[53]

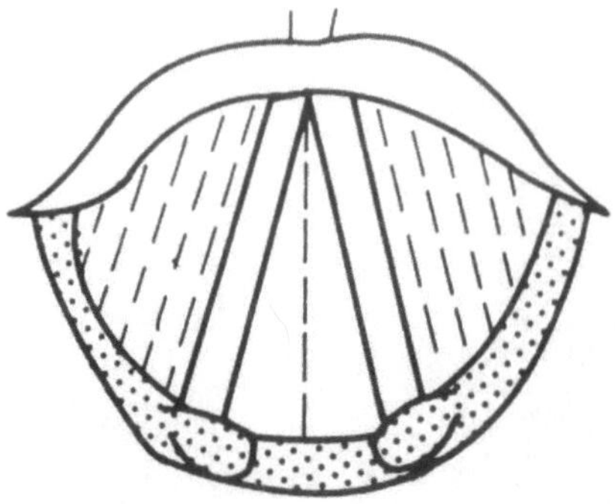

Figure 17.18. Bilateral vocal cord paralysis in paramedian position indicates bilateral inferior laryngeal nerve palsy. (Reprinted with permission from Jacobson L. Bilateral vocal cord paralysis. Anesthesia 1979;34:1022, Fig. 2.)

Treatment of inferior laryngeal nerve injury should include waiting at least 6 months for spontaneous recovery of function or natural adaptation to occur. If this fails, or if the patient has problems with aspiration of swallowed

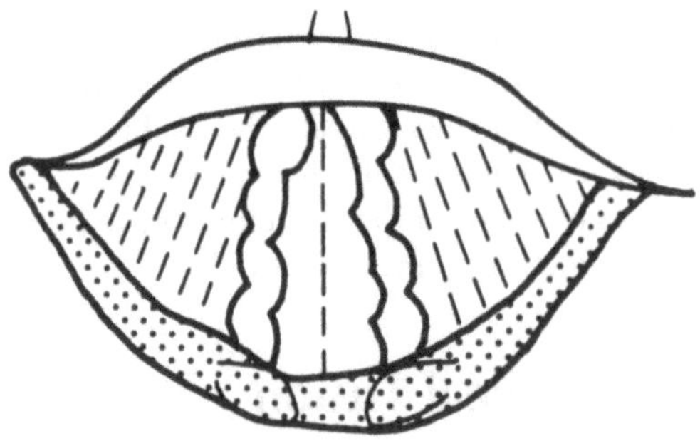

Figure 17.19. Laxity of vocal cords indicates loss of tensing function of cricothyroid muscles because of laryngeal nerve palsy. (Reprinted with permission from Jacobson L. Bilateral vocal cord paralysis. Anesthesia 1979;34:1022, Fig. 4.)

material into the lungs, then stiffening of the involved vocal cord with Teflon paste injection can cure the symptoms in 80% of patients.[53]

Thoracic Duct

This important structure enters the neck on the left side between the vertebral column and esophagus. It passes in a medial to lateral direction behind the carotid artery to enter the left subclavian vein[53,57] (Fig. 17.20). It is usually vulnerable only in approaches to the lower cervical or upper thoracic spine, and in these situations a right-sided approach may be preferable.[57] If this structure is divided it should be ligated proximally and distally in order to prevent a chylothorax.[58]

Thyroid Arteries

The superior thyroid artery exits the carotid sheath and travels medially toward the thyroid gland and larynx in the company of the superior laryngeal nerve at the level of C3. This vessel is rarely involved in anterior approaches. The inferior thyroid artery is usually a small branch that travels from the subclavian artery upward and medially posterior to the carotid sheath. It is often in the middle of the field of dissection during approaches to the lower cervical vertebrae, and is commonly ligated with impunity.[57] Failure to ligate the inferior thyroid artery can lead to significant bleeding during the surgery or to postoperative hematoma.

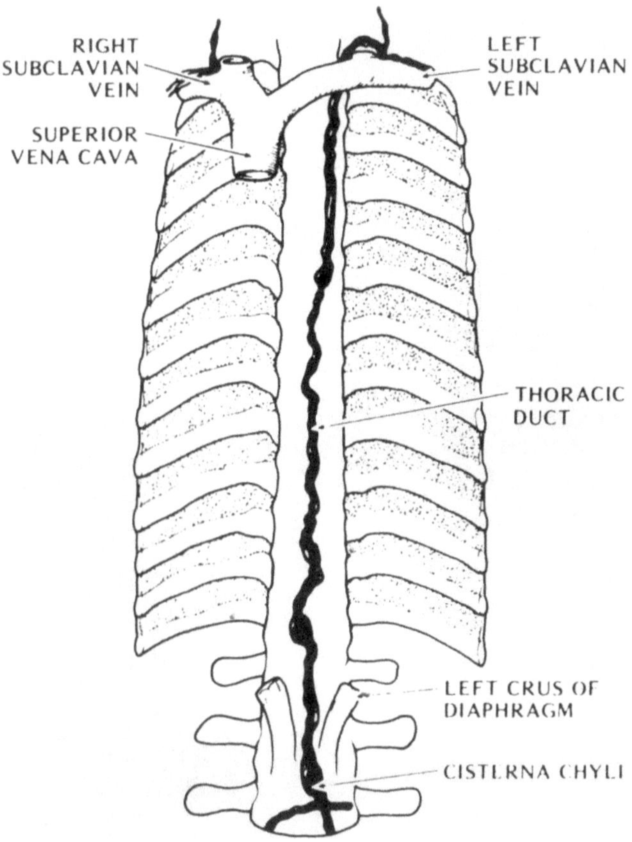

Figure 17.20. Course of thoracic duct from diaphragm to left subclavian vein. (Reprinted with permission from Propst-Procter SL, Rinsky LA, Bleck EE. The cisterma chyli in orthopaedic surgery. Spine 1983;8:790, Fig. 3.)[73]

Carotid Sheath

The carotid sheath lies deep to the sternocleidomastoid muscle just lateral to the area of dissection during an anterior approach to the cervical spine. Within the sheath is contained the internal jugular vein, common carotid artery, and the vagus nerve. Laceration of the contents of the carotid sheath is extremely rare.

Sympathetic Chain

The cervical sympathetic chain lies on the anterior surface of the longus capitus and longus colli muscles posterior to the carotid sheath. Damage to these nerves can result in a Horner's syndrome that is usually not permanent.[3] The incidence of persistent Horner's syndrome was reviewed by Barber and others and found to be 1% or less.[2,59]

Soft-Tissue Injuries to the Trachea and Esophagus

Esophageal or pharyngeal perforation is a serious and fortunately rare complication of anterior cervical spine fusions that occurs in only about 1 of 500 procedures.[3] During the procedure, the esophagus must be retracted laterally away from the front of the vertebral bodies along with the trachea and larynx. Damage can occur from sharp retractors or inadequate retraction with accidental cutting of multiple structures including the esophageal wall. Often, the perforation is not recognized until the postoperative period when the patient develops a retropharyngeal abscess or a tracheoesophageal fistula.

The usual treatment involves early operative closure of the fistula, but an unusual circumstance was reported where an esophagocutaneous fistula was successfully treated conservatively with only gastrostomy feeding.[60] In a review of 20 tracheoesophageal fistulas, all from nonmalignant causes, Hilgenberg and Grillo recommended direct repair of the esophagus with tracheal resection and repair.[61] Treatment of these difficulties and serious lesions often requires consultation with head and neck surgeons.

Spinal Fluid Leak

Spinal fluid leaks after anterior cervical fusion fortunately are rare, with few cases present in the literature. In the experience of the authors, the incidence is somewhat more common after complete vertebrectomies for fractures, although it is sometimes difficult to tell if the leak is iatrogenic or secondary to the injury. Tew and Mayfield[3] suggested that leaks were caused by damage by the high-speed burr during bone removal and could not be repaired, but leaks could be stopped by placing fascial graft posterior to the bone graft.

Major Neurological Injury

Significant neurological injury may occur during anterior spine fusions, but fortunately is rare. Kraus[64] reported on 10 cases and found that, in about one-half, the injury could be directly attributed to graft or instruments that inadvertently protruded into the canal. The frequency of this complication is certainly less than 1%[2,62] (although one author[63] reported 2 cases of 110), but at least one review suggested that removal of posterior osteophytes may contribute to this injury by requiring the passage of instruments near the spinal cord.[64] The need to remove these osteophytes is still a controversial issue, but at least the incidence of this very serious injury appears to be low. Treatment of serious neurological injury after anterior fusion should include an immediate search for a cause such as graft material within the canal. If a cause can be found, then removal of the offending material seems appropriate.

Degenerative Changes Above or Below Fusion

Degenerative changes above and below fusion masses in the cervical spine have been reported by several au-

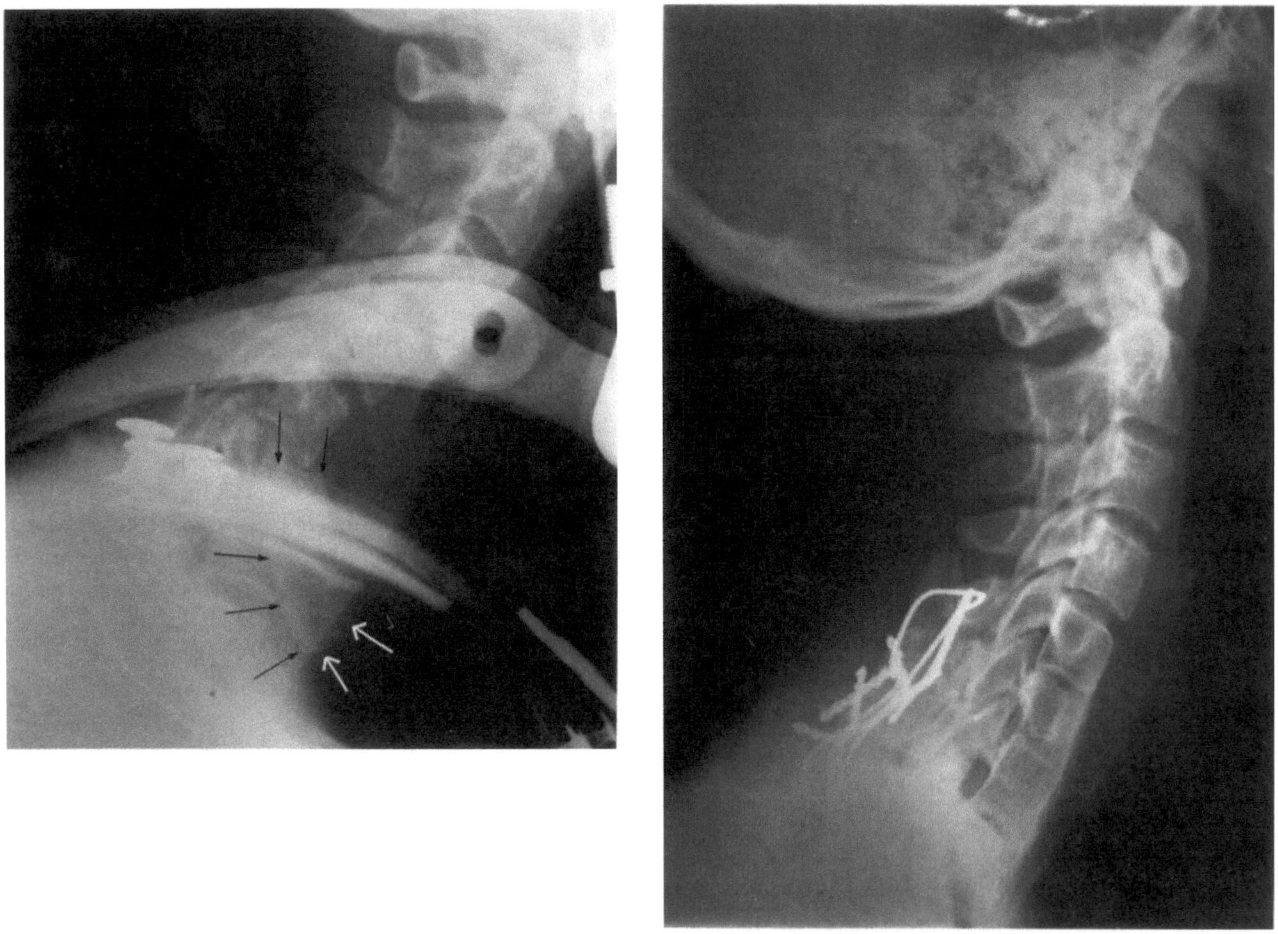
A B

Figure 17.21. **A.** Displacement of anterior strut graft (*arrows*) anteriorly causing dysphagia. **B.** Several months after graft revision, excellent alignment and solid fusion are seen.

thors.[65–67]. Presumably these degenerative changes result from altered biomechanics caused by the fused rigid segment, which puts additional stress on the normal segments above and below. Like changes in other regions of the spine the significance of these findings is not clear, but it is interesting to note that most of these patients remain asymptomatic.[65] However, at least one author suggested that newly developed spondylosis in adjacent segments led to neurological deterioration in several patients.[63]

Graft Extrusion

Extrusion of graft usually occurs anteriorly away from the spinal cord. It can be associated with dysphagia (Fig. 17.21), kyphotic instability, and persistent neurological symptoms. Review of the literature indicates an incidence from less than 1% to 13%.[2,30,20,66] The patients often complain of dysphagia, but reoperation is not usually necessary unless persistent esophageal or tracheal compression occurs.[3,68] The incidence of graft dislodgement is related to the patients diagnosis (i.e., trauma with unstable spine versus rigid arthritic spine), method of postoperative immobilization, and length and type of graft.

Nonunion

Just as in other areas of the spine, nonunion of an anterior cervical fusion is difficult to adequately evaluate. The incidence of nonunion, identified by radiography has been reported to be as high as 21%[69]; however, most of these patients only had minor symptoms. The average incidence in the literature is in the range of 0% to 5%.[2,3,20] Certainly there are patients with symptomatic nonunions that benefit from prolonged immobilization or revision surgery, but they are rare.

Graft collapse is similarly difficult to interpret (Fig. 17.22). The incidence of graft collapse appears to be somewhat higher for allograft than autograft.[20] Collapse of the graft is more significant if it occurs in a patient who has had multiple vertebral resections with a long anterior strut than if in a patient with a single interbody graft. The

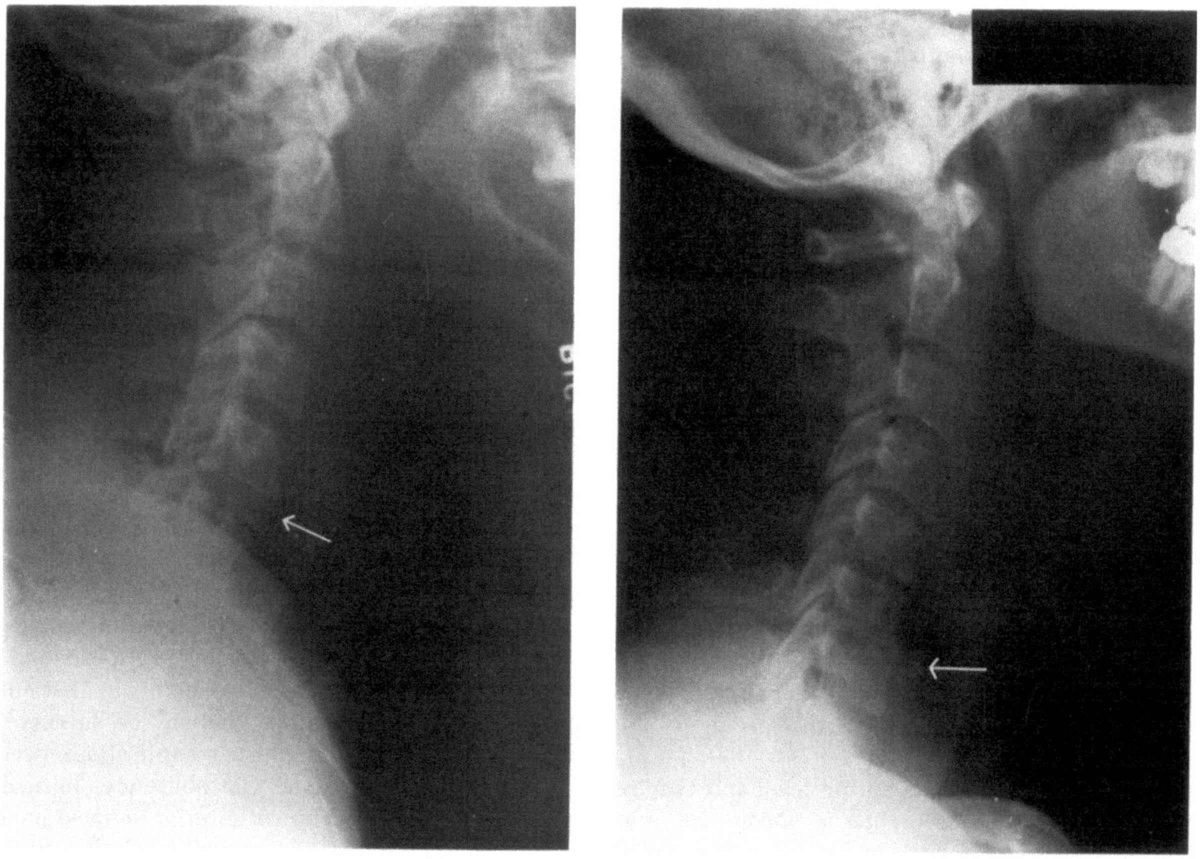

A B

Figure 17.22. Immediate postoperative view (**A**) of interbody tricortical iliac crest graft at C5–C6 (*arrow*) that collapsed (**B**) and extruded several months later.

former patient is at much greater risk for developing an angulatory deformity. Depending on the situation, treatment may require revision of the graft.

Retropharyngeal Edema

Retropharyngeal edema can be a quite serious complication if it leads to unobserved airway compromise. Fortunately, when it occurs it is usually mild and clears rapidly. The incidence is approximately 2%. Far more serious airway compromise was reported by Tew and Mayfield[3] secondary to a hematoma in 1 case of 500 reviewed. The patient required a tracheostomy to maintain an airway. This case highlights the importance of careful intraoperative hemostasis, wound drainage, and postoperative observation.

Posterior Cervical Fusions

Posterior cervical fusions are commonly performed for instability secondary to trauma or systemic arthritides; however, they are usually relatively free of serious complications.

The most common complication of posterior cervical fusion is unintended superior or inferior extension of the fusion mass. In a review of 98 of these procedures, Capen et al.[66] found 74% to have this complication. Traditionally, this is believed to be present to a greater extent in young patients, but is an extremely common phenomenon in all patients. The extent of the fusion can be limited somewhat by only exposing the segments that are going to be fused; however, when instrumentation is used, it is often difficult to perform a limited exposure.

The most frequent serious complications are related to the use of instrumentation in this region. Wires are commonly passed beneath lamina or through spinous processes. This must be performed with great care to avoid durotomy or neurological compromise. In a review of 12 high cervical fusions, Thompson and Meyer[70] found 17% of their patients had parasthesias postoperatively, probably associated with passage of wires into the spinal canal. In contrast, passage of wires through spinous processes should be almost completely without complication if proper landmarks are observed and all burr holes are kept above the posterior spinolaminar line. Wire breakage and nonunion are rare complications that occur in only 1% or 2% of cases.[66]

Significant bleeding depends on the level and type of surgery. Vertebral artery laceration is uncommon, but when it occurs is usually related to fusions in the area of the ring of C1 where the artery travels unprotected toward the midline in its course toward the occiput. It is far more common to experience significant muscular arterial or venous bleeding. This bleeding is usually amenable to packing with prompt resolution. Taking care to remain in the avascular midline plane will usually avoid this problem, although dissection out laterally over the facets will almost always result in some bleeding. Using electrocautery for the exposure can be very helpful, but great care must be taken not to plunge the tip of the cautery deeper than can be directly visualized.

Anterior Thoracolumbar Fusion

Literature outlining complications of anterior thoracolumbar fusions is limited, and most reports refer to the lumbar rather than the thoracic spine. As with any surgical procedure, the surgeon must be intimately familiar with local anatomy and variants. This is particularly important in anterior thoracic and lumbar approaches where the orthopaedic or neurological surgeon is working in unfamiliar territory near structures such as the spleen or thoracic duct that can be easily damaged.[71–73] Analysis of anterior thoracolumbar fusions will be segregated into (1) technical complications that encompass the approach, development of the bed, and graft insertion; and (2) those complications indigenous to the graft or the host.

Approaches in the lumbar area may be anterior transperitoneal, which is most useful for the L3–S1 areas, or retroperitoneal from either the right or left sides. This latter approach is desirable from the thoracolumbar junction to L5 and may be carried more proximally into the retropleural space. For the transperitoneal approach to L3, L4, L5, the abdominal contents must be avoided and not perforated. Usually the abdominal contents are retracted to the patient's right side to allow access through the parietal and visceral peritoneum. Great care must be taken not to entrap or damage the left ureter that runs longitudinally in this area. In addition, the bifurcation of the aorta at L4 with its accompanying inferior vena cava must not be damaged. Of course, the vena cava lies inferiorly and somewhat to the patient's right in relationship to the aorta. Structurally the aorta and common iliac vessels are more resistant to damage and somewhat easier to repair. In distinction, the vena cava and iliac veins are more delicate and more difficult to repair. Persistent pressure on these vessels may predispose to thrombosis, laceration, A-V fistulae, or aneurysm. Patients with previous local infection, irradiation, or surgery appear to be at greater risk for such complications because of the presence of scar tissue that obliterates normal tissue planes. A rare complication of anterior thoracic and lumbar fusions is symptomatic retroperitoneal fibrosis. Hematoma, infection, and metallic implants appear to predispose to this condition.[74,75] Treatment is usually directed toward relieving urinary obstruction.

The next layer of dissection brings the operator to the fine willowy superior hypogastric plexus (Fig. 17.23). Violation of this plexus may result in retrograde ejaculation. The prevalence of this complication is variable and difficult to accurately determine. In addition, great confusion exists in the literature because of inexact use of the terms impotence and sterility. Flynn and Price's conclusion, after surveying the English and French literature and personally contacting experienced surgeons around the world, was that impotence is no more common with anterior spine fusion operations than all other operations on the spine.[76,77] Most surgeons reported that cases of impotence disappeared with time and psychotherapy or a combination thereof. Sterility in males has been attributed to loss of the autonomic nerve supply to the internal vesicle sphincter, which causes retrograde ejaculation into the bladder. Flynn reported this to occur most infrequently (0.42%). The anatomic location of the nerve supply is such that fibers that innervate the venous plexuses of the penis are not usually affected, so impotence (failure to obtain and maintain an erection) is not a problem.[76] In addition, Ditunno[78] reported retrograde ejaculation does not necessarily result in sterility. If the male voids postcoitively, the sperm may be transferred intravaginally and not be lost or lose functional potential. Nonetheless, care should be taken not to damage the superior hypogastric plexus, and Goldner et al.[79] suggested injection of saline solution into the prevertebral (sacral) tissues to aid in outlining nerve filaments. Indiscriminate use of electrocoagulation to control bleeding in the prevertebral tissues should be avoided for fear of disruption of neural elements.

Attempts to completely clear the disc space as suggested by Sacks have the potential to damage neural elements of the cauda equina.[80] More specifically, attempting to remove posteriorly sequestrated disc material from an anterior exposure may result in damage to fibers of the cauda equina. In addition, total removal of a sequestrated fragment may be impossible because local bony configuration limits surgical access.

Union of the fusion mass in anterior fusion is extremely difficult to ascertain. All asssessment modalities clinically available today leave a large subjective element. Tools for assessment include routine radiographs[62] (Fig. 17.24), planar tomography, CAT with reformatting, and bone

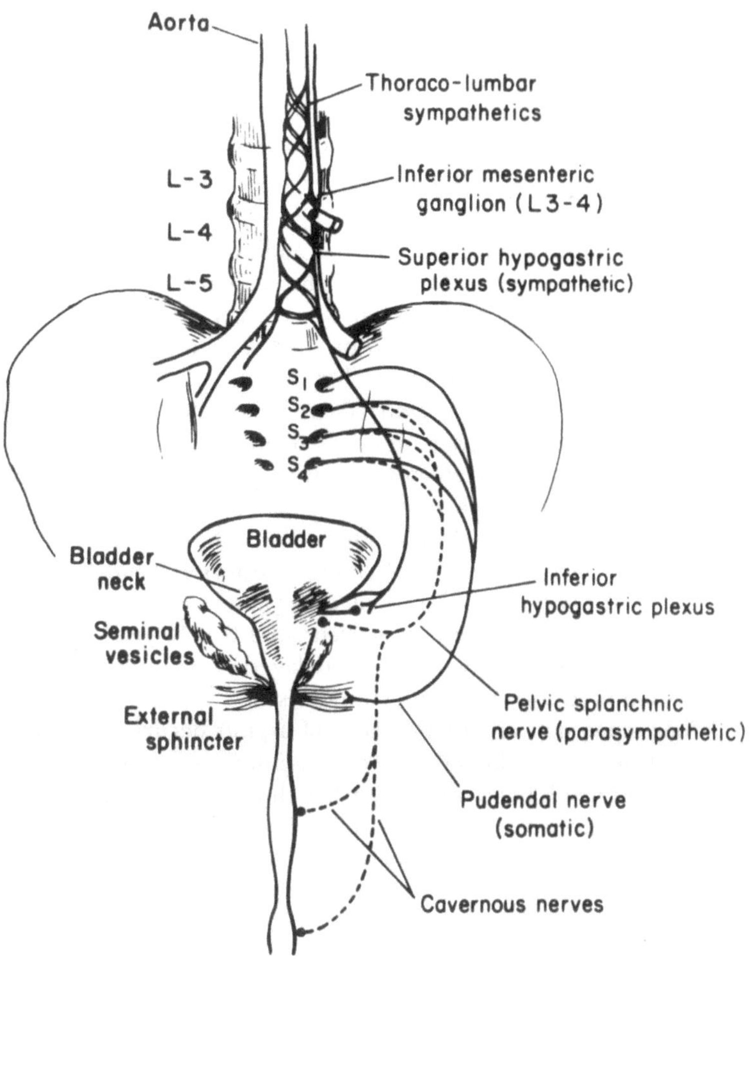

Figure 17.23. Location of superior hypogastric plexus anterior to lumbar vertebral bodies. (Reprinted with permission from Flynn JC, Price CT. Sexual complications of anterior fusion of the lumbar spine. Spine 1984;9:490, Fig. 1.)

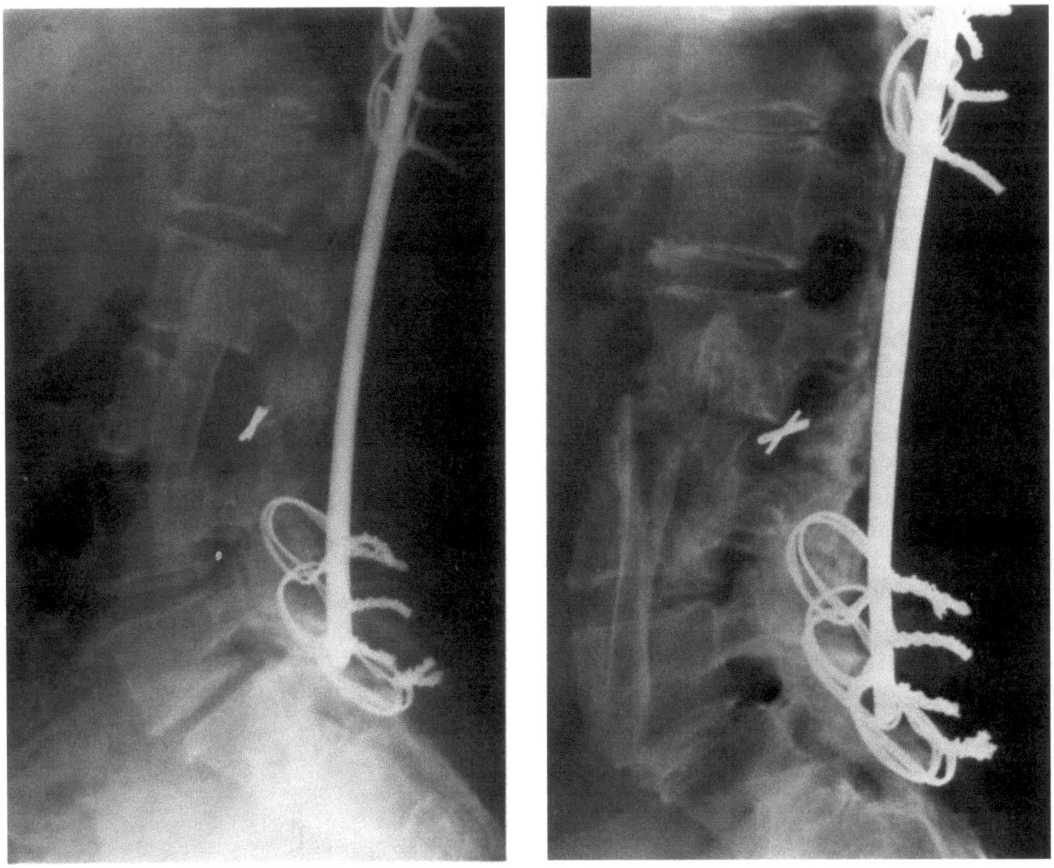

A B

Figure 17.24. **A.** Immediate postoperative view after anterior iliac crest strut graft. **B.** Same patient after failure of second grafting procedure. A vascularized fibular transfer was ultimately required because of compromise of graft bed by irradiation.

scan. Radiographs during forced flexion and extension may help demonstrate motion in the specific segment. Flynn and Hoque suggested that motion is lost early and then later trabeculae cross the joint to produce a solid fusion. Not all levels complete the cycle.[81,82]

Using autogenous fibular graft, about 50% unite, while autogenous iliac crest graft proceeds to union in about 75% of cases. Times for union to occur vary greatly from 0.7 to 15 years. An average fusion time is approximately 2 to 3 years. Goldner et al.,[79] Bunnell et al.,[83] Flynn and Hoque,[81] and others noted that prior posterior pseudarthrosis often will unite after union of the anterior fusion. An extraarticular arthrodesis may occur after 5 to 10 years at the site of a previously diagnosed delayed or nonunion of an attempted intraarticular arthrodesis.

When nonunion or dislodgement of a graft occurs, it does not necessarily follow that reoperation is necessary. A judgment needs to be made regarding the risk of sudden collapse, progressive loss of correction, and compromise of adjacent structures. If the patient is deemed to be at high risk then additional intervention is necessary. This intervention can take the form of bracing, revision of the anterior graft, or augmentation of the anterior fusion with a posterior fusion. It is particularly important to consider the viability of the bed into which the graft is inserted. For the vast majority of anterior fusions, autogenous iliac crest produces excellent incorporation. However, when local factors such as multiple operations, infection, irradiation, or chemotherapy compromise the paraspinal tissues, it may be necessary to use a graft with its own blood supply such as a vascularized fibula or rib transplant.

Pain as a postoperative complaint also is an indeterminate variable. Beetham,[84] Freebody et al.,[62] and Flynn and Hoque[81] noted this to be present with and without a solid vertebral fusion. Clinical success for private patients to return to work with or without solid fusion was 3 to 6 months, whereas compensation patients required 6 to 12 months to return to work. Maximum clinical improvement after 2 to 4 years frequently does not correlate with solid radiographic union. Long-term radiographic follow-up after as long as 15 years frequently demonstrated healing of interspaces previously not known to be united without associated alteration of the patient's clinical complaints of pain. Instability above or below fused segments has not been studied in great detail. One author reported that 3 of 24 patients fused anteriorly for spondylolisthesis developed instability at the interspace above the fusion.[77]

Incisional hernia may represent a complication of anterior thoracolumbar fusion as with any other abdominal procedure. Its presence may result from many factors including quality of the tissues, experience of the surgeon, and the technique of closure.

The use of anterior instrumentation in the thoracic and lumbar spine remains controversial.[85] Recent reports and the authors' personal experience have documented cases of fatal or nearly fatal major vessel laceration after placement of these devices.[86] Different surgeons have suggested ways to avoid this problem, including instrumenting in the area of either the aorta or the vena cava, but there is no clear consensus. It is also not clear at the present time how great the risks are with the different types of anterior devices, and without this information it is difficult to make an informed decision about risks versus benefits of such use. The authors no longer use these devices.

Posterior Spine Fusions in the Thoracic and Lumbar Spine

The two main indications for posterior fusion in the thoracic and lumbar spine are scoliosis and trauma. Many of the complications of this procedure are similar to those that occur after lumbosacral fusions for degenerative disease. However, the addition of instrumentation in almost all these cases produces additional morbidity. For a review of these types of instrumentation the reader is referred to standard scoliosis texts.[87]

One area of interest with respect to these fusions involves the biomechanical effects of these long fusion masses. Several reports have documented pain after fusions that extend into the lumbar spine causing loss of the normal lumbar lordosis.[4,88,89] These patients may even require corrective osteotomies to reduce pain and improve ability to walk in an upright position. As a result, appropriate forms of fixation should be used to preserve lumbar lordosis.

Similarly, Ginsburg et al.[48] have shown that long fusions extending into the lower lumbar spine are associated with increased back pain. It appears that the more motion segments that can be left uninstrumented, the less likely it is that the patient will have back pain. Leaving segments unfused but instrumented (rod-long, fuse short) does not seem to be adequate as these patients develop degenerative changes of the unfused segments and full motion does not appear to return after removal of instrumentation.[90,91] In spite of the problems with back pain, true instability at the ends of a long fusion is a rare event.[92–94]

The problem of spinal stenosis that is discussed in greater detail next with regard to fusions in the lower lumbar spine does not seem to be as significant in thoracolumbar fusions. For some reason, straight posterior fusions at these levels very rarely cause spinal stenosis.[95]

The incidence of pseudarthrosis in posterior thoracolumbar fusions depends on several factors including the type of bone graft used, quality of the bed, nutritional states of the patient, the presence of instrumentation, and the method for determining the presence of a pseudarthrosis. Without instrumentation, the presence of pseudarthrosis diagnosed by radiographs has been reported to be as high as 68%. With instrumentation, it is more commonly in the range of 2% to 25%.[96–100] Reexploration appears to be a more accurate way to diagnose pseudarthrosis than radiographs.

A great variety of complications are associated with posterior instrumentation in the thoracolumbar spine, such as hook dislodgement, neural compromise from sublaminar wire passage, and rod breakage[101,102] (Fig. 17.25). These topics are very complex and specific to each indication for their use and type of instrumentation. They are also changing at a rapid rate because of the proliferation

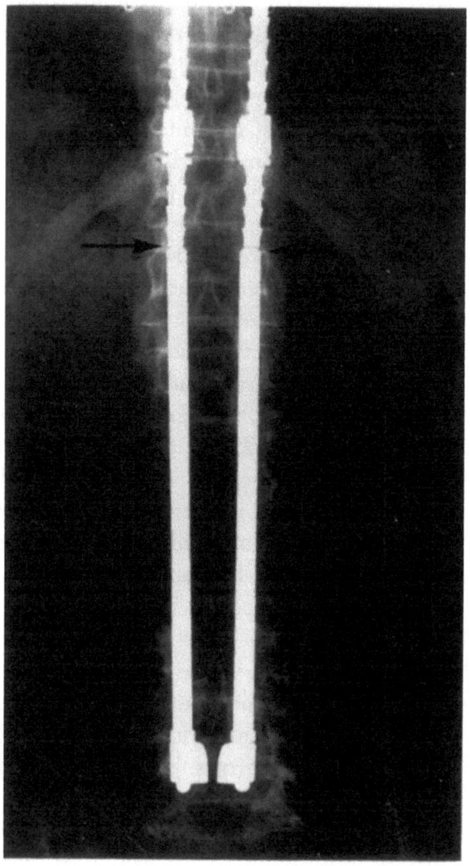

Figure 17.25. Bilateral fracture of Harrington rods (*arrows*).

of various types of instrumentation. The reader is encouraged to become familiar with the advantages, disadvantages, and indications for each type of instrumentation that he/she chooses to use, and to be aware of new developments that occur in a span of time that is too rapid for any book to remain current.

Lumbar and Lumbosacral Spine Fusions from the Posterior Approach

Lumbar spine fusions from the posterior approach include true posterior interlaminar fusions, posterolateral intertransverse process fusions, and posterior lumbar interbody fusions. These fusions can be performed with and without instrumentation. Posterior spine fusions of all types are the most commonly performed procedure for spine stabilization. Fortunately, they have a relatively low complication rate compared with other types of fusions, although there are certainly differences among the different types.

The rate of union after posterior spine fusions without instrumentation appears to be related to the type of fusion performed as well as the number of vertebrae involved. Intertransverse process fusions were shown by Prothero et al.[6] to have a lower pseudarthrosis rate than interlaminar fusions. The rates were 10% and 15%, respectively. Similarly, Macnab reviewed more than 500 fusions and found similar rates of 7% and 17%, respectively. Several authors have also shown that the rate of nonunion increases with the number of vertebrae that are fused.[103–106]

Posterior lumbar interbody fusions (PLIF) remain an area of great controversy; many surgeons have strong opinions about the merits of this procedure, although there is relatively little evidence in the literature. Lin reported a 12% pseudarthrosis rate with this procedure, but without concurrent controls this number is difficult to interpret.[107]

The problem of assessing the rate and impact of pseudarthrosis is further complicated by poor correlation with symptoms (Fig. 17.26). In a study of 58 intertransverse fusions, Dawson showed no significant correlation between pseudarthrosis and economic or functional recovery. Dawson et al. also found that floating fusions (where the fusion mass did not extend to the sacrum) had a significantly higher rate of pseudarthrosis. The importance of this is difficult to assess because of poor correlation with symptoms.[104,105,108]

In summary, at the present time intertransverse fusions are believed to be superior to posterior interlaminar fusions with respect to pseudarthrosis. In spite of strong advocates on either side, posterior lumbar interbody fusions have not been shown to provide any additional improvement in fusion rate when compared with intertransverse fusions, and as is discussed next, PLIF have a significantly higher potential risk of complications.

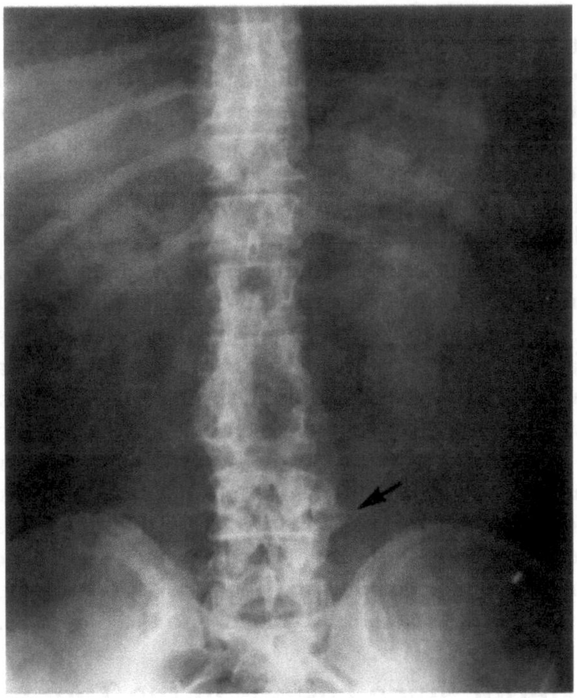

Figure 17.26. Pseudarthrosis of lumbar intertransverse fusion (*arrow*).

Intertransverse and posterior interlaminar fusions have an extremely low risk of neurological or dural complications because it is not necessary to open the neural canal for either of these procedures. For those surgeons who

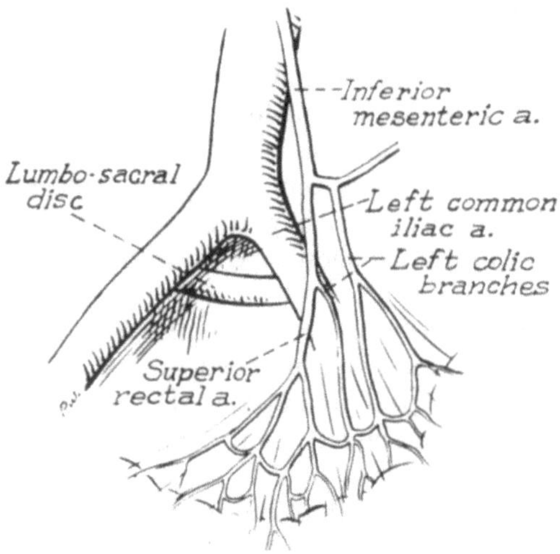

Figure 17.27. Illustration of relationship of L5–S1 disc space to overlying anterior arterial structures. (Reprinted with permission from Birkeland IW, Taylor TKF. Major vascular injuries in lumbar disc surgery. J Bone Joint Surg 1969;51B:4, Fig. 1.)

perform their fusions through a midline posterior approach there is, of course, some risk of inadvertently entering the neural canal during the approach, particularly if there is an unrecognized spina bifida occulta. However, this should be a relatively rare complication.

Posterior lumbar interbody fusions, always require significant manipulation of the neural elements. In a review of the PLIF procedure, although no statistics are provided, Lin[107] discussed the problems of graft protrusion into the neural canal, dural laceration, and epidural venous bleeding. Certainly, these complications should be almost unheard of in posterior interlaminar or intertransverse fusions. Moreover, PLIF requires a complete discectomy from posterior, which puts the anteriorly placed structures at risk. Although the PLIF literature is sparse with respect to these complications, the discectomy literature is replete with reports of significant complications including death from penetration of the anterior longitudinal ligament with damage to intraabdominal structures (Fig. 17.27). These reports include damage to major vascular structures as well as the ureters. Review of these articles should be mandatory for anyone who performs PLIF procedures.[109–113]

As in other areas of the spine, posterior lumbar and lumbosacral spine fusions produce altered biomechanics. Several reports have documented acquired spondylolysis or spondylolisthesis above the fused segment especially from interlaminar fusions.[105,114,115] This fusion technique produces damage to the pars interarticularis as well as the posterior ligament complex that may predispose to fatigue fracture and instability. In one report, the incidence of spondylolysis acquisita was 1% in 380 interlaminar fusions and 0% in 260 intertransverse fusions.[116]

Several biomechanical studies have documented the effects of fusions on the adjacent spinal segments in vitro.[37,117] In one such study, intertransverse fusions were found to have the least adverse effects on adjacent vertebra when compared with anterior or interlaminar fusion.[117]

Postfusion stenosis is another area in which intertransverse fusions appear to be superior to posterior fusions. For reasons not clearly defined, fusions applied to the posterior lamina, spinous process, and medial facets

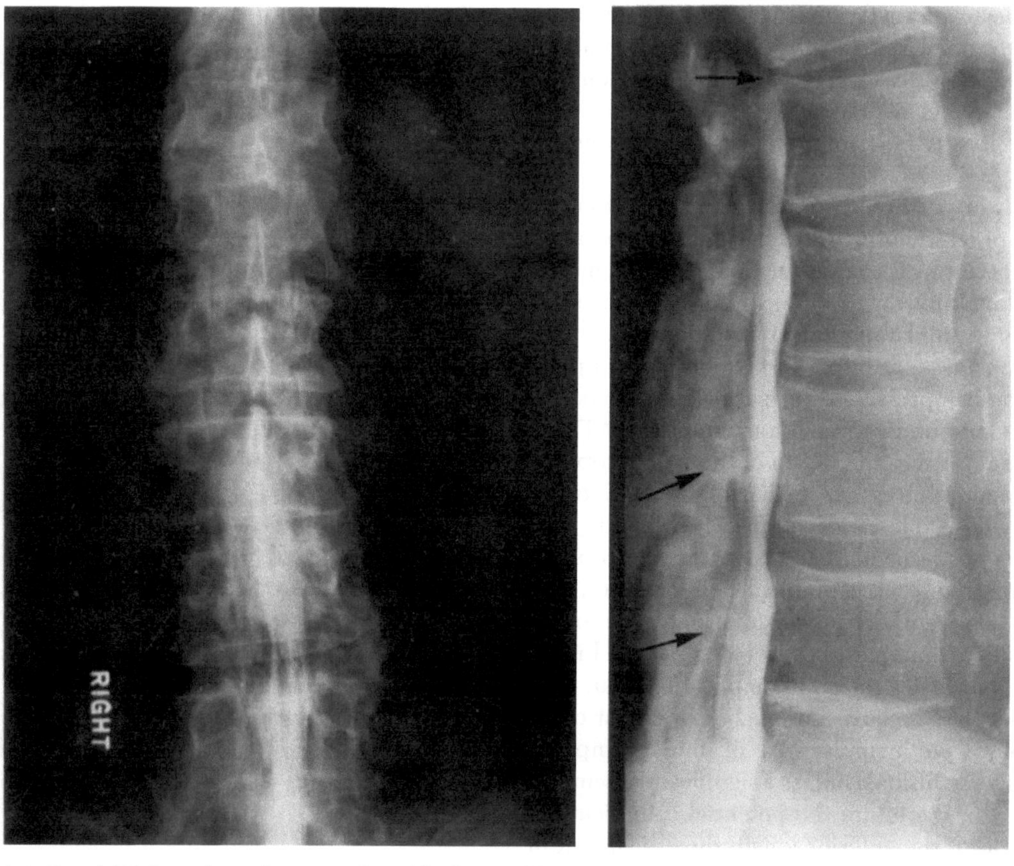

A B

Figure 17.28. (**A**) A–P and (**B**) lateral myelograms show blockage of flow of contrast medium at superior edge of previous posterior spine fusion (*superior arrow*). Note dense posterior hypertrophied bone located posteriorly on lateral view (*inferior arrows*).

in the lumbosacral spine have a high propensity to hypertrophy with time (Fig. 17.28). The hypertrophic process is circumferential in direction, causing compromise of the neural canal and neural foramen. Through an insidious process the fusion mass expands and is particularly bothersome to the patient by its intrusion at the interspace at the upper end of the canal. At this point a combination of hypertrophied ligamentum flavum and fusion mass compresses the neural elements. Presentation of the entity frequently is associated with a delay of a decade or more after the fusion is performed. One is always impressed by the sheer volume of bone present over the posterior elements in this entity, particularly if the patient is one for whom you were the initial operating surgeon. The bone frequently has hypertrophied two- to fourfold or more times the volume of autograft that was initially applied to achieve arthrodesis.

In a review of 380 posterior fusions and 260 intertransverse fusions, Macnab discovered 34 cases of stenosis, all of which occurred in the posterior fusion group.[116] This was supported by Brodsky's observations in 231 patients with postoperative spinal stenosis.[118] These patients developed concentric stenosis at the top of the fusion mass. The stenosis was contributed to by disc space collapse, bony hypertrophy of the grafted lamina, ligamentum infolding, intraluminal spurs, and scar tissue formation. The incidence of stenosis several years after interlaminar fusion is in the range of 9% to 15%.[108,116] Brodsky[118] suggested that it was best to avoid laminar fusions for this reason.

The diagnosis of postfusion stenosis, similar to that for other types of spinal stenosis, is made using a combination of clinical history, physical examination, and diagnostic imaging. Myelography may demonstrate a spectrum of findings including mild thinning of the contrast column above the fusion mass, a wasp waist lesion, or complete obstruction. The compression is primarily from the posterior direction. Computerized axial tomography (CAT) can dramatically demonstrate the depth of the hypertrophied fusion mass. Magnetic resonance imaging is a relatively new modality whose role is not yet clearly defined.

In summary, posterior lumbar fusions for appropriate indications can produce acceptable levels of union and complications. The authors advocate use of the intertransverse fusion technique because of apparent higher rates of union and lower rates of complication than with interlaminar fusion. Similarly, although in the best of reports PLIF may have a similar rate of union compared with intertransverse fusions, unless a significant advantage is demonstrated in the future the potential complications from penetration of the anterior longitudinal ligament or manipulation of the neural elements mitigate against its use.

Posterior Spine Fusions with Instrumentation in the Lumbar Spine

A variety of instrumentation systems are used in the lumbar and lumbosacral spine to provide additional fixation. At the present time the role of these devices is still being determined. Most of the devices that are currently being advocated involve fixation to the vertebral body by threading a screw down the pedicle. Although no statistics are yet available, the potential complications can be quite significant.

Insertion of these devices requires absolute certainty about the landmarks to avoid inserting screws into the neural canal or foramen. In some of these systems, it is necessary to penetrate the anterior cortex to provide secure fixation particularly in the sacrum. Great care must be taken to not produce the vascular and ureteral complications discussed previously with respect to discectomy. As the role of these devices becomes clearer, the complication rates should also become more apparent, and only then can an intelligent decision be made regarding their use (Fig. 17.29).

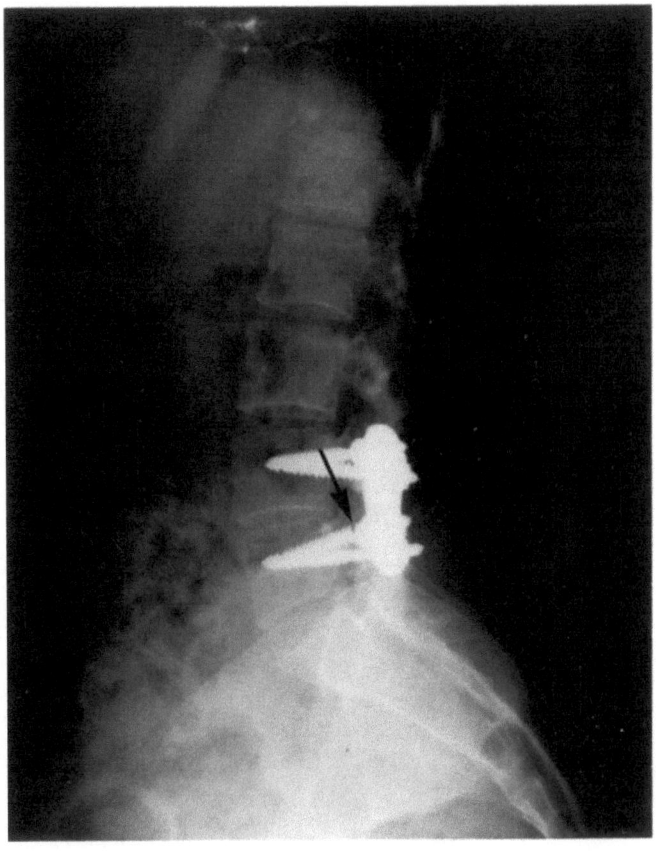

Figure 17.29. Failure of pedicular screws used to augment lumbar spine fusion (*arrow*).

References

1. Simchen E, Stein H, Sacks TG, Shapiro M, Michel J. Multivariate analysis of determinants of postoperative wound infection in orthopaedic patients. J Hosp Infect 1984;5:137.
2. Barber FA, Anterior cervical fusion. Rocky Mountain Med J 1978;75:29.
3. Tew JM, Mayfield FH. Complications of surgery of the anterior cervical spine. In: Clinical Neurosurgery. Baltimore: Williams & Wilkins, 1976:424.
4. Kostuik JP, Hall BB. Spinal fusions to the sacrum in adults and scoliosis. Spine 1983;8:489.
5. Watkins MB. Posterolateral fusion in pseudarthrosis and posterior element defects of the lumbosacral spine. Clin Orthop Rel Res 1964;35:80.
6. Prothero SR, Parkes JC, Stinchfield EE. Complications after low-back fusion in 1000 patients. J Bone Joint Surg 1966;48A:57.
7. Lonstein J, Winter R, Moe J, Gaines D. Wound infection with Harrington instrumentation and spine fusion for scoliosis. Clin Orthop Rel Res 1973;96:222.
8. Altemeier WA, Alexander JW. Retroperitoneal abscesses. Arch Surg 1961;83:512.
9. Meyers MA. Dynamic Radiology of the Abdomen. New York: Springer-Verlag, 1982:110.
10. Simons GW, Sty JR, Starshak RJ. Retroperitoneal and retrofascial abscesses. J Bone Joint Surg 1983;65A:1041.
11. Mayfield FH, Kurokawa K. Watertight closure of spinal dura mater. J Neurosurg 1975;43:639.
12. Urist MR, Dawson E. Intertransverse process fusion with the aid of chemosterilized autolyzed antigen-extracted allogeneic (AAA) bone. Clin Orthop Rel Res 1981;154:97.
13. Burwell RG. Studies in the transplantation of bone. J Bone Joint Surg 1966;48B:532.
14. Burwell RG. Studies in the transplantation of bone. J Bone Joint Surg 1963;45B:386.
15. Goldberg VM, Lance EM. Revascularization and accretion in transplantation. J Bone Joint Surg 1972;54A:807.
16. Goldberg VM, Stevenson S. Natural history of autografts and allografts. Clin Orthop Rel Res 1987;225:7.
17. Heiple KG, Chase SW, Herndon CH. A comparative study of the healing process following different types of bone transplantation. J Bone Joint Surg 1963;45A:1593.
18. May VR, Mauck WR. Exploration of the spine for pseudarthrosis following spinal fusion in the treatment of scoliosis. Clin Orthop Rel Res 1967;53:115.
19. Stabler CL, Eismont FJ, Brown MD, Green BA, Malinin TI. Failure of posterior cervical fusions using cadaveric bone graft in children. J Bone Joint Surg 1985;67A:370.
20. Brown MD, Malinin TI, David PB. A roentgenographic evaluation of frozen allografts versus autografts in anterior cervical spine fusions. Clin Orthop Rel Res 1976;119:231.
21a. Nasca RJ, Whelchel JD. Use of cryopreserved bone in spinal surgery. Spine 1987;12:222.
21b. Ray RD, Holloway JA. Vascularization of bone grafts and implants. Clin Orthop 1957;87:43.
22. Albrektsson T. The healing of autologous bone grafts after varying degrees of surgical trauma. J Bone Joint Surg 1980;62B:403.
23. Watson-Jones R. Transplantation of bone. In: Fracture and Joint Injuries. Ed. 4. Baltimore: Williams & Wilkins, 1955.
24. Heppenstall RB. Bone grafting. In: Fracture Treatment and Healing. Philadelphia: Saunders, 1980:97–112.
25. Cockin J. Autologous bone grafting—complications at the donor site. Abstract. J Bone Joint Surg 1971;53B:153.
26. Frymoyer JW, Howe J, Kuhlmann D. The long-term effects of spinal fusion on the sacroiliac joints and ilium. Clin Orthop Rel Res 1978;134:196.
27. Coventry MB, Tapper EM. Pelvic instability. J Bone Joint Surg 1972;54A:83.
28. Lichtblau S. Dislocation of the sacro-iliac joint. J Bone Joint Surg 1962;44A:193.
29. Escalas F, DeWald RL. Combined traumatic arteriovenous fistula and ureteral injury: a complication of iliac bone-grafting. J Bone Joint Surg 1977;59A:270.
30. Kahn B. Superior gluteal artery laceration, a complication of iliac bone graft surgery. Clin Orthop Rel Res 1979; 140:204.
31. Cotler HB. Personal communication.
32. Cowley SP, Anderson LD. Brief note: hernias through donor sites for iliac-bone grafts. J Bone Joint Surg 1983; 65A:1023.
33. Froimson AI, Cummings AG. Iliac hernia following hip arthrodesis. Clin Orthop Rel Res 1971;80:89.
34. Lotem M, Maor P, Haimoff H, Woloch Y. Lumbar hernia at an iliac bone graft donor site. Clin Orthop Rel Res 1971;80:130.
35. Oldfield MC. Iliac hernia after bone-grafting. Lancet 1:810.
36. Prytek LJ, Kelly CC. Management of herniation through large iliac bone defects. Clin Orthop Rel Res 1960;152:998.
37. Quinnell RC, Stockdale HR. Some experimental observations of the influence of a single lumbar floating fusion on the remaining lumbar spine. Spine 1981;6:263.
38. Bosworth DM. Repair of herniae through iliac-crest defects. J Bone Joint Surg 1955;37A:1069.
39. Hsu K, Zucherman JF, White AH. Bone grafts and implants in spine surgery. In: White AH, Rothman RH, Ray CD, eds. Lumbar Spine Surgery. St. Louis: Mosby, 1987:434–458.
40. Hollingshead WH. Anatomy for Surgeons. Volume 3, The back and limbs. Philadelphia: Harper and Row, 1982.
41. Chow SP, Leong JCY, Srmlt AM, Yau ACMC. Anterior spinal fusion for deranged lumbar intervertebral disc. Spine 1980;5:452.
42. Weikel AM, Habal MB. Meralgia paresthetica: a complication of iliac bone procurement. Plast Reconstr Surg 1977; 60:572.
43. Bernardt M. Ueber isolirt im geriete des n. cutaneus femoris externis Norkommends parasthesiea. Neurol Zentralbl 1895;12:242.
44. Hollingshead WH. Textbook of Anatomy. Philadelphia: Harper and Row, 1974.
45. Smith SE, DeLee JC, Ramamurthy S. Ilioguinal neuralgia

following iliac bone-grafting. J Bone Joint Surg 1984; 66A:1306.
46. Drury BJ. Clinical evaluation of back and leg pain due to irritation of the superior cluneal nerve. Abst. J Bone Joint Surg 1967;49A:199.
47. Frymoyer JW, Hanley E, Howe J, Kuhlmann D, Matteri R. Disc excision and spine fusion in the management of lumbar disc disease. Spine 1978;3:1.
48. Ginsburg HH, Goldstein LA, Robinson SC, Haake PW, Devanny JR, Chan DPK, Suk SI. Back pain in postoperative idiopathic scoliosis. Abstract Spine 1979;4:518.
49. MacEwen GD. Personal communication.
50. Enneking, WF. Personal communication.
51. Friedlaender GE. Current concepts review: bone grafts. J Bone Joint Surg 1987;69A:786.
52. Friedlaender GE, Tross RB, Doganis AC, Kirkwood JM, Baron R. Effects of chemotherapeutic agents on bone. J Bone Joint Surg 1984;66A:602.
53. Bulger RF, Rejowski JE, Beatty RA. Vocal cord paralysis associated with anterior cervical fusion: considerations for prevention and treatment. J Neurosurg 1985;62:657.
54a. Sanders G, Uyeda RY, Karlan MS. Nonrecurrent inferior laryngeal nerves and their association with a recurrent branch. Am J Surg 1983;146:501.
54b. Heeneman H. Vocal cord paralysis following approaches to the anterior cervical spine. Laryngoscope 1973;83:17.
55. Meurman Y. Operative mediofixation of the vocal cord in complete unilateral paralysis. AMA Arch Otolaryngol 1952;55:544.
56. Jacobson L. Bilateral vocal cord paralysis. Anesthesia 1979;34:1020.
57. Johnson RM, Southwick WO. Function and surgical anatomy of the neck. In: Rothman RH, Simeone FA, eds. The Spine. Philadelphia: Saunders, 1982:67–187.
58. Lindskog GE, Liebow AA, Glenn WWL. Thoracic and Cardiovascular Surgery with Related Pathology. New York: Appleton Century Crofts, 1962:439–440.
59. Flynn TB. Neurologic complications of anterior cervical interbody fusion. Spine 1982;7:536.
60. Balmaseda MT, Pellioni DJ. Esophagocutaneous fistula in spinal cord injury: a complication of anterior cervical fusion. Arch Phys Med Rehabil 1985;66:783.
61. Hilgenberg AD, Grillo HC. Acquired nonmalignant tracheoesophageal fistula. J Thorac Cardiovasc Surg 1983; 85:492.
62. Freebody D, Bendall R, Taylor RD. Anterior transperitoneal lumbar fusion. J Bone Joint Surg 1971;53B:617.
63. Yonenobu K, Okada K, Fuji T, Fujiwara K, Yamashita K, Ono K. Causes of neurologic deterioration following surgical treatment of cervical myelopathy. Spine 1986; 11:818.
64. Kraus DR, Stauffer ES. Spinal cord injury as a complication of elective anterior cervical fusion. Clin Orthop Rel Res 1975;112:130.
65. Braunstein EM, Hunter LY, Bailey RW. Long-term radiographic changes following anterior cervical fusion. Clin Radiol 1980;31:201.
66. Capen DA, Garland DE, Waters RL. Surgical stabilization of the cervical spine: a comparative analysis of anterior and posterior spine fusions. Clin Orth Rel Res 1985;196:229.
67. Hunter LY, Braunstein EM, Bailey RW. Radiographic changes following anterior cervical fusion. Spine 1980;5:399.
68. Welsh LW, Welsh JJ, Chinnici JC. Dysphagia due to cervical spine surgery. Ann Otol Rhinol Laryngol 1987;96:112.
69. Brodsky AE. Cervical angina. Spine 1985;10:699.
70. Thompson RA, Meyer TJ. Posterior surgical stabilization for atlantoaxial subluxation in rheumatoid arthritis. Spine 1985;10:597.
71. Colletta AJ, Mayer PJ. Chylothorax: an unusual complication of anterior thoracic interbody spinal fusion. Spine 1982;7:46.
72. Hodge WA, DeWald RL. Splenic injury complicating the anterior thoracoabdominal surgical approach for scoliosis. J Bone Joint Surg 1983;65A:396.
73. Propst-Proctor SL, Rinsky LA, Bleck EE. The cisterna chyli in orthopaedic surgery. Spine 1983;8:787.
74. Chan FL, Chow SP. Retroperitoneal fibrosis after anterior spinal fusion. Clin Radiol 1983;34:331.
75. Cleveland RH, Gilsanz V, Lebowitz RL, Wilkinson RH. Hydronephrosis from retroperitoneal fibrosis after anterior spine fusion. J Bone Joint Surg 1978;60A:996.
76. Flynn JC, Price CT. Sexual complications of anterior fusion of the lumbar spine. Spine 1984;9:489.
77. van Rens JG, van Horn JR. Long-term results in lumbosacral interbody fusion for spondylolisthesis. Acta Orthop Scand 1982;53:383.
78. Ditunno JF. Personal communication.
79. Goldner JL, McCollum DE, Urbaniak JR. Anterior disc excision and interbody spine fusion for chronic low back pain. In: American Academy of Orthopaedic Surgeons, Symposium on the Spine. St. Louis: Mosby, 1969:111.
80. Sacks S. Anterior interbody fusion of the lumbar spine. J Bone Joint Surg 1965;47B:211.
81. Flynn JC, Hoque MA. Anterior fusion of the lumbar spine. J Bone Joint Surg 1979;61A:1143.
82. Stauffer RN, Coventry MB. Anterior interbody lumbar spine fusion. Analysis of Mayo Clinic series. J Bone Joint Surg 1972;54A:756.
83. Bunnell WP, MacEwen GD, Riser W. Anterior spinal fusion—experimental evaluation of technique. Orthop Trans 1977;1:129.
84. Beetham R. Anterior spinal surgery in Ballarat. In: Proceedings of the Australian Orthopaedic Association. J Bone Joint Surg 1978;52B:392.
85. Dwyer AF. Experience of anterior correction of scoliosis. Clin Orthop Rel Res 1973;93:191.
86. Woolsey RM. Aortic laceration after anterior spinal fusion. Surg Neurol 1986;25:267.
87. Bradford DS, Lonstein JE, Moe JH, Ogilvie JW, Winter RB. Moe's Textbook of Scoliosis and Other Spinal Deformities. Philadelphia: Saunders, 1987.
88. Grobler LJ, Winter RB, Lonstein JE, Moe JH, Bradford DS. Loss of lumbar lordosis following surgical correction of thoracolumbar deformities: its recognition, treatment and prevention. J Bone Joint Surg 1980;62B:277.
89. Moe JH, Denis F. The iatrogenic loss of lumbar lordosis. Abstract Orthop Trans 1977;1:131.

90. Hasday CA, Passoff TL, Perry J. Gait abnormalities arising from iatrogenic loss of lumbar lordosis secondary to Harrington instrumentation in lumbar fractures. Spine 1983;8:501.
91. Kahanovitz N, Arnoczky SP, Levine DB, Otis JP. The effects of internal fixation of the articular cartilage of unfused canine facet joint cartilage. Spine 1984;9:268.
92. Barrack RL, Whitecloud TS, Skinner HB. Spondylolysis after spinal instrumentation in osteogenesis imperfecta. South Med J 1984;77:1453.
93. Drennan JC, King EW. Cervical dislocation following fusion of the upper thoracic spine for scoliosis. J Bone Joint Surg 1978;60A:1003.
94. Friedman RJ, Micheli LJ. Acquired spondylolisthesis following scoliosis surgery. Clin Orthop Rel Res 1984;190:132.
95. Eismont FJ, Simeone FA. Bone overgrowth (hypertrophy) as a cause of late paraparesis after scoliosis fusion. J Bone Joint Surg 1981;63A:1016.
96. Aurori BF, Weierman RJ, Lowell HA, Nadel CI, Parsons JR. Pseudarthrosis after spinal fusion for scoliosis. Clin Orthop Rel Res 1985;199:153.
97. Goldstein LA. Treatment of idiopathic scoliosis by Harrington instrumentation and spinal fusion. J Bone Joint Surg 1969;51A:209.
98. Hall JE, Gillespie R. Idiopathic scoliosis treated by Harrington instrumentation and spinal fusion. J Bone Joint Surg 1971;53A:198.
99. McMaster MJ, James JIP. Pseudarthrosis after spinal fusion for scoliosis. J Bone Joint Surg 1976;58B:305.
100. Moe JH, Valuska JW. Evaluation of treatment of scoliosis by Harrington instrumentation. J Bone Joint Surg 50A:848.
101. Bowen JR, Ferrer J. Spinal stenosis caused by a Harrington hook in neuromuscular disease. Clin Orthop Rel Res 1983;180:179.
102. Court-Brown CM, McMaster MJ. Pseudarthrosis: a late cause of paraparesis after scoliosis surgery. J Bone Joint Surg 1982;64B:1246.
103. Cleveland M, Bosworth DM, Thompson FR. Pseudarthrosis in the lumbosacral spine. J Bone Joint Surg 1948; 30A:302.
104. Dawson EG, Lotysch M, Urist MR. Intertransverse process lumbar arthrodesis with autogenous bone graft. Clin Orthop Rel Res 1981;154:90.
105. DePalma AF, Rothman RH. The nature of pseudarthrosis. Clin Orthop Rel Res 1968;59:113.
106. Thompson WA, Ralston EL. Pseudarthrosis following spine fusion. J Bone Joint Surg 1949;31A:400.
107. Lin PM. Posterior lumbar interbody fusion technique: Complications and pitfalls. Clin Orth Rel Res 1985;193:90.
108. Lehmann TR, Spratt KF, Tozzi JE, Weinstein JN, Reinarz SJ, El-Khoury GY, Colby H. Long term follow-up of lower lumbar fusion patients. Spine 1987;12:97.
109. Birkeland IW, Taylor TKF. Major vascular injuries in lumbar disc surgery. J Bone Joint Surg 1969;51B:4.
110. Borski AA, Smith RA. Ureteral injury in lumbar-disc operation. J Neurosurg 1960;17:925.
111. DeSaussure RL. Vascular injury coincident to disc surgery. J Neurosurg 1959;16:222.
112. Sandoz I, Hodges CV. Ureteral injury incident to lumbar disk operation. J Urol 1965;93:687.
113. Spittell JA, Palumbo PJ, Love JG, Ellis FH. Arteriovenous fistula complicating lumbar-disk surgery. N Engl J Med 1963;268:1162.
114. Brunet JA, Willey JJ. Acquired spondylolysis after spinal fusion. J Bone Joint Surg 1984;66B:720.
115. Wiltse LL, Newman PH, Macnab I. Classification of spondylolysis and spondylolisthesis. Clin Orthop Rel Res 1976;117:23.
116. Macnab I, Dall D. The blood supply of the lumbar spine and its application to the technique of intertransverse lumbar fusion. J Bone Joint Surg 1971;53B:628.
117. Lee CK, Langrana NA. Lumbosacral spinal fusion. Spine 1984;9:574.
118. Brodsky AE. Post-laminectomy and post-fusion stenosis of the lumbar spine. Clin Orthop Rel Res 1976;115:130.

VI
The Future

18

The Future of Spinal Fusions

John J. Gartland

Attempting to describe the future of spinal fusion as an orthopaedic surgical procedure is a provocative assignment, because it offers a writer an opportunity to exercise predictive ability. How many orthopaedic surgeons interested in spinal disorders would not agree that the near future might include a scene such as the following? A young adult patient is playing a gentle set of tennis attired in loose-fitting togs. The tennis clothing, despite the looseness, reveals several protuberances underneath. Few spectators realize the protuberances represent the rods of a spinal external fixation device inserted a few weeks before during the performance of a spinal fusion operation. While resting and sipping a cool drink between sets, the young adult patient sits hooked up to an electrical source.

Possible—yes; probable—no, at least to this observer. Not that it might not be attempted; it is the chance of a successful outcome that seems somewhat uncertain at the time of this writing.

To be able to discuss the future of any subject with any degree of intellectual accuracy, one has to be certain a past occurred and a present exists. A strong case can be made to support the contention that a past history for spinal fusion occurred, as attested by the description of the history of spinal fusion by Wiltse. The publications of Ollier, Hadra, Lange, Hibbs, and Albee describe the early efforts that led, ultimately, to the almost routine performance of a surgical effort known as a spinal fusion operation. The clinical experiences of those orthopaedists whose practices encompassed the past 50 years should be sufficient to persuade even the most skeptical that spinal fusion was once listed among the classical orthopaedic surgical procedures. The past history of spinal fusion is solid enough and in no way interferes with the sighting of a future. Rather, it is the present status of spinal fusion that is troublesome and contributes a certain opaqueness to a clear sighting of its future status.

Once considered a prototypical orthopaedic operation, spinal fusion seems regarded with a degree of suspicion today. What seemed to be clear-cut indications for its performance yesterday seem less obvious today. Operative treatment for derangements of the lumbar spine is still very much in an evolutionary state. Indications for surgical intervention, decision of appropriate surgical technique, and patient management remain controversial, and much has yet to be learned before the fundamental principles underlying the procedure are universally accepted, much less forecasted for future use.

A rational view would dictate that a firm future for spinal fusion rests squarely on appreciating and solving the multitude of problems besetting its present status. For all the thousands of spinal fusion operations performed in the past, a technique that guarantees a successful outcome to the vast majority of patients still cannot be identified with certainty. The spine has been approached from every conceivable direction with no clear indication as to which is the best approach. Techniques learned from surgery for tuberculosis and scoliosis have been applied to the surgical correction of lumbar derangements. Not all such techniques were found to be applicable; a plethora of new techniques and technical solutions, many of which were later discovered to have been founded on faulty biomechanical principles, have attempted to fill the gap.

Bone graft material used to augment the actual process of spine fusion has had an interesting history of its own and is not without its present problems. In 1867, Ollier described a method of bone transplantation using an osteoperiosteal graft. This experiment marks the actual beginning of the process that might make it possible to join segments of the spine to arrest disease and alleviate pain. The next major forward steps came in 1911 with the contributions of Hibbs and Albee. Hibbs used local bone from the patient as graft material, and Albee used a motor saw to cut a cortical graft from the patient's tibia. Since then, advocates of fibula, rib, and ilium as the site of bone graft material have presented their cases, but the supporting data have not yet convinced everyone that the final answer lies with any one particular site of bone graft harvest.

It could have been anticipated that proponents of heterogenous bone material would appear. A period has been recorded when lyophilized bone from calves was used as graft material. It ultimately proved a failure in spinal fusion because, by becoming invaded by fibrous tissue, it did not ossify or become incorporated into the underlying bone. Various types of allografts have been advocated more recently, but have yet to be proved equal to autografts. At this time, it would appear that autogenous corticocancellous bone graft material from the ilium is favored.

Bone graft failure remains a major reason for an unsuccessful spinal fusion. The answer to bone graft failure, like unsuccessful fracture healing, lies in the laboratory with delineation of the cellular details of bone healing. It is critical that the unknown factors underlying the conflict between mechanical and biological properties of bone graft material be clarified. It is interesting to note that present-day clinicians, impatient for a laboratory solution, have sought peripheral solutions through the use of internal fixation devices and adjunctive electrical stimulation with, as yet, no conclusive evidence that use of these peripheral solutions improves fusion rates.

The present status of spinal fusion is troublesome because many technical problems remain unsolved and successful patient outcomes are far from certain. The reasons for this present troublesome state are many and varied, but bear directly on a reasonable discussion of a future status for this surgical procedure. In some instances, new knowledge has cast doubt on indications for the procedure for which a former clinical consensus existed; such consensus has been based, however, on anecdotal evidence for the most part. In other instances, conclusions derived from data generated in clinical studies have been uncertain and contradictory because of faulty study design. A fuller discussion of current problems and controversies may allow a better understanding of what would be required to ensure a future status for this surgical procedure that could be accompanied by more successful patient outcomes. The accomplishment of better patient outcomes, not concentration on technique, must be the focus if spinal fusion is to have a future that is brighter than its present status.

Current Problems and Controversies

Controversies exist in spinal surgery that require clarification or resolution before a future role for spinal fusion can be defined realistically. General agreement on the indications for the procedure do not exist. Reported success rates for the operation vary widely from optimistically high to disturbingly low. The reported outcomes for lumbar spine surgery, for example, would seem to be significantly manipulated by the criteria selected for the assessment of end results. Interpreting the results of surgical treatment for lumbar spine disorders is difficult because different types of outcome rating scales are used. In some studies admission criteria are not identified, making the need for the surgical procedure difficult to assess. The design of many reported studies is sufficiently flawed to question the scientific validity of the results.

Indications

At the present time there appears to be agreement on the indication for spinal fusion in some spinal conditions, but not in others. A case in point is the uncertain role for spinal fusion following discectomy at the lumbosacral joint.

At this time, few would doubt the value of spinal fusion in the treatment of unstable thoracolumbar fractures, particularly when the results obtained by spinal canal decompression are compared to the results now obtained by open reduction, fusion, and stabilization. Follow-up studies have demonstrated that surgical treatment significantly improved fracture reduction and considerably reduced the immobilization and hospital times for these patients. Reflecting the seriousness of these injuries and putting the role of spinal fusion in sharper perspective, however, longer follow-up studies suggest no apparent differences between nonoperative treatment and surgical stabilization regarding the final neurological and rehabilitation status of examined patients.

The role of spinal fusion in the surgical treatment of spinal stenosis has not yet been totally clarified. The realization that a thickened posterior midline fusion can, of itself, cause spinal stenosis has been disturbing. Still unsettled is the occurrence and frequency of postoperative instability after surgical decompression for spinal stenosis and, if it does occur, whether it is symptomatic enough to warrant the addition of spinal fusion to the decompression procedure. There seems to be agreement that extensive laminectomy in patients with degenerative spondylolisthesis does result in sufficient postoperative instability to warrant the addition of spinal fusion to the decompression procedure. The indication for the addition of spinal fusion in other patients operated on for spinal stenosis is less clear.

A traditional role for spinal fusion has been in the patient identified as having low back instability. Characteristic roentgenographic changes such as disc space narrowing and facet joint degeneration have been said to be confirming findings. In fact, except for spondylolisthesis, no agreement presently exists on the definition of lumbar instability, how it can be identified, and what is the best treatment for it once identified. The presently used classification of degenerative segmental instability is based on current understanding of spinal degeneration and the biomechanical behavior of spinal motion segments. Unfortunately, these concepts are not proved by existing biomechanical knowledge or surgical outcome studies. The identification of an instability state and the tailoring of a specific fusion technique to the type of instability may be one means of reducing an unacceptably high failure rate in the surgical management of degenerative diseases of the lumbar spine.

One of the most interesting indications for spinal fusion that needs to be clarified in the future is its role following surgical excision of an intervertebral disc. There was a time most orthopaedists were convinced that patients who had partial laminectomy and disc excision at the lumbosacral interspace had better outcomes if lumbosacral fusion was included in the surgical procedure. However, the data upon which this conviction was based were largely anecdotal and do not appear to have stood the test of time. It must also be noted that the increase in surgical time and associated patient morbidity, along with the fear of pseudarthrosis, tempered the enthusiasm of many for associated spinal fusion.

Biomechanical studies have demonstrated an inherent stability associated with the lumbosacral joint that has lent added credence to those denying the need for spinal fusion after lumbosacral joint discectomy. The weight of present opinion lies with the view that an associated spinal fusion is not necessary after routine removal of a disc. Review of published large series comparing the results of discectomy alone with discectomy and fusion show the results to be very little, if any, better with discectomy and fusion for most patients. This slight possible advantage for fusion, when evaluated against the risk of pseudarthrosis, has not been sufficient to persuade most to fuse the lumbosacral joint following discectomy. Most would agree that fusion is indicated if the patient is deemed to have an associated instability. However, as pointed out, neither the definition nor the identification of lumbar instability has yet been agreed.

Surgical Techniques

It seems to this observer that surgical techniques developed for thoracolumbar spine problems are based on firmer data than the multitude of techniques proposed for lumbar spine problems.

Much of the past experience for thoracolumbar surgery, including fusion techniques, is derived from tuberculosis and scoliosis surgery. Internal fixation devices, originally designed for use in scoliosis surgery, were adapted for use in spine fracture and neoplasm surgery, but not all proved useful. As a result new devices have been developed especially for use in spine fracture surgery. Two controversies remaining in thoracolumbar spinal fracture surgery that await solution are (1) should the decompression be from an anterior or posterior direction? and (2) how long a segment of vertebrae should be fused?

A clear surgical solution to lumbar spine problems remains elusive, and a large part of the future for spinal fusion rests on a better understanding in this area. Because of dissatisfaction with the results achieved by conventional surgical treatment, novel surgical approaches and alterations in technique have been suggested to secure arthrodesis of lumbar vertebral segments considered unstable. However, the prognosis that the patient can be offered for a successful result by surgical treatment remains guarded. A useful and successful future for spinal fusion will depend, in the final analysis, on markedly improving that prognosis for patients. Many of the surgical techniques described for use in the lumbar spine seemed logical and useful on initial review, only to be discarded in light of eventual critical reappraisal. Even though a plethora of choices of techniques are available for lumbar spine fusions, none has yet proven itself ideal.

The distressingly high failure rate with posterior lumbar fusion awakened interest in attempting to achieve a more acceptable fusion rate with vertebral interbody fusion approached by either an anterior or posterior route. Enthusiasm for anterior interbody fusion peaked during the 1960s, but rapidly diminished when better follow-up studies demonstrated low fusion rates. At the present time anterior interbody fusion for lumbar spine disorders must be regarded as a technically unsolved problem.

Reported results with posterior lumbar interbody fusion are better than those obtained through the anterior route, but there appears to be only scattered enthusiasm for its adoption as the primary technique of choice for lumbar spine fusion. In addition, consensus does not exist on the type of bone graft material to use, with bone dowels, chip grafts, and unicortical and bicortical autologous grafts each having their champions. Current available data would suggest posterolateral fusion as the most efficient spinal fusion technique for the majority of lumbar spine problems. Some biomechanical data suggest that less motion of solidly arthrodesed lumbar segments occurs with posterolateral fusion than with either anterior interbody fusion or strictly posterior fusions. This suggests success for this technique for preventing irritating intrasegmental motion postoperatively for successfully fused patients.

Dissatisfaction with the results obtained by current lumbar spine fusion techniques has led to the introduction of different forms of internal fixation devices as internal stabilizers to help attain a higher successful lumbar fusion rate. The evidence to date is inconclusive that any of these devices is effective in improving fusion rates. In addition, the devices carry complications of their own, such as pulling loose from their attachment to bone.

Interest now exists in the role of electricity in augmenting the consolidation of a spinal fusion. Preliminary studies tend to indicate that electrical stimulation does cause increased osteoblastic activity in the spine and could increase the chance of a successful fusion. Electrical stimulation as an asset to spinal fusion continues to be used, but as yet no convincing proof exists that such use improves fusion rates over that obtained with autogenous bone grafting alone.

Future Directions

Because orthopaedics is a surgically oriented discipline that concentrates on operative procedures and techniques, it would be an easy task to predict a future status for spinal fusion replete with imaginative indications and novel techniques applied to the vertebral columns of countless patients. Realism intrudes, however.

If the current problems relating to patient selection, bone graft failure, surgical techniques, and design validity of published studies are not addressed with the serious intent of arriving at valid and effective solutions, it is difficult to foresee how the future of spinal fusion can be very much different from its present status. A brighter future for spinal fusion lies not in the design of better internal fixation devices, but in the solution of its present problems. The future goal that should be strived for is the delineation of a spinal fusion technique that achieves a success rate as close to 100% as is humanly possible in those patients in whom the operation is truly indicated.

In designing future studies to evaluate the utility and effectiveness of spinal fusion, orthopaedic surgeons with an interest in the spine must keep another consideration in mind. That consideration is the influence now wielded by those paying health care costs in this country. There is a growing recognition among health policy makers that new approaches must be developed to meet the continuing demand for expensive health care services. One of the approaches could be tying payment for expensive orthopaedic health care services to demonstrated efficacy in improving the health and quality of life of patients receiving the service. Most of the published studies on spinal fusion to date have focused primarily on procedural value or technical efficiency instead of on patient health outcomes.

Little data currently exist to support justification of payment for expensive orthopaedic health care services such as spinal fusion. Not only are such data almost nonexistent at the present time, there is virtually no agreement on what constitutes important parameters of outcome. It seems clear that a significant future direction is better study design to improve the scientific validity of spinal fusion clinical studies. The reports of such research should focus more on patient health outcome instead of concentrating primarily on procedural values or technical efficiency.

Orthopaedic surgeons with an interest in the spine need to develop agreement on patient selection for this operative procedure. Currently there is such agreement on the indications for spinal fusion in certain spinal conditions but not in others. Agreement on indications for spinal fusion is needed in the surgical treatment for spinal stenosis, lumbar instability, lumbar spine degenerative processes, and clarification of its role, if any, following lumbar discectomy. Agreement on specific and exact indications for each diagnosis is probably neither required nor desirable. What would be most helpful, and also improve the design validity of future clinical end-result studies, is agreement on suitably similar indications for each diagnosis in which spinal fusion might be an appropriate treatment option.

A more meaningful future role for spinal fusion, as far as future patients are concerned, will depend on improving the rate of successful fusion. Many of the surgical techniques promulgated to effect fusion of two or more vertebrae initially seemed logical and useful, only to be discarded when later critical analysis indicated a high failure rate. Often what appeared to be a successful fusion on conventional radiographs turned out to be a failure when examined by biplanar radiography or CT scan.

It seems likely that better solutions to bone graft failure and spinal fusion nonunion will come from laboratory study rather than from clinical tinkering with existing techniques. Bone graft healing, as a cellular process, has many basic similarities to fracture healing, although some differences are mediated by cellular responses to immune system triggers. The process by which fractures heal is now being investigated in orthopaedic laboratories. Once the chemical nature of the bone-inducing substance and its mechanism of action, the chemical composition of the organic matrix of bone, the organic matrix elements necessary for normal bone repair, and the mechanisms of cellular control of bone mineralization are known, this information can be shared and utilized for improving the union rate of spinal fusions. It seems logical to suggest that an approach such as this promises to improve the future status of spinal fusion more than the design of alternate internal fixation devices that promise to continue to pull loose in osteoporotic bone.

Finally, when the secrets of bone graft transplantation and the biological secrets of bone repair are fully understood and the clinical results of spinal fusion greatly improved for patients, it remains for those orthopaedic surgeons with an interest in the spine to design studies that, when reported, are scientifically valid. Much of the present literature on techniques and results for spinal fusion does not fulfill the criteria considered necessary by clinical scientists for scientific validity. A tendency exists in surgical disciplines to attribute the origin of much knowledge to prior experience. This perception often results in enthusiastic reporting of specific treatments evaluated by retrospective analyses of large series of patients presented to readers without proper appreciation of study design strategies that enhance scientific validity. Such reports are usually also flawed by observer bias and frequently by skill bias.

Future reports dealing with spinal fusion techniques and results would be more valid and meaningful if the study design included such strategies as agreed-upon indications, admission criteria, treatment responses, and patient health outcomes, awareness of the strengths supplied to the study by inclusion of a concurrent control group, and appreciation of the flaws introduced by statistical errors such as observer and skill bias.

Published reports of orthopaedic surgical treatments frequently compare postsurgical outcomes to presurgical conditions. This is a natural comparison for most surgeons as it mirrors the situation encountered in practice. Unfortunately, it is not the comparison actually needed to truly measure the effectiveness of a surgical treatment. Ideally, to properly appreciate the value of a reported treatment, readers need an evaluation of postsurgical outcomes compared to patient conditions encountered in the absence of the reported surgical treatment.

Spinal fusion would seem to be an important surgical procedure with a potential to benefit countless patients. If it is to have a significant and useful future, those orthopaedic surgeons interested in the spine must continue to strive to accomplish three goals: (1) determine what patients would benefit from the operation; (2) determine how to ensure that those patients operated on enjoy a successful outcome; and (3) publish reports in a form that is scientifically valid so that knowledge of which treatments are truly effective will increase.

Index

MIX
Papier aus verantwortungsvollen Quellen
Paper from responsible sources
FSC® C105338

FSC
www.fsc.org

If you have any concerns about our products,
you can contact us on
ProductSafety@springernature.com

In case Publisher is established outside the EU,
the EU authorized representative is:
Springer Nature Customer Service Center GmbH
Europaplatz 3, 69115 Heidelberg, Germany

Printed by Libri Plureos GmbH
in Hamburg, Germany